THIRD EDITION

Mosby's
DENTAL
DICTIONARY

ELSEVIER
MOSBY

ELSEVIER
MOSBY

3251 Riverport Lane
St. Louis, Missouri 63043

MOSBY'S DENTAL DICTIONARY, THIRD EDITION   ISBN: 978-0-323-10012-0
Copyright © 2014 by Mosby, an imprint of Elsevier Inc.
Copyright © 2008, 2004 by Mosby, Inc., an affiliate of Elsevier Inc.

Notices

Knowledge and best practice in this field are constantly changing. As new research and experience broaden our understanding, changes in research methods, professional practices, or medical treatment may become necessary.

Practitioners and researchers must always rely on their own experience and knowledge in evaluating and using any information, methods, compounds, or experiments described herein. In using such information or methods they should be mindful of their own safety and the safety of others, including parties for whom they have a professional responsibility.

With respect to any drug or pharmaceutical products identified, readers are advised to check the most current information provided (i) on procedures featured or (ii) by the manufacturer of each product to be administered, to verify the recommended dose or formula, the method and duration of administration, and contraindications. It is the responsibility of practitioners, relying on their own experience and knowledge of their patients, to make diagnoses, to determine dosages and the best treatment for each individual patient, and to take all appropriate safety precautions.

To the fullest extent of the law, neither the Publisher nor the authors, contributors, or editors, assume any liability for any injury and/or damage to persons or property as a matter of products liability, negligence or otherwise, or from any use or operation of any methods, products, instructions, or ideas contained in the material herein.

ISBN: 978-0-323-10012-0

Vice President and Content Strategy Director: Linda Duncan
Executive Content Strategist: Kathy Falk
Senior Content Development Specialist: Courtney Sprehe
Publishing Services Manager: Julie Eddy
Senior Project Manager: Marquita Parker
Design Direction: Ashley Eberts

Printed in China

Last digit is the print number: 9   8   7   6   5   4   3   2   1

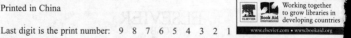

Working together
to grow libraries in
developing countries

www.elsevier.com • www.bookaid.org

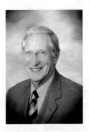

This third edition of *Mosby's Dental Dictionary* is dedicated to William F. Bird, DDS, MPH, DrPH, FACD, who passed away July 2012. Throughout his career, Dr. Bird was a well-respected author and educator who was always willing to lend his time and talents to a project that would help further the scope of dental education. Whether serving as a co-author on *Dental Materials: Clinical Applications for Dental Assistants and Dental Hygienists* or contributing to one of many other projects, his leadership, knowledge, strong work ethic, and unwavering commitment to excellence not only made the work better but also made working with him a pleasure. We will miss you, Bill...

The Publishers

Editorial Board

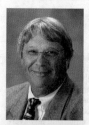
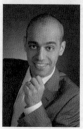
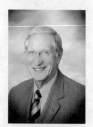
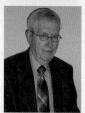

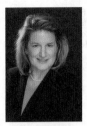
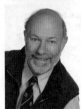
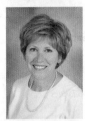
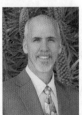

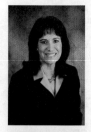
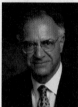
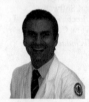

About the Dictionary

NEW TO THE EDITION

- **Best of the best.** The best of Elsevier's authors (and leaders in their fields) scrutinizing the dictionary with an eye towards their particular area of expertise for what terms needed to be deleted, added, or expanded.
- **Updated art program.** The art program has been thoroughly revised to relate specifically to the practice of dentistry.
- **Companion website.** The new website offers a wealth of additional material, including audio pronunciations, additional images, videos, and animations. Icons make it easy to identify when there is supplemental material on the website:

[image icon]	This icon indicates that a corresponding image for the term appears on the website.
[video icon]	This icon indicates that there is corresponding video or animation for the term on the website.
(an-ti-bi-ot′ik)	A bold pronunciation indicates that there is an audio pronunciation for the term on the website.

KEY FEATURES

- Comprehensive coverage, with over 10,000 terms covering all areas of dentistry
- Pocket-sized, durable, chair-side/computer-side reference
- Colored thumb bleeds aid in locating definitions
- A variety of appendices provide information on anesthesia color codes, oral structures, tooth designations systems, implants, and much more!

Contents

Pronunciation Guide

VOWEL SOUNDS
Print Key Words

a	hat
ä	father
aø	play, fate, feign
e	flesh
eø	she, sweet
er	air, ferry
i	sit
ī	eye, kind, mine
ir	ear, weird
o	proper
oø	nose, coal
T	saw, fawn
oi	coin, (German) feuer
oo	moon, move
o̽o̽	put, book
ou	out
u	cup, love
Y	(German) grün, Führer; (French) tu
ur	fur, first
ə	ago, career
œ	(German) schön, Goethe'
N	This symbol does not represent a sound, but indicates that the preceding vowel is nasal, as in (French) bon.

CONSONANTS
Print Key Words

b	book
ch	chew, watch
d	day, dead
f	fast, phone, enough
g	good
h	happy
j	jump, gem
k	cook, quick
l	late
m	mammal
n	noon
ng	sing, drink
ng-g	finger
p	pulp
r	ready, rely
s	sassy
sh	shine, sure, lotion
t	to
th	thin (voiceless)
th	than, with (voiced)

v	valve
w	work
y	yes
z	zeal, has
zh	azure, vision
(h)w	**wh**en, **wh**ile
kh	(Scottish) lo**ch**, (German) Ba**ch**
kh	(German) i**ch**
nyə	o**ni**on, (Spanish) se**ñor**, (French) Boulo**gne**

a nativitate (ä′nətiv′itāt, -tä′tā), *adj* the state of existing at birth or from infancy; denotes a congenital disability.

A point, *n* See point, A.

A-P discrepancy, *n* See anterior-posterior discrepancy.

A:G ratio, *n* See ratio, A:G.

aa, *adv* an abbreviation for the Greek term ana, used in prescription writing, meaning "of each."

A-alpha fibers, *n.pl* See fibers, nerve.

ab (antecedent), *prep* beforehand; a notice given previously or a condition existing earlier.

abacavir, *n brand name:* Ziagen; *drug class:* a nucleoside; *action:* reverse transcriptase inhibitor; *use:* treat HIV infection.

abacterial (ā′baktir′ē-əl), *adj* nonbacterial; free from bacteria.

abandonment (of a patient), *n* the withdrawing of a patient from treatment without giving reasonable notice or providing a competent replacement.

abatement (əbāt′ment), *n* a decrease in severity of pain or symptoms.

Abbé-Estlander operation (ab′ē-est′landur), *n* See operation, Abbé-Estlander.

abciximab, *n brand name:* ReoPro; *drug class:* monoclonal antibody (fab fragment); *action:* binds to integrin glycoprotein (GP IIb/IIIa) receptors on platelets; *uses:* reduce platelet aggregation, reduce risk of myocardial infarction.

abdomen, *n* the portion of the body between the thorax and the pelvis.

abdominal thrust, *n* See Heimlich maneuver.

abduct (abdukt′), *v* to draw away from the median line or from a neighboring part or limb.

abduction (abduk′shən), *n* the process of abducting; opposite of adduction.

aberrant (aber′ənt), *adj* deviating from the usual or normal course, location, or action.

A-beta fibers, See fibers, nerve.

abfraction (abfrak′shən), *n* a mechanism that explains the loss of dentin tissue and tooth enamel caused by flexure and ultimate material fatigue of susceptible teeth at locations away from the point of loading. The breakdown is dependent on the magnitude, duration, frequency, and location of the forces.

abfraction area, *n* the part of the tooth, most commonly the cervical area, that is affected by the loss of dentin and enamel caused by flexure and material fatigue.

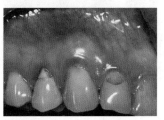

Abfraction area. (Bath Balogh/Fehrenbach, 2011)

ablation (ablā′shən), *n* an amputation or excision of any part of the body, or a removal of a growth or harmful substance.

abnormal (abnôr′məl), *adj* departing from the norm, however defined; departing from the mean of a distribution (statistics); departing from the usual, from a state of integration or adjustment.

abnormal tooth mobility, *n* excessive movement of a tooth within its socket as a result of changes in the supporting tissues caused by injury or disease.

abrade (əbrād), *v* to wear away by friction.

abrasion (əbrā′zhən), *n* **I.** the abnormal wearing away of a substance or tissue by a mechanical process. *n* **2.** the pathologic wearing away of tooth structure by an external mechanical source, most commonly incorrect toothbrushing methods.

abrasion, dentifrice, *n* the wearing away of the cementum and dentin of an exposed root by an abrasive-containing dentifrice.

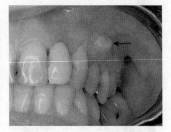

Abscess. (Regezi/Sciubba/Jordan, 2012)

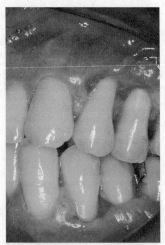

Abrasion caused by dentifrice. (Newman/Takei/Klokkevold, 2012)

abrasion resistance, n See resistance, abrasion.

abrasive (əbrā′siv), n a substance used for grinding or polishing that will wear away a material or tissue.

abrasive disk, n See disk, abrasive.

abrasive, finishing, n the application of abrasive materials in order to eliminate surface imperfections.

abrasive point, rotary, n See point, abrasive, rotary.

abrasive polishing agent, n a paste containing sharp-edged particles that are moved over the surface of a material with varying pressure and speed. The movement abrades the surface with microscopic scratches, which creates a polished finish. See also dentifrice and polishing.

abrasive strip, n See strip, abrasive.

abrasive system, n the materials used for polishing and cleansing. Common materials include calcium carbonate (calcite, chalk, whiting), diamond particles (for porcelain), some aluminum derivatives (not for enamel), rouge (jeweler's rouge; applied to gold and precious metal alloys), and tin oxide (putty powder, stannic oxide).

abscess (ab′ses), n a localized accumulation of suppuration in a confined space formed by tissue disintegration.

abscess, alveolar, n See periapical abscess.

abscess, apical, n See periapical abscess.

abscess, dentoalveolar, n See periapical abscess.

abscess, gingival, n a superficial periodontal abscess occurring within the free gingival sulcus surrounding the tooth, frequently caused by the impaction of food or another object into a periodontal pocket.

abscess, lateral, n See periodontal abscess.

abscess, periapical (per′ēā′pikəl), n an abscess involving the apical region of the root, alveolus, and surrounding bone as a result of pulpal disease.

abscess, pericoronal, n See pericoronitis.

abscess, periodontal, n an abscess involving the attachment tissues and alveolar bone as a result of periodontal disease.

abscess, periradicular (per′ērədik′y ələr), n an abscess involving the periradicular region of the root, alveolus, and surrounding bone as a result of pulpal disease.

abscess, pulpal, n an abscess occurring within pulpal tissue.

abscess, staphylococcal (staf′əlōkok ′əl), n an abscess caused by the bacteria *S. aureus,* an infectious agent that can be transmitted via saliva and other discharges of the body. The incubation period is 4 to 10 days; the duration of the abscess varies and is indefinite. The bacteria are communicable throughout the drainage period of the lesions and while the carrier state continues.

absolute refractory period, n during nerve conduction, the interval during which a second action potential absolutely cannot be initiated to restimulate the nerve membrane, no matter how large a stimulus is applied.

absorb (əbzôrb′), v **1.** to suck up or be removed. v **2.** to incorporate or assimilate a liquid or gas into tissue or cells.

absorbable gelatin sponge, n *brand name:* Gelfoam; *drug class:* hemostatic; *action:* absorbs blood and provides area for clot formation; *use:* hemostasis during and following surgery.

absorbefacient (abzôr′bifā′shənt), *adj/n* causing absorption, or an agent that promotes absorption.

absorbent (abzôrb′ənt), *adj* a substance that causes absorption of diseased tissue; taking up by suction.

absorptiometry, dual energy radiograph, n the standard technique that uses two radiographic beams to diagnose osteoporosis and to assess the efficacy of treatment.

absorption (abzôrp′shən), n **1.** the passage of a substance into the interior of another by solution or penetration. n **2.** the taking up of fluids or other substances by the skin, mucous surfaces, absorbent vessels, or dental materials so that they are removed. n **3.** the process by which radiation imparts some or all of its energy to any material through which it passes.

absorption coefficient, n the ratio of the linear rate of change of intensity of roentgen rays in a given homogeneous material to the intensity at a given point within the same mass.

absorption, drug, n the process by which a drug enters the body, such as a local anesthetic being taken up by the blood stream after injection. The faster the absorption, the higher the chance of systemic toxicity and the lower the duration of effectiveness. The rate is altered by route of administration, use of vasoconstrictors, and patient factors.

abstinence (ab′stənəns), n selfrestraint, especially from harmful substances or morally questionable behaviors. See also withdrawal.

abstraction (abstrak′shən), n teeth or other maxillary and mandibular structures that are inferior to (below) their normal position; away from the occlusal plane.

abuse, n the improper use of program benefits, resources, and/or services by either dental professionals, institutions, or patients.

abuse, child, n See child abuse.

abuse, drug, n the misuse of legal or illegal substances with the intent to alter the user's feelings, behavior, or perception.

abuse, elder, n the behavior or treatment toward an elderly person, by another person in a position of care, that has the purpose or effect of harming the elderly person's wellbeing. Such harm may include economic, physical, sexual, or mental abuse.

abuse, nitrous oxide, n the deliberate inhalation of nitrous oxide to produce mood-altering effects. A type of substance abuse.

abuse, sexual, n sexual acts performed with children or with nonconsenting adults in a criminal manner.

abuse, substance, n the misuse of legal or illegal substances with the intent to alter some aspect of the user's experience. May include medications, illicit drugs, legal substances with potential mood-altering effects (such as alcohol or tobacco), or substances whose primary use may not be for human consumption (such as inhalants).

abutment (əbut′mənt), n a tooth, root, or implant used for support and retention of a fixed or removable prosthesis. See also pontic.

abutment, angulated **(ang′gyəlātid),** n an abutment whose body is not parallel to the long axis of the implant. It is utilized when the implant is at a different inclination in relation to the proposed prosthesis.

abutment, custom, n a custom-made post attached to the superior part of the metal dental implant that protrudes through the gingival tissues and onto which the restoration is fitted; either machined or cast, and used in situations where prefabricated abutments cannot be used.

abutment, healing, n a cylinder or screw used during the second stage of dental restoration. This serves two purposes: to allow gingival tissues to heal prior to the placement of the permanent abutment, and to maintain proper spacing in the oral cavity before the final restoration (prosthesis) is placed.

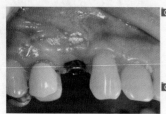

Healing abutment. (Perry/Beemsterboer, 2007.)

abutment, intermediate, n an abutment located between the abutments that form the ends of the prosthesis.

abutment, multiple, n abutments splinted together as a unit to support and retain a fixed prosthesis.

abutment, prefabricated, n a machine-manufactured post attached to the superior part of a dental implant that protrudes through the gingival tissues and onto which a restoration is fitted.

abutment, preparable, n a dental implant abutment that can be prepared and changed from the manufacturer's original design.

abutment, screw, n a screw that secures an abutment to an implant. It is usually torqued to a final seating position.

abutment, UCLA, n a cast component used to create a custom abutment for a prosthesis. Also known as a *castable abutment.*

a.c., adv the abbreviation for *ante cibum,* a Latin phrase meaning "before eating."

Academy of General Dentistry (AGD), *n.pr* a nonprofit, international organization dedicated to serving the needs and representing the general interests of dental professionals.

acamprosate, *n brand name:* Campral; *drug class:* a gamma-aminobutyric acid (GABA) analogue; *action:* blocks a certain class of glutamate receptors in the brain; *use:* reduce relapse in alcoholics

acanthesthesia (əkan'thesthē'zēə, -zhə), *n* a form of paresthesia experienced as numbness, tingling, or "pins and needles." See also paresthesia.

acanthion (əkan'thēon), *n* the tip of the anterior nasal spine.

acantholysis (ak'anthol'isis), *n* the loosening, separation, or disassociation of individual prickle cells within the epithelium from their neighbor, often seen in conditions such as pemphigus vulgaris and keratosis follicularis.

acanthosis (ak'ənthō'sis), *n* an increase in the number of cells in the prickle cell layer of stratified squamous epithelium, with thickening of the entire epithelial cell layer and a broadening and fusing of rete pegs.

acapnia (akap'nēə), *n* a condition characterized by diminished carbon dioxide in the blood.

acarbia (akär'bēə), *n* a condition in which the blood bicarbonate level is decreased.

acarbose, *n brand name:* Precose, Prandase; *drug class:* oligosaccharide, glucosidase enzyme inhibitor; *action:* inhibits α-glucosidase enzyme in the GI tract to slow the breakdown of carbohydrates to glucose; *use:* a single drug (or in combination with others) used when diet control is ineffective in controlling blood glucose levels, such as with type 2 diabetes mellitus.

acatalasemia (a'katələsē'mēə), *n* a congenital lack of the enzyme catalase in blood and other tissues that leads to a progressive necrosis of the oral tissues Also known as *acatalasia* or *Takahara's disease.*

accelerator (aksel'ərātur), *n* **1.** a substance that increases rapidity of action or function. *n* **2.** a catalyst or other substance that hastens a chemical reaction (e.g., NaCl added to water and plaster to hasten the set). *n* **3.** a film-developing solution of potassium hydroxide or sodium carbonate used to enlarge the emulsion and to establish an alkaline medium.

accelerator, platelet thrombin, n See factor, platelet 2.

accelerator, prothrombin conversion, I **(prōthrom'bin kənvur'zhən),** *n* (factor V, labile factor, plasma accelerator globulin, proaccelerin, serum accelerator globulin), a substance that is considered by some to be a factor in serum and plasma that catalyzes the conversion of inactive prothrombin to an active form.

accelerator, prothrombin conversion, II, n (extrinsic thromboplastin, factor

VII, serum prothrombin conversion accelerator [SPCA], stable factor), a substance that is considered by some to be one of the factors in the blood that accelerates the conversion of active prothrombin to thrombin by thromboplastin. Vitamin K deficiency reduces the activity of this factor.

accelerator, serum, n See factor V.

accelerin (aksel′ərin), n See factor V.

acceptability, n an overall assessment of the dental care available to a person or group; includes accessibility, cost, quality, results, convenience, and attitudes of dental professionals and patients.

acceptance, n the act of a person to whom something is offered or tendered by another, whereby he receives that which is offered with the intention of retaining it. A contract is not valid without the acceptance of an offer by the party to whom the offer is made, either expressly or by conduct.

acceptance, absolute, n an express and positive agreement to pay a bill according to its text.

acceptance, conditional, n an agreement to pay a bill on the fulfillment of a condition.

acceptance, implied, n an acceptance interpreted by law from the acts or conduct of the patient.

access (ak′ses), n I. the means of approach. n 2. a surgical preparation of hard or soft tissue to allow entrance to a treatment site and adequate space for visualization and instrumentation of the field.

access, cavity, n a coronal opening required for effective cleaning, shaping, and filling of the pulp space.

access, computer, n I. the process of transferring information into or out of a storage location. n 2. the time required to begin and complete the read and write functions of a specified piece of data.

access flap, n a periodontal surgical technique that provides visualization of the root in conjunction with curettage and root planing. Types of access flaps include supracrestal, subcrestal-full thickness, and partial thickness flaps. See also flaps, periodontal.

access, form, n the surgical removal of tooth structure sufficient for visualization and instrumentation of a restorative preparation.

access to care, n ability of a person to receive health/dental care services based on availability of personnel, supplies, and person's ability to pay for those services.

accessibility standards (akses′abil′itē), n.pl the requirements designed by the Americans with Disabilities Act (ADA), by which public places must provide disabled individuals with barrier-free access to buildings, forms of communication, and modes of transportation such as dental offices and clinics.

accessory (akses′ərē), adj providing complementary or supplementary assistance.

accessory root, n See root, accessory.

accident, n I. an unusual, unforeseen event. n 2. an unusual or unexpected result attending the performance of a usual or necessary act or event. n 3. occurring without intent or happening by chance. The term does not have a precise legal definition but is generally used to indicate that an occurrence was not the result of negligence.

accident, cerebrovascular (CVA) (ser′əbrōvas′kyələr), (stroke) n apoplexy resulting from hemorrhage into the brain or occlusion of the cerebral vessels from an embolism or thrombosis. It can result in paralysis (mainly one side), speech difficulties, and difficulty in maintaining personal hygiene, including oral care.

accident, unavoidable, n an accident not occasioned, either remotely or directly, by the want of such care or skill as the law holds every person bound to exercise; occurring without fault or negligence.

accident prevention, n a set of precautionary measures taken to avoid possible bodily harm. Devices that can be especially important in preventing damage to the orofacial area are seat belts and bicycle helmets; the use of these should be encouraged in all patients.

accidental exposure management, n a set of regulations followed in case of inadvertent exposure to hazardous materials.

account, n a basic storage unit in an accounting system. Individual accounts accept debit and credit entries that reflect the different types of transactions made by the practice.

account book, *n* a book in which the financial transactions of a business or profession are entered. Such books may be admitted as evidence.

account, open, *n* a straightforward arrangement between the dental provider and the patient for the handling of financial payments due the dental provider and owed by the patient.

account, payable, *n* a dollar amount owed to creditors for items or services purchased from them.

accountability, *n* an obligation to periodically disclose appropriate information in adequate detail and consistent form to all contractually involved parties.

accreditation (əkred'itā'shən), *n* a process of formal recognition of a school or institution attesting to the required ability and performance in an area of education, training, or practice. In dentistry, this process is controlled by the Commission on Dental Accreditation (CODA).

accretions (əkrē'shənz), *n.pl* an older term for accumulations of foreign material such as plaque, materia alba, calculus, and other debris on teeth. Now called deposits.

accrual, *n* continually recurring short-term liabilities. Examples are accrued wages, taxes, and interest.

accrued needs, *n.pl* the amount of treatment needed by an individual or a group at any given time. In dental plans, usually refers to conditions present at the time of enrollment. Synonym: accumulated needs.

acebutolol HCl (as'əbyōō'təlôl), *n* brand names: Monitan, Sectral; *drug class:* antihypertensive, selective β₁ receptor blocker; *action:* produces fall in blood pressure without reflex tachycardia; *uses:* mild-to-moderate hypertension, ventricular dysrhythmias.

acellular (āsel'yələr), *adj* not composed of or having cells.

acenesthesia (əsen'esthē'zēə, -zhə), *n* the loss, or lack, of the normal perception of one's own body; absence of the feelings of a physical existence, a symptom that is common with many psychiatric disorders.

acentric relation (āsen'trik), *n* See relation, jaw, eccentric.

acesulfame-K, *n* a synthetic nonnutritive sweetener.

acetabulum (as'ətab'yələm), *n* a cup-shaped attachment site located laterally on the hip bone for the head of the femur.

acetaminophen (əsē'təmin'əfin), *n* brand names: Tylenol, Anacin-3; *drug class:* nonnarcotic analgesic; *action:* thought to block initiation of pain impulses by inhibition of prostaglandin synthesis, especially in the central nervous sysem; *uses:* mild-to moderate pain, fever; also used in combination with narcotic analgesics such as with oxycodone as Percocet, Tylox, or Roxicet.

acetate (as'ətāt), *n* **1.** a salt of acetic acid. *n* **2.** a short form for cellulose acetate, the film base for radiographs.

acetazolamide/acetazolamide sodium (əsē'təzō'ləmīd sō'dēəm), *n* brand name: Diamox; *drug class:* diuretic; carbonic anhydrase inhibitor; *action:* inhibits carbonic anhydrase activity in proximal renal tubular cells to decrease reabsorption of water, sodium, potassium, bicarbonate; *uses:* open-angle glaucoma, epilepsy, edema.

acetic acid, *n* a clear, colorless, pungent liquid that is miscible with water, alcohol, glycerin, and ether and that constitutes 3% to 5% of vinegar.

acetohexamide, *n* brand names: Dimelor, Dymelor; *drug class:* sulfonylurea; antidiabetic; *action:* causes functioning β cells in the pancreas to release insulin, leading to a drop in blood glucose level; *use:* stable type 2 diabetes mellitus.

acetone (as'ətōn), *n* Dimethylketone; **1.** an organic solvent. *n* **2.** in the body, a chemical that is formed when the body uses fat instead of glucose for energy. The formation of acetone means that cells lack insulin or cannot effectively use available insulin to burn glucose for energy. It passes through the body into the urine as ketone bodies. *n* **3.** the simplest ketone. It is normally present in urine in small amounts but can increase in those who have diabetes mellitus. Results in having "fruity" acetone breath.

acetone abuse, *n* a deliberate inhalation of acetone to produce moodaltering effects. See also huffing.

acetone breath, *n* a characteristic "fruity" or acetone breath odor that occurs with a life-threatening condition of diabetic ketoacidosis. See diabetic ketoacidosis and acetone.

acetyl groups, *n.pl* in chemistry, a functional group containing a methyl group attached to a carbonyl group (CH_3-CO); an important group in many chemicals.

acetylcholine (as'ətilkō'lēn, əsē'til), *n* an acetate ester of choline that serves as a neurohumoral agent in the transmission of an impulse in autonomic ganglia, cholinergic neuroeffector junctions, skeletal neuromuscular junctions, and certain synapses in the central nervous system.

acetylcysteine (əsē'tlsis'tēn), *n brand name:* Mucomyst; *drug class:* mucolytic; *action:* decreases viscosity of pulmonary secretions by breaking disulfide links of mucoproteins; protects the liver by preventing the loss of glutathione; *uses:* acetaminophen toxicity, bronchitis, pneumonia, cystic fibrosis, emphysema, atelectasis tuberculosis, and complications of thoracic surgery. Also called *N-acetylcysteine.*

achlorhydria (ā'klôrhī'drēə), *n* the absence of free hydrochloric acid in the stomach, even with histamine stimulation.

achondroplasia (ākon'drōplā'zēə, -zhə), *n* a hereditary disturbance of endochondral bone formation transmitted as a mendelian dominant factor and resulting in dwarfism. Malocclusion and prognathism may occur.

achromatopsia (əkrōmətōp'sēə), *n* the condition of total color blindness.

Achromycin V, *n.pr* a brand name for the antibiotic tetracycline hydrochloride.

achylia (ākē'lēə), *n* the absence or lack of hydrochloric acid and the enzyme pepsinogen in the stomach.

acid (as'id), *n* a chemical substance that, in an aqueous solution, undergoes dissociation with the formation of hydrogen ions; pH levels range from 0 to 6.9. Opposite: base. See also pH and acidic.

acid, acetic, *n* the acid of vinegar, sometimes used as a solvent for the

removal of calculus from a removable dental prosthesis. See also solvent.

acid, ascorbic, *n* See vitamin C.

acid, carbolic, *n* See phenol.

acid, cevitamic, *n* See vitamin C.

acid conditioning, *n* the use of acid (such as phosphoric acid) to prepare the tooth surface for bonding of dental adhesives or enamel sealants.

acid etchant, *n* an application of phosphoric acid used to prepare enamel surfaces to aid enamel sealant placement.

acid etching, *n* the process of treating the tooth enamel, generally with phosphoric acid, by removal of approximately 3-10 μm of enamel rod to provide retention for enamel sealant, restorative material, or orthodontic bracket.

acid, folic, *n* See vitamin B complex.

acid, hydroxypropionic (hī'drō ok'sēprōpēon'ik), *n* referring to either of two chemical compounds: 3-hydroxypropionic acid (hydracrylic acid) and 2-hydroxypropanoic acid (lactic acid).

acid, lactic (2-hydroxypropanoic acid), *n* a monobasic acid, $C_3H_6O_3$, formed as an end product in the intermediary metabolism of carbohydrates. The accumulation of lactic acid in the tissues is in part responsible for the lowering of pH levels during inflammatory states; that is, the drop in pH level is believed to increase bone loss level.

acid, nicotinic, *n* **1.** a vitamin of the B complex group and its vitamer, niacinamide, specific for the treatment of pellagra. Niacinamide functions as a constituent of coenzyme I (DPN) and coenzyme II (TPN). Nicotinic acid is found in lean meats, liver, yeast, milk, and leafy green vegetables. *n* **2.** an acid (C_5H_4N [COOH]) that forms part of the B complex group of vitamins. It acts as a cofactor in intermediary carbohydrate metabolism. It is a constituent of certain coenzymes that function in oxidative-reductive metabolic systems. With niacinamide, it is a pellagra-preventive factor. Also called *niacin, P.-P. factor, pyridine 3-carboxylic acid, vitamin P.-P.*

acid, orthophosphoric (ôr'thō fosfôr'ik), *n* See acid, phosphoric.

acid, pantothenic (pan'tōthen'ik), *n* a vitamin of the B complex group, the importance of which has not been established. It is a constituent of coenzyme A.

acid phosphatase, n an enzyme found in the kidneys, serum, semen, and prostate gland. It is elevated in serum blood levels in individuals with prostate cancer and in individuals who have recently experienced trauma.

acid, phosphoric (H_3PO_4, orthophosphoric acid), n the principal ingredient of silicate and zinc phosphate cement liquids.

acid, pteroylglutamic, n See vitamin B complex.

acid salt, n a salt containing one or more replaceable hydrogen ions.

acid, strong, n an acid that is completely ionized in aqueous solution.

acid-base balance, *n* the balance of acid to base necessary to keep the blood pH level normal (between 7.35 and 7.43).

acidemia (as'idē'mēə), n a decreased pH level of the blood, irrespective of changes in the blood bicarbonate.

acidemia, isovaleric, *n* a genetic disorder of amino acid metabolism in which isovaleric acid accumulates in the blood and urine at abnormally high levels; may respond to a low-protein diet and the administration of synthetic amino acids. See also homocystinuria.

acidic (ə'sidik), *adj* having the properties of an acid; acid-forming properties.

acidifier (əsid'ifī'ur), *n* a chemical ingredient (acetic acid) that maintains the required acidity of the fixer and stop-bath solutions in the photographic development process.

acidogenic (əsidə'jenik), *adj* generating acid or acidity. See also acid and acidic.

acidophilic (as'idōfil'ik), *adj* **1.** readily stained with acid dyes. *adj* **2.** growing well in an acid medium.

acidosis (as'idō'sis), *n* a pathologic disturbance of the acid-base balance of the body characterized by an excess of acid or inadequate base. Causes include acid ingestion, increased acid production such as that seen in diabetes mellitus or starvation, or loss of base through the kidneys or intestine.

acidosis, compensated, n a condition of acidosis in which the body pH level is maintained within the normal range through compensatory mechanisms involving the kidneys or lungs.

acidosis, respiratory, n an acidemia resulting from retention of an excess of CO_2 caused by hypoventilation.

acidosis, uncompensated, n an acidosis in which compensatory mechanisms are unable to maintain the body pH level within the normal range.

acidulated phosphate fluoride, *n* a topical agent with a low pH that is used in the prevention of dental caries.

Acinetobacter (əsin'ətōbak'tər), n a genus of nonmotile, aerobic bacteria of the family *Neisseriaceae* that often occurs in clinical specimens.

acinus (*pl.* acini) **(as'inəs),** *n* **1.** a saclike cavity present in a gland or the lungs. *n* **2.** a group of secretory cells of the salivary gland.

acinus, serous (as'inəs sēr'əs), n a group of serous cells producing serous secretory product such as in the salivary glands.

acne, *n* an inflammatory, papulopustular skin eruption occurring most often in or near the sebaceous glands on the face, neck, shoulders, and upper back.

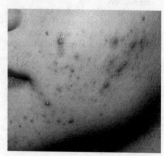

Acne. (Swartz, 2010)

acne rosacea, n a condition of the facial skin typically indicated by blushing, swelling, and the appearance of broken blood vessels in a "spider web" pattern that may lead to severe scarring of the skin surface. Etiology is not fully understood.

acne vulgaris, *n* a common form of acne seen predominantly in adolescents and young adults. Probably an effect of the rise of androgenic hormones.

acoustic turbulence, *n* agitation observed in fluids by mechanical vibrations of an ultrasonic tip; used to disrupt bacterial cell walls.

acquired centric relation (sen′trik), *n* See relation, centric, and relation, jaw, eccentric.

acquired immunity, *n* any form of immunity that is not innate and is obtained during life. It may be naturally or artificially acquired and actively or passively induced.

acquired immunodeficiency syndrome (AIDS), *n* a disease caused by a retrovirus known as human immunodeficiency virus type 1 (HIV-1). A related but distinct retrovirus (HIV-2) has recently appeared in a limited number of patients in the United States. Patients are considered to have AIDS when one or more indicator diseases, as defined by the Centers for Disease Control and Prevention (CDC), are present. See also human immunodeficiency virus (HIV). The CDC has classified stages of the disease as follows:

Group I: acute HIV infection, *n* a group who within one month of exposure develops the first clinical evidence of HIV infection, which may appear as an acute retroviral syndrome. This is a mononucleosis-like syndrome with symptoms including fever, rash, diarrhea, lymphadenopathy, myalgia, arthralgia, and fatigue. Development of antibodies usually follows.

Group II: asymptomatic HIV infection, *n* a group in which most persons develop antibodies to the HIV within 6 to 12 weeks after exposure. Although individuals may remain asymptomatic for months or years, they can transmit the virus.

Group III: persistent generalized lymphadenopathy (PGL), *n* a group who develops persistent generalized lymphadenopathy that lasts longer than 3 months. See also lymphadenopathy, persistent generalized.

Group IV: HIV-associated diseases, *n* a group who is clinically variable

and has signs and symptoms of HIV infection other than or in addition to lymphadenopathy. Based on clinical findings, patients in Group IV may be assigned to one or more of the following subgroups: (A) constitutional disease, also known as wasting syndrome. This subgroup is characterized by fever that lasts more than one month, involuntary weight loss of greater than 10% for baseline, or diarrhea persisting for more than one month, (B) neurological disease, (C) secondary infectious disease, (D) secondary cancers, and (E) other conditions resulting from HIV infections.

acridine (ak′ridēn), *n* a dibenzo-pyridine compound used in the synthesis of dyes and drugs. In dentistry, has been used to research dental deposits.

acroanesthesia (ak′rōan′esthē′zēə, -zhə), *n* anesthesia of the extremities.

acrocephalia (ak′rōəsefal′ēə), *n* a deformity of the head characterized by a superior and anterior bulge of the frontal bones and a flat occiput. Synonym: *oxycephalia.*

acrodermatitis (ak′rōder′mətī′ tis), *n* an eruption of the skin of the hands and feet caused by a parasitic mite, which is a member of the order Acarina.

acrodynia (ak′rōdī′nēə), *n* (erythredema polyneuropathy, Feer's syndrome, pink disease, Swift's syndrome, Selter's disease), a disease that occurs in infants and young children in which manifestations occur with the eruption of the primary teeth. Symptoms include raw-beef hands and feet, superficial sensory loss, photophobia, tachycardia, muscular hypotonia, changes in temperament, stomatitis, periodontitis, and premature loss of teeth. The etiology has been related to mercury and deficiency of vitamin B6 and essential fatty acids. See also erythredema polyneuropathy.

acroesthesia (ak′rōesthē′zēə, -zhə), *n* **1.** increased sensitivity. *n* **2.** pain in the extremities.

acromegaly (akrəmeg′əlē), *n* (Marie's disease), a condition caused by hyperfunction of the pituitary gland in adults. Characterized by enlargement of the skeletal extremities, including the feet, hands, mandible, and nose.

acrosclerosis (ak'rōsklerō'sis), *n* a special form of scleroderma that affects the extremities, head, and face and is associated with Raynaud's phenomenon. There may be significant thickening of the periodontal ligament.

acrylic (əkril'ik), *adj* formed from acrylic acid (e.g., acrylic resin, acrylic resin denture, and acrylic resin tooth). See also denture, acrylic resin; and tooth, acrylic resin.

acrylic resin, n See resin, acrylic.

ACTH (adrenocorticotropic hormone) (ədrē'nōkor'tikōtrō'pik hor'mōn), *n* a hormone produced by basophilic cells of the anterior lobe of the pituitary gland that exerts a reciprocal regulating influence on the production of corticosteroids by the adrenal cortex.

actinic cheilitis (aktin'ik), *n* See cheilitis, actinic.

Actinobacillus **(ak'tənōbəsil'is),** *n* a genus of nonmobile, gram-negative aerobic and facultatively anaerobic bacteria of the family Brucellaceae.

Actinomyces **(ak'tənōmī'sēz),** *n.pl* filamentous microorganisms that have been implicated in the formation of dental calculus and serve as a mode of attachment of dental calculus to the tooth surface. These microorganisms have also been found in pathologic lesions of the alveolar processes (actinomycosis).

A. israelii **(ak'tənōmī'sēz izrā'lē),** *n. pl* a normally occurring oral bacteria that aggressively causes infection (actinomycosis) when oral health is compromised.

A. naeslundii **(ak'tənōmī'sēz nāzlun'dē),** *n* a specific strain of bacteria resident in open sores in the oral cavity.

A. viscosus, n a species of *Actinomyces* occurring in high numbers in the dental plaque, cemental caries, and tonsillar crypts.

🔲 **actinomycosis (ak'tinōmikō'sis),** *n* (lumpy jaw), an infection of humans and some animal species caused by species of *Actinomyces,* which are gram-positive, filamentous, micro-aerophilic microorganisms.

action, *n* the coordinated movement of a group of muscles, relative to the resting position of the body.

action potential, *n* **1.** an electric impulse consisting of a selfpropagating series of polarizations and depolarizations, transmitted across the cell membranes of a nerve fiber during the transmission of a nerve impulse and across the cell membranes of a muscle cell during contraction. *n* **2.** the electrical potential developed in a muscle or nerve during activity.

activate (ak'tivāt), *v* in orthodontics, to adjust an appliance so that it will exert effective force on the teeth and jaws.

activated resin, *n* See resin, autopolymer.

activator (ak'tivātur), *n* **1.** an alkali, sodium carbonate, which is a component of photographic developing solution that softens and swells the gelatin of the film emulsion and provides the necessary alkaline medium for the developing agents to react with the sensitized silver halide crystals. *n* **2.** in orthodontics, a removable orthodontic appliance intended to function as a passive transmitter and sometimes stimulator of the forces of the perioral muscles. One in the orofacial myofunctional category of appliances also known by such names as *Andresen, Bimler, Monobloc,* and *Frankel.*

active, *adj* in orthodontics, pertaining to the condition of an orthodontic appliance that has been adjusted to apply effective force to the teeth or jaws.

active reciprocation, n See reciprocation, active.

acts, practice, *n.pl* the statutory requirements of a state for the education, training, examination, credentialing, supervision, and accountability of dental professionals.

acuity (əkyōōitē), *n* sharpness; clearness; keenness.

acuity, auditory, n the sensitivity of the auditory apparatus; sharpness of hearing. The ability to hear a given tone with respect to the degree of intensity required to produce a sensation that is just perceptible.

acuity, visual, n sharpness, acuteness, clearness of vision. Visual acuity may be defective because of optical or neurologic dysfunction.

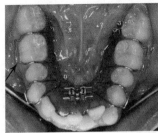

acupuncture (ak′yəpunk′chər), *n* a method of producing analgesia or altering the function of a system of the body by inserting fine, wire-thin needles into the skin at specific sites along a series of lines or channels called meridians. The needles may be twirled, energized electrically, or warmed.

acute, *adj* pertaining to a traumatic, pathologic, or physiologic phenomenon or process having a short and relatively severe course. Antonym: chronic.

Adams' clasp. (Courtesy Dr. Flavio Uribe)

acute phase reactions, *n.pl* the abnormalities in the blood associated with acute and chronic inflammatory and necrotic processes and detected by a variety of tests, including erythrocyte sedimentation rate, C-reactive protein, serum hexosamine, serum mucoprotein, and serum nonglucosamine polysaccharides.

acyanotic (āsī′yənot′ik), *adj* refers to the absence of cyanosis, or deficient oxygenation of blood. Typically used in reference to types of congenital heart defects that do not prevent blood from being properly oxygenated by the lungs.

acyclovir (āsī′klōvir), *n brand name:* Zovirax; *drug class:* antiviral. *Uses:* may be used topically and systemically. Drug of choice in simple mucocutaneous herpes simplex, in immunocompromised patients with initial herpes genitalis. Active against herpes viruses such as herpes zoster or varicella (chickenpox).

ADA Seal of Acceptance, *n.pr* the insignia of the American Dental Association's Council on Scientific Affairs, given to products used in all aspects of oral health and maintenance. Designed to help the public and dental professionals make informed decisions about safe and effective dental products.

adamantinoma (adəman′tinō′mə), *n* See ameloblastoma.

adamantoblastoma (adəman′tōblastō′mə), *n* See ameloblastoma.

Adams' clasp, *n* a retention clasp to stabilize removable appliances by engaging the mesiobuccal and distobuccal surfaces of molar teeth.

adaptation, *n* **1.** an alteration that an organ or organism undergoes to adjust to its environment. *n* **2.** a close approximation of a tissue flap, an appliance, or a restorative material to natural tissue. *n* **3.** an accurate adjustment of a band or a shell to a tooth. *n* **4.** a condition in reflex activity marked by a decline in the frequency of impulses when sensory stimuli are repeated several times.

adaptation, instrument, *n* the process of manually adjusting and positioning the functional end, edge, or surface of a dental instrument for safe and effective use according to its purpose and relative to the shape of the tooth.

adapter, band, *n* an instrument used as an aid in fitting an orthodontic band to a tooth.

adaptive functioning, *n* the relative ability of a person to effectively interact with society on all levels and care for one's self; affected by one's willingness to practice skills and pursue opportunities for improvement on all levels. Often used to describe levels of mental retardation.

addict (ad′ikt), *n* an individual who has become physiologically or psychologically dependent on a chemical such as alcohol or other drugs. Normal social, occupational, and other life functions are disrupted.

addiction (ədik′shən), *n* the state of being addicted. Addiction is generally considered a condition involving 3 factors: (1) a compulsive use of a substance known to the user to be harmful, (2) a craving for the substance, and (3) a tendency to relapse after a period of not using of the substance.

A

addictive (ədik′tiv), *adj* pertaining to a drug whose repeated use may produce addiction.

Addison's disease, *n.pr* See disease, Addison's.

Addison-Biermer anemia (ad′isən-bir′mur), *n.pr* See anemia, pernicious.

additive, *n* an ingredient added to a food, drug, or other preparation to produce a desired result, such as color or consistency, unrelated to the primary purpose of the preparation.

adduct (ədukt′), *v* to draw toward the center or midline.

adduction (əduk′shən), *n* the process of bringing two objects toward each other; the opposite of abduction.

A-delta fibers, *n.pl* See fiber, nerve.

adenine (ad′ənēn), *n* a component of the nucleic acids, DNA and RNA, and a constituent of cyclic AMP and the adenosine portion of AMP, ADP, and ATP.

adenitis (ad′əni′tis), *n* an inflammation of glandular tissue, often accompanied by pain.

adenocarcinoma (ad′ənōkarsinō′mə), *n* a large group of malignant epithelial cell tumors of the glands. Specific tumors are diagnosed and named by the cell type of the tissue affected.

adenocarcinoma, acinic cell, n a cancer of the salivary glands, primarily the parotid gland.

adenocarcinoma, polymorphous low-grade (PLGA) (pol′ēmor′fəs), n a cancer of the salivary glands, primarily in the minor salivary glands.

adenoidectomy (ad′ənoidek′təmē), *n* the removal of the lymphoid tissue in the nasopharynx, usually in conjunction with the surgical removal of the palatine tonsils.

adenoids (ad′ənoidz′), *adj* See tonsil, pharyngeal.

adenoid facies, n an older term used to describe patients who exhibit a long, narrow face, short upper lip, oral cavity breathing, and a hyperactive swallowing pattern. Newer term is *long face syndrome.*

adenoma (ad′ənō′mə), *n* a benign epithelial neoplasm or tumor with a basic glandular (acinar) structure, suggesting derivation from glandular tissue.

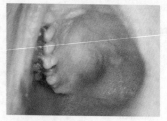

Adenoma. (Regezi/Sciubba/Jordan, 2012)

adenoma, acidophilic, n See oncocytoma.

adenoma, oxyphilic, n See oncocytoma.

adenomatosis oris (ad′ənōmətō′sis), *n* an enlargement of the mucous glands of the lip without secretion or inflammation.

adenopathy (ad′ənop′əthē), *n* an enlargement or increase in size of glandular organs or tissues usually resulting from disease processes.

adenosine (əden′əsēn′), *n* a compound derived from nucleic acid, composed of adenine and a sugar, D-ribose. Major molecular component of nucleotides and the nucleic acids.

adenosine monophosphate (AMP), n an ester, composed of adenine, D-ribose, and phosphoric acid, that affects energy release in work done by a muscle.

adenosine triphosphate (ATP), n a compound consisting of the nucleotide adenosine attached through its ribose group to three phosphoric acid molecules. Stores energy in muscles, which is released when it is hydrolized to adenosine diphosphate.

adenoviridae (ad′ənōvēr′idē), n a family of unenveloped, 20-sided DNA viruses found in mammals (Mastadenovirus) and birds (Aviadenovirus). The human variety can cause a number of diseases, from conjunctivitis to urinary tract infection.

adequacy, velopharyngeal, *n* a functional closure of the velum to the postpharyngeal wall that restricts air and sound from entering the nasopharyngeal and nasal cavities.

adequate intake *(AI),* *n* the consumption and absorption of sufficient food, vitamins, and essential minerals necessary to maintain health. See also dietary reference intakes; estimated average dietary requirement; recommended dietary allowances; and upper intake levels, tolerable.

ADH, *n* See hormone, antidiuretic.

adhesion (adh′zhən), *n* **1.** the attraction of unlike molecules for one another. *n* **2.** the molecular attraction existing between surfaces in close contact. *n* **3.** the condition in which a material sticks to itself or another material. *n* **4.** the abnormal joining of tissues, generally by fibrous connective tissue, to each other after repair of an injury.

adhesion, bacterial, n a microbial surface antigen that frequently exists in the form of filamentous projections and binds to specific receptors on epithelial cell membranes.

adhesion, sublabial, n the abnormal union of the sublabial mucosa of the upper lip to the alveolar process; usually present in a unilateral or bilateral cleft of the lip.

adhesive, *n* an intermediate material that causes two materials to stick together; a luting agent.

adhesives, bonding, for desensitization, n sealant materials applied to the open ends of dentinal tubules that block the stimuli linked to tooth sensitivity.

adhesive foil, n See foil, adhesive.

adipose tissue (ad′əpōs′), *n* a connective tissue composed of a collection of fat cells.

adjudicate (əjōō′dikāt′), *v* the final step in dental peer review at which the dental peer review committee renders a formal, nonlegal decision on a case.

adjunct (aj′ungkt), *n* a drug or other substance that serves a supplemental purpose in therapy.

adjust (əjust′), *v* to make correspondent, comfortable, or to fit.

adjustment (əjust′ment), *n* a modification of a restoration or of a denture after insertion in the oral cavity.

adjustment, in orthodontics, n change of elastic ligatures or elastic chain and arch wire if needed, once in every 4-6 weeks.

adjustment, occlusal, n a grinding of the occluding surfaces of teeth to develop harmonious relationships between each other, their supporting structures, muscles of mastication, and temporomandibular joints.

adjuvant (aj′əvənt), *n* an auxiliary active ingredient that supports the action of the basic drug. See also basis.

administration, *n* the giving of, dispensing of, or application of medicines, drugs, or remedies to relieve or cure an illness.

administration, buccal, n the delivery of a medication by application to the buccal mucosa.

administration, inhalation, n the delivery of a medication by breathing it.

administration, intranasal, n the delivery of a medication into the nasal cavity.

administration, oral, n the delivery of a medication by oral cavity.

administration, rectal, n the delivery of a medication through the rectum.

administration, sublingual, n the delivery of a medication by placing it under the ventral surface of the tongue for dissolution and absorption through the mucous membrane.

administration, topical, n the delivery of a medication by application to the skin or mucous membrane.

administrative costs, *n.pl* the overhead expenses incurred in the operation of a dental benefits program, excluding costs of dental services provided.

administrative services only (ASO), *n* an arrangement in which a third party, for a fee, processes claims and handles paperwork for a self-funded group. This frequently includes almost all insurance company services, including actuarial services, underwriting, and benefit description, and excluding assumption of risk.

administrator, *n* a person who manages or directs a dental benefits program on behalf of the program's sponsor. See also third-party administrator and dental benefits organization.

admission, *n* the voluntary concession or admission that a fact or allegation is true.

admission, hospital, n **1.** a full stay. The formal acceptance by a hospital or other inpatient health care facility of a patient who is to be provided with room, board, and continuous nursing service in an area of the hospital or facility where patients generally reside at least overnight. *n* **2.** a surgicenter with short stays. Day bed only with nursing; patient does not stay overnight. *n* **3.** an outpatient admission. Pertains to a patient who enters the hospital but requires no bed; the patient enters for treatment and leaves after treatment.

adnexa (adnek'sə), *n* the conjoined anatomic parts, or tissues adjacent to or contained within a nearby space.

adolescence, *n* the period of development between the onset of puberty and adulthood. This period is generally marked by the appearance of secondary sex characteristics, usually from 11 to 13 years of age, and spans the teen years.

adolescent growth spurt, *n* a period of rapid increase in height, weight, and muscle mass, which for boys takes place at age 12 to 16 and for girls at age 11 to 14. See also adolescence.

adrenal cortex (ədrē'nəl kor'teks), *n* the greater portion of the adrenal gland fused with the gland's medulla and producing mineralocorticoids, androgens, and glucocorticoids, hormones essential to homeostasis. The outer cortex is normally a deep yellow; the inner part is dark red or brown.

adrenal corticoid (ədrē'nəl kor'təkoid'), *n* See corticoid, adrenal.

adrenal crisis, *n* See crisis, adrenal.

adrenal steroids, *n.pl* See corticoid, adrenal.

adrenalectomy (ədrē'nəlek'tə mē), *n* the surgical removal of one or both of the adrenal glands or the resection of a portion of one or both of the adrenal glands.

Adrenalin (ədren'əlin), *n* the brand name for epinephrine. See also epinephrine.

adrenaline (ədren'əlin), *n* the British term for epinephrine.

adrenergic (ad'rinur'jik), *adj* **1.** transmitted by norepinephrine or activated by norepinephrine or the other sympathomimetic agents. *n* **2.** a term applied to nerve fibers that liberate epinephrine or norepinephrine at a synapse when a nerve impulse passes. *n* **3.** a drug that mimics the action of adrenergic nerves.

adrenergic agonists, *n.pl* drugs that mimic the actions of norepinephrine, a neurotransmitter, resulting in stimulation of the sympathetic nervous system.

adrenergic blocking agent, *n* See agent, adrenergic blocking.

adrenergic fibers, *n.pl* See fibers, adrenergic.

adrenergic receptors, *n.pl* See receptors, adrenergic.

adrenic (ədrē'nik), *adj* pertaining to the adrenal gland.

adrenocortical insufficiency (ədrē' nōkôr'tikəl), *n* an acute or chronic adrenocortical hypofunction, as in Waterhouse-Friderichsen syndrome or Addison's disease. See also hypoadrenocorticalism.

adrenocorticotropin (ədrē'nō kôr'tikōtrō'pin), *n* See ACTH.

adrenolytic (ədrē'nōlit'ik), *adj* capable of impeding the action of epinephrine, levarterenol (norepinephrine), or both (sympatholytic).

adrenolytic agent, *n* See agent, adrenergic blocking.

adrenotropic (ədrē'nōtrōp'ik), *adj* having a special affinity for the adrenal gland.

adsorb, *v* to attract molecules of a substance to the surface of another solid substance.

adsorbent (adsor'bənt), *adj* a substance that adsorbs, such as activated charcoal and clay.

adsorption, *n* a natural process whereby molecules of a gas or liquid adhere to the surface of a solid.

adult, *n* **1.** a person who has the fully developed characteristics of a mature person. *n* **2.** a person who has reached full legal age.

adumbration (ad'əmbrā'shən), *n* a geometric lack of sharpness of the radiograph shadow. See also penumbra, geometric.

advances, *n.pl* monies paid before the scheduled time of payment.

adverse drug effect, *n* a harmful, unintended reaction to a drug administered at normal dosage.

adverse reaction, *n* a harmful, unintended effect of a medication, diagnostic test, or therapeutic intervention.

adverse reactions, *n.pl* an unwanted or unexpected negative reaction to a medication or treatment that is used in an approved manner.

adverse selection, *n* a statistical condition within a group when there is a greater demand for dental services and/or more services necessary than the average expected for that group.

advertising, *n* a paid form of nonpersonal presentation and promotion of ideas, goods, or services by an identified sponsor.

aeration (erā´shən), *n* the passage of air or gases into liquid (e.g., the passage of oxygen from pulmonary alveoli into the blood).

aerobe, *n* a microorganism able to live and grow in the presence of free oxygen. An aerobe may be facultative or obligate.

aerobiosis (er´ōbīō´sis), *n* life occurring in the presence of oxygen.

aerodontalgia   (er´ōdontal´jə), *n* pulpal pain with decreased barometric pressure.

Aeromonas **(er´ōmō´nas),** *n* a genus of bacteria usually found in water.

aerosol (er´əsôl), *n* **1.** the suspension of materials in a gas or vapor (e.g., saliva vaporized in air-water spray from a high-speed handpiece). *n* **2.** a substance dispensed as a constituent of a gas or vapor suspension.

aesthetic factors, *n.pl* See esthetic dentistry.

affect (af´ekt), *n* **1.** the feeling of pleasantness or unpleasantness produced by a stimulus. *n* **2.** the emotional complex influencing a mental state. *n* **3.** the feeling experienced in connection with an emotion.

affective domain, *n* the area of learning involved in appreciation, interests, and attitudes.

afferent (af´ərənt), *adj* conveying from a periphery to a center.

afferent impulse, *n* an impulse that arises in the periphery and is carried into the central nervous system. An afferent nerve conducts the impulse from the site of origin to the central nervous system.

afferent nerves, *n.pl* See nerves, afferent, in pulp. See also afferent impulse.

afferent nervous system, *n.* the sensory nerves, a subdivision of the peripheral nervous system. Afferent nerves receive sensory input.

affiliation (əfil´ēā´shən), *n* the incorporation or formation of a partnership by dental professionals for the purpose of practicing the profession of dentistry.

afflux (af´luks), *n* the rush of blood to a body part.

affricative (əfrik´ətiv), *n* a fricative speech sound initiated by a plosive.

aflatoxins   (af´lətok´sins), *n.pl* a group of carcinogenic and toxic factors produced by *Aspergillus flavus* food molds.

afterperception, the perception of a sensation after the stimulus producing it has ceased. (not current)

agar, hydrocolloid (ä´gär), *n* a reversible hydrocolloid made from agar-agar.

age, *n* the period of time a person has existed or an object has existed.

age, biological, *n* the age determined by physiology rather than chronology. Factors include changes in the physical structure of the body as well as changes in the performance of motor skills and sensory awareness.

age, chronologic, *n* age determined by the passage of time since birth.

age, dental, *n* age determined based on the eruption stage of dentition.

age determination, *n* (by teeth), an estimate of age from the stage of tooth development and/or pattern of wear.

age distribution, *n* a grouping of the persons within a population on the basis of birth date.

age factors, *n.pl* variables affected by time since birth.

age hardening, *n* See hardening, age.

age of onset, *n* the chronologic age of the patient at which the disease, affliction, or disability appeared.

age, psychological, *n* a subjectively experienced age based on a person's behavior, or "how old they feel."

age, skeletal, *n* the age based on skeletal measurements relative to chronological skeletal development.

aged, *n* a state of having grown older or more mature than others of the population. See also geriatrics.

agenesis (ājen´əsis), *n* the defective development or congenital absence of parts.

agent(s), *n/n.pl* **1.** a person or product that causes action. *n* **2.** a person authorized to act for, or in place of, another.

agent, adrenergic blocking, *n* a drug that blocks the action of the neurohormones norepinephrine and/or epinephrine or of adrenergic drugs at sympathetic neuroeffectors.

agent, adrenolytic blocking (ədrē′nə lit′ik), *n* an uncertain term sometimes used in reference to adrenergic blocking agents.

agent, anesthetic, *n* a drug that produces local or general loss of sensation.

agent, antianxiety, *n* any medication prescribed to relieve anxiety disorder symptoms, primarily stress and insomnia. The most common forms are benzodiazepine derivatives.

agent, antiarrhythmic (an′tiərith′ mik), *n* a substance used to prevent or relieve an irregular rhythm of heartbeat. Also called *antidysrhythmic.*

agent, antigingivitis, *n* compound that inhibits, controls, or kills organisms associated with the formation of gingivitis.

agent, antihypertensive, *n* a medication used to lower elevated blood pressure (e.g., diuretics, beta-blockers, and vasodilators).

agent, antiinflammatory, *n* a drug that reduces inflammation.

agent, antimanic, *n* a substance used to treat various nervous system and psychiatric disorders; possible effects on fetal development include sluggishness, oxygen deficiency, and physical malformations.

agent, antiparasitic, *n* an antimicrobe that specifically targets pathogenic microorganisms.

agent, blocking, *n* an agent that occupies or usurps the receptor site normally occupied by a drug or a biochemical intermediary (e.g., acetylcholine or epinephrine).

agent, bonding, *n* a substance used to bond fillings and tooth restorations to the tooth surface.

agent, chemotherapeutic (kē′mō therəpyōō′tik), *n* a chemical of natural or synthetic origin used for its specific action against disease, usually against infection.

agent, cholinergic blocking (kō′lə ner′jik), *n* **1.** a drug that inhibits the action of acetylcholine or cholinergic drugs at the postganglionic

cholinergic neuroeffectors. *n* **2.** an anticholinergic agent.

agent, cleaning, *n* an abrasive substance contained in toothpastes, gels, and powders that polishes teeth and aids in the removal of stains and plaque biofilm. See also abrasion, dentifrice.

agent, coloring, *n* any substance contained in toothpastes, gels, and powders purely to make the product more appealing.

agent, coupling, *n* a substance or material that binds to both resin and reinforcement material and helps join them to make a composite.

agent, ganglionic blocking (gang′lēo n′ik), *n* a drug that prevents passage of nerve impulses at the synapses between preganglionic and postganglionic neurons.

agent, myoneural blocking (mī′ōnŏŏ r′əl), *n* a drug that prevents transmission of nerve impulses at the junction of the nerve and the muscle.

agent, oxidizing, *n* an agent that provides oxygen in reaction with another substance or, in the broader and more definitive chemical sense, a chemical capable of accepting electrons and thereby decreasing the negative charge on an atom of the substance being oxidized.

agent, polishing, *n* an abrasive that produces a smooth, lustrous finish.

agent, postganglionic sympathetic blocking, *n* a medication used to treat hypertension by blocking the release of the naturally occurring hormone norepinephrine.

agent, reducing, *n* a category of chemicals used in film processing that brings out the gray tones of an image by creating black metallic silver from silver halide crystals.

agent, wetting, *n* any agent that will reduce the surface tension of water. Generally used in investing wax patterns.

agent, whitening, *n* a bleaching substance applied to teeth to lighten their appearance.

agents, antiadrenergic, centrally acting (an′tēad′rəner′jik), *n.pl* antihypertensive drugs used to lower blood pressure, specifically those that operate by stimulating α-receptors in the central nervous system and arterioles.

agents, antianginal, n. pl medications used to treat heart disease; they alleviate pain associated with angina such as by lowering blood pressure during systole. See also vasodilator.

agents, oxygenating, n.pl substances, such as hydrogen peroxide, that, when used as mouthrinses, release oxygen into gingival tissues and reduce inflammation. The process has not proved to reduce the bacteria causing the inflammation. Long-term use may cause tissue damage.

agents, sympathetic, n.pl medications that stimulate the sympathetic nervous system by imitating the actions of naturally occurring norepinephrine and epinephrine. They may be used to treat cardiac arrest, nasal congestion, asthma, glaucoma, and attention deficit hyperactivity disorder and may cause anxiety, loss of appetite, and arrythmias. Also called *adrenergic agents.*

age-related macular degeneration (AMD), n the loss of central (as opposed to peripheral) vision caused by diminished functioning of the macula of the retina. In those age 60 years and older, it is the most common cause of blindness.

ageusia (əgōō′sēə), n a loss or impairment of the sense of taste.

agglutination (əglōō′tinä′shən), n the aggregation or clumping together of cells as a result of their interaction with specific antibodies called agglutinins, commonly used in blood typing and in identifying or estimating the strength of immunoglobulins or immune sera.

agglutinin (əglōō′tinin), n 1. a specific kind of antibody whose interaction with antigens is manifested as agglutination. n 2. an antibody that agglutinates red blood cells or renders them agglutinable.

aging, n in human development, the process of growing old. Physically, aging is marked by the reduction in the ability of cells to function normally or to produce new body cells at an optimal rate.

aging schedule, n a report showing how long accounts receivable have been outstanding. It gives the percentage of receivables not past due and the percentage past due by 1 month, 2 months, or other periods.

agitation, n 1. the shaking of a substance, either for mixing ingredients or to remove debris or buildup from an object within the substance, such as a removable oral prosthetic. n 2. the intentional, usually mild, disturbance of the skin, mucosa, or other surface (e.g., with a wooden interdental cleaner or probe instrument) to determine if infection or disease is present. If agitated surfaces bruise or bleed easily, or are otherwise disrupted (e.g., develop a lesion), the presence of a pathologic condition should be suspected. n 3. a psychosomatic condition represented by uncontrollable or excessive body movements. The psychologic aspect may often indicate the presence of unresolved stress.

aglossia (aglôs′ēə), n a developmental anomaly in which a portion or all of the tongue is absent.

agnathia (agnath′ēə), n an absence of the mandible.

agnosia (agnō′zēə, -zhə), n a loss of ability to recognize common objects (that is, a loss of ability to understand the significance of sensory stimuli [e.g., tactile, auditory, or visual] resulting from brain damage).

agonist (ag′ənist), n 1. an organ, gland, muscle, or nerve center that is so connected physiologically with another that the two function simultaneously in forwarding a given process, such as when two muscles pull on the same skeletal member and receive a nervous excitation at the same time. Opposite: antagonist. n 2. a drug or other substance having a selective receptor affinity that produces a predictable response in a cell.

agony, n severe pain or extreme suffering.

agoraphobia (ag′ərəfō′bēə), n an anxiety disorder characterized by a fear of being in an open, crowded, or public place where escape may be difficult or help may not be available if needed.

agranulocytosis (āgran′yŏŏlō sītō′sis), n a decrease in the number of granulocytes in peripheral blood resulting from bone marrow depression by drugs and chemicals or replacement by a neoplasm. Oral lesions are ulceronecrotic, involving the gingivae, tongue, buccal mucosa, or lips. Regional lymphadenopathy and lymphadenitis are prevalent.

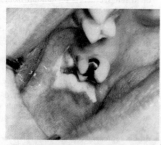

Agranulocytosis.   (Sapp/Eversole/
Wysocki, 2004)

agreement, *n* the coming together in accord of two minds on a given proposition.

AH-26, *n* an epoxy resin root canal sealer.

AHF, *n* the abbreviation for antihemophilic factor. See also factor VIII.

aid, *n* assistance; support.

aid in physiotherapy, *n* an agent used by the patient to cleanse the teeth and oral tissues and provide pseudofunctional stimulation of the gingival tissues to maintain periodontal health.

aid, speech therapy, *n* a restoration, appliance, or electronic device used to improve speech.

aid, visual, *n* a model, drawing, or photograph used to help the patient understand proposed treatment.

AIDS, *n* the abbreviation for acquired immunodeficiency syndrome. See also human immunodeficiency virus (HIV).

air, *n* the invisible, odorless, gaseous mixture that makes up the earth's atmosphere.

air, ambient, *n* the encircling or enveloping environment; surrounding air.

air chamber, *n* See chamber, relief.

air, complemental, *n* See volume, inspiratory reserve.

air, functional residual, *n* See capacity, functional residual.

air, minimal, *n* the volume of air in the air sacs themselves (part of the residual air).

air reserve, *n* See volume, expiratory reserve.

air, residual, *n* See volume, residual.

air, supplemental, *n* See volume, expiratory reserve.

air syringe, *n* See syringe, air.

air, tidal, *n* See volume, tidal.

air turbine handpiece, *n* See handpiece, air turbine.

air application in calculus identification, *n* See calculus, identification of, by air application.

air bubbles on radiographic film, *n* See film fault, white spots.

air embolism, *n* an obstruction of a blood vessel caused by the entrance of air into the bloodstream. See also embolism.

air tip, *n* a part of a compressed air-water syringe, with an angled end that facilitates dental examination procedures.

air-powder polishing, *n* a technique for plaque and stain removal in which sodium bicarbonate particles and water are propeled against the teeth in a regulated flow using air and water pressure. Also called *air abrasive* or *airbrasive.*

airborne, *adj* carried through the air. In health care settings, viruses or bacteria may become airborne (e.g., when someone sneezes or coughs).

airborne contaminants, *n.pl* materials in the atmosphere that can affect the health of persons in the same or a nearby environment. Also referred to as *air pollution.*

airway, *n* **1.** a clear passageway for air into and out of the lungs. *n* **2.** a device for securing unobstructed respiration during general anesthesia or in states of unconsciousness.

airway, chin lift, *n* a method of opening the trachea of an individual by manually changing the position of his or her head in order to perform rescue breathing.

airway obstruction, *n* an abnormal condition of the respiratory pathway characterized by a mechanical impediment to the delivery or to the absorption of oxygen in the lungs, as in choking, bronchospasm, obstructive lung disease, or laryngospasm.

airway obstruction, chest thrust, *n* an alternate method of removing an obstacle lodged in the airway by compressing the sternum; used when pregnancy or a patient's body size render the Heimlich maneuver impossible or inappropriate. See also Heimlich maneuver.

airway obstruction, infant chest thrust, n a method of removing an obstacle lodged in the airway of an infant by placing the child facedown along the forearm and striking the child's back with the opposite hand. See also Heimlich maneuver.

airway resistance, n the ratio of pressure difference between the oral cavity, nose, or other airway opening and the alveoli to the simultaneously measured resulting volumetric gas flow rate.

akinesia (ā′kənē′zhə), n a loss of controllable motion and feelings of exhaustion. It is a common consequence of Parkinson's disease, causing dopamine loss in the direct pathway of movement.

ala (ā′lə), n winglike cutaneous-covered cartilaginous structure on the lateral aspect of the external naris of the nose.

alanine (al′ənēn), n a nonessential amino acid found in many proteins in the body. It is metabolized in the liver to produce pyruvate and glutamate.

ALARA concept, n an acronym for "As Low As Reasonably Achievable"; it pertains to radiation exposure encountered when exposing radiographs. This idea requires that every possible precaution is taken to minimize radiation levels when exposing the patient or clinician to radiation.

alarm reaction, n See reaction, alarm; and syndrome, general adaptation.

Albers-Schönberg disease (al′berz-shœn′berg), n.pr See osteopetrosis.

Albright's syndrome, n.pr See syndrome, McCune-Albright.

albumin (albyōō′min), n the primary protein of plasma (4.5% g) that aids in maintaining capillary osmotic pressure.

albuminuria (albyōō′minyōō′rēə), n (hyperproteinuria, proteinuria, proteuria), the presence of clinically detectable amounts of protein in the urine. Usually less than 100 mg/24 hr may be found normally by special methods. The usual protein is albumin, although globulins, Bence Jones protein, and fibrinogen may be present and may exceed the amount of albumin. The condition may be caused by prerenal or renal disease or by inflammation of the urinary tract.

albuterol, n brand names: Proventil, Proventil Repetabs, Nova-Salmol, Ventodisk, Ventolin, Ventolin Rotacaps; drug class: β₂ adrenergic receptor agonist; action: causes bronchodilation; uses: to treat asthma, to reverse bronchospasm.

Alcaligenes (al′kəlij′ənēz), n.pl (literally, "alkali-generating") aerobic, gram-negative eubacteria, commonly found in invertebrate intestinal tracts and normally occurring on the skin.

alcohol (al′kəhôl), n a transparent, colorless liquid that is mobile and volatile. Alcohols are organic compounds formed from hydrocarbons by the substitution of hydroxyl radicals for the same number of hydrogen atoms.

alcohol, absolute, n an alcohol containing no more than 1% H_2O.

alcohol abuse, n the frequent intake of large amounts of alcohol, typically distinguished by decreased health and physical and social functioning impairment. See also alcoholism.

alcohol blood level, n See blood alcohol concentration.

alcohol dependence, n a mental and physical need to consume alcohol in order to prevent the pains of withdrawal and obtain certain results; causes a limited capacity to control actions during consumption of alcohol. See also alcohol abuse.

alcohol hallucinosis (həlōō′sənō′sis), n a complication of the last stage of withdrawal from alcohol, occurring within 48 hours of sudden decrease or halt of increased consumption after a lengthy period of dependence. It is indicated by severely impairing visual and auditory hallucinations similar to schizophrenia symptoms that may persist for weeks or months.

alcohol withdrawal delirium, n a complication of the last stage of withdrawal from alcohol, occurring within 1 week of sudden decrease or halt of increased consumption after a lengthy period of dependence; indicated by dramatic auditory, visual, and tactile hallucinations, confusion, delusions, disorientation, tremors, nervous actions, sweating, and rapid heartbeat. Also called *DTs* or *delirium tremens*.

alcoholic group therapy, *n* an association of men and women devoted to helping each other treat alcohol dependence. Participants and facilitators may use psychotherapy, behavior therapy, and the recruitment of family members and friends to achieve objectives.

alcoholic, recovering, *n* a person who is attempting to refrain from the compulsive consumption of alcohol and thereby escape the physiologic, psychologic, and social impairments associated with it.

Alcoholics Anonymous (AA), *n.pr* a group program in which the members help themselves and each other defeat alcoholism.

alcoholism, *n* the continued extreme dependence on excessive amounts of alcohol, accompanied by a cumulative pattern of deviant behaviors. The most frequent consequences are chronic gastritis, central nervous system depression, and cirrhosis of the liver, each of which can compromise the delivery of dental care. Oral cancer and increased levels of periodontal disease are also risks.

aldehyde (al′dəhīd′), *n* a large category of organic compounds derived from a corresponding alcohol by the removal of two hydrogen atoms, as in the conversion of ethyl alcohol to acetaldehyde.

aldesleukin (al′dəslōō′kin), *n* (interleukin-2, IL-2), *brand name:* Proleukin; *drug class:* antineoplastic; *action:* enhancement of lymphocyte mitogenesis and stimulation of IL-2 dependent cell lines; *use:* metastatic renal cell carcinoma in adults.

aldosterone (aldos′tərōn), *n* an adrenal corticosteroid hormone that acts primarily to accelerate the exchange of potassium for sodium in the renal tubules and other cells. It is a potent mineralocorticoid but also has some regulatory effect on carbohydrate metabolism.

aldosteronism, primary (aldos′tərō′nizəm), *n* a hyperadrenal syndrome caused by abnormal elaboration of aldosterone and characterized by excessive loss of potassium and resultant muscle weakness. The symptoms

suggest tetany. The condition is often associated with an adenoma or cortical hyperplasia of the adrenal glands.

alendronate sodium (əlen′drənāt′ sō′dēəm), *n brand name:* Fosamax; *drug class:* amino biphosphonate; *action:* acts as an inhibitor of bone resorption by inhibiting osteoclast activity; *uses:* osteoporosis in postmenopausal women, Paget's disease of bone.

alfentanyl, *n brand name:* Alfenta; *drug class:* opioid analgesic; *actions:* agonist at opioid receptors, analgesic action; *uses:* analgesia, used as an adjunct to anesthesia prior to and during surgery (especially cardiac surgery).

alganesthesia (algan′esthē′zhə), *n* the absence of a normal sense of pain.

algesia (aljē′zēə), *n* sensitivity to pain; hyperesthesia; a sense of pain.

algesic (aljē′sik), *adj* painful.

algesimetry (aljəsim′etrē), *n* the measurement of response to painful stimuli.

algetic (aljet′ik), *adj* painful.

alginate (al′jināt), *n* a salt of alginic acid (e.g., sodium alginate), which, when mixed with water in accurate proportions, forms an irreversible hydrocolloid gel used for making impressions or molds of the dentition. See also hydrocolloid, irreversible.

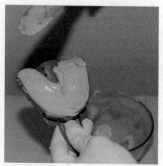

Mixed alginate. (Garg, 2010)

algorithm (al′gərith′əm), *n* an explicit protocol with well-defined rules to be followed in solving a complex problem.

align (əlīn), *v* to move the teeth into their proper positions to conform to the line of occlusion.

align, in orthodontics, *n* the first step in biomechanical execution of orthodontic treatment sequence to relieve crowding .

alignment, tooth (əlīn′ment), *n* the arrangement of the teeth in relationship to their supporting bone (alveolar process), adjacent teeth, and opposing dentition.

aliskiren, *n* *brand name:* Tecturna; *drug class:* renin inhibitor; *action:* inhibits the rate-limiting step in the renin-angiotensin system; *use:* hypertension.

alkali (al′kəlī), *n* a strong water-soluble base. A chemical substance that, in aqueous solution, undergoes dissociation, resulting in the formation of hydroxyl (OH) ions.

alkaline (al′kəlin), *adj* having the reductions of an alkali. A pH level of 7.1 to 14 designates an alkaline solution. See also basic.

alkaline diet, *n* See diet, alkaline.

alkaline phosphatase, *n* an enzyme present in bone, the kidneys, the intestines, plasma, and teeth. It may be elevated in the serum in some diseases associated with disturbances in bone, liver, or other tissues.

alkaline reserve, *n* See reserve, alkaline.

alkaloid (al′kəloid), *n* the many nitrogen-containing organic bases derived from plants. They are bitter and physiologically active. A number are useful therapeutic agents.

alkaloid, synthetic, *n* a synthetically prepared compound having the chemical characteristics of the alkaloids.

alkalosis (alkəlō′sis), *n* a disturbance of acid-base balance and water balance, characterized by an excess of alkali or a deficiency of acids.

alkalosis, compensated, *n* a condition in which the blood bicarbonate is usually higher than normal but compensatory mechanisms have kept the pH level within normal range. See also alkalosis, uncompensated.

alkalosis, hypochloremic, *n* a metabolic abnormality caused by an increase in blood bicarbonate after significant chloride loss.

alkalosis, respiratory, *n* alkalemia produced by hypoventilation. Plasma bicarbonate is therefore decreased in respiratory alkalosis but raised in metabolic alkalosis.

alkalosis, uncompensated, *n* alkalemia usually accompanied by an increased blood bicarbonate.

allele (əlēl′), *n* (allelomorph), one or more genes occupying the same location in a chromosome but differing because of a mutational change of one.

allergen (al′urjen), *n* a substance capable of producing an allergic response or antigen. Common allergens are pollens, dust, drugs, and foods. See also antigen.

allergy (al′urjē), *n* a hypersensitive reaction to an allergen; an antigen-antibody reaction is manifested in several forms—anaphylaxis, asthma, hay fever, urticaria, angioedema, dermatitis, and stomatitis.

allergy, cross-reactive, *n* a condition in which a patient allergic to one medication will experience an allergic reaction to all other medications possessing a similar chemical structure (e.g., cross-sensitivity between penicillin derivatives, cephalosporins, and carbapenems). See also resistance, cross.

allergy, "spontaneous" clinical, *n* See atopy.

allied health personnel, *n.pl* the health care professionals, other than physicians, dental professionals, clinical psychologists, pharmacists, and nurses, with education, training, and experience to serve as members of the health care delivery team.

allochiria (al′ōkī′rēə, al′ōkir′ēə), *n* the tactile sensation experienced at the side opposite its origin.

allogenic, *adj* from individuals of the same species. Tissue transplanted from one person to another is said to be allogenic.

allografts (al′əgrafts), *n.pl* the transplantation of tissue between genetically nonidentical individuals of the same species. Also known as *homoplastic grafts* or *homografts*.

alloplast (al′lōplast), *n* inorganic material used as a bone substitute or an implant.

alloplastic (al′ōplas′tik), *adj* nonbiologic material such as metal, ceramic, and plastic.

alloplasty (al′ōplas′tē), *n* a plastic surgery procedure in which material not from the human body is used.

allopurinol (al'əpyŏō'rinol), *n brand names:* Lopurin, Zyloprim; *drug class:* antigout drug; *actions:* inhibits the enzyme xanthine oxidase, reducing uric acid synthesis; *uses:* chronic gout, hyperuricemia associated with malignancies.

allowable benefits, *n.pl* necessary, reasonable, and customary items of service or treatments covered in whole or in part under an insurance plan.

allowable charge, *n* the maximum dollar amount on which benefit payment is based for each dental procedure.

allowable expenses, *n.pl* the dollar amounts allowable for each dental procedure covered by a dental insurance policy.

alloxan (əlok'san), *n* a substance, mesoxalyl urea, capable of producing experimental diabetes by destroying the islet cells of the pancreas.

alloy (al'oi), *n* **1.** a solution composed of two metals dissolved in each other when in the liquid state. *n* **2.** the product of the fusion of two or more metals.

alloy, amalgam **(əmal'gəm),** *n* the alloy or product of the fusion of several metals, usually supplied as filings, that is mixed with mercury to produce dental amalgam. Colloquial term is *silver fillings*.

alloy, cobalt-chromium, *n* (chrome-cobalt amalgam), a base metal alloy. Used in dentistry for metallic denture bases and partial dentures. Also used in orthodontics as an archwire. Four types (color coded) based on level of resilience. Also known as *Elgiloy.*

alloy, dental amalgam, *n* See amalgam.

alloy, dental gold, *n* an alloy in which the principal ingredient is gold.

alloy, eutectic, *n* any combination of metals the melting point of which is lower than that of any of the individual metals of which it consists. An alloy in which the components are mutually soluble in the solid state. A eutectic alloy has a nonhomogeneous grain structure and is therefore likely to be brittle and subject to tarnishing and corrosion.

alloy, nickel-chromium, *n* a stainless steel.

almotriptan, *n brand name:* Axert; *drug class:* serotonin 5-HT$_{1B/1D}$

receptor agonist; *action:* inhibits neurovascular inflammation in the dura matter and other actions in the brain; *use:* migraine.

alopecia (al'əpē'shə), *n* the loss of hair (baldness). Various types with varying causes.

alpha-adrenergic receptor blockers (al'fə-ad'rəner'jik), *n.pl* drugs that block α-adrenergic receptors, which in turn inhibits sympathetic autonomic nervous system and drug stimulation of those receptors. Uses include, hypertension, benign prostate hyperplasia, peripheral vascular disease, reversal of soft tissue anesthesia after local anesthesia. See also agent, adrenergic receptor blocking.

alpha-amylase (al'fə-am'əlās'), *n* a starch-splitting enzyme that is a major protein component of saliva and pancreatic juice.

alpha-estradiol (al'fə-estrədī'ôl), *n* an estrogenic steroid, prepared by dehydrogenation of estrone, which is one of the factors responsible for the maintenance of the epithelial integrity of the oral tissues. A deficiency results in epithelial desquamation.

alpha-glucosidase inhibitors (al'fə-glōōkō'sidās'), *n.pl* an orally administered agent used in the treatment of type 2 diabetes mellitus. Examples include acarbose, which slows the digestion and absorption of glucose into the bloodstream.

alpha-hemihydrate (al'fə-hem'ēhī'drāt), *n* a physical form of the hemihydrate of calcium sulfate (CaSO$_4$)-H$_2$O; dental artificial stone.

alpha-interferon, *n* See interferon, alpha.

alpha-tocopherol, *n* See vitamin E.

alphabet, international phonetic, *n* a set of internationally agreed upon alphabetical symbols, one for each sound; supplements the existing alphabet to fill out needed representation of sounds.

alphanumeric, *adj* pertaining to a character set that contains letters and numerals and usually other special characters.

alprazolam (alprāz'əlam'), *n brand names:* Xanax, Apo-Alpraz, Novo-Alprazol, Nu-Alpraz; *drug class:* benzodiazepine; *action:* produces CNS depression; *uses:* anxiety, panic disorders, anxiety with depressive symptoms.

alprostadil (alpros'tədil'), *n brand names:* Caverject, Prostin VR Pediatric; *drug class:* prostaglandin E$_1$; *action:* induces erection by relaxation of trabecular smooth muscle and by dilation of cavernosal arteries; *uses:* treatment of erectile dysfunction caused by neurogenic, vasculogenic, psychogenetic, or mixed etiology. Also used to maintain promote of the *ductus arteriosus* in neonates.

alteplase (tissue plasminogin activator [t-PA]), *n brand name:* Activase; *drug class:* fibrinolytic; *action:* binds to fibrin and cleaves plasminogen to produce plasmin; *uses:* breaks down blood clots after myocardial infarction, ischemic stroke, or pulmonary embolism.

alternate benefit, *n* a provision in a dental plan contract that allows the third-party payer to determine the benefit based on an alternative procedure that is generally less expensive than the one provided or proposed.

alternate treatment, *n* the contract provisions that authorize the insurance carrier to determine the amount of benefits payable, giving consideration to alternate procedures, services, or courses of treatment that may be performed to accomplish the desired result. The attending dental provider and the patient have the option of which procedure to use, although payment for the procedure may be based on the alternate treatment principle.

alternative benefit plan, *n* a plan other than a traditional (fee-for-service, freedom of choice) indemnity or service corporation plan for reimbursing a participating dental provider for providing treatment to an enrolled patient population.

alternative delivery system, *n* an arrangement for the provision of dental services in other than the traditional way (e.g., licensed dental provider providing treatment in a fee-for-service dental office).

alternative treatment plan, *n* a compromise plan of treatment deviating from the ideal plan in scope and financial investment.

altitude, *n* pertaining to any location on earth with reference to a fixed surface point, which is usually sea level. The higher the altitude, the lower the oxygen concentration and the greater the ultraviolet radiation, both of which can cause health problems.

altretamine (altret'əmēn'), *n brand name:* Hexalen; *drug class:* antineoplastic; *action:* products of metabolism interact with tissue macromolecules, including DNA, which may be responsible for cytotoxicity; *use:* palliative treatment of recurrent, persistent ovarian cancer.

alumina (əlōōminə), *n* aluminum oxide, an abrasive sometimes used as a polishing agent.

aluminum, *n* a widely used metallic element and the third most abundant of all the elements. Aluminum is a principal component of many compounds used in antacids, antiseptics, astringents, and styptics. Aluminum hydroxychloride is the most commonly used agent in antiperspirants.

aluminum carbonate gel, *n brand name:* Basajel; *drug class:* antacid; *actions:* neutralizes gastric acidity, binds phosphates in GI tract; *uses:* antacid, prevention of phosphate stones, phosphate binder in chronic renal failure.

aluminum filters/disks, *n.pl* the extremely thin (0.05 cm) pieces of aluminum that are placed over the aperture of the radiographic tube to eliminate x-rays over a certain wavelength.

aluminum hydroxide, *n brand names:* AlternaGEL, Alu-Cap, Alu-Tab, Amphojel, Dialume; *drug class:* antacid; *action:* neutralizes gastric acidity, binds phosphates in GI tract; *uses:* antacid, hyperphosphatemia in chronic renal failure.

aluminum oxide, *n* a metallic oxide that includes alpha single crystal (an inert, biocompatible strong ceramic material used in the fabrication of some endosseous implants) and polycrystal (a constituent of dental porcelain that increases viscosity and strength).

Aluwax (al'yəwaks), *n* a commercially prepared wax wafer containing aluminum that is used to register jaw relationship.

alveolalgia (al'vēōlal'jēə), *n* See socket, dry.

alveolar (alvē'ōlär), *adj* pertaining to an alveolus.

alveolar bone loss, *n* See bone loss, periodontal.

alveolar crest, n See crest, alveolar.

alveolar crest group, n a portion of the alveodental ligament that originates in the alveolar crest and fans out to insert into the cervical cementum.

alveolar process, n See process, alveolar.

alveolar ridge, n See ridge, alveolar.

alveolar ridge augmentation, n a surgical procedure to improve the shape and size of the alveolar ridge(s) in preparation to receive and retain a dental prosthesis.

alveolectomy **(al'vēəlek'təmē),** n the excision of a portion of the alveolar process to aid in the removal of teeth, modification of the contour after the removal of teeth, and preparation of the oral cavity for dentures.

alveolitis **(al'vēəlī'tis),** n the inflammation of the alveolus, commonly occurring in a tooth socket after extraction.

alveoloplasty **(alvē'əlōplas'tē),** n the surgical shaping and smoothing of the margins of the tooth socket after extraction of the tooth, generally in preparation for the placement of a prosthesis.

alveolus **(alvē'əlus),** n **1.** an air sac of the lungs formed by terminal dilations of the bronchioles. n **2.** the socket in the bone in which a tooth is attached by means of the periodontal ligament.

Alzheimer's disease, *n.pr* a presenile dementia characterized by confusion, memory failure, disorientation, restlessness, agnosia, hallucinosis, speech disturbances, and the inability to carry out purposeful movement. The disease usually begins in later middle life with slight defects in memory and behavior that become progressively more severe.

▣ **amalgam** **(əmal'gəm),** n (dental amalgam alloy), an alloy, one of the constituents of which is mercury.

amalgam, bonded, n **1.** a composite of tooth-colored acrylic resin and finely ground glasslike particles that is bonded or adhered to the tooth during dental restoration. The advantage is ▣ that less of the tooth structure needs to be removed during the restoration, resulting in a smaller filling compared with traditional amalgams. n **2.** a composite filling.

amalgam carrier, n See carrier, amalgam.

amalgam carver, n See carver, amalgam.

amalgam condenser, n See condenser, amalgam.

amalgam, copper, n an alloy composed principally of copper and mercury. See also amalgam.

amalgam, dental, n an amalgam used for dental restorations and dyes.

amalgam matrix, n See matrix, amalgam.

amalgam pigmentation, n See amalgam tattoo.

amalgam plugger, n See condenser, amalgam.

amalgam, silver, n a dental amalgam, the main constituent of which is silver. The ADA composition specifications are as follows: silver, 65% minimum; tin, 25% minimum; copper, 6% maximum; zinc, 2% maximum.

amalgam squeeze cloth, n a piece of linen used to hold plastic amalgam from which excess mercury is to be squeezed. Used with hand trituration.

amalgam tattoo, n a solitary discrete gray, blue, or black discoloration of tissue usually located in the gingiva, alveolar ridge, or buccal mucosa caused by small amounts of dental amalgam that became embedded under the surface. The asymptomatic lesion is static and requires no treatment. If doubt exists about the lesion or if the lesion is unsightly, excisional biopsy is recommended.

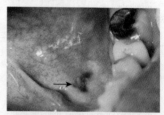

Amalgam tattoo. (Regezi/Sciubba/Jordan, 2012)

amalgam well, n a small, bowl-shaped container that holds mixed amalgam prior to its being loaded into the amalgam carrier.

amalgamation **(əmal'gəmā'shən),** n the formation of an alloy by mixing mercury with another metal or other metals. See also trituration.

amalgamation amalgamator **(əmal ′gəmātur),** *n* a mechanical device used to triturate the ingredients of dental amalgam into a plastic mass. See also trituration.

amantadine, *n* an antiviral drug that prevents uncoating and replication of the influenza A virus; most effectively used in the early stages of exposure. It is used as an alternate drug in the treatment of parkinsonism. Several mechanisms, including blocking re-uptake of dopamine, have been proposed.

ambu bag, *n* a flexible reservoir bag connected by flexible tubing and a non-rebreathing valve to a face mask or endotracheal tube and used for artificial ventilation. It is self-inflating with room air or from an oxygen source.

ambulatory (am′byələtôr′ē), *adj* capable of walking; not bedridden.

ambulatory care, *n* the health services provided on an outpatient basis to those who can visit a health care facility and return home the same day.

ambulatory surgery, *n* the surgical care provided to persons who do not require overnight nursing care.

amcinonide, *n brand name:* Cyclocort; *drug class:* topical fluorinated corticosteroid; *actions:* antipruritic, antiinflammatory; *uses:* psoriasis, eczema, contact dermatitis, pruritus.

amelia (əmel′ēə, əmē′lēə), *n* a congenital abnormality characterized by the absence of one or more limbs.

ameloblast (am′əlōblast′), *n* an epithelial cell associated with the enamel organ that, during tooth development, secretes enamel matrix.

ameloblast atrophy, *n* a wasting of or decrease in the epithelial cells, which form tooth enamel; may occur as the result of a deficiency in vitamin A. See also atrophy, periodontal.

ameloblastic fibroma, *n* See fibroma, ameloblastic.

ameloblastic fibro-odontoma (am′əlōblas′tik fī′brō-ō′dontō′mə), *n* an aggressive, generally benign tumor of the oral tissues, most commonly occurring in the posterior mandible. It is generally associated with developing teeth and thus is usually found in children or adolescents.

ameloblastic sarcoma (am′əlō blas′tik sarkō′mə), *n* See sarcoma, ameloblastic.

ameloblastoma (am′əlōblastō′mə), *n* an epithelial neoplasm with a basic structure resembling the enamel organ and suggesting derivation from ameloblastic cells. It is usually benign but aggressive. Also called *adamantinoblastoma* or *adamantinoma.*

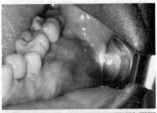
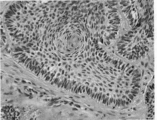
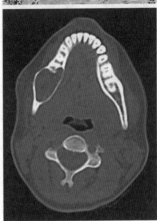

Ameloblastoma. (Top, Fehrenbach/Herring, 2012; middle/bottom, courtesy Dr. James Sciubba)

ameloblastoma, acanthomatous, *n* a type that differs from the simple form in that the central cells within the cell nests are squamous and may be keratinized rather than stellate. The peripheries of the cell nests are composed of ameloblastic cells. See also ameloblastoma.

amelogenesis (am′əlōjen′əsis), *n* the process during which the enamel matrix is formed by ameloblasts. See also ameloblast.

amelogenesis imperfecta, *n* a broad category of developmental disturbances in the structural formation of enamel. The disease is divided into four main types (type 1, Hypoplastic; type 2, Hypomaturation; type 3, Hypocalcified; type 4, mixed) and 15 subtypes, which range from mild to severe.

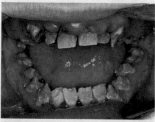

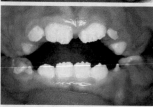

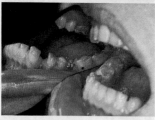

Amelogenesis imperfecta. (Regezi/Sciubba/Jordan, 2012)

amenorrhea (əmen′ōrē′ə), *n* the absence or abnormal cessation of the menstrual cycle.

American Academy of Oral and Maxillofacial Radiology (AAOMR), *n.pr* a professional association committed to ethical, evidence-based, and high quality oral and maxillofacial diagnostic services to the public.

American Academy of Oral Medicine (AAOM), *n.pr* nonprofit professional association of dental professionals specializing in the practice of Oral Medicine. Oral Medicine is the discipline of dentistry concerned with the oral health care of medically compromised patients and with the diagnosis and non-surgical management of medically-related disorders or conditions affecting the oral and maxillofacial region.

American Academy of Periodontology (AAP), *n.pr* a nonprofit professional association of dental professionals specializing in the prevention, diagnosis, and treatment of diseases affecting the periodontium and in the placement and maintenance of dental implants.

American Association of Endodontists (AAE), *n.pr* a professional association committed to excellence and quality in the art and science of endodontics and to the highest standard of patient care.

American Association of Oral and Maxillofacial Surgeons (AAOMS), *n.pr* professional association representing oral and maxillofacial surgeons in the United States. It supports its members' ability to practice their specialty through education, research, and advocacy. Its members must comply with rigorous continuing education requirements and submit to periodic office examinations, ensuring the public that all office procedures and personnel meet stringent national standards.

American Association of Orthodontics (AAO), *n.pr* a nonprofit professional association of dental professionals specialized in the treatment of malocclusions. Its headquarters is in Saint Louis, Missouri.

American Cancer Society (ACS), *n.pr* a national advocacy and fundraising organization, headquartered in Atlanta, Georgia, that is dedicated to raising public awareness about cancer and to providing support for cancer patients and their families.

American Dental Association (ADA), *n.pr* a nonprofit professional association whose membership is dental professionals in the United

States. Its purpose is to assist its members in providing the highest professional and ethical care to the citizens of the United States and to serve as an advocate for the advancement of the profession.

**American Dental Hygienists Association *(ADHA), n.pr* a nonprofit professional association of dental hygienists in the United States created to assist its members in providing the highest professional and ethical care to the citizens of the United States and to serve as an advocate for the advancement of the profession.

**American Heart Association *(AHA), n.pr* a national voluntary health agency that has the goal of increasing public and medical awareness of cardiovascular diseases and stroke, and thereby reducing the number of associated deaths and disabilities. It also provides dentistry with guidelines on the management of patients with various cardiovascular diseases, such as prevention of infective endocarditis.

**American Hospital Association *(AHA), n.pr* a nonprofit national organization of individuals, institutions, and organizations engaged in direct patient care. The association works to promote the improvement of health care services.

**American manual alphabet, *n.pr* a representation of alphabet letters using a variety of finger positions.

**American Medical Association *(AMA), n.pr* a nonprofit professional association of physicians in the United States, including all medical specialties. Its purpose is to assist its members in providing the highest professional and ethical medical care to the citizens of the United States and to serve as an advocate for the advancement of the profession.

**American National Standards Institute *(ANSI), n.pr* a private non-profit organization of manufacturers designed to develop voluntary standards for American products.

**American Sign Language *(ASL), n. pr* a mode of communication using gestures and visuals with a unique grammatical structure. ASL is used by individuals with limited or no hearing ability and by those who communicate regularly with such individuals.

**Americans with Disabilities Act *(ADA), n.pr* a federal law that defines a private dental office as a place of public accommodation, thereby requiring that dental offices serve persons with disabilities.

amide (am′īd), *n* 1. an ammonia-derived organic compound formed through the displacement of a hydrogen atom by an acyl radical. *n* **2.** an ammonia-derived inorganic compound formed through the replacement of an acid's hydroxyl group (OH) with that of an amino group such as $-NH_2$. *n* **3.** a type of local anesthetic agent. See also anesthetic, amide.

**amikacin, *n* brand name:* Amikin; *drug class:* aminoglycoside antibiotic; *action:* binds to 30S ribosomal subunit in aerobic bacteria causing misreading of genetic code and inhibition of protein synthesis, bactericidal effect; *uses:* aerobic gram negative bacterial infections, sometimes for tuberculosis.

**amiloride HCl (əmil′ərīd′), *n* brand name:* Midamor; *drug class:* potassium-sparing diuretic; *action:* acts primarily on the collecting duct, increasing the retention of potassium; *uses:* edema in chronic heart failure in combination with other diuretics, for hypertension, with INH solution for cystic fibrosis.

**amines (əmēnz′), *n.pl* organic compounds that contain nitrogen.

**amino acid, *n* an organic acid in which one of the CH hydrogen atoms has been replaced by NH_2. Amino acids are the building blocks of proteins.

amino acid, essential, n the group of amino acids that cannot be synthesized by the organism but are required by the organism. They must be supplied by the diet. Isoleucine, leucine, lysine, methionine, phenylalanine, threonine, tryptophan, and valine are essential for adults; these eight plus arginine and histidine are considered essential for infants and children.

amino acid, glucogenic (glōōkō jen′ik), n the group of amino acids that produce enzymes that may be converted to glucose if necessary.

amino acid, ketogenic (kē′tōjen′ik), n an amino acid that produces ketone bodies following chemical alteration of its carbon skeleton.

amino acid, nonessential, *n* the group of amino acids that can be synthesized by the organism and are not required in the diet.

amino acid pool, *n* an accumulation of amino acids in the liver and blood that adjusts to meet the body's need for protein and amino acids.

aminocaproic acid (əmē′nōkəprō′ik), *n brand name:* Amicar; *drug class:* hemostatic; *action:* inhibits fibrinolysis by inhibiting plasminogen and plasminogen activator substances; *uses:* hemorrhage from hyperfibrinolysis; adjunctive therapy in hemophilia; unapproved, hemorrhage following dental surgery in hemophilia.

aminoglutethimide (əmē′nōglōōte th′əmĭd), *n brand name:* Cytadren; *drug class:* antineoplastic, adrenal steroid inhibitor; *action:* acts by inhibiting the enzymatic conversion of cholesterol to pregnenolone, thereby blocking synthesis of all adrenal steroids; *uses:* suppression of adrenal function in Cushing's syndrome, metastatic breast cancer, adrenal cancer.

aminoglycosides (əmē′nōglī′kəs īdz′), *n.pl* the bactericidal antibiotics obtained from *Streptomyces* or *Micromonospora* species that inhibit protein synthesis in bacterial ribosomes and are effective against aerobic gram-negative bacilli.

aminophylline (theophylline ethylenediamine), *n brand name:* Phyllocontin; *drug class:* xanthine; *action:* relaxes smooth muscle of the respiratory system; *uses:* bronchial asthma, bronchospasm, Cheyne-Stokes respirations.

amiodarone HCl (əmē′ōdərōn′), *n brand name:* Cordarone; *drug class:* antidysrhythmic (drug class III); *action:* prolongs action potential duration and effective refractory period; *uses:* atrial fibrillation, ventricular tachycardia.

amitriptyline HCl (am′itrip′təlēn), *n brand names:* Apo-Amitriptyline, Elavil, Emitrip, Endep, Enovil, Levate, Novotriptyn; *drug class:* tricyclic antidepressant; *action:* inhibits both norepinephrine and serotonin (5-HT) uptake into nerve terminals; *use:* major depression.

amlodipine besylate (amlō′dipēn bes′əlāt), *n brand name:* Norvasc; *drug class:* calcium channel blocker; *actions:* inhibits calcium ion influx across cell membranes of smooth muscle cells, myocardial cells, and the cells of the SA and AV nodes; produces relaxation of peripheral blood vessels and dilates coronary arteries; decreases SA/AV node conduction; *uses:* hypertension as a single agent or in combination with other antihypertensives, chronic stable angina pectoris, vasospastic angina.

ammeter (am′ētur), *n* a contraction of amperemeter. An apparatus that measures the amperage of an electric current.

ammonia (əmō′nyə), *n* a colorless aromatic gas consisting of nitrogen and hydrogen, produced by the decomposition of nitrogenous organic matter. Some of its many uses are as an aromatic stimulant, a detergent, and an emulsifier.

ammonia thiosulfate (əmō′nyə thīōsul′fāt), *n* an ingredient of the photographic fixing solution that acts as a solvent for silver halides.

ammoniacal silver nitrate, *n* See silver nitrate, ammoniacal.

ammonium chloride, *n* the chlorine salt of the ammonium ion. It is a popular deliquescent agent (i.e., it attracts and absorbs water from the atmosphere).

amnesia (amnē′zēə, -zhə), *n* the lack or loss of memory.

amnesiac (amnē′zēak), *n* a person affected by amnesia.

amniocentesis, *n* a prenatal diagnostic procedure in which the amniotic fluid is sampled.

amniotic cavity, *n* the fluid filled cavity that faces the epiblast layer.

amniotic fluid (am′nēot′ik), *n* a serum within the amniotic sac in which the embryo is immersed and cushioned.

amniotic sac, *n* a thin membrane that completely surrounds the embryo and contains a protective fluid in which the embryo is immersed. Also called the *amnion.*

amobarbital/amobarbital sodium (am′ōbär′bital), *n brand name:* Amytal; *drug class:* a little-used barbiturate sedative-hypnotic (Controlled Substance Schedule II); *action:* nonselective depression of CNS ranging from sedation to hypnosis to anesthesia to coma, depending on dose administered; *uses:* sedation, preanesthetic sedation, insommia, hypnotic.

amoeba (əmē′bə), *n* a Rhizopod protozoa that uses extensions of its cytoplasm, called pseudopodia, to move. Some varieties of amoebae are implicated in human infection. Also spelled *ameba(s).*

amorphous (āmôr′fus, əmôr′fus), *adj* having no specific space lattice; possibly the molecules being distributed at random.

amortization (amərtəzāshən), *n* a generic term that includes various specific practices, such as depreciation, depletion, write-off of intangibles, prepaid expenses, and deferred charges.

amoxapine (əmok′səpēn), *n brand name:* Asendin; *drug class:* tricyclic antidepressant; *action:* inhibits both norepinephrine and serotonin (5-HT) uptake in brain; *uses:* depression.

amoxicillin trihydrate (əmok′sə sil′in trīhī′drāt), *n brand names:* Amoxil, Apo-Amoxi, Novamoxin, Nu-Amoxi and others; *drug class:* aminopenicillin; *action:* has an extended spectrum and interferes with cell wall replication of susceptible organisms; *uses:* sinus infections, pneumonia, otitis media, skin, urinary tract infections. This is a drug of choice for antibiotic premedication for patients at risk for bacterial endocarditis unless there is an allergy to penicillin-related antibiotics.

amoxicillin/clavulanate potassium, *n brand names:* Augmentin, Clavulin; *drug class:* aminopenicillin with a β-lactamase inhibitor; *action:* interferes with cell wall replication of susceptible organisms; *uses:* sinus infections, pneumonia, otitis media, skin, urinary tract infections; effective for strains of *E. coli, H. influenzae, S. pneumoniae,* and β-lactamase-producing organisms.

amoxapine, *n brand name:* ascendin; *drug class:* antidepressant, antipsychotic; *actions:* blocks reuptake of norepinephrine and serotonin, blocks dopamine and serotonin 5-HT$_{2A}$ receptors; *uses:* depression, psychosis.

ampere (am′pir), *n* (Amp), a unit of measurement of the quantity of electric current, equal to a flow of 1 coulomb per second or 6.25 time 10^{18}

electrons per second. The current produced by 1 volt acting through a resistance of 1 ohm.

amphetamines (amfet′əmēnz′), *n. pl* a group of nervous system stimulants that are subject to abuse because of their ability to reduce appetite and produce wakefulness and euphoria. Abuse of amphetamines may lead to compulsive behavior, paranoia, hallucinations, and suicidal tendencies.

amphotericin B, topical (am′fə ter′əsin), *n brand name:* Fungizone; *drug class:* polyene antifungal; *action:* increases cell membrane permeability in susceptible organisms by binding to sterols; *uses:* cutaneous, mucocutaneous infections caused by *Candida;* infections caused by several systemic fungi.

ampicillin (am′pisil′in), *n* an aminopenicillin, similar in uses and almost identical in spectrum to amoxicillin.

amprenavir, *n brand name:* Agenerase; *drug class:* anti-HIV drug; *action:* HIV protease inhibition; *use:* HIV infection.

amputation neuroma, *n* See neuroma, traumatic.

amputation, root, *n* the removal of a root of a multirooted tooth.

amyl nitrate, *n brand name:* Amyl nitrate; *drug class:* organic nitrite; *actions:* dilates blood vessels, converts hemoglobin to methemoglobin; *uses:* angina pectoris, treatment of cyanide poisoning.

amylase (am′ilās), *n* an enzymatic protein essential for changing starches into sugars. See also alpha amylase.

amyloid (am′əloid′), *n* a starchlike protein-carbohydrate complex that is deposited abnormally in some tissues during certain chronic disease states, such as amyloidosis, rheumatoid arthritis, and tuberculosis.

amyloidosis (am′iloidō′sis), *n* a condition in which amyloid, a glycoprotein, is deposited intercellularly in tissues and organs. Four types of amyloidosis are recognized, two of which, primary amyloidosis and amyloid tumor, frequently produce nodules in the tongue and gingiva.

amyloidosis, primary, *n* a type occurring without a known predisposing cause. Amyloid deposits are found in the tongue, lips, skeletal muscles, and other mesodermal structures. The disease may be manifested by poly-neuropathy, purpura, hepatospleno-megaly, heart failure, and the nephrotic syndrome.

amyloidosis, secondary, *n* a type occurring secondary to chronic dis-eases such as tuberculosis, leprosy, rheumatoid arthritis, multiple myeloma, and prolonged bacterial infections. Amyloid deposits are found in parenchymal organs. The disease is usually manifested by pro-teinuria and hepatosplenomegaly.

amyotonia (ā′mīōtō′nēə), *n* an abnormal flaccidity or flabbiness of a muscle or group of muscles.

amyotrophic lateral sclerosis (ALS) (ā′mīətrŏ′fik lat′ərəl sklərō′sis), *n* a degenerative disease of the motor neurons, characterized by atrophy of the muscles of the hands, forearms, and legs, and spreading to involve most of the body. Colloquial term is *Lou Gehrig's disease.*

anabolic steroids, *n.pl* a group of compounds derived from testosterone or prepared synthetically to promote general growth. Anabolic steroids are used in the treatment of aplastic anemia, anemias associated with renal failure, myeloid metaplasia, and leu-kemia. Anabolic steroids are subject to abuse to promote muscle mass in athletes.

anabolism (ənab′əlizəm), *n* the con-structive process by which substances are converted from simple to complex forms by living cells; constructive metabolism.

anaerobe (an′ərōb), *n* a microorgan-ism that can exist and grow only in the partial or complete absence of molec-ular oxygen.

anaerobe, facultative (fak′ultātiv), *n* an organism that can grow in the absence or presence of oxygen.

analeptic (an′əlep′tik), *n* **1.** an agent that acts to overcome depression of the central nervous system. *n* **2.** a strong central nervous system stimu-lant that is used to restore conscious-ness, especially from a drug-induced coma.

analgesia (an′əljē′zēə), *n* an insensi-bility to pain without loss of con-sciousness; a state in which painful stimuli are not perceived or inter-preted as pain; usually induced by a drug, although trauma or a disease

process may produce a general or regional analgesia.

analgesia, diagnostic, *n* the adminis-tration of a local anesthetic to deter-mine the location, source, or cause of pain.

analgesia, endotracheal (en′dōtrā′k ēəl), *n* an inhalation technique in which the anesthetic agent and respi-ratory gases are passed through a tube inserted in the trachea via either the nose or oral cavity.

analgesia, infiltration, *n* the arrest of the sensory responses of nerve endings at the surgical site by injec-tions of an anesthetic at that site.

analgesia, insufflation, *n* the deliv-ery of anesthetic gases or vapors directly to the airway of a patient while he or she is breathing room air. Insufflation is usually an open drop method.

analgesia, intranasal, *n* the delivery of an analgesic agent to the membrane of the nose by either topical applica-tion or insufflation.

analgesia, nonnarcotic, *n* drugs that relieve pain by an action other than binding to opioid receptors. Most inhibit cyclooxygenase. Generally, nonnarcotic analgesics do not produce tolerance or dependence.

analgesia, patient-controlled, *n* mechanisms by which the patient can administer and/or control the applica-tion of an analgesic agent to an area. One such mechanism is the use of transcutaneous electric nerve stimula-tion (TENS) to control facial pain. The TENS unit is a variable controlled device designed to deliver a con-trolled electrical stimulus to the skin surface overlying a painful muscle.

analgesia, regional, *n* the reversible loss of pain sensation over an area by blocking the afferent conduction of its innervation with a local anesthetic agent.

analgesic (anəljē′zik), *adj* (anal-getic), **1.** the property of a drug that enables it to raise the pain threshold (e.g., nitrous oxide). *n* **2.** an analgesic may act peripherally or on the central nervous system to raise the pain threshold.

analgetic (anəljet′ik), *adj* See analgesic.

analgia (anal′jēə), *n* an absence of pain.

analysis (ənal′isis), *n* a separation into component parts.

analysis, anthropometric **(an′thrəpə met′rik),** *n* a study of the human body that uses such tools as body mass index, basal metabolic rate, bioelectrical impedance, and dual energy radiograph absorptiometry, along with measurements of skinfold thickness and arm muscle circumference, to assess the structure, form, and composition of the body for purposes of comparison.

analysis, bite mark, *n* a technique in forensic dentistry for comparing a bite mark to a dental cast for purposes of identifying the person who made the mark.

analysis, cephalometric **(sef′əlō met′rik),** *n* the evaluation of the growth pattern or morphologic conoval of teeth, modification of the contour after the removal of teeth, and preparation of the oral cavity for dentures.

analysis, dietary, *n* a comparison of an individual's typical food choices with those recommended in the Food Guide Pyramid and MyPlate; deviations are noted, and recommendations are given.

analysis, occlusal, *n* a study of the relations of the occlusal surfaces of the opposing teeth and their functional harmony.

analysis, space, *n* a space analysis done on study casts comparing the amount of space available with the amount of space required to align the teeth.

analyzing rod, *n* See rod, analyzing.

anamnesis (an′amnē′sis), *n* a history of disease or injury based on the patient's memory or recall at the time of dental and/or medical interview and examination.

anaphase, *n* the third phase of mitosis, which involves separation of the two chromatids of each chromosome where they are joined at their centromeres and migration to opposite poles of the cell.

anaphylactic (an′əfilak′tik), *adj* pertaining to anaphylaxis.

anaphylactoid (an′əfilak′toid), *adj* resembling anaphylaxis; pertaining to a reaction, the symptoms of which resemble those of the anaphylactic response.

anaphylaxis (an′əfilak′sis), *n* a violent allergic reaction characterized by sudden collapse, shock, or respiratory and circulatory failure after exposure to an allergen.

anaplasia (an′əplā′zhə), *n* a regressive change in cells toward a more primitive or embryonic cell type. It is a prominent characteristic of malignancy in tumors.

anasarca (an′sär′kə), *n* (dropsy), generalized edema.

anastomosis (pl. anastomoses) (ənas′təmō′sis), *n* the joining together of two blood vessels or other tubular structures to furnish a direct or indirect communication between the two structures.

anastomosis graft, *n* the connection of two autogenous tubular structures as a part of reconstructive surgery.

anastrozole, *n* brand name: Arimidex; drug class: preventors of the synthesis of estrogens; action: aromatase inhibitor; use: advanced breast cancer in postmenopausal women.

anatomic (anətom′ik), *adj* pertaining to the anatomy of a structure.

anatomic dead space, *n* the actual capacity of the respiratory passages that extend from the nostrils to and including the terminal bronchioles.

anatomic form, *n* See form, anatomic.

anatomic height of contour, *n* See contour, height of.

anatomic impression, *n* See impression, anatomic.

anatomic landmark, *n* See landmark, anatomic.

anatomic nomenclature, *n* a system of names of anatomic structures.

anatomic position, *n* the body at an erect position, with arms at sides, palms and toes directed forward, and with eyes looking forward.

anatomic teeth, *n.pl* See tooth, anatomic.

anatomic root, *n* See root.

anatomical crown, *n* See crown, anatomical.

anatomy (ənat′ōmē), *n* the science of the form, structure, and parts of animal organisms.

anatomy, dental, *n* the science of the structure of the teeth and the relationship of their parts. The study involves macroscopic and microscopic components.

A

anatomy, head and neck, *n* the study of the head and neck regions of the body.

anatomy, radiographic, *n* the images on a radiographic film of the combined anatomic structures through which the roentgen rays (radiographs) have passed.

ANB angle, *n* a cephalometric measurement of the antero-posterior relationship of the maxilla with the mandible in reference to the cranial base.

anchorage, *n* **1.** the supporting base for orthodontic forces applied to stimulate tooth movement. *n* **2.** the area of application of the reciprocal forces generated when corrective forces are applied to teeth. Anchorage units may be one tooth or more or may include a portion of the neck or cranium.

anchorage bends, *n.pl* bends placed in an orthodontic wire to enhance the resistance to the anterior displacement of teeth during orthodontic treatment; primarily used in the Tweed and Begg techniques.

anchorage, cervical, *n* an extraoral anchorage based at the back of the neck.

anchorage, cranial, *n* an extraoral anchorage based at the back of the skull.

anchorage, extraoral, *n* in orthodontics, an orthodontic anchorage based outside the oral cavity. Dental attachments are typically linked to a wire bow or hooks extending between the lips and attached elastically to a cap, a strap around the neck, or another extraoral device.

anchorage, facial, *n* an extraoral anchorage based on the face, usually the chin or forehead.

anchorage, intermaxillary, *n* an anchorage based in the opposite jaw.

anchorage, intramaxillary, *n* an anchorage based on teeth within the same jaw.

anchorage, intraoral, *n* an anchorage based within the oral cavity (intermaxillary, intramaxillary, or myofunctional).

anchorage, occipital, *n* a cranial anchorage based in the occipital area.

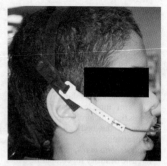

Occipital anchorage. (Courtesy Dr. Flavio Uribe)

anchorage, reciprocal, *n* two or more teeth moving in opposite directions and pitted against each other by the appliance. Usually the resistance to each other is equal and opposite.

anchorage, simple, *n* the use of a tooth as a resistance unit without tipping control.

anchorage, skeletal, *n* anchorage derived from endosseous dental implants, mini-implants, miniplates attached with screws to basal bone, or from miniscrews placed in the alveolar process of the maxilla or mandible.

anchorage, stationary, *n* resistance to bodily movement of one group of teeth against tipping.

Andresen appliance, *n.pr* See appliance, Andresen.

androgen (an′drōjen), *n* a substance that possesses masculinizing qualities, such as testosterone.

anemia (ənē′mēə), *n* a term indicating that the concentration of hemoglobin or the number of red blood cells is below the accepted normal value with respect to age and gender. In true anemia the total concentration of hemoglobin, or the total number of erythrocytes, is below normal regardless of concentration values. Symptoms, which may not be evident, include weakness, pallor, anorexia, and those related to the cause of the anemia.

anemia, Addison-Biermer, *n.pr* See anemia, pernicious.

anemia, aplastic, *n* a type characterized by a decrease in all marrow elements, including platelets, red blood cells, and granulocytes.

anemia, Biermer's, *n.pr* See anemia, pernicious.

anemia, Cooley's, *n.pr* See thalassemia major.

anemia, displacement, *n* See anemia, myelophthisic.

anemia, erythroblastic, *n* See thalassemia major.

anemia, hemolytic, *n* a type characterized by an increased rate of destruction of red blood cells, reticulocytosis, hyperbilirubinemia, and/or increased urinary and fecal urobilinogen, and, generally, splenic enlargement. Hereditary ones include congenital hemolytic jaundice, sickle cell anemia, oval cell anemia, and thalassemia. Included are paroxysmal nocturnal hemoglobinuria and those caused by immune mechanisms (erythroblastosis fetalis), transfusions of incompatible blood, infections, drugs, and poisons. Autoimmune ones are acquired hemolytic anemias associated with antibody-like substances that may not be true autoantibodies or even antibodies; they may be primary (idiopathic), or they may be secondary to lymphoma, lymphatic leukemia, disseminated lupus erythematosus, or sensitization to drugs and pollens.

anemia, hemorrhagic **(hem′əraj′ik),** *n* a type caused by deficiency in red blood cells and/or hemoglobin resulting from excessive bleeding.

anemia, hyperchromic, *n* a type in which the erythrocytes have an increased level of hemoglobin per volume of red blood cells.

anemia, hypochromic, *n* a type caused by impaired hemoglobin synthesis resulting from a deficiency of iron or pyridoxine and from chronic lead poisoning.

anemia, iron deficiency, *n* a type resulting from a deficiency of iron, characterized by hypochromic microcytic erythrocytes and a normoblastic reaction of the bone marrow. Iron deficiency may result from an increased demand during growth or repeated pregnancies; chronic or recurrent hemorrhage such as from menstrual abnormalities, hemorrhoids, or peptic ulcer; a low intake of

iron; or impaired absorption, as often occurs with chronic diarrhea.

anemia, macrocytic normochromic **(mak′rəsit′ik nor′məkrō′mik),** *n* a type related to a failure of nucleoprotein synthesis caused by a deficiency of vitamin B_{12}, folic acid, or related substances.

anemia, Mediterranean, *n* See thalassemia major.

anemia, megaloblastic, *n* a type characterized by hyperplastic bone marrow changes and maturation arrest resulting from a dietary deficiency, impaired absorption, impaired storage and modification, or impaired use of one or more hematopoietic factors. Included are pernicious anemia, nutritional macrocytic anemias associated with gastrointestinal disturbances, anemias associated with impaired liver function (e.g., macrocytic anemia of pregnancy), hypothyroidism, leukemia, and achrestic anemia.

anemia, microcytic hypochromic, *n* a type in which the mean corpuscular volume (MCV), mean corpuscular hemoglobin (MCH) content, and mean corpuscular hemoglobin concentration (MCHC) are all low (e.g., iron deficiency anemia, hereditary leptocytosis, hemoglobin C anemia, and anemias resulting from pyridoxine deficiency and chronic lead poisoning).

anemia, myelophthisic **(mī′əlo ffthizik),** *n* (displacement anemia), a type resulting from displacement or crowding out of erythropoietic cells of the bone marrow by foreign tissue, as in leukemia, metastatic carcinoma, lymphoblastoma, multiple myeloma, osteoradionecrosis, and xanthomatosis.

anemia, normocytic normochromic **(nor′məsit′ik nor′məkrō′mik),** *n* a type associated with disturbances of red cell formation and related to endocrine deficiencies, chronic inflammation, and carcinomatosis.

anemia, nutritional macrocytic, *n* macrocytic normochromic type occurring as a result of a deficiency of substances necessary for deoxyribonucleic acid synthesis; e.g., vitamin and folic acid deficiency may result from a lack of intrinsic factors, sprue, or regional enteritis or with chronic alcoholism, as a result of a diet deficient in meats and vegetables, and in diseases causing intestinal malabsorption.

anemia, oval cell, *n* See elliptocytosis.

anemia, pernicious (per'nishəs), *n* (Addison-Biermer anemia), a macrocytic normochromic (megaloblastic) type associated with achlorhydria and lack of a gastric intrinsic factor necessary for the binding and absorption of vitamin B_{12}, erythrocyte maturing factor. In addition to hematologic findings, atrophic glossitis and gastrointestinal and nervous disorders occur.

anemia, physiologic, *n* a type characterized by lowered blood values resulting from an increase in plasma volume that occurs most markedly during the sixth and seventh months of pregnancy.

anemia, sickle cell, *n* (drepanocythemia, sicklemia), a hereditary hemolytic type in which the presence of an abnormal hemoglobin (hemoglobin S) results in distorted, sickle shaped erythrocytes. Manifestations include episodic crises of muscle, joint, and abdominal pain; neurologic symptoms; and leg ulcers. Sickle cell anemia occurs almost exclusively in African Americans. See also trait, sickle cell.

anemia, spherocytic (sfē'rōsit'ik), *n* See jaundice, congenital hemolytic.

anergy (an'urjē), *n* in terms of hypersensitivity, an inability to react to specific antigens (e.g., lack of reaction to intradermally injected antigens in measles, Hodgkin's sarcoma, and overwhelming tuberculosis).

anesthesia (an'esthē'zēə, an'esthē 'zhə), *n* the loss of feeling or sensation, especially loss of tactile sensibility, with or without loss of consciousness, resulting from the use of certain drugs or gases that serve as inhibitory neurotransmitters.

anesthesia, nerve block, *n* local anesthesia induced by injecting the local anesthetic drug close to the nerve trunk, at some distance from the operative field.

anesthesia, conduction, *n* a local anesthesia induced by injecting the local anesthetic agent close to the nerve trunk, at some distance from the operative field.

anesthesia, general, *n* an irregular, reversible depression of the cells of the higher centers of the central nervous system that makes the patient unconscious and insensible to pain.

anesthesia, glove, *n* an anesthesia with a distribution corresponding to the part of the skin covered by a glove.

anesthesia, infiltration, *n* a local anesthesia induced by injecting the anesthetic agent directly into or around the tissues to be anesthetized (e.g., used for operative procedures on the maxillary premolars, anterior teeth, and mandibular incisors). Also called *field block.*

anesthesia, intraosseous, *n* the local anesthesia produced by the injection of a local anesthetic agent into the cancellous portion of a bone.

anesthesia, intrapulpal, *n* the injection of a local anesthetic agent directly into pulpal tissue.

anesthesia, local, *n* (regional anesthesia), the loss of pain sensation over a specific area of the anatomy without loss of consciousness.

anesthesia, periodontal ligament, *n* a supplemental injection used when pulpal anesthesia is indicated on a single tooth, mainly in the mandibular arch.

anesthesia, regional, *n* a term used for local anesthesia. See also anesthesia, local.

anesthesia, topical, *n* a form of local anesthetic agent with which the surface free nerve endings in accessible structures are rendered incapable of stimulation by applying a suitable solution directly to the surface of the area. Used on the surface soft tissue before a local anesthetic injection to anesthetize surface soft tissues for minor operative procedures.

anesthesiologist (an'əsthē'zēol'ə jist), *n* a physician specializing in the administration of anesthetics.

anesthesiology (an'isthē'zēol'ōjē), *n* the branch of medicine concerned with the relief of pain and the administration of medication to relieve pain during surgery or other invasive procedures.

anesthetic (an'esthet'ik), *n* a drug that produces loss of feeling or sensation generally or locally.

anesthetic, aerosol spray topical, *n* application of an aerosol spray directly on the surface of a mucous membrane, resulting in loss of nerve conduction.

anesthetic   agent, *n* See agent, anesthetic.

anesthetic, allergy to, *n* hypersensitivity to a local agent, which is fairly common with esters but rarely occurs with amides. Allergy to bisulfites in vasoconstrictors also needs to be considered, as well as agents containing sulfites.

anesthetic, amide, *n* a local anesthetic agent made from a specific class of chemical compounds that are primarily broken down by the liver and are generally considered more effective and longer-lasting than esters. This type of anesthetic rarely causes allergic reactions.

anesthetic, antioxidants in, *n* a preservative substance added by the manufacturer to a local anesthetic cartridge containing a vasoconstrictor. Metabisulfite and sodium bisulfite are the most commonly used antioxidants.

anesthetic, cartridge, *n* a capsulelike vessel containing the local anesthetic solution that is inserted into the syringe in preparation for an injection. Older term is *carpule.*

anesthetic, ester, *n* a short-acting local anesthetic agent made from a specific class of chemical compounds that are broken down by blood enzymes. They are less effective than amide anesthetics and more likely to cause allergic reactions. No longer used as an injection in the United States but still used as a topical agent. See also benzocaine.

anesthetic,   hydrophilic   group **(hī'drōfil'ik),** *n* a portion of a local anesthetic agent's chemical structure, with strong water-soluble properties that enable the diffusion of the agent through the water portions of the tissues to the final destination in the nerves. Typically described in opposition to the lipophilic portion of a local anesthetic agent.

anesthetic,   intermediate   chain linkage, *n* the connecting linkage between the lipophilic and hydrophilic portions of a local anesthetic agent's chemical structure. Local anesthetic agent's classification is performed on the basis of whether the intermediate chain is made up of an ester or an amide. See also ester and amide.

anesthetic, lipophilic group **(lip'ōfi l'ik),** *n* a portion of a local anesthetic agent's chemical structure, with its fat-soluble properties that enable the agent to pass through the lipid-membrane of the tissues in order to reach the nerve destination. Typically described in opposition to the hydrophilic portion of the local anesthetic agent.

anesthetic, local, *n* a drug that, when injected into the tissues and absorbed into a nerve, will temporarily interrupt its property of conduction. See also anesthetic, ester; and anesthetics, amide.

anesthetic, topical, *n* a drug applied to the surface of the skin or mucosal tissues that produces local insensibility to pain. See also benzocaine.

anesthetist (ənes'thətist), *n* a person who administers anesthetics.

anesthetize (ənes'thətīz), *v* to place under anesthesia.

aneurysm (an'yŏŏrizəm), *n* a localized dilation of an artery in which one or more layers of the vessel walls are distended.

aneurysm,   arteriovenous, *n* See shunt, arteriovenous.

angiitis, visceral (an'jēī'tis), *n* See disease, collagen.

angina (anjīnə), *n* a spasmodic, choking pain. The term is sometimes applied to the disease producing the pain (e.g., Ludwig's angina).

angina, agranulocytic **(ā'gran'yəlōs it'ik),** *n* See agranulocytosis.

angina, Ludwig's, *n.pr* a cellulitis involving the submandibular space and characterized clinically by a firm swelling of the floor of the oral cavity, with elevation of the tongue.

angina,   monocytic, *n* a "sore throat" associated with infectious mononucleosis.

angina pectoris, *n* a symptom of cardiovascular diseases; characterized by a severe, viselike pain behind the sternum that sometimes radiates to the arms, neck, or mandible. It also includes a sense of constriction or pressure of the chest. Angina pectoris is caused by exertion or excitement and is relieved by rest.

angina, Vincent's, *n* an outdated term for involvement of the pharynx by the spread of necrotizing ulcero-membranous gingivitis. See also gingivitis, necrotizing ulcerative.

angioedema (angioneurotic edema, Quincke's disease) (an'jē ōədē'mə), *n* the spontaneous swelling of the lips, cheeks, eyelids, tongue, soft palate, pharynx, and glottis, frequently associated with allergy to food or drugs and lasting from several hours to several days. Involvement of the glottis results in obstruction of the airway.

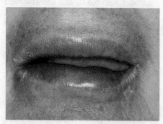

Angiodema. (Regezi/Sciubba/Jordan, 2012)

angiography (an'jēog'rəfē), *n* the radiographic visualization of the internal anatomy of the heart and blood vessels after the intravascular introduction of radiopaque contrast medium.

angioma (an'jēō'mə), *n* a benign tumor of vascular nature. See also hemangioma and lymphangioma.

angiomatosis, Sturge-Weber (an'jē ōmətō'sis sturj'-web'ər), *n.pr* an encephalofacial angiomatosis characterized by cutaneous facial cerebral angiomatosis, ipsilateral gyriform calcifications of the brain, mental retardation, seizures, contralateral hemiplegia, and ocular involvement. The facial lesions (port wine stain) may present along with intraoral angiomas on the buccal mucosa and gingival tissues.

angioneurotic edema (an'jēōnyŏōr ot'ik), *n* See edema, angioneurotic.

angioplasty (an'jēəplas'tē), *n* a medical procedure used to treat angina or blockage of the coronary arteries. The procedure involves the insertion of a balloon-tipped catheter into the body through a small incision, usually in the groin. The catheter is guided to the blockage using radiographs and injected dye. Once the blockage is reached, the balloon on the catheter is gently inflated to open the blood vessel. Also called *percutaneous transluminal coronary angioplasty (PTCA).*

angle, *n* the degree of divergence of two or more lines or planes that meet each other; the space between such lines. Measured in degrees of an arc.

angle, bayonet former, *n* a hoe-shaped, paired cutting instrument; biangled with the blade parallel with the axis of the shaft. The cutting edge is not perpendicular to the axis of the blade. Used to accentuate angles in an "invisible" class 3 cavity.

angle, Bennett, *n* the angle formed by the sagittal plane and the path of the advancing condyle during lateral mandibular movement, as viewed in the horizontal plane.

angle board, *n* a device used to facilitate the establishment of reproducible angular relationships between the head of a patient, the beam of radiation, and the receptor.

angle, cavosurface (kā'vōsur'fəs), *n* the angle in a prepared cavity, formed by the junction of the wall of the cavity with the surface of the tooth.

angle, contact, *n* the angle at which a liquid or vapor meets a solid surface (e.g., the angle at which a droplet of water rests on an oily surface).

angle, cranial base, *n* the angle formed by a line representing the floor of the anterior cranial fossa intersecting a line representing the axis of the clivus of the base of the skull. Also known as a *saddle angle.*

angle, cusp, *n* **1.** the angle made by the slopes of a cusp with the plane that passes through the tip of the cusp and is perpendicular to a line bisecting the cusp; measured mesiodistally or buccolingually. Half of the included angle between the buccolingual or mesiodistal cusp inclines. *n* **2.** the angle made by the slopes of a cusp with a perpendicular line bisecting the cusp; measured mesiodistally or buccolingually.

angle, facial, *n* an anthropometric expression of the degree of protrusion of the lower face, assessed by measuring the inclination of the facial plane relative to a horizontal reference plane.

angle, former, *n* a paired, hoeshaped cutting instrument that has the cutting edge at an angle other than a right angle in relation to the axis of the blade.

angle, Frankfort-mandibular incisor (FMIA) (frank'fərt-mandib'yələr insī'zər), *n* a measure of the mandibular incisor inclination to the Frankfort horizontal plane.

angle, incisal (insī'zal), *n* the degree of slope between the axis-orbital plane and the palatal discluding skidway of the maxillary incisor.

angle, incisal guidance, *n* the angle formed with the occlusal plane by drawing a line in the sagittal plane between the incisal edges of the maxillary and mandibular central incisors when the teeth are in centric occlusion.

angle, incisal guide, *n* the inclination of the incisal guide on the articulator.

angle, incisor, mandibular plane (IMPA), *n* angle formed between the mandibular plane and the long axis of lower incisors.

angle, interincisal, *n* angle formed between the long axis of maxillary and mandibular central incisors.

angle, lateral incisal guide, *n* the inclination of the incisal guide in the frontal plane.

angle, line, *n* an angle formed by the junction of the two walls along a line; designated by combining the names of the walls forming the angle.

angle, occlusal rest, *n* the angle formed by the occlusal rest with the upright minor connector.

angle of mandible, *n* an angle at the intersection of the posterior and inferior borders of the ramus.

angle, point, *n* an angle formed by the junction of three walls at a common point; designated by combining the names of the walls forming the angle.

angle, prophylaxis (prōfəlak'sis), *n* the term for an angled instrument that holds a rubber cup or bristle brush used to polish teeth. It may be either contra- or right-angled. May also be called a *prophy angle.*

angle, protrusive incisional guide, *n* the inclination of the incisal guide in the sagittal plane.

angle, rest, *n* See angle, occlusal rest.

angle, symphyseal (sim'fisē'əl), *n* the angle of the chin, which may be protruding straight or receding, according to type.

Angle's classification of malocclusion (modified), *n.pr* a classification of the different forms of malocclusion. See also malocclusion.

Class I, *n.pr* the normal anteroposterior relationship of the mandible to the maxillae. The mesiobuccal cusp of the permanent maxillary first molar occludes in the buccal groove of the permanent mandibular first molar.

Type I, *n.pr* dentition in linguoversion.

Type II, *n.pr* with narrow arches; labioversion of the maxillary anterior teeth and linguoversion of the mandibular anterior teeth.

Type III, *n.pr* with linguoversion of the maxillary anterior teeth; crowded; lack of development in the proximal region.

Class II, *n.pr* the posterior relationship of the mandible to the maxillae. The mesiobuccal cusp of the permanent maxillary first molar occludes mesial to the buccal groove of the permanent mandibular first molar.

Division 1, *n.pr* with labioversion of the maxillary teeth.

Subdivision, *n.pr* signifies a unilateral condition.

Division 2, *n.pr* with linguoversion of the maxillary central incisor teeth.

Subdivision, *n.pr* signifies a unilateral condition.

Class III, *n.pr* the anterior relationship of the mandible to the maxillae, may have a subdivision. The mesiobuccal cusp of the permanent maxillary first molar occludes distal to the buccal groove of the permanent mandibular first molar.

Type I, *n.pr* with good alignment generally but arch relationship abnormal.

Type II, *n.pr* with good alignment of the maxillary anterior teeth but linguoversion of the mandibular anterior teeth.

Type III, *n.pr* an underdeveloped maxillary arch; linguoversion of maxillary anterior teeth; good mandibular alignment.

angled shank, *n* an adaptation to the design of a handheld instrument in order to allow easier access to posterior teeth or to individual tooth surfaces which might otherwise be difficult to reach. See also instrument, hand.

angstrom (Å) unit (ang'strəm), *n* See unit, angstrom.

angular cheilitis (kīlī'təs), *n* a disease that most often occurs among the elderly but is caused by parasitic fungi, along with bacterial involvement, or a deficiency in vitamin B rather than age; angular cheilitis appears as skin lesions on the lips, particularly as breaks in the tissue at the corners of the oral cavity (commissures). Often occurs in conjunction with reduced mobility and strength in the oral cavity.

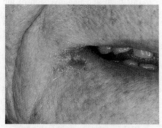

Angular cheilitis. (Ibsen/Phelan, 2009)

angular cheilosis, *n* See cheilosis, angular.

angulation (instrumental) (ang′gyō ōlā′shən), *n* the angle formed between the blade of an instrument and a tooth or tissue to provide increased access and more effective treatment.

angulation, bisecting error, *n* See bisecting-the-angle error.

angulation, bisecting-angle technique, *n* an intraoral radiographic technique used to expose periapical images. The beam of radiation is directed perpendicular to the imaginary bisector formed between the receptor and the long axis of the tooth.

angulation for air-powder polishing, *n* the correct angle at which the polisher's handpiece must be positioned in order to reduce the backflow of aerosol spray during treatment. The position varies according to tooth position and surface.

angulation, horizontal, *n* the direction of the position-indicating device (PID) in a horizontal plane, allowing radiation to open the contact areas between teeth.

angulation, mandibular midline projection, *n* the proper angle to expose a mandibular midline radiograph. The position-indicating device should be pointed at the end of the chin at a −55°

angle to the receptor for a view of the incisal region. To view the floor of the oral cavity, the position-indicating device should be perpendicular to the receptor, directly below the chin.

angulation, maxillary midline projection, *n* the proper angle to expose a maxillary midline radiograph. The position-indicating device should be aimed at a +65° angle to the receptor at the bridge of the nose.

angulation of central ray/beam, *n* the horizontal and vertical angles at which the central ray is aimed. Incorrect horizontal angulation causes overlapped images, excessive vertical angulation causes foreshortening. Insufficient little vertical angulation causes elongation of the image.

angulation, vertical, *n* the direction of the position-indicating device (PID) in a vertical plane.

angulation (radiographic), *n* the direction of the primary beam of radiation in relation to object and receptor.

anhidrosis (an′hīdrō′sis), *n* a severe deficiency in the production of sweat; may be associated with hypodontia or anodontia in ectodermal dysplasia.

anhidrotic ectodermal dysplasia (an′hīdrot′ik ek′tōder′məl displā′zhə), *n* See hypohidrotic ectodermal dysplasia.

anhydrous (anhī′drus), *adj* without water.

anion (an′īən), *n* a negatively charged ion.

anion, local anesthetic, *n* base form of the local anesthetic that is lipid soluble and penetrates the nerve.

anionic detergent (an′īon′ik), *n* See detergent, anionic.

anirodia (an′irō′dēə), *n* the absence of the iris. Usually a congenital condition.

anisocytosis (anī′sōsītō′sis), *n* a wide variation in cell size, especially of red blood cells.

anisognathous (an′īsogī′nathəs), *adj* having maxillary and mandibular dental arches or jaws that are of different sizes.

anisotropy (an′āsôt′rəpē), *n* the condition of not having properties or characteristics that are the same in all directions.

ankyloglossia (ang′kilōglôs′ēə), *n* an abnormally short lingual frenum that limits movement of the tongue.

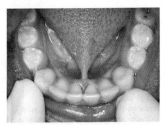

Ankyloglossia. (Zitelli/McIntire/Nowak, 2012)

ankylosis (ang'kilō'sis), *n* **I.** an abnormal fixation or immobility of a joint. *n* **2.** in dentistry, referring to the immobility of the periodontal ligament connection of a tooth to the alveolar bone as a result of bony fusion or a disease state.

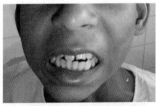

Ankylosis. (Mehrotraa, 2008)

ankylosis, bony, *n* a joining of bone with tooth or bone with bone that causes total loss of movement. See also tooth, ankylosed.

ankylosis, false, *n* an inability to open the oral cavity because of trismus rather than disease of the joint.

ankylosis, fibrous, *n* the fixation of a joint by fibrous tissue.

ankylosis of tooth, *n* See tooth, ankylosed.

anlage (on'lägə), *n* the first cells in the embryo that form any distinct part or organ.

anneal (anēl'), *n* (homogenizing heat treatment, softening heat treatment), the softening of a metal by controlled heating and cooling.

anneal foil, *n* a process of subjecting noncohesive foil to heat to volatilize a protective gaseous coating on its surface, thus leaving the surface clean, making it cohesive.

anneal glass, *n* a process of regulated heating and subsequent cooling to remove strain hardening or work hardening of glass.

anneal metal, *n* a process of regulated heating and subsequent cooling to remove strain hardening or work hardening of metal.

announcement, *n* a communication, usually printed, that states office policies or practice limitations to the public and profession.

annual reports, *n.pl* the statistical, fiscal, and descriptive yearly reports used to inform a constituency of the status of the institution or organization.

annual statement, *n* the report of an insurer or carrier showing assets and liabilities, receipts and disbursements, and other information for a specified 12-month period (fiscal or calendar year).

anochromasia (an'ōkrōmā'zēə, -zhə), *n* a variation in the staining quality of cells, particularly of degenerating red blood cells.

anociassociation (ənō'sēəsōsēā 'shən), *n* the blocking of neuroses, fear, pain, and harmful influences or associations to prevent shock.

anode (an'ōd), *n* the electrically positive terminal of a roentgen ray (radiographic) tube; a tungsten block embedded in a copper stem and set at an angle of 20° or 45° to the cathode. The anode emits x-ray photons from the point of impact of the electronic stream from the cathode.

anode, rotating, *n* an anode that rotates during x-ray production to present a constantly different focal spot to the electron stream and to permit use of small focal spots or higher tube voltages without overheating the tube.

anodontia (an'ōdon'tēə), *n* (aplasia of dentition), the complete failure of teeth to form; the total absence of teeth.

anodyne (an'ōdīn), *n* an agent or drug that relieves pain; milder than analgesia.

anomaly (ənom'əlē), *n* an aberration or deviation from normal anatomic growth, development, or function.

anomaly, dental, *n* an abnormality in which a tooth or teeth have deviated from normal in form, function, or position.

A

anomaly, developmental **(divel′əp men′təl),** *n* **1.** an abnormality originating in fetal development. *n* **2.** deficiencies or imperfections occurring in the teeth as a consequence of irregular tooth growth.

anomaly, dysgnathic **(disnath′ik),** *n* an older term for an abnormality that extends beyond the teeth and includes the maxillae, the mandible, or both.

anomaly, eugnathic **(yōōnath′ik),** *n* an older term for an abnormality limited to the teeth and their immediate alveolar supports.

anomaly, gestant **(jes′tənt),** *n* See odontoma.

anomaly, maxillofacial, *n* a distortion of normal development of the face and jaws; a dysgnathic anomaly.

anomaly, oral, *n* an abnormal structure of the oral cavity other than of the teeth.

anomaly, orofacial, *n* a term indicating an oral or facial abnormality.

anomaly, root, *n* a general term for describing any deviation from normal found in a tooth root.

anophaxia (anōfax′ēə), *n* a tendency for one eye to turn upward.

anophthalmos (an′opthal′məs), *n* a congenital absence of all tissues of the eyes.

anorexia (anōrek′sēə), *n* the partial or complete loss of appetite for food.

anorexia nervosa, *n* a psychoneurotic disorder characterized by a prolonged refusal to eat, resulting in emaciation, amenorrhea in women, emotional disturbance concerning body image, and an abnormal fear of becoming fat. See also disorder, body dysmorphic.

anoxemia (an′oksē′mēə), *n* a deficient aeration of the blood; a total lack of oxygen content in the blood.

anoxia (anok′sēə), *n* a condition of total lack of oxygen; a term frequently misused as a synonym for hypoxia.

anoxic hypoxia, *n* See hypoxia, anoxic.

antagonist(s) (antagə′nist), *n* **1.** a drug that counteracts, blocks, or abolishes the action of another drug. *n* **2.** a muscle that acts in opposition to the action of another muscle (e.g., flexor vs. extensor). *n* **3.** a tooth in one jaw that occludes with a tooth in the other jaw.

antagonist, narcotic, *n* a drug that acts specifically to reverse depression of the central nervous system caused by an opioid.

antagonists, insulin, *n.pl* the circulating hormonal and nonhormonal substances that stimulate glyconeogenesis (e.g., 11-oxysteroids and S hormones).

ante cibum (an′tē sī′bum), *adv* See a.c.

antegonial notch (an′təgō′nēəl), *n* the notch or concavity usually present at the junction between the ramus and body of the mandible, near the anterior margin of the masseter muscle attachment.

anterior, *adj* **1.** situated in front of. *adj* **2.** a term used to denote the incisor and canine teeth or the forward region of the oral cavity. *adj* **3.** the forward position.

anterior cervical triangle, *n* See triangle, anterior cervical.

anterior cranial base, *n* the anterior cranial fossa, sometimes identified by related landmarks such as the sella turcica and nasion.

anterior determinants of occlusion, *n.pl* See occlusion, anterior determinants of cusp.

anterior discrepancy, *n* a difference (as in tooth size or another characteristic) between the members of a pair of corresponding teeth in the anterior sextant.

anterior faucial tonsillar pillar, *n* the anterior lateral folds of tissue created by underlying muscle.

anterior guide, *n* See guide, anterior.

anterior nasal spine, *n* See spine, anterior nasal.

anterior palatal bar, *n* See connector, anterior palatal major.

anterior tooth arrangement, *n* See arrangement, tooth, anterior.

anterior-posterior discrepancy (antē′rēər-postē′rēər), *n* an anterior-posterior morphologic imbalance between the maxilla and mandible and consequently between structures attached to either.

anterior-posterior spread, *n* a calculation of the greatest amount of cantilever allowed for a dental implant within its bilateral distal ranges. It is measured by determining the distance from the center of the most posterior to the center of the most anterior implants and multiplying by 1.5.

anterocclusion (an′terōklōō′zhən), *n* a malocclusion of the teeth, in which the mandibular teeth are in a position anterior to their normal position relative to the teeth in the maxillary arch.

anteroposterior plane of space, *n* See sagittal plane.

anteversion (an′tivur′shən), *n* the tipping or tilting of teeth or other maxillary and mandibular structures too far forward (anterior) from the normal or generally accepted standard.

anthelmintic (an′thelmin′tik), *n* a drug that acts against parasitic worms, especially intestinal worms.

anthrax (an′thraks), *n* an infectious disease in herbivorous animals caused by a spore-forming *Bacillus* organism. Primary lesions in human beings may be on the lips or cheeks.

anthrocyclanins (an′thrōsī′kləninz), *n.pl* a group of floral pigments existing as glycosides that may be used as hematoxylin substitutes.

anthropology, *n* the science of human beings ranging from physical characteristics to cultural, social, and environmental aspects.

anthropology, cultural, *n* the study of the interpersonal and community mores of a society or isolate.

anthropology, physical, *n* the study of the physical attributes of a society or isolate.

anthropometry (an′thrəpom′ətrē), *n* the measurement of the body and its parts.

anti-HAV, *n* a passively acquired antibody to the hepatitis A virus that provides protective immunity against recurrences of the infection. It may be detected in the blood of infected individuals within 14 days after they show the first symptoms of hepatitis A.

anti-HBc, IgM, *n* an antibody to the core antigen of the hepatitis B virus. Its presence in the blood indicates a previous infection with the hepatitis B virus.

anti-HBe, *n* an antibody to the e antigen of the hepatitis B virus. Its detection in the blood indicates the presence of a low-titer hepatitis B infection and decreased ability of the infected person to pass the virus on to another person.

anti-HBs, *n* an antibody to the surface antigen of the hepatitis B virus; indicative of either active immunity to the hepatitis B virus as a result of prior infection or passive immunity from

the presence of hepatitis B immunoglobulin in the blood. It may also be an immune response triggered as the result of having received vaccination against the hepatitis B virus.

anti-HCV, *n* an antibody to the hepatitis C virus. Its presence in the blood is indicative of an active or chronic hepatitis C infection.

anti-HDV, *n* an antibody to the hepatitis D virus. Its presence in the blood is indicative of a hepatitis D infection that may be either active, chronic, or under control.

anti-HSV antibodies, *n.pl* an immunoglobulin contained in the fluid of the gingival sulcus that may or may not provide immunity to recurrent attacks of the herpes simplex virus.

anti-retraction device, *n* valves used to prevent aspiration of patient materials into dental handpieces and waterlines.

antibiotic (an′tibīot′ik), *n* an organic substance produced by one of several microorganisms, especially certain molds, that is capable, in low concentration, of destroying or inhibiting the growth of certain other microorganisms.

antibiotic, oral reactions to, *n* the manifestations on the oral mucous membrane of reactions to antibiotics; characterized by glossitis, angular cheilosis, and/or a hairy tongue. Reactions may result from an imbalance of oral flora produced by the antibiotics or from hypersensitivity to the antibiotics.

antibiotic prophylaxis (prōfəlak′sis), *n* the use of an antibiotic to protect a patient from an anticipated bacterial invasion associated with a medical or dental invasive procedure, particularly patients with a compromised cardiovascular system and risk of bacterial endocarditis. *Primary antibiotic prophylaxis* is used to prevent infection of a prosthetic device at the time of insertion; *secondary antibiotic prophylaxis* is used to prevent infection from treatment related bacteremias or post-operative infection.

antibiotic, subgingival placement, *n* the administration of antimicrobials in the subgingival region to control bacterial infections and manage periodontal disease.

antibiotic therapy, *n* See therapy, antibiotic.

antibody (an'tibodē), *n* **1.** a specific substance that is produced by an animal as a reaction to the presence of an antigen and that reacts specifically with an antigen in some observable way. *n* **2.** an immunoglobulin (preferred term), essential to the immune system, produced by lymphoid tissue in response to bacteria, viruses, or other antigenic substances. Each type is identified by its action, agglutinins, bacteriolysins, opsonins, and precipitins. See also immunoglobulins.

antibody, antinuclear, n an antibody having an affinity for the cell nuclei.

antibody formation, n the response of the lymphatic system to the presence of foreign substances in the body such as bacteria, viruses, food substances, pollens, and other antigens.

antibody, monoclonal **(mon'ō klon'əl),** n an antibody produced by a clone or genetically homogeneous population of hybrid cells.

antibody, specificity, n the lymphatic system produces antibodies specific to each antigen. Viruses have the capacity to alter an antigen's genetic makeup, thereby creating a mutant antigen that requires new antibodies to combat it.

antibody-mediated hypersensitivity, *n* **1.** an anaphylactic (Type I) reaction, also known as "immediate"; allergen-induced IgE antibodies remember the target antigen and proliferate against it, producing mediators such as histamines. *n* **2.** a cytotoxic (Type II) reaction; antigens and antibodies come together on the surface of a cell, causing lysis of the cell or other cell membrane damage. *n* **3.** an immune complex (Type III) reaction; a complex of antigens and antibodies that is attracted to tissue.

anticariogenic (an'tiker'ēōjen'ik), *adj* describing foods, chemicals, or other agents that tend to contribute favorably to dental health by remineralizing teeth and discouraging the acid that causes dental caries.

anticariogenic agents (an'tiker'ēōj en'ik), *n.pl* substances that inhibit or arrest dental caries formation. See also fluorides, sealants.

anticholinergic (an'tīkō'linur'jik), *n* (parasympatholytic, cholinolytic), a drug that acts to inhibit the effects of the neurohormone acetylcholine by binding to cholinergic receptors. A cholinergic blocking agent.

anticholinesterase (an'tīkō'lines'tə rās), *n* a drug or chemical that inhibits or inactivates the enzyme cholinesterase, resulting in the actions produced by the accumulation of acetylcholine at cholinergic sites.

anticoagulant (an'tīkōag'yələnt), *n* a drug that delays or prevents coagulation of blood.

anticonvulsive (an'tīkonvul'siv), *adj* relieving or preventing convulsion.

antidepressants, *n.pl* agents used to counteract or treat depression.

antidepressants, tricyclic (TCA), n. pl a classification of antidepressant drugs used to treat a variety of psychiatric conditions, including mental depression, social phobia, and mood, panic, or obsessive-compulsive disorders, neuropathic pain, and other conditions.

antidiabetes mellitus agents (an'tē dī'əbē'tēz məli'təs), *n.pl* drugs, particularly insulin, used to combat diabetes mellitus; also drugs that combat the common side effects of diabetes mellitus, hypoglycemia, and hyperglycemia. See also diabetes.

antidiarrheals (an'tēdī'ərē'əlz), *n.pl* drugs that combat diarrhea.

antidote (an'tidōt), *n* a substance that acts to antagonize the toxic effects of a drug, especially in overdose, or of a poison. See also poison.

antiemetic (an'tēəmet'ik, an'tīəme t'ik), *n* drug used to prevent, stop, or relieve nausea and emesis (vomiting).

antiepileptic drugs, *n.pl* agents that inhibit or control seizures associated with epilepsy or other conditions.

antifibrinolytics (an'tēfī'brənoli t'iks), *n* a type of substance that prevents the breakdown of fibrin in blood clots. Used to prevent excessive bleeding.

antiflux, *n* a material that prevents and confines the flow of solder (e.g., graphite).

antifungal agents, *n.pl* agents that inhibit, control, or kill fungi. The most common yeastlike fungus occurring in or near the oral cavity is *Candida albicans.*

antigen (an'tijen), *n* a substance, usually a protein, that elicits the formation of antibodies that react with it when exposed to an individual or species to which it is foreign. See also immunogens.

antigen, human leukocyte (HLA), *n* the group of genes contained within the major histocompatibility complex (MHC), these antigen-bearing proteins are encoded by multiple genetic loci on human chromosome 6 and are found on the outer regions of the cellular structure.

antigenic drift (an'tējen'ik), *n* the ability of viruses to alter their genetic makeup, thereby creating mutant antigens and bypassing the antibody barrier of the host.

antihemophilic factor (an'tīhē'mōf il'ik), *n* See factor VIII.

antihistamine (an'tīhis'təmin), *n* a drug that blocks histamine receptors. Common usage limits this term to blockers of histamine H₁ receptors. Some antihistamines have topical anesthetic and sedative effects, as well as a drying effect on the nasal mucosa.

antihistaminic (an'tīhistəmin'ik), *adj* referring to action of an antihistamine.

antihypertensive drugs, *n.pl* agents that lower or reduce high blood pressure.

antiinflammatory agents, *n.pl* compounds that counteract or reduce inflammation.

antimicrobial, systemic, *n* an antimicrobial agent, usually in the form of an antibiotic, that is generally administered orally and absorbed from the bloodstream through the intestine. They move from the circulatory system to the tissues e.g., the periodontal pocket through the gingival sulcus fluid.

antimony (an'təmō'nē), *n* a bluish crystalline metallic element occurring in nature both free and as salts. Antimony compounds are used in the treatment of filariasis, leishmaniasis, and other parasitic diseases. Antimony is also used as an emetic.

antineoplastic agent, *n* a drug that prevents the development, maturation, or spread of neoplastic cells.

antiodontalgic, *adj* pertaining to a toothache remedy.

antioxidants, *n.pl* agents that reduce or prevent oxidation, such as occurs in the deterioration of fats, oils, and non-precious metals.

antiphlogistic (an'tīflōjis'tik), *adj* an older term for antiinflammatory or antipyretic.

antiplaque agents, *n.pl* compounds that inhibit, control, or kill organisms associated with plaque formation.

antipruritic (an'tīprōōrit'ik), *adj* relieving or preventing itching.

antipsychotics (an'tēsīkot'iks), *n.pl* medications used to decrease hallucinations, delusions, and other symptoms associated with schizophrenia and other psychotic disorders; enables functioning in daily life for individuals.

antipyretic (an'tīpīret'ik), *n* a drug that reduces fever primarily through action on the hypothalamus, thereby resulting in a lowering of the hypothalamic set-point and increasing heat dissipation through augmented peripheral blood flow and sweating.

antisepsis (an'tīsep'sis), *n* the prevention of infection of a body surface, usually skin or oral mucosa, through the application of an antimicrobial agent.

antiseptic (an'tisep'tik), *n* an antimicrobial agent for application to a body surface, usually skin or oral mucosa, in an attempt to prevent or minimize infection at the area of application.

antisialic (an'tīsīal'ik), *adj* act of inhibiting salivary flow.

antisialogogue (an'tīsīal'əgog), *n* a drug that reduces, slows, or prevents the flow of saliva.

antispasmodic (an'tīspazmod'ik), *n* (antispastic), a drug that relieves muscle spasms.

antispastic, *adj* See antispasmodic.

antistreptolysin O (an'tīstreptol 'sin), *n* an antibody against streptolysin O, a hemolysin produced by group A streptococci. A high titer is supporting evidence of rheumatic fever.

antithermic, *adj* reducing temperature. See also antipyretic.

antitoxin (an'tētok'sin), *n* a subgroup of antisera usually prepared from the serum of horses immunized against a particular toxin-producing organism, such as botulism antitoxin and diphtheria antitoxin given prophylactically to prevent those infections.

antitragus (an'titrā'gus), *n* the structure located opposite the tragus, a cartilaginous prominence in front of the external opening of the ear.

antitussive (an'tītus'iv), *n* a drug that relieves or prevents cough.

antrodynia (an'trōdǐ'nēə), *n* an older term for pain in the maxillary antrum.

antrostomy (antros'təmē), *n* a surgical opening into an antrum, either through the medial wall into the nose or through the lateral wall into the oral cavity.

antrum (an'trum), *n* a general term for cavity or chamber that may have specific meaning in referencing certain organs or sites in the body. For example, referring to paranasal sinuses, the maxillary sinus can be referred to as a maxillary antrum.

antrum, maxillary, n See sinus, maxillary.

antrum of Highmore, n.pl See sinus, maxillary.

ANUG, *n* the abbreviation for acute necrotizing ulcerative gingivitis. An obsolete term. See gingivitis, necrotizing ulcerative.

anxiety, *n* a condition of heightened and often disruptive tension accompanied by an ill-defined and distressing aura of impending harm or injury. It can disrupt physiologic functions through its effect on the autonomic nervous system. The patient may assume a tense posture, show excessive vigilance, move the hands and feet restlessly, and speak with a strained, uneven voice. The pupils may be widely dilated, giving the appearance of unrestrained fright, and the hands and face may perspire excessively. In extremely acute forms the patient may have generalized visceral reactions of respiratory, cardiac, vascular, and gastrointestinal dysfunction. The dental professional must recognize the existence of it, seek its etiology and relation to dental treatment, and determine ways that the patient's defenses against it can be used to facilitate rather than inhibit treatment.

anxiety control, n the combination of measures that are used to eliminate patient apprehension and control pain during the performance of a dental procedure. The determination of the appropriate measures to be taken depends on the patient's overall periodontal health and tolerance for pain, as well as the specific treatment to be delivered.

anxiety neurosis, n an extreme manifestation of anxiety characterized by acute anxiety attacks (sympathetic overreactivity) and phobias, causing avoidance of the anxiety-provoking situations.

anxiolytic medication (angk'seōli t'ik), *n* a drug used to decrease emotional stress or anxiety. Also called *antianxiety agent.*

aorta (āor'tə), *n* the main arterial trunk of the systemic circulation. Consists of four parts: the ascending aorta, the arch of the aorta, the thoracic portion of the descending aorta, and the abdominal portion of the descending aorta. Gives rise to the common carotid and subclavian arteries on the left side and to the brachiocephalic artery on the right side.

aortic aneurysm, *n* a localized dilation or ballooning of the wall of the aorta caused by atherosclerosis, hypertension, or a combination.

aortic valve, *n* a valve in the heart between the left ventricle and the aorta; also known as the tricuspid valve.

apathism (ap'əthizm), *n* the state of being slow in responding to stimuli.

apatite (ap'ətīt), *n* the inorganic mineral substance of teeth and bone. See also carbonate hydroxyapatite.

APC, *n* See aspirin, phenacetin, caffeine.

Apert syndrome, *n.pr* See syndrome, Apert.

apertognathia (əpur'tōnath'ēə), *n* an occlusion characterized by a vertical separation between the maxillary and mandibular anterior teeth. Commonly called an *open bite.*

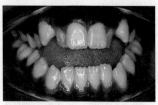

Apertognathia. (Courtesy Dr. Flavio Uribe)

aperture, *n* an opening such as in bone.

aperture, piriform, n the anterior opening of the nasal cavity.

apertures, posterior nasal, n.pl the posterior openings of the nasal cavity.

apex, *n* **I.** the pointed end of a conical structure. *n* **2.** the end of the root.

apex blunderbuss, *n* an open or everted apex of a tooth, resembling the divergent form of the barrel of a blunderbuss rifle.

apex of nose, *n* the tip of nose.

apex of tongue, *n* the tip of tongue.

apexification (āpek'sifikā'shən), *n* the process of induced root development or apical closure of the root by hard tissue deposition.

apexigraph (āpek'sigraf), *n* a device for determining the position of the apex of a tooth root.

APF, *n* the abbreviation for *acidulated phosphate fluoride.*

aphagia (əfā'jēə), *n* the inability to swallow.

aphasia (əfa'zhə), *n* a loss of power of expression through speech, writing, or signs of comprehension of spoken or written language resulting from disease or injury of the brain centers.

aphtha (af'thə), *n* (aphthous stomatitis), **I.** a small ulcer on the mucous membrane. **(-hae)** *n.pl* **2.** vesicles that undergo subsequent ulceration and are surrounded by a raised erythematous area.

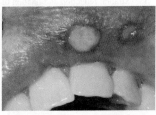

Aphtha. (Neville et al, 2009)

aphtha, Bednar's **(bed'närz),** *n.pr* (pterygoid ulcer), an ulcer on the soft palate near the greater palatine foramen; seen in newborns.

aphtha, Mikulicz' **(mik'ulich),** *n.pr* a recurrent ulceration of the oral mucosa, resembling herpes. See also periadenitis mucosa necrotica recurrens.

aphtha, recurrent, *n* See stomatitis, herpetic; and ulcer, aphthous, recurrent.

aphtha, recurrent scarring, See periadenitis mucosa necrotica recurrens.

aphthosis (afthō'sis), *n* a clinical manifestation of apthae.

aphthous (af'thus), *adj* characterized by aphthae or aphthosis.

aphthous fever, *n* a fever associated with aphthosis.

aphthous pharyngitis **(af'thus far'injī'tis),** *n* aphthosis of the pharynx.

aphthous stomatitis, *n* See aphtha and stomatitis, aphthous.

apical (ap'ikəl), *adj* pertaining to the end portion of the root.

apical curettage, *n* the surgical removal of diseased tissue surrounding a root apex.

apical fiber, *n* See fiber, apical.

apical foramen, *n* See foramen, apical.

apical group, *n* the portion of the alveolodental group of the periodontal ligament that radiates apically from the cementum.

apical third, *adj* the inferior third of a tooth's root or root canal.

apicectomy, See apicoectomy.

apicoectomy (ap'ikōek'təmē), *n* (apicectomy, apicetomy, root amputation, root resection), the surgical removal of the apex or apical portion of a root.

Apicomplexa protozoa **(ap'ikom plek'sə),** *n* a parasitic group that sometimes needs multiple hosts to survive. Some varieties are implicated in diarrhea and malaria.

aplasia (əplā'zhə), *n* a lack of origin or development (e.g., aplasia of dentition associated with ectodermal dysplasia).

aplasia of dentition, *n* See anodontia.

apnea (apnē'ə, ap'nēə), *n* a temporary cessation of respiratory movements.

apnea, sleep, *n* temporary cessation of breathing during sleep.

apneumatic (apnōōmat'ik), *adj* free from air; used to describe something accomplished with the exclusion of air, such as an apneumatic operation.

apoplexy (ap'ōplek'sē), *n* a sudden loss or decrease of neurologic function often caused by cerebrovascular accident (CVA).

apoptosis (ap'ətō'sis), *n* cell reduction by fragmentation into membrane-bound particles that are phagocytosed by other cells.

apostematosa, cheilitis glandularis (kīlī'təs glan'jəlar'is), *n* See cheilitis glandularis apostematosa.

apothecaries' system (əpoth'əka r'ēz), *n* See system, apothecaries'.

apoxesis (ap'əksē'sis), *n* See curettage, apical.

apparatus (ap'ərat'us), *n* **I.** an arrangement of a number of parts that act together to perform some special function. *n* **2.** a device.

apparatus, attachment, n an older term for the tissues that invest and support the teeth for function and include gingivae, cementum of the tooth, periodontal ligament, and alveolar bone. Now commonly called *periodontium.*

apparatus, branchial, n See branchial apparatus.

apparatus, masticating, n an older term for the structures involved in chewing (i.e., the teeth, mandibular musculature, mandible and its temporomandibular joints, accessory mandibular and facial musculature, and tongue), which are controlled by an exquisitely functioning neuromuscular mechanism. See also system, stomatognathic.

appellant (əpel'ənt), *n* the party who, dissatisfied with the disposition of a case on the trial level, appeals to a higher court.

appendicitis (əpen'disi'tis), *n* an inflammation of the vermiform appendix, usually acute, which, if undiagnosed and not surgically removed, leads rapidly to perforation and peritonitis.

appendix (əpen'diks), *n* **I.** an accessory part of a main structure or text; *n* **2.** the term generally refers to the *vermiform appendix,* which is located at the junction of the small and large intestines.

appetite suppressant, *n* an agent that diminishes the desire for eating.

appliance (əpli'əns), *n* a device used to provide function or therapeutic effect. See also restoration.

appliance, Andresen removable orthodontic, n.pr an appliance intended to function as a passive transmitter and sometimes stimulator of the forces of the perioral muscles. One of the activator types of orthodontic appliances that induces or directs oral forces to contribute to improved tooth position and jaw relationship.

appliance, Begg fixed orthodontic, n.pr an appliance based on a modified ribbon-arch attachment.

appliance, Bimler removable orthodontic, n.pr an activator-type appliance.

appliance, chin cup extraoral orthodontic, n an extraoral traction appliance used to restrain the forward positioning of the mandible and/or the forward growth of the mandible.

appliance, Crozat removable orthodontic, n.pr a wrought wire appliance originally introduced by George Crozat.

appliance, edgewise fixed orthodontic, n an orthodontic appliance characterized by attachment brackets with a rectangular slot for engagement of a round or rectangular arch wire.

appliance, extraoral orthodontic, n a device that uses a portion of the face, neck, or back of the head as a base from which to deliver traction force to the teeth or jaws.

appliance, fixed orthodontic, n an appliance that is cemented to the teeth or attached by an adhesive material.

appliance, fracture, n (biphase pin fixation, external pin fixation, Stader splint), any one of the various devices for extraoral reduction and fixation of fractures in which pins, clamps, or screws are placed in the fractured segments, the fractured parts are aligned, and then the pins, clamps, or screws are joined with metal bars or rigid plastic connectors (e.g., the Stader splint or Roger-Anderson pin-fixation appliance).

appliance, Frankel removable orthodontic, n.pr an activator-type appliance.

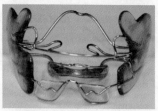

Frankel appliance. (Courtesy Dr. Flavio Uribe)

appliance, Hawley retaining orthodontic, n.pr See retainer.

appliance, hay rake fixed orthodontic, n a device used to limit abnormal swallowing excursions of the tongue. In this manner, harmful effects of tongue thrusting are mitigated until the patient learns a new swallowing pattern.

appliance, intraoral orthodontic (in'trəor'əl ôr'thədän'tik), *n* a device placed inside the oral cavity to correct or alleviate a malocclusion.

appliance, Kloehn cervical extraoral orthodontic (kloen ser'vikəl ek'strəôr'əl ôr'thədän'tik), *n.pr* the classical cervical extraoral traction appliance. Uses a relatively light and flexible (0.045 inch; 1.15 mm) inner arch rigidly attached to a long outer bow (0.071 inch outer bow).

appliance, labiolingual fixed orthodontic (lā'bēōling'gwəl fikst ôr'thədän'tik), *n* an appliance using the maxillary and mandibular first permanent molars as anchorage, with labial arches 0.036 to 0.040 inch (0.090 to 0.10 cm) in diameter introduced into horizontal buccal tubes attached to the anchor bands and lingual arches of the same diameter fitted into vertical or horizontal tubes fastened to the lingual side of the anchor bands.

appliance, obturator (ob'tərātər), *n* a dental prosthesis used to close an opening such as cleft palate.

appliance, orthodontic, n a device used for influencing tooth position. Orthodontic appliances may be classified as fixed or removable, active or retaining, and intraoral or extraoral.

appliance, pin and tube fixed orthodontic, n a labial arch with vertical posts that insert into tubes attached to bands on the teeth.

appliance, prosthetic (prosthet'ik), *n* an older term referring to a complete or partial denture for children when groups of teeth are lost or are congenitally missing. Used to maintain space or masticatory function or for aesthetic reasons.

appliance, removable orthodontic, n an appliance designed so that it can be removed and replaced by the patient.

appliance, retaining orthodontic, n an orthodontic device used to hold the teeth in place, following orthodontic

tooth movement, until the occlusion is stabilized.

appliance, straight-wire fixed orthodontic, n a variation of the edgewise appliance in which an effort is made to obviate the need for many archwire adjustments by reorientation of the arch-wire slots.

appliance, therapeutic, n a vehicle used to transport and retain some agent for therapeutic purposes (e.g., a radium carrier).

appliance, twin-wire fixed orthodontic, n an orthodontic appliance typically using a pair of 0.010-inch (0.25-mm) wires to form the midsection of the arch wire.

appliance, universal fixed orthodontic, n an orthodontic appliance developed by S.R. Atkinson, combining some of the principles of edgewise and ribbon-arch appliances with very light arch wires.

application program, *n* a standard and frequently used computer program tailored to medical and dental needs. It may be supplied to the user by the manufacturer, purchased from a software house, or written by the user.

applicator, *n* a device for applying medication; usually a slender rod of glass or wood, used with a pledget of cotton on the end.

appointment, *n* a mutually agreed-on time reserved for the patient to receive treatment.

appointment book, n a ledger or table of workdays divided into segments of time to enable the dental staff to reserve specified lengths of time for patient treatment. Now appointments are usually on the computer, but the computer program is still referred to using this term.

appointment card, n a small card given to the patient as a reminder of the time reserved for the appointment. Even if sent via e-mail, it is still referred to as this.

apposition (ap'əzish'ən), *n* **1.** the condition of being placed or fitted together; juxtaposition; coaptation. *n* **2.** a layered formation of a firm or hard tissue such as cartilage, bone, enamel, dentin, and cementum.

appropriate, *adj* **1.** the determination that the service provided is suited for the condition. *adj* **2.** being suitable for a particular person, group, community, condition, occasion, and/or place. *adj* **3.** proper.

appropriate, space, *n* interdisciplinary approach to create or uniformly distribute space orthodontically prior to final prosthodontic restoration.

Appropriatech, *n.pr* an approach to providing complete dentures with simplified procedures and the fewest clinical visits.

approved services, *n.pl* **1.** all services provided in a dental plan. In some plans, authorization must be obtained before approved service is provided; other plans make exception for treatment of emergency needs; still others require no prior authorization for any treatment approved under the program. *n.pl* **2.** dental services that meet quality standards maintained in a dental plan.

approximal (əprôk′səməl), *adj* (approximating), contiguous; adjacent; next to each other.

approximating, *adj* See approximal.

apraclonidine (ap′rəklon′idēn), *n* *brand name:* Iopidine; *drug class:* selective α₂-adrenergic agonist; *action:* reduces intraocular pressure; *use:* control or prevention of increases in intraocular pressure related to laser surgery of eye.

apraxia (əprak′sēə), *n* a loss of ability to execute a purposeful, goal-oriented, or skilled act resulting from selective damage to certain high-level brain centers, either sensory, motor, or both.

aprepitant, *n* *brand name:* Emend; *drug class:* antiemetic; *action:* neurokinin 1 receptor antagonist; *use:* prevent nausea and vomiting resulting 🔊 from chemotherapy.

apron, *n* a piece of clothing worn in front of the body for protection.

apron band, *n* a labioincisal or gingival extension of an orthodontic band that aids in retention of the band and in proper positioning of the bracket.

🔊 *apron, lead,* *n* an apron made of materials containing metallic lead or lead compounds used to protect patient tissues from scatter radiation.

apron, lingual, *n* See connector, linguoplate major.

apron, rubber dam, *n* a small strip of rubber dam, perforated to fit over an implant abutment that is used to

inhibit introduction of cement into the periimplant space.

aprotinin (āprō′tənin), *n* a protease and kallikrein inhibitor useful in controlling inflammation and blood loss resulting from cardiopulmonary bypass surgery.

aqueous (ā′kwēus), *adj* containing or relating to water.

arachidonic acid (ar′əkədon′ik), *n* an essential fatty acid that is a component of lecithin and a precursor in the biosynthesis of prostaglandins and leukotrienes.

Arachnia *propionica* (ərak′nēə prō′pēon′ikə), *n* an opportunistic, naturally occurring organism in the body, especially in body cavities and on the skin. It is sometimes implicated in actinomycosis, especially in open wounds.

arboviruses (ar′bōvī′rəsəz), *n.pl* an acronym for hemophagic *arthropod-borne viruses,* passed on to the host by a bite; implicated in viral encephalitis. The term is not accepted as an official taxonomic nomenclature.

ARC, *n* the abbreviation for *AIDS-related complex.* See also acquired immunodeficiency syndrome.

arc, reflex, *n* a system of nerves used in a reflex or involuntary act, consisting primarily of an afferent nerve with sensory receptor, a nerve center, and an efferent nerve that stimulates the effector muscle or gland.

arch (pl. es), *n* a structure with a curved outline, such as bone.

arch anterior, *n* an arch of the atlas or first cervical vertebra.

arch bar, *n* See bar, arch.

arch, basal, *n* See base, apical.

arch, branchial, *n* See branchial arches. Also known as the *pharyngeal arches.*

arch, dental, *n* the composite structure of the dentition and alveolar ridge or the remains thereof after the loss of some or all of the natural teeth.

arch, dental, contraction, *n* See contraction.

arch, dentulous dental (den′chələs), *n* a dental arch containing natural teeth.

arch, edentulous dental (ē′den′chə ləs), *n* a dental arch from which all natural teeth are missing. Also called the *residual alveolar ridge.*

arch expansion, *n* See expansion.

arch form, See form, arch.

arch, high labial, *n* a labial arch wire adapted so that it lies gingival to the anterior tooth crowns; it has auxiliary springs extending downward in contact with the teeth to be moved.

arch, inferior dental, *n* See arch, lower.

arch length, *n* the distance from a line perpendicular to the mesial surface of the permanent first molars to the contact point of the central incisors. Often used interchangeably with arch perimeter.

arch length, available, *n* the space available for all teeth.

arch length, deficiency, *n* the difference between required and available arch length.

arch length, required, *n* the sum of the mesiodistal widths of all teeth.

arch, lower, *n* the archlike curve of the cutting edges and surfaces of the teeth on the mandible. Also known as the *inferior dental arch.*

arch, ovoid, *n* an arch that curves continuously from the molars on one side to the molars on the opposite side so that two such arches placed back to back describe an oval.

arch, palatine, *n* (glossopalatine arch), the pillars of the fauces; the two arches of mucous membrane enclosing the muscles at the sides of the passage from the oral cavity to the pharynx.

arch, partially edentulous dental, *n* a dental arch from which one or more but not all teeth are missing.

arch, passive lingual, *n* an orthodontic appliance effective in maintaining space and preserving arch length when bilateral primary molars are prematurely lost.

arch, perimeter, *n* the length of the dental arch usually measured through the point of contacts around the arch from the mesial of the first molar to the mesial of the contralateral molar. Often used interchangeably with *arch length.*

arch, pharyngeal, *n* See arch, branchial.

arch, posterior, *n* an arch on the first cervical vertebra.

arch, removable lingual, *n* an arch wire designed to fit the lingual surface of the teeth. It has two posts soldered on each end that fit snugly into the

vertical tubes of the molar anchor bands.

arch, stationary lingual, *n* an arch wire designed to fit the lingual surface of the teeth and soldered to the anchor bands.

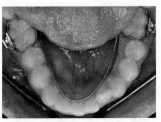

Stationary lingual arch wire. (Courtesy Dr. Flavio Uribe)

arch, tapering, *n* a dental arch that converges from molars to central incisors to such an extent that lines passing through the central grooves of the molars and premolars intersect within 1 inch (2.5 cm) anterior to the central incisors.

arch, trapezoidal **(trap′ǝzoid′ǝl),** *n* an arch that has the same convergence as a tapering arch but to a lesser degree. The anterior teeth are somewhat square to abruptly rounded from canine tip to canine tip. The canines act as corners of the arch.

arch, U-shaped, *n* a dental arch in which there is little difference in diameter (width) between the first premolars and the last molars; the curve from canine to canine is abrupt, so a dental arch in the shape of a capital U is formed.

arch width, *n* the width of a dental arch. The width, which varies in all diameters between the right and left opposites, is determined by direct measurement between the canines, between the first molars, and between the second premolars. These intercanine, interpremolar, and intermolar distances can be cited as arch width.

arch wire, *n* a wire applied to two or more teeth through fixed attachments to cause or guide orthodontic tooth movement.

arch wire, full, *n* a wire extending from the molar region of one side of an arch to the other.

arch wire, sectional, n a wire extending to only a few teeth, usually on one side or in the anterior segment.

architecture, n in medicine and dentistry, usually refers to the framework of a structure or system.

architecture, gingival, n See gingival architecture.

archive (ar′kīv), n the storage of older, rarely required data or patient information in a cheaper and/or more compact form.

arcus senilis (är′kəs senil′is), n an opaque, grayish-white ring at the periphery of the cornea occurring in older adults.

area, n region.

area, apical, n See base, apical.

area, basal seat, n (denture-bearing area, denture-supporting area, stress-bearing area, stress-supporting area), the portion of the oral structures available to support a denture.

area, contact, n See point, contact.

area, denture-bearing, n See area, basal seat.

area, denture-supporting, n See area, basal seat.

area, impression, n the surface of the oral structures recorded in an impression.

area, pear-shaped, n See pad, retromolar.

area, post dam, n See area, posterior palatal seal.

area, posterior palatal seal, n the soft tissues along the junction of the hard and soft palates on which compression, within the physiologic limits of the tissues, can be applied by a denture to aid in its retention.

area, postpalatal seal (post′pal′ətəl), n See area, posterior palatal seal.

area, pressure, n an area of excessive displacement of soft tissue by a prosthesis.

area, recipient, n the portion of the body on which a skin, bone, tooth, or other graft is placed.

area, relief, n the portion of the surface of the oral cavity under prosthesis on which pressures are reduced or eliminated.

area, rest (rest seat), n the prepared surface of a tooth or fixed restoration into which the rest fits, giving support to a removable partial denture.

area, rugae (rōō′jē), n (rugae zone), that portion of the hard palate in which rugae are found.

area, saddle, n See area, basal seat.

area, stress-bearing, n See area, basal seat.

area, stress-supporting, n See area, basal seat.

area, supporting, n the areas of the maxillary and mandibular edentulous ridges best suited to carry the forces of mastication when the dentures are in use. See also area, basal seat.

area, work, n the entire space in which the dental practitioner moves and works while treating a patient. This includes the instrument tray and dental chair, unit, and light.

Arenaviridae (ərē′nəvī′ridē), n a grouping of enveloped, helix-shaped RNA viruses implicated in a relatively benign form of meningitis (lymphoctyic choriomeningitis; severe encephalitic forms do occur rarely) that affects young adults.

arginine, n an essential amino acid for infants and children. See also amino acid.

Argyll Robertson pupil (ärgil′), n.pr See pupil, Argyll Robertson.

argyria, local (ärjir′ēə), n a localized blue pigmentation of the oral mucosa from the deposition of silver amalgam in the submucosal connective tissue.

argyrosis (ärjirō′sis), n a pathologic bluish-black pigmentation in a tissue resulting from the deposition of an insoluble albuminate of silver.

ariboflavinosis (ərī′bōflāvinō′sis), n a nutritional disease resulting from a deficiency of riboflavin (vitamin B_2); characterized by angular cheilosis, seborrheic dermatitis, a magenta tongue, and ocular disturbance.

aripiprazole, n *brand name:* Abilify; *drug class:* antipsychotic (atypical); *actions:* dopamine D_2 receptor partial agonist, an inhibitor at several other receptors including serotonin 5-HT_{2A} receptors; *uses:* schizophrenia, bipolar disease, adjunct in treating depression.

Arkansas stone (är′kənsô), n See stone, Arkansas.

arm, n an extension or projection of a removable partial denture framework.

arm, ADD-, cantilever, n an end of wire engaged to one tooth or a group of teeth with one point contact to bring about desired tooth movement.

arm, neutral position of, n a body position to be assumed while treating a patient that prevents cumulative trauma to the arm; incorporates proper placement of the wrist, elbow, and shoulder.

arm, reciprocal, n a clasp arm used on a removable partial denture to oppose any force arising from an opposing clasp arm on the same tooth. See also arm, retention.

arm, retention, n an extension or projection that is part of a removable partial denture and is used to aid in the retention and stabilization of the restoration. See also retainer divet.

arm, truss, n See connector, minor.

arm, upright, n See connector, minor.

armamentarium (är'məmenter'ē əm), n the equipment and materials of the clinician.

arrangement, n the pattern into which a group of things is organized.

arrangement, financial, n an agreement between the dental provider and patient on the method of handling the patient's account.

arrangement, tooth, n the placement of teeth on a denture or temporary base with definite objectives in mind.

arrest lines, n the smooth, stained microscopic lines noted in cartilage, bone, and cementum due to apposition occurring in these tissues.

arrhythmia (ərith'mēə), n a variation from the normal rhythm of the heart.

arteriole (ärtir'ēōl), n a smaller arterial branch off an artery and connecting to a capillary.

arteriosclerosis (ärtir'ēōsklerō'sis), n a term applied to a group of diseases that affect the elasticity of the blood vessels. It may refer to atherosclerosis or hyperplastic arteriosclerosis. These degenerative processes generally affect only the tunica media and tunica intima. The effect is narrowing of the lumen of a blood vessel, causing rupture of the blood vessel or ischemia of an area of tissue that the vessel supplies.

arteriosclerotic heart disease (ärt ir'ēōsklerot'ik), n See disease, heart, arteriosclerotic.

arteriovenous shunt (ärtir'ēōvē' nus), n See shunt, arteriovenous.

arteritis (ärtərī'tis), n an inflammatory condition of the inner layers or the outer coat of one or more arteries. It may occur as a separate clinical entity or accompanying another disorder, such as rheumatoid arthritis, rheumatic fever, or systemic lupus erythematosus.

arteritis, temporal, n an inflammation of the temporal artery that produces a nodular, tortuous swelling of the temporal artery accompanied by a burning, throbbing pain, initially in the teeth, temporomandibular joint, and eye, but ultimately localized over the artery. This disorder occurs primarily in persons over 55 years of age.

artery (är'tərē), n a blood vessel through which the blood passes away from the heart to the various structures. There are three layers: the inner coat (tunica intima), composed of an inner endothelial lining, connective tissue, and an outer layer of elastic tissue (inner elastic membrane); the middle coat (tunica media), composed mainly of muscle tissue; and the outer coat (tunica adventitia), composed mainly of connective tissue. The structure of the three layers varies with the location, size, and purpose of the blood vessel.

artery, angular, n an arterial branch that is a termination of the facial artery and supplies the tissues along the side of the nose.

artery, anterior superior alveolar, n the arterial branch from the infraorbital artery that gives rise to the dental and alveolar branches, which supply the pulp tissue and periodontium of the anterior maxillary teeth.

artery arthograms, n.pl radiographs of a joint, usually with the introduction of a contrast compound into the joint capsule. In dentistry, an arthogram usually involves the temporomandibular joint.

artery, ascending palatine, n an arterial branch from the facial artery that supplies the palatine muscles and tonsils.

artery, ascending pharyngeal, n the medial arterial branch from the external carotid artery that supplies the pharyngeal walls, soft palate, and brain tissue.

artery, brachiocephalic, n the artery that branches directly off the aorta on the right side of the body and gives rise to the right common carotid and subclavian arteries.

artery, buccal, n the arterial branch from the maxillary artery that supplies the buccinator muscle and cheek tissues.

artery, common carotid, *n* the artery that travels in the carotid sheath, up the neck ,to branch into the internal and external carotid arteries.

artery(ies), deep temporal, *n/n.pl* the arterial branches from the maxillary artery that supply the temporalis muscle.

artery, external carotid, *n* an artery that arises from the common carotid artery and supplies the extracranial tissues of the head and neck, including the oral cavity.

artery, facial, *n* See facial artery.

artery, greater palatine, *n* an arterial branch from the maxillary artery that travels to the palate.

artery, incisive, *n* an arterial branch from the inferior alveolar artery that divides into the dental and alveolar branches to supply the pulp tissue and periodontium of the mandibular anterior teeth.

artery, inferior alveolar, *n* an arterial branch from the maxillary artery that supplies the mandibular posterior teeth and branches into the mental and incisive arteries.

artery, inferior labia, *n* an arterial branch from the facial artery that supplies the lower lip tissues.

artery, infraorbital, *n* an arterial branch from the maxillary artery that gives off the anterior superior alveolar artery and branches to the orbit.

artery, internal carotid, *n* an artery off the common carotid artery that gives rise to the ophthalmic artery and supplies the intracranial structures.

artery, large, *n* an elastic artery with an abundant supply of elastic tissue and a great reduction of smooth muscle. The tunica intima is thick, and the endothelial cells are round or polygonal. The tunica media is the thickest of the three layers. It contains few smooth muscle fibers, and its outer border has a special concentration of elastic fibers—the external elastic membrane. The tunica adventitia is relatively thin and ill defined and is continuous with the loose connective tissue surrounding the vessel.

artery, lesser palatine, *n* the arterial branch from the maxillary artery that travels to the soft palate.

artery, lingual, *n* anterior artery, branching from the external carotid artery, which supplies tissues superior to the hyoid bone, as well as, the tongue and floor of the mouth.

artery, masseteric, *n* the arterial branch from the maxillary artery that supplies the masseter muscle.

artery, maxillary, *n* See maxillary artery.

artery, medium-sized, *n* most of the arteries in the body (e.g., facial, maxillary, radial, ulnar, and popliteal). Thick muscular bands are found in the tunica media. Thin elastic fibers course circularly in the tunica media and run longitudinally in the tunica adventitia. The tunica adventitia is as thick as the tunica media, and its outer layer gradually blends with the connective tissue that supports the artery and surrounding structures.

artery, mental, *n* the mental branch of the inferior alveolar artery, running from the mandibular canal to the apical foramen of the teeth.

artery, middle temporal, *n* an arterial branch from the superficial temporal artery that supplies the temporalis muscle.

artery, mylohyoid, *n* an arterial branch from the inferior alveolar artery that supplies the floor of the mouth and the mylohyoid muscle.

artery, occipital, *n* the posterior arterial branch from the external carotid artery that supplies the suprahyoid and sternocleidomastoid muscles and posterior scalp tissues.

artery, ophthalmic, *n* an arterial branch that supplies the eye, orbit, and lacrimal gland.

artery, posterior auricular, *n* the posterior arterial branch from the external carotid artery that supplies the tissues around the ear.

artery, posterior superior alveolar, *n* the artery that originates from the maxillary artery; its branches supply the maxillary molars and maxillary sinus.

artery, pterygoid, *n* an arterial branch of the maxillary artery that supplies the pterygoid muscles.

artery, sphenopalatine, *n* the terminal arterial branch from the maxillary artery that supplies the nose, including a branch through the incisive foramen.

artery, stylomastoid, *n* an artery that is a branch from the posterior auricular artery and supplies the mastoid air cells.

artery, subclavian, *n* an artery that arises from the aorta on the left and the brachiocephalic artery on the right and gives off branches to supply both intracranial and extracranial structures, as well as, the arms.

artery, sublingual, *n* an arterial branch from the lingual artery that supplies the sublingual salivary glands, floor of the mouth, and mylohyoid muscles.

artery, submental, *n* an arterial branch from the facial artery that supplies the submandibular lymph nodes, submandibular salivary glands, and mylohyoid and digastric muscles.

artery, superficial, *n* the terminal arterial branch from the external carotid artery that arises in the parotid salivary gland and gives off the transverse facial and middle temporal arteries, as well as, frontal and parietal branches.

artery, superior labial, *n* an arterial branch from the facial artery that supplies the upper lip tissues.

artery, superior thyroid, *n* an anterior arterial branch from the external carotid artery that supplies the tissues inferior to the hyoid bone, including the thyroid gland.

artery, transverse facial, *n* an arterial branch from the superficial temporal artery that supplies the parotid salivary gland.

arthralgia (ärthral′jēə), *n* pain in a joint or joints.

arthritis (ärthrī′tis), *n* any of a number of types of inflammation of a joint or joints.

arthritis, allergic, *n* an arthralgia, swelling, and stiffness of joints associated with food and drug allergies and serum sickness.

arthritis, atrophic, *n* See arthritis, rheumatoid.

arthritis, bacterial, *n* See arthritis, infective.

arthritis, hypertrophic (hī′per trō′fik), *n* See osteoarthritis.

arthritis, infective, *n* (bacterial arthritis), a primary and secondary bacterial infection of the joints (e.g., by staphylococcal, gonococcal, streptococcal, or pneumococcal organisms).

arthritis, juvenile idiopathic (rheumatoid), *n* a form of rheumatoid arthritis, usually affecting the larger joints of children less than 16 years of age and often accompanied by systemic manifestations. Because bone growth in children is dependent on the epiphyseal plates of the distal epiphyses, skeletal development may be impaired if these structures are damaged.

arthritis, rheumatic (rōōmat′ik), *n* an acute polyarticular and migratory arthritis of unknown cause but assumed to be related to group A streptococcal infection of the upper respiratory tract.

arthritis, rheumatoid (rōō′mətoid), *n* a chronic destructive inflammation of the joints caused by an autoimmunity with unknown etiology, with associated systemic manifestations such as weakness, weight loss, anemia, leukopenia, splenomegaly, lymphadenopathy, and the formation of subcutaneous nodules. Chronic synovitis and regressive changes in the articular cartilage occur with pain, swelling, deformity, limitation of motion, and occasionally ankylosis of the joints. Small joints are principally affected, with onset in the third or fourth decade of life.

arthritis, senile, *n* an arthritis occurring in persons of advanced age.

arthritis, specific infectious, *n* an arthritis caused by direct invasion and subsequent infection of joint structures by microorganisms from the bloodstream. Nearly all pathogenic bacteria have been isolated as etiologic agents.

arthritis, traumatic, *n* an acute or chronic inflammation of a joint as a result of acute or chronic injury.

Arthrobacter, *n* a genus of a strictly aerobic gram-positive bacteria found in soil and present in dental caries.

arthroplasty (är′thrəplas′tē), *n* the surgical correction of a joint abnormality.

arthroplasty, gap, *n* See gap arthroplasty.

arthroplasty, interposition, *n* See interposition arthroplasty.

arthroscope (ar′thrōskōp′), *n* an instrument used to view the inside of a joint.

arthrostomy (ärthros′təmē), *n* the surgical formation of an opening into a joint.

articaine (ar′tikān′), *n* a local anesthetic drug of the amide group that is used to anesthetize the treatment site during a dental procedure. It is the only amide local anesthetic drug that has an extra ester linkage, which causes the drug to be 95% hydrolyzed in the plasma and only 5% metabolized in the liver.

articular cartilage, *n* See cartilage, articular.

articular eminence (artik′yələr em′ənəns), *n* a raised area located on the articulated surface of the temporal bone; in conjunction with the condyle of the mandible it allows for the opening and closing of the jaw.

articular fossa, *n* See fossa, articular.

articulare (artik′yəlār′), *n* the point of intersection of the dorsal contour of the mandibular condyle and the temporal bone.

articulate (ärtik′yōōlāt), *v* **1.** to arrange or place in connected sequence. See also arrangement, tooth. *v* **2.** to connect by articulating strips, paper, or cloth coated with ink-containing or dye-containing wax, used for marking or locating occlusal contacts.

articulating paper, *n* a paper treated with brightly colored material, such as dye or wax, that marks the points of contact made by the teeth when a patient bites or grinds on it.

articulating surface of the condyle, *n* the head of mandibular condyle involved in the temporomandibular joint.

articulation (ärtik′yōōlā′shən), *n* **1.** a joint where the bones are joined together. See also joint. *n* **2.** the relationship of cusps of teeth during the jaw movement.

articulation, anatomic, n a rigid or movable junction of a bony part.

articulation, articulator, n the use of a device that incorporates artificial temporomandibular joints that permit the orientation of casts in a manner duplicating or simulating various positions or movements of the mandible.

articulation, balanced, n the simultaneous contacting of the maxillary and mandibular teeth as they glide over each other when the mandible is moved from centric relation to the various eccentric relations. See also occlusion, balanced.

articulation, mandibular, n See articulation, temporomandibular.

articulation, temporomandibular **(tem′pərōmandib′yələr),** *n* (temporomandibular joint, mandibular joint), **1.** the joint formed by the two condyles of the mandible. *n* **2.** the bilateral articulation between the glenoid or mandibular fossae of the temporal bones and condyles (condyloid processes) of the mandible.

articulation, temporomandibular, capsule, n the ligamentous covering of the temporomandibular joint.

articulation, temporomandibular, collagen disease, n a rheumatoid arthritis in which the joint may be so involved because of bone changes that the mandibular condyle is fused to the articular fossa in the base of the cranium.

articulation, temporomandibular, hormonal disturbances, n.pl hormonal disorders that frequently affect growth patterns of the skeleton, involving the temporomandibular joint (e.g., acromegaly).

articulation, temporomandibular, neuromuscular disorders, n.pl neuromuscular disorders involving the temporomandibular joint in which the patient is unable to maintain appropriate patterns of mandibular closure consistent with good dental occlusion. The natural teeth degenerate rapidly and are frequently lost prematurely; when dentures are substituted, they cause the residual tissues to deteriorate rapidly. In addition to the chronic masticatory disability, the deglutitive mechanism functions poorly because of incoordinated lip and tongue action.

articulation, temporomandibular, pain-dysfunction syndrome, n See temporomandibular joint disorder.

articulator, adjustable (ärti k′yōōlātur), *n* an articulator that may be adjusted to permit movement of the casts into various recorded eccentric relationships.

articulator, fully-adjustable, n a design in which all nine elements of the articulator can be programmed from patient records.

articulator, semi-adjustable, n design in which some, but not all, anterior incisal and posterior condylar controls can be modified.

articulator, Arcon, *n.pr* a type of articulator where the condylar controls are on the upper member as opposed to the lower member of earlier designs. This design allows for casts to have the same condylar controls when remounted.

articulator, crescent, *n* a device used in creating dental prostheses and evaluating casts. It represents the temporomandibular joints and simulates jaw movement.

articulator, disposable, n a simple plastic hinge that is bonded to dental models.

articulator, plasterless, n a design that uses adjustable clamps to hold two dental models and a universal ball joint and shaft to relate the clamps.

artifact (är′təfakt), *n* a blemish or foreign substance in the radiographic image that is not present in the actual image of the object.

artificial intelligence (AI), *n* a system that makes it possible for a machine to perform functions similar to human intelligence. Computer technology produces many systems and functions that mimic and surpass some human capabilities, such as the ability to play chess.

artificial organs, *n.pl* the devices used to support life because of the failure or limited capacity of the human organ. The most effective is the artificial kidney, which consists of a set of tubes that pass the blood through a dialysate solution where wastes are removed by osmosis and diffusion. See also hemodialysis.

artificial respiration, *n* See respiration, artificial.

artificial stone, *n* See stone, artificial.

arytenoepiglottic (er′ətē′nōep′iglo t′ik), *adj* pertaining to the arytenoid cartilage and the epiglottis.

ASA classification, *n* See health, ASA classification.

asbestos (asbes′təs), *n* a group of fibrous impure magnesium silicate minerals. Inhalation of the fibers can lead to pulmonary fibrosis.

◯ *Ascaris* **(as′kəris),** *n* a genus of large parasitic intestinal roundworms such as *A. lumbricoides*.

Aschheim-Zondek (AZ) test (ash′hīm tson′dek), *n* See test, pregnancy.

ascites (əsī′tēz), *n* an abnormal accumulation of serous fluid, containing large amounts of protein and electrolytes, in the peritoneal cavity. Ascites is a complication of cirrhosis, congestive heart failure, nephrosis, malignant neoplastic disease, and various fungal and parasitic diseases.

ascorbic acid (vitamin C), *n* generic; many brand names; *drug class:* vitamin C, water-soluble vitamin; *actions:* needed for wound healing, collagen synthesis, antioxidant, carbohydrate metabolism; *uses:* vitamin C deficiency, scurvy, delayed wound and bone healing, chronic disease, urine acidification, before gastrectomy.

asepsis (əsep′sis), *n* the condition of being without infection; of being free of viable pathogenic microorganisms.

asepsis, chain of, n a series of tasks, each step of which is performed in a bacteria-free environment, which serves to maintain the sterility of the entire process.

aseptic (əsep′tik), *adj* not producing microorganisms or free from microorganisms.

asialia (əsēā′lēə), *n* See asialorrhea.

asialorrhea (əsī′əlōrē′ə), *n* (asialia), a decrease in or lack of salivary flow. See also hyposalivation.

asparaginase (L-asparaginase), *n* *brand names:* Elspar, Oncaspar; *drug class:* antineoplastic; *action:* catalyzes the metabolism of L-asparagine resulting in inhibition of protein synthesis in lymphocytes; *use:* acute lymphocytic leukemia.

asparagine, *n* a nonessential amino acid found in many proteins in the body.

aspartame (as′pərtām), *n,* a low-calorie sweetening agent about 200 times as sweet as sucrose. Brand name: *NutriSweet.*

aspect, buccal (buk′əl), *n* the facial surface or cheek side of posterior teeth.

◯ **aspergillosis (asp′pərjəlōsis),** *n* an infection caused by a fungus of the genus *Aspergillus.* Most commonly affects the lungs and sinuses but is capable of causing inflammatory, granulomatous lesions on or in any organ.

Aspergillus, n a genus of fungi that is a common contaminant in the laboratory and a cause of nosocomial infection. See also aspergillosis.

asphyxia (asfik′sēə), *n* a condition of suffocation resulting from restriction of oxygen intake and interference with the elimination of carbon dioxide.

aspirate (as'pirāt), *v* **1.** to draw or breathe in. *v* **2.** to remove materials by vacuum. *n* **3.** a phonetic unit whose identifying characteristic is the sound generated by the passage of air through a relatively open channel; the sound of *h;* a sound followed by or combined with the sound of *h.*

aspirated materials, managing, *n* steps taken to keep a patient from ingesting tools or materials during treatment, (e.g., a rubber dam). See also risk management.

aspiration (as'pirā'shən), *n* **1.** the act of breathing or drawing in. *n* **2.** the removal of fluids, gases, or solids from a cavity by means of a vacuum pump.

aspiration biopsy, n See aspiration, fine needle (FNA).

aspiration, fine needle (FNA), n the procedure of obtaining a biopsy specimen by aspiration through a needle; used for diagnosing bone or deep soft tissue lesions. Also known as a *needle biopsy.*

aspiration pneumonia, n pneumonia produced by aspiration of foreign material into the lungs.

aspiration test, n the procedure used during local anesthetic injections by applying negative pressure on the anesthetic syringe prior to the deposition of the anesthetic to determine if the tip of the needle rests within a blood vessel, observed by absence or entry of blood into the cartridge.

aspirator (as'pərātur), *n* a device used for removal of fluids, gases, or solids from a cavity by vacuum.

aspirin, *n brand names:* ASA, Aspirin, Ecotrin; *drug class:* nonnarcotic analgesic salicylate; *actions:* inhibits prostaglandin synthesis, possesses analgesic, antiinflammatory, antipyretic and antiplatelet properties; *uses:* mild to moderate pain or fever, in low dose to reduce platelet aggregation. It was the first discovered member of the class of drugs known as nonsteroidal antiinflammatory drugs (NSAIDs), not all of which are salicylates, although they all have similar effects and a similar action mechanism. Its primary undesirable side effects, especially in stronger doses, are gastrointestinal distress (including ulcers and stomach bleeding) and tinnitus. Another side effect, caused by its anticoagulant properties, is increased bleeding.

aspirin burn, n See burn, aspirin.

assault, *n* an intentional, unlawful offer of bodily injury to another by force or unlawfully directing force toward another person to create a reasonable fear of imminent danger, coupled with the apparent ability to do the harm threatened if not prevented. A completed assault is a battery. In a medical setting, the unconsented touching of the body would be an assault and battery.

assessment, *n* the qualified opinion of a healthcare provider, informed by patient feedback and examination results, with regard to a specific health issue, whether critical, pending, or routine.

assessment, extraoral, n a preliminary examination of the head, neck, and face, usually made in conjunction with an intraoral examination, to recognize anomalies that might impact the patient's health; may require observation, listening, touch, and smell.

assessment, risk, n process of evaluating a potential hazard, likelihood of suffering, or any adverse effects.

assessment stroke, n the light movement of an instrument against a tooth to detect calculus, caries, overhangs, or other surface irregularities; the movement of a probe to determine pocket depth. Also called *exploratory stroke.*

assets, *n.pl* everything a business owns or that is owned. Cash, investments, money due, materials, and inventories are current assets. Buildings and equipment are fixed assets.

assignment of benefits, *n* a procedure whereby a beneficiary or patient authorizes the administrator of the program to forward payment for a covered procedure directly to the treating dental professional.

assistant, *n* an agent or employee.

assistant, dental, n an auxiliary to the dental operator. See also certified dental assistant.

assistant's stool, n an adjustable chair with additional base support and footrest used to maintain the comfort of the individual assisting the clinician during an examination.

association, *n* a connection, union, joining, or combination of things.

asthenia (asthē'nēə), *n* the loss of vitality or strength; a condition of debility; weakness.

asthenic (asthēn'ik), *adj* describing an individual with a long, slender appearance who is thin and flat-chested and has long limbs and a short trunk; comparable to the ectomorph in Sheldon's classification.

asthma (az'mə), *n* a condition characterized by paroxysmal wheezing or coughing and difficulty in breathing resulting from bronchospasms. Frequently has an allergic basis and occasionally an emotional origin. See also status asthmaticus.

asthma, cardiac, *n* a condition characterized by shortness of breath (paroxysmal dyspnea), sonorous rales, and expiratory wheezes that resemble bronchial asthma; related to cardiac failure.

astigmatism (əstig'mətizəm), *n* a defective curvature of the refractive surfaces of the eye, resulting in a condition in which a ray of light is not focused sharply on the retina but is spread over a more or less diffuse area.

astringent (əstrin'jənt), *n* styptic; an agent that checks the secretions of mucous membranes and contracts and hardens tissues, limiting the secretions of glands.

astrocytes (as'trōsī'ts), *n* a large, star-shaped cell found in certain tissues of the nervous system. A mass of astrocytes is called astroglia. See also astrocytoma.

astrocytoma (as'trōsītō'mə), *n* a primary tumor of the brain composed of astrocytes and characterized by slow growth, cyst formation, invasion of surrounding structures, and often, the development of a highly malignant glioblastoma within the primary tumor mass.

asymmetric (āsimet'rik), *adj* unevenly arranged; out of balance; not the same on both sides; not a mirror image on both sides.

asymmetry, *n* an inharmonious relationship between the maxillary and mandibular teeth during closure or functional jaw movements or facial features.

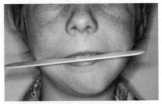

Facial asymmetry. (Proffit/Fields/Sarver, 2013)

asymptomatic, *n* the absence of any evidence or symptoms of illness or condition.

asymptomatic carrier, *n* an individual who serves as host for an infectious agent but who does not show any apparent signs of the illness; may serve as a source of infection for others.

asynergy (āsin'urjē), *n* a lack of muscular coordination in special functions (e.g., hand-to-oral cavity movements for feeding).

asystole (āsis'təlē), *n* the faulty contraction of the ventricles of the heart, resulting in incomplete or imperfect systole.

ataxia (ātak'sēə), *n* a muscular incoordination characterized by irregular muscle activity.

ataxia, locomotor, *n* See tabes dorsalis.

atelectasis (at'ilek'təsis), *n* the complete or partial collapse of a lung.

atenolol (əten'əlōl), *n brand names:* Nova-Atenol, Tenormin; *drug class:* antihypertensive, selective β₁ adrenergic receptor blocker; *action:* produces fall in blood pressure and a reduction in heart rate; *uses:* acute myocardial infarction, mild to moderate hypertension, prophylaxis of angina pectoris, certain arrhythmias.

atheroma (ath'ərō'mə), *n* a fatty, fibrous deposit developing on the artery lining. Also called *atheromatous plaque.*

atherosclerosis (ath'ərōsklərō'sis), *n* a degenerative disease principally affecting the aorta and its major branches, the coronary artery, and the larger cerebral arteries. The arterial changes include narrowing of the lumen of the vessels; weakening of the arterioles, leading to rupture; an increased tendency toward development of atheromatous plaques; and

A

thrombi. Atherosclerosis is a common cause of myocardial infarctions and cerebrovascular accident.

athetosis (ath′ətō′sis), *n* a neuromuscular impairment in which extensive twisting and swaying spasms of the skeletal musculature interfere with voluntary control of movement; the spasms are especially conspicuous and disconcerting during emotional stress and on initiation of conscious voluntary acts.

athiaminosis (əthī′əminō′sis), *n* a deficiency of thiamine. See also beriberi.

athletic (athlet′ik), *adj* pertaining to a bodily constitution characterized by a strong, muscular, robust appearance.

athletic injuries, n.pl injuries sustained by persons while engaged in sports, more frequently while engaged in contact sports such as football.

atlantooccipital joint (atlan′ toksip′itl), *n* condyloid joint formed by the articulation of the atlas of the vertebral column with the occipital bone of the skull.

◻ atlas, *n* the first cervical vertebra articulating superiorly with the occipital bone and inferiorly with the axis (second cervical vertebra).

atmosphere (atm), *n* the natural body of air, composed of approximately 20% oxygen, 78% nitrogen, and 2% carbon dioxide and other gases.

atom (at′əm), *n* the smallest part of an element capable of entering into a chemical reaction.

atomic (ətom′ik), *adj* pertaining to the atom.

atomic energy, n See energy, atomic.

atomic mass number, n (symbol: A), the total number of nucleons (protons and neutrons) of which an atom is composed.

atomic number (Z), n **1.** the number of electrons outside the nucleus of a neutral atom. *n* **2.** the number of protons in the nucleus.

atomic structure theory, n the theory that matter is composed of a vast number of particles, or atoms, bound together by a force of attraction of electrical charges.

atomic weight, n the weight of one atom of an element as compared with the weight of an atom of hydrogen.

atomizer (at′əmīzur), *n* a device for changing a jet of liquid into a spray.

atonia, in cerebral palsy (ātō′nēə), *n* an inability to stand or lift the head and diminished capacity to speak or swallow caused by weak muscular tone.

atonic, *adj* lacking rigidity or regular tone.

atopy (ā′tōpē), *n* (atopic hypersensitivity, "spontaneous" clinical allergy), a group of "allergic" disorders showing a marked familial distribution; although the susceptibility appears to be inherited, contact with the antigen must occur before hypersensitivity can develop. Disorders include asthma or hay fever resulting from pollens and gastrointestinal tract and skin reactions resulting from food.

atovaquone (ətō′vəkōn′), *n brand name:* Mepron; *drug class:* antipneumocystic; *action:* unknown, may inhibit synthesis of ATP and nucleic acids; *use:* treatment of *Pneumocystis jiroveci (carinii)* pneumonia in patients who are intolerant of trimethoprim-sulfamethoxazole.

atracurium, *n brand name:* Tracrium; *drug class:* competitive nondepolarizing peripheral neuromuscular blocker; *action:* competes with acetylcholine at nicotinic receptors located at the skeletal neuromuscular junction, causes muscle paralysis; *use:* muscle relaxation during general anesthesia.

atraumatic restorative treatment (ART), *n* the removal of dental caries with only hand instruments and restoring the tooth by filling the resulting cavity with an adhesive restorative material.

atresia (ətrē′zēə), *n* the congenital absence or occlusion of a normal opening of one or more ducts in an organ.

atresia, aural, n the absence of closure of the auditory canal.

atrial fibrillation, *n* a heart condition characterized by rapid and irregular contractions of the atria.

atrophy (at′rōfē), *n/v* a progressive, acquired decrease in the size of a normally developed cell, tissue, or organ. Atrophy may result from a decrease in cell size, number of cells, or both.

atrophy, adipose (ad′əpōz), n an atrophy resulting from a reduction in fatty tissue.

atrophy, alveolar, n a depletion of the size of the alveolar process of the jaws from disuse, overuse, or pathologic disturbance of the bone.

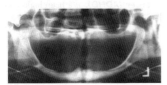

Alveolar atrophy. (White/Pharoah, 2009)

atrophy, bone, *n* **1.** the bone resorption internally (in density) and externally (in form) (e.g., of residual ridges). *n* **2.** a loss of bone substance or volume. Atrophy of bone ordinarily occurs without a corresponding change in the volume or external dimensions of bone, but the mass of bone tissue may be reduced by as much as 75%. The internal architecture of the bone gradually becomes attenuated and finally disappears. Atrophied bone is brittle and has a more spongy consistency than normal bone. In cross-section the cortex is thin, and the periosteal surface is smooth and unchanged, but the intramedullary substance is composed of a yellow, fatty, cancellous bone tissue. Bone atrophy may be systemic, regional, or local.

atrophy, central papillary, *n* a lesion on the central dorsum of the tongue, possibly caused by a fungal infection, not a developmental disorder; it may be raised or flat. Formerly called *median rhomboid glossitis.*

atrophy, diffuse alveolar, *n* See periodontosis.

atrophy, facial, *n* the failure of facial development. If it is bilateral, it may produce brachygnathia; unilateral types, although rare, are more common than the bilateral type. Causes include physical injury, neurovascular disease, and paralysis.

atrophy, gerodontic mucosal (jerōdon′tik myōōkō′səl), *n* an oral degeneration in which the tissue of the epithelium in the oral cavity thins and loses some of its vascular structure and elasticity.

atrophy, muscular, *n* a wasting of muscle tissue, especially resulting from lack of use. There are numerous causes for simple atrophy of muscle,

such as chronic malnutrition, immobilization, and denervation.

atrophy, of disuse, *n* an atrophy resulting from a lack of function of a tissue, organ, or body part.

atrophy, periodontal, *n* the quantitative degenerative changes that occur in the periodontium of a tooth as a result of disease or disuse. When a tooth loses its antagonist, osteoporotic changes in the supporting bone, an afunctional change in the direction of periodontal fibers, and a narrowing of the periodontal ligament.

atrophy, postmenopausal, *n* a thinning of the oral mucosa after menopause.

atrophy, pressure, *n* the tissue destruction and reduction in size as a consequence of prolonged or continued pressure on a local area or group of cells.

atrophy, pressure, by epithelial attachment, *n* a theoretical type of atrophy. The theory, advanced to explain destruction of gingival fibers during gingival inflammation, states that gingival fiber degeneration is produced by pressure exerted by the proliferating pocket epithelium. It is now generally conceded that proteolytic substances produced in the tissues during inflammation are responsible for gingival fiber destruction; subsequently, the epithelium can proliferate apically.

atrophy, senile, *n* the atrophy or diminution of all tissues characteristic of advanced age.

atropine (at′rōpēn), *n* an alkaloid that inhibits muscarinic cholinergic receptors antagonizing the effects of nerve stimulation that leads to muscarinc receptor stimulation and inhibiting the effects of muscarinc receptor agonists such as pilocarpine. Atropine acts directly on the effector cells, preventing the action but not the liberation of acetylcholine. It suppresses sweat in addition to parasympathetic nerve stimulation.

atropine sulfate, *n brand name:* Sal-Tropine; *drug class:* anticholinergic; *action:* inhibits muscarinic actions of acetylcholine at postganglionic cholinergic neuroeffector sites; *use:* reduction of salivary and bronchial secretions.

attached gingiva, *n* See gingiva, attached.

attachment, *n* **1.** a fastener, connector, associated part. *n* **2.** a mechanical device for retention and stabilization of a dental prosthesis.

attachment, abnormal frenum **(frē'nəm),** *n* the insertions of labial, buccal, or lingual frena capable of initiating or continuing periodontal disease, such as creating diastemata between teeth, limiting lip or tongue movement.

attachment, epithelial (EA), *n* the epithelial-derived tissue device that connects the junctional epithelium to the tooth surface.

attachment, gingival, *n* the fibrous attachment of the gingival tissues to the teeth.

attachment, intracoronal, *n* (precision attachment, slotted attachment). See retainer, intracoronal.

attachment level, clinical (CAL), *n* the amount of space between attached periodontal tissues and a fixed point, usually the cementoenamel junction. A measurement used to assess the stability of attachment as part of a periodontal maintenance program.

attachment loss, *n* See loss of attachment (LOA).

attachment, migration of epithelial, *n* the apical progression of the epithelial attachment along the tooth root.

attachment, orthodontic, *n* a device, secured to the crown of a tooth, that serves as a means of attaching the arch wire to the tooth.

attachment, parallel, *n* a prefabricated device for attaching a denture base to an abutment tooth. Retention is provided by friction between the parallel walls of the two parts of the attachment.

attachment, precision, *n* See retainer, intracoronal.

attachment, slotted, *n* See retainer, intracoronal.

attack, heart, *n* See myocardial infarction.

attending dental professional's statement, *n* a form used to report dental procedures to a third-party payer. The claim form was developed by the American Dental Association. Also called *dental claim form.*

attention, *n* the element of cognitive functioning in which the mental focus is maintained on a specific issue, object, or activity. The length of time of such focus is called *attention span.*

attention deficit hyperactivity disorder (ADHD), *n* a neurologic disorder that manifests itself as excessive movement, irritability, immaturity, and an inability to concentrate or control impulses. It affects learning and skill acquisition.

attenuation (əten'yōōā'shən), *n* **1.** to make thinner, weaker, or less virulent. *n* **2.** the process by which a beam of radiation is reduced in energy when passing through certain types of material.

attrition (ətrish'ən), *n* the normal loss of tooth substance resulting from friction caused by physiologic forces.

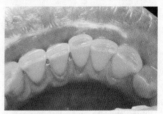

Attrition. (Ibsen/Phelan, 2009)

attritional occlusion (ətrish'ənəl əklōō'zhən), *n* See occlusion, attritional.

atypical (ātip'ikəl), *adj* pertaining to deviation from the basic or typical.

Au, *n* See unit, angstrom.

audioanalgesia, *n* the use of music, white noise, or other sounds to decrease the perception of pain. It is commonly used during dental work.

audiogram (ô'dēəgram), *n* a graphic summary of the measurement of hearing loss showing the number of decibels lost at each frequency tested.

audiologist, *n* individual trained to identify, diagnose, measure, and rehabilitate hearing impairments.

audiology (ô'dēol'əjē), *n* the study of the entire field of hearing, including the anatomy and function of the ear; impairment of hearing; and evaluation, education or reeducation, and treatment of persons with hearing loss.

audiometer (ôdēom'ətər), *n* a device for testing hearing; calibrated to register hearing loss in terms of decibels.

audit, *n* **1.** an examination of records or accounts to check accuracy. *n* **2.** a posttreatment record review or clinical examination to verify information reported on claims.

audit trail, *n* security-relevant chronological record, set of records, or destination and source of records that provide documentary evidence of the sequence of activities that have affected at any time a specific operation, procedure, or event.

audit of treatment, *n* **1.** an administrative or professional review of a participating dental professional's treatment recommendations (peer audit). *n* **2.** the review of reimbursement claims for service performed (postaudit).

auditory stimuli, *n.pl* in dentistry, the irregularities or deposits on the surface of a tooth that may be detected by ear of both patient and clinician during examination and probing. As an example, the movement of an instrument across clean enamel makes no sound, while calculus and metallic restorations are noisy when scraped.

augmentation (ôg′mentā′shən), *n* **1.** assistance to respiration by the application of intermittent pressure on inspiration. *n* **2.** an increase in size beyond the existing size, such as an implant placed over the mandibular or maxillary ridges.

aura, *n* the brief period of heightened sensory activity that immediately precedes the onset of a seizure. It may be characterized by numbness, nausea, or unusual sensitivity to light, odor, or sound.

aural (ôr′əl), *adj* relating to the ear.

auranofin (ôran′əfin), *n brand name:* Ridaura; *drug class:* gold salt; *action:* specific antiinflammatory action unknown; *uses:* rheumatoid arthritis.

Aureomycin (ô′rēōmī′sin), *n* the brand name for chlortetracycline.

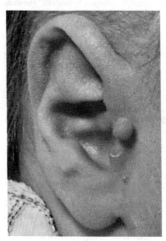

auricle (ô′rikəl), *n* **1.** the oval flap of the external part of the ear. *n* **2.** atrium, the chamber of the heart that receives the blood: on the right, from the general circulation, and on the left, from the pulmonary circulation.

auricular fibrillation (ôrik′yələr fib′rilā′shən), *n* See fibrillation, auricular.

auricular tags, *n* the rudimentary appendages of auricular tissue on the face along the line of union of the first branchial arch.

Auricular tags. (Zitelli/McIntire/Nowak, 2012)

auriculotemporal syndrome (ôrik′ yəlōtem′pərəl), *n* See syndrome, Frey.

aurothioglucose/gold sodium thiomalate (ôr′othī′ōglōō′kōs thī′ōmal′āt), *n brand name:* Solganal/ Myochrysine; *drug class:* antiinflammatory gold compound; *action:* unknown; may decrease phagocytosis, lysosomal activity, prostaglandin synthesis; *uses:* rheumatoid arthritis; juvenile arthritis.

auscultation (ôskultā′shən), *n* the examination procedure of listening for sounds produced by the body to detect or judge an abnormal condition.

auscultatory gap (ôskul′tətôrē), *n* a pause that occurs during the auscultatory method of measuring blood pressure. Noted as the silent period that is present when the sound of systolic pressure diminishes and returns at a lower pressure point. Many errors in recording low blood pressure are attributed to the auscultatory gap.

authorization, *n* a written consent to release protected health information.

autism, *n* a developmental disorder usually appearing in children before the age of 3 that is characterized by communication, behavioral, and sensory impairments, including the inability to interact with others in a socially acceptable manner. The condition may require a special approach when working with the patient as well as when instructing in oral care.

autoantibody, *n* an immunoglobulin produced by the immune system that is directed against one or more of the host's own proteins. Many autoimmune diseases in humans, most notably lupus erythematosus, are caused by such antibodies.

autoclave (ô'tōklāv), *n* a device for effecting sterilization by steam under pressure. It uses steam heated to 121° C (250° F), at 103 kPa (15 psi) above atmospheric pressure, for 15 minutes. The steam and pressure transfer sufficient heat into organisms to kill them.

autocure, *v* hardened or set by a chemical reaction of two materials.

autogenous (ôtoj'ənəs), *adj* self-originated; springing from within.

autogenous bone graft, *n* See graft, autogenous bone.

autograft, *n* See graft, autogenous.

autograft, free gingival, *n* a procedure in which a graft is attached to an exposed area of a tooth's root. The graft is normally obtained from the palate of the oral cavity.

autoimmune (ô'tōimyōōn'), *adj* the development of an immune response to one's own tissues.

autoimmune disease, n May also be called *autoimmune disorder.* See disease, autoimmune, and autoantibody.

autologous (ôtol'əgəs), *adj* in biology, refers to tissues, cells, or proteins that are transplanted from one part of a patient's body to another. In dentistry, autologous bone grafts are used in the reconstruction of the mandible and the reconstruction of alveolar defects prior to dental implants.

automatic condenser, *n* See condenser, mechanical.

automatic mallet, *n* See condenser, mechanical.

automatic processor, *n* a device that automates all film processing steps. It requires less processing time, equipment and space and time and temperatures are automatically controlled.

automation, *n* the use of a machine designed to follow repeatedly and automatically a predetermined sequence of individual operations. Automation is used extensively in preparing tissue for microscopic examination.

automatism (ôtom'ətiz'əm), *n* a tendency to take extra or superfluous doses of a drug when under its influence.

automatrix, *n* a system designed to establish a temporary wall for tooth restoration without the use of a retainer.

autonomic, *n* See autonomic nervous system.

autonomic drugs, n agents that act on the autonomic nervous system.

autonomic dysreflexia/hyperreflexia (ôtənom'ik disrēflek'sēə hī'per rəflek'sēə), n an emergent, typically life-threatening, medical condition resulting from a dramatic increase in blood pressure occurring in individuals with traumatic lesions at or above T6. Symptoms may include a throbbing headache, blushing, chills, sweating, stuffy nose, and fidgetiness.

autonomic nervous system (ANS), n a subdivision of the efferent peripheral nervous system that regulates involuntary vital function, including the activity of the cardiac muscle, the smooth muscle, and the glands. Has two parts: the sympathetic nervous system, which accelerates heart rate, constricts blood vessels, and raises blood pressure; and the parasympathetic nervous system, which slows heart rate, increases intestinal peristalsis and gland activity, and relaxes sphincters. See also peripheral nervous system.

autonomic nervous system, fibers of, in pulp, n.pl the nerve fibers of the sympathetic autonomic system that enter the pulp tissue and function in regulating blood flow.

autonomic symptoms, n the indications of pathology of or trauma to the autonomic nervous system, including paleness, sweating, blushing, dilation of pupils, irregular cardiac rhythm, and lack of bladder control.

autopolymer (ô'tōpol'imur), *n* a resin to which certain chemicals have been added to initiate and propagate polymerization without addition of heat.

autopolymer resin, n See resin, autopolymer.

autopolymerization (ô'tō pol'imərizā'shən), *n* (cold-curing), the accomplishment of polymerization by chemical means without external application of heat or light.

autoprothrombin I (ô'tōprōthrom'bin), *n* See factor VII.

autoprothrombin II, *n* See factor IX.

autopsy, *n* a postmortem examination performed to confirm or determine the cause of death.

autoradiography (ô'tōrādēog'rə fē), *n* **1.** a photographic recording of radiation from radioactive material, obtained by placing the surface of the radioactive material in close proximity to a photographic emulsion. *n* **2.** the use of radioactive substances introduced into tissue followed by the placement of a photographic plate on the surface of the tissue preparation, usually employed in cytology and histology.

autosomal dominant disorders (ôtəsō'məl), *n.pl* the genetic disorders that are transmitted by a dominant gene within an autosomal chromosome as opposed to a sex chromosome.

autosomal recessive disorders, *n. pl* the genetic disorders carried by a recessive gene within an autosomal chromosome as opposed to a sex chromosome.

autotransformer, *n* a transformer with a single winding, having a large number of connections, or taps. Used to deliver a precise voltage to the high-tension primary circuit.

autotransplant, *n* See graft, autogenous.

auxiliary (ôksil'yərē), *adj* supporting or assisting; supplementary; secondary.

auxiliary personnel, n.pl a group of dental professionals that work in a dental office or clinic with a dentist includes dental hygienists who are formally trained and may be licensed or certified by state authorities. It also includes dental assistants, laboratory technicians, and other auxiliaries, who may or may not be formally trained, certified, or licensed.

auxiliary wires, n.pl the orthodontic wires that support or augment the action of the main or primary arch wire in an orthodontic appliance. The Begg technique and the segmental

technique make frequent and regular use of auxiliary wires.

AV, *n* **1.** the abbreviation for *atrioventricular. n* **2.** the abbreviation for *auriculoventricular.*

average life (mean life), *n* the average of the individual lives of all of the atoms of a particular radioactive substance; 1.443 times radioactive half-life. See also half-life.

avidin (av'idin), *n* a glycoprotein in nondenatured egg whites (raw) that binds biotin and prevents its absorption, causing biotin depletion.

avitaminosis (āvī'təminō'sis), *n* a disease or condition resulting from a deficiency of one or more vitamins in the diet (e.g., scurvy, resulting from ascorbic acid deficiency and beriberi, resulting from a thiamine deficiency).

avitaminosis, fat-soluble, n a disease resulting from deficiency of the fat-soluble vitamins (i.e., A, D, E, and K).

avoidance behavior, *n* a conscious or unconscious defense mechanism by which a person tries to escape from unpleasant situations or feelings, such as anxiety and pain.

avoirdupois system (av'ərdəpioz'), *n* See system, avoirdupois.

avulse, *v* to tear off forcibly, as when a tooth is lost in an accident.

avulsed tooth, *n* See tooth, evulsed.

avulsion (əvul'shən), *n* the sudden tearing out, or away, of tissue as a result of a traumatic episode.

avulsion, nerve, n the operation of tearing a nerve from its central origin by traction.

avulsion, tooth, n the displacement of a tooth from its alveolar housing; may be partial or complete.

axial filaments (ak'sēəl), *n.pl* the means of mobility for the spirochete-type bacteria.

axial inclination, *n* See inclination, axial.

axial plane, *n* See plane, axial.

axial wall plane, *n* See plane, axial wall.

axilla, *n* a pyramid-shaped space forming the underside of the shoulder between the upper part of the arm and the side of the chest.

axiopulpal (ak'sēōpul'pəl), *adj* relating to the angle formed by the axial and pulpal walls of a prepared cavity.

axis (ak'sis), *n* **1.** a straight line around which a body may rotate. *n* **2.** the second cervical vertebra, which articulates with the first (atlas) and third cervical vertebrae.

axis, cephalometric, n See axis, Y.

axis, condylar, n an imaginary line through the two mandibular condyles around which the mandible may rotate during a part of the opening movement.

axis, condylar, determination, n the location of the condylar axis by fixing a face-bow rigidly to the mandibular teeth, having the patient open and close the jaws, and recording the most posterosuperior points of pure rotation with tattoo ink on the outer skin. See also face-bow and hinge-bow.

axis, condyle, n one of three axes of the jaw condyles: (1) the hinge axis, an intercondyle imaginary line across the face through both condyles; whenever either condyle is chosen to be a rotator, it will display (2) a vertical axis, and (3) a sagittal axis. The hinge axis is a moving center for the opening and closing movements. The vertical axis is the center for the horizontal components of orbital movements. The sagittal axis is the center for the vertical components of orbital movements.

axis, hinge, -orbital plane, n a craniofacial plane determined by three tattooed points. Two are located with one on each side of the face at the point of exit through the skin in front of the tragus of the imagined extended rearmost mandibular hinge axis. The third point is located on the right side of the nose at the level of the orbital rim just beneath the pupil when the patient is gazing directly forward. This plane corresponds to the anthropologic Frankfort plane.

axis, horizontal, n See axis, hinge.

axis, long, n an imaginary line passing longitudinally through the center of a body.

axis, mandibular, n See axis, condylar.

axis of preparation, n the path taken by a restoration as it slides on or off the preparation.

axis, opening, n See axis, condylar.

axis, orbital movements of, n.pl the movements projected on the axis-orbital plane in gathering the input data for an articulator.

axis, sagittal, n the imaginary line around which the working condyle rotates in the frontal plane during

lateral mandibular movement. The sagittal and vertical axes function concurrently.

axis shift, n the imprecise term used before the nine different directional-ized laterotrusions were discovered and named.

axis, vertical, n the imaginary line around which the working condyle rotates in the horizontal plane during lateral mandibular movement. The sagittal and vertical axes function concurrently.

axis, Y, n (cephalometric axis), the angle of a line connecting the sella turcica and the gnathion and related to a horizontal plane. An indicator of downward and forward growth of the mandible.

axon (ak′son), *n* an extension of a nerve cell body that conducts impulses away from the cell. Generally there is only one axon to a cell.

azatadine maleate (əzat′ədēn mā′lēāt), *n brand name:* Optimine; *drug class:* antihistamine; *action:* decreases allergic response by blocking histamine; *uses:* allergy symptoms, rhinitis, chronic urticaria, pruritus.

azathioprine (az′əthiōprēn), *n brand name:* Imuran; *drug class:* immunosuppressant; *action:* inhibits purine synthesis in cells, thereby preventing RNA and DNA synthesis; *uses:* renal transplants to prevent graft rejection, refractory rheumatoid arthritis, bone marrow transplants, glomerulonephritis.

azelaic acid (az′əla′ik), *n brand name:* Azelex; *drug class:* a naturally occurring straight-chain dicarboxylic acid; *action:* has antimicrobial activity against *P. acnes* and *S. epidermidis; use:* topical therapy of mild-to-moderate inflammatory acne vulgaris.

azelastine *n brand names:* Astelin, Azalex; *drug class:* topical antihistamine; *action:* blocks histamine H_1 receptors; *use:* treat nasal allergies.

azidothymidine *(AZT)* (əzid′ōthi′m ədēn), *n brand name:* Retrovir; *drug class:* antiviral thymidine analog; *action:* a drug used to inhibit the human immunodeficiency virus.

azithromycin (əzith′rōmī′sin), *n brand name:* Zithromax; *drug class:* macrolide antibiotic; *action:* binds to 50S ribosomal subunits of susceptible bacteria and suppresses protein synthesis, similar spectrum of activity to erythromycin; *uses:* infections of the upper and lower respiratory tract, uncomplicated skin infections, alternative antibiotic in prophylaxis related to a dental procedure.

AZT, *n* the abbreviation for *azidothymidine.* See also azidothymidine.

Azteonam, *n brand names:* Azactam, Cayston; *drug class:* monocyclic Beta-lactam antibiotic; *action:* inhibits cell wall synthesis; *uses:* abdominal, lower respiratory tract, urinary tact, septicemia, cause by a number of gram negative bacteria.

B point, *n* See point, B.

Babesia microti, *n.pl* the parasitic protozoan microbes from the Apicomplexa phylum, spread primarily by ticks. They are implicated in babesiosis, a disease with malaria-like manifestations.

babesiosis (bəbē′zē o′sis), *n* a disease caused by *B. microti* that is evidenced by malaria-like symptoms. Also called *babesiasis* or *piroplas mosis.*

baby bottle tooth decay, *n* a dental condition that occurs in children from 1 to 3 years of age as a result of being given a bottle at bedtime, resulting in prolonged exposure of the teeth to milk, formula, or juice with a high sugar content. Dental caries results from the breakdown of sugars to lactic acid and other decay-causing substances. Newer term is *early childhood caries.*

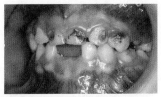

Baby bottle tooth decay. (Dean/Avery/McDonald, 2011)

bacampicillin HCl (bəkam′pəsil′in), *n brand names:* Penglobe, Spectrobid; *drug class:* an aminopenicillin that has an extended spectrum; *action:* interferes with cell-wall replication of suspectible organisms; *uses:* respiratory tract, skin, and urinary tract infections; effective for gram-positive cocci.

bacillary dysentery (bas′iler′ē), *n* a gastrointestinal tract infection contracted from food or water contaminated by infected individuals. Also called *shigellosis.* See also *Shigella.*

Bacillus (bəsil′əs), *n* a genus of gram-positive, spore-producing bacteria in the family Bacillaceae, order Eubacteriales.

B. anthracis, *n* causes anthrax. The spores of this organism, if inhaled, can cause a pulmonary form; the spores can live for many years in animal products such as hides and wool, as well as in the soil.

B. stearothermophilus (stēer′ōthur mof′əlus), *n* a type of biologic spore, the absence of which is tested for to verify proper sterilization of equipment in the dental environment; used with steam autoclave sterilizing or chemical vapor sterilizer methods.

bacitracin, topical, *n brand names:* Baciguent, Bacitin; *drug class:* local antiinfective produced by gram-positive, spore-forming organism of the *B. lichen formis* group; *action:* blocks bacterial cell-wall synthesis; *use:* topical for nonserious infections caused by staphylococci and streptococci.

back, *n* the posterior or dorsal portion of the trunk of the body between the neck and the pelvis. The skeletal portion of the back includes the thoracic and lumbar vertebrae and both scapulae. The nerves that innervate the muscles of the back include some branches of the dorsal primary divisions of the spinal nerves, the lateral branches of the dorsal primary division of the middle and lower cervical nerves, and some branches of the ventral primary division of the spinal nerves.

back pain, *n* a pain in the lumbar, lumbosacral, or cervical regions of the back, varying in sharpness and intensity. Causes may include muscle strain or pressure on the root of a nerve.

back-action clasp, *n* See clasp, back-action.

backing, *n* a metal support used to attach a facing to a prosthesis.

baclofen (bak′lōfen′), *n brand name:* Lioresal; *drug class:* central-acting skeletal muscle relaxant; *action:* stimulates GABA$_B$ receptors in the central nervous system; *uses:* treatment for skeletal muscle spasticity in multiple sclerosis and spinal cord injury, occasionaly for trigeminal neuralgia.

bacteremia (bak′tirē′mēə), *n* **1.** the presence of bacteria in the bloodstream. It may be transient, intermittent, or continuous. Transient bacteremia may result from dental procedures such as extraction and adult prophylaxis, or it may accompany the early phases of many infections. Continuous bacteremia is a feature of endocarditis. *n* **2.** the presence of bacteria in the blood (e.g., as occurs during adult prophylaxis of a patient with the risk of complications caused by bacteremia).

bacteria, *n.pl* **1.** small, unicellular microorganisms of the kingdom Monera. The genera vary morphologically, being spheric (cocci), rod-shaped (bacilli), spiral (spirochetes), or comma-shaped (vibrios). *n* **2.** the phylum in which these microorganisms are classified.

bacteria, aerobic, n.pl bacteria that require the presence of oxygen to live and grow.

bacteria, anaerobic, n.pl bacteria that can survive and grow without the presence of free oxygen in their immediate environment. See also anaerobe, facultative.

bacteria, chromogenic (krō′mə jen′ik), n a microorganism that reacts with the iron in saliva to create a stain on the surface of the teeth. The color of the stain is indicative of the color, or chroma, of the bacteria (e.g., a green stain is caused by bacteria such as *Penicillium* and *Aspergillus*).

bacteria, resident (oral), n.pl the microorganisms that are normally in the oral flora of an individual.

bacterial culture, *n* See culture, bacterial.

bacterial spore, *n* a bacteria that, because of its thick outer wall, is easily able to survive in hostile environments otherwise not conducive to bacterial growth and reproduction.

bacterial toxin, *n* any poisonous substance produced by a bacterium. Two general types are common: those formed within the cell (endotoxins) and those formed within the cell and excreted (exotoxins).

bactericidal *adj* the ability of a drug to kill bacteria.

bactericide (baktir′isīd), *n* a substance that kills bacteria. See also bacteriophage.

bacteriology, *n* the scientific study of bacteria.

bacteriolytic action (baktir′ēō lit′ik), *n* the breaking down of bacteria by an enzyme or other agent (e.g., by antibacterial factors in saliva).

bacteriophage, *n* any virus that causes lysis of host bacteria.

bacteriostatic (baktir′eōstat′ik), *adj* preventing bacteria from growing and multiplying but possibly not killing them.

Bacteroides (bak′təroi′dēz), *n* a genus of *Schizomycetes* with rod-shaped, highly pleomorphic, gram-negative, nonspore-forming obligate anaerobic bacteria.

B. endodontalis (en′dōdon′təlis), n a strain of *B. melaninogenicus* associated with pulpal infections.

B. forsythus (forsith′əs), n a recently identified strain found in periodontal pockets.

B. fragilis (frəjil′is), n the most common and virulent strain, normally found in the oral cavity, upper respiratory system, colon, and genital tract.

B. gingivalis (jin′jəval′is), n a strain of *B. melaninogenicus* associated with acute periodontitis.

B. intermedius, n a strain of *B. melaninogenicus* associated with acute necrotizing ulcerative gingivitis.

B. melaninogenicus (melaninō jenikəs), n a small, diplobacillus, also known as *B. melaninogenicum,* found in the oral cavity and pharynx; sometimes associated with periodontitis.

bad-faith insurance practices, *n.pl* **1.** the failure to deal with a beneficiary of a dental benefits plan fairly and in good faith. *n.pl* **2.** an activity that impairs the right of the beneficiary to receive the appropriate benefits of a dental benefits plan or receive them in a timely manner (e.g., evaluating claims based on standards significantly at variance with the standards of the community, failure to investigate a claim for benefits properly, and unreasonably and purposely delaying or withholding payment of a claim).

badge, film, *n* See film badge.

bailment, *n* the delivery of personal property by one person to another in trust for a specific purpose with an expressed or implied contract that after the purpose has been fulfilled the property shall be returned, duly accounted for, or kept until reclaimed.

balance, *n* **1.** equilibrium or harmony. *n* **2.** in dentistry, an occlusal equilibrium or facial esthetic harmony.

balance, acid-base, *n* in metabolism, the balance of acid to base necessary to keep the blood pH level normal (between 7.35 and 7.43).

balance billing, *n* the billing of a patient for the difference between the dental professional's actual charge and the amount reimbursed under the patient's dental benefits plan.

balance sheet, *n* a condensed statement showing the nature and amount of a company's assets, liabilities, and capital on a given date. In dollar amounts the balance sheet shows the assets the company owns, the money it owes, and the ownership interest in the company of its stockholders.

balanced articulation, *n* See occlusion, balanced.

balanced bite, See occlusion, balanced.

balanced occlusion, *n* See occlusion, balanced.

balancing contacts, *n.pl* the contacts of teeth on the side opposite the bolus side. See also contact, balancing.

balancing interference, *n* a situation in which teeth are in contact on the balancing side during lateral occlusion.

balancing occlusal surfaces, See surfaces, occlusal, balancing.

balancing side, *n* the side opposite the working side of the dentition or denture.

balloon payment, *n* a final payment larger than the preceding payments when a debt is not fully amortized.

balloon, sinus, *n* a hollow rubber structure expandable with liquid or air that is used to support depressed

fractures of the walls of the maxillary sinus.

BANA, *n.pr* an acronym for *benzol-arginine napthylamide.* See also benzol-arginine naphthylamide.

band, *n* **1.** a cord, tie, chain, or metal collar by which something is bound. *n* **2.** a contrasting strip or strip of material running through or along the edge of a material.

band adapter, *n* See adapter, band.

band, adjustable orthodontic, *n* a band provided with an adjusting screw to permit alteration in size.

band, apron, *n* See apron band.

band, orthodontic, *n* a thin metal ring, usually stainless steel, that secures orthodontic attachments to a tooth. The band, with orthodontic attachments welded or soldered to it, is closely adapted to fit the contours of the tooth and then is cemented into place.

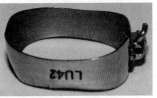

Orthodontic band. (Courtesy Dr. Flavio Uribe)

band, pusher, *n* an instrument used to adapt the metal band to the tooth.

band remover, *n* an instrument used to remove bands from the teeth.

band, rubber, *n* See elastic.

band, slip, *n* a band formed when a metal is placed under a load and one grain tends to slip or slide on another.

band, striated **(strī´ātəd),** *n* See striations, muscle.

bandage, *n* a strip of material wrapped about or applied to any body part.

bandage, Barton's, *n.pr* a figure-eight bandage passing below the mandible and around the cranial bone to give upward support to the mandible.

bandage, thyroid, *n* a large bandage consisting principally of a towel applied around the neck that exerts moderate pressure to the anterolateral part of the neck.

band and loop, *n.* an appliance consisting of a wire loop soldered to a band and designed to prevent space loss in a dental arch when a tooth has been lost prematurely.

bank plan, *n* a financial arrangement made between the dental professional, patient, and bank for financing dental accounts; the bank provides the capital for a rate of interest that enables the patient to pay the dental account over a longer period than would otherwise be possible—usually 12 to 18 months.

bankruptcy, *n* the legal process by which a person, business, or corporation is declared to be insolvent and unable to pay creditors.

bar, *n* a metal segment of greater length than width. See also bar, connector.

bar, anterior palatal, *n* See connector, major, anterior palatal.

bar, arch, *n* any one of several types of wires, bars, and splints conforming to the arch of the teeth and used for the treatment of fractures of the jaws and the stabilization of injured teeth (e.g., *Erich, Jelenko, Niro,* or *Winter*).

bar, buccal, *n* an orthodontic appliance auxiliary consisting of a rigid metal wire extending from the buccal side of the molar band anteriorly.

bar clasp, *n* See clasp, bar.

bar, connector, *n* a connector of greater thickness and reduced width as compared with a platelike connector, which has greater width and is thinner.

bar, fixable-removable cross-arch, *n* See connector, cross-arch bar splint.

bar, Gilson fixable-removable, n.pr See connector, cross-arch bar splint.

bar, Kennedy, *n* See connector, minor, secondary lingual bar.

bar, labial, *n* a major connector located labial (or buccal) to the dental arch that joins bilateral parts of a mandibular removable partial denture.

bar, lingual, *n* a major connector located lingual to the dental arch that joins bilateral parts of a mandibular removable partial denture. May also be the orthodontic splinting on the lingual of either the maxillary or mandibular anterior teeth to maintain position of the teeth over time. See also connector, major, lingual bar.

bar, palatal, *n* a major connector that crosses the palate and unites bilateral parts of a maxillary removable partial denture. See also connector, major.

bar, posterior palatal, *n* See connector, major, posterior palatal.

bar, secondary lingual, *n* See connector, minor, secondary lingual bar.

bar, transpalatal in orthodontics, *n* a rigid wire connecting two teeth across the arch, generally the first maxillary molars. Used to expand, constrict, or maintain intermolar width and also to enhance posterior anchorage.

barb-, a combining form used to indicate derivatives of barbituric acid.

barbiturate (bärbich′ŏŏrāt), *n* a derivative of barbituric acid that acts as a sedative or hypnotic. Barbiturates are controlled substances that have addictive potentials. Use in dentistry as a sedative medication has declined greatly, the benzodiazepines are now generally used.

barbiturates, ultrashort-acting, n.pl drugs administered to bring on rapid anesthesia (e.g., thiopental sodium [Pentathol] and methehexital sodium [Brevital]); rapid onset is countered by an abbreviated period of duration.

barium *(Ba)* **(ber′ēəm),** *n* a pale yellow, metallic element classified with the alkaline earths.

barium sulfate, *n* a white, finely ground, tasteless powder that is insoluble in water, solvents, and solutions of acids and alkalis; used in radiography as a contrast medium because of its opacity to roentgen rays and as a protective barrier in plaster walls.

barodontalgia (barōdontal′jēə), *n* sudden, sharp tooth pain that may occur in response to a decrease in atmospheric pressure such as that experienced during flight at high altitudes. Also called *aerodontalgia.*

barosinusitis (bar′ōsī′nəsī′təs), *n* the painful symptoms related to the maxillary sinus resulting from a change in barometric pressure.

barrier, protective, *n* a material of a composition that greatly absorbs radiation (e.g., lead or concrete).

barrier techniques, *n.pl* protocols used in infection control to prevent cross-contamination between health care worker and patient, between patient and health care worker, and between patients. Strict barrier techniques are recommended by the

Centers for Disease Control and Prevention (CDC) and the American Dental Association (ADA).

basal (baz'əl), *adj* **1.** describing the minimal functions necessary for life. *adj* **2.** located at or forming the base of a structure. *n* **3.** the fundamental structures from which an organism is derived.

basal bone, *n* the bone which supports and is continuous with the alveolar process. Also referred to as the *apical base.*

basal lamina, *n* a layer composed of the lamina densa and the lamina lucida. It is an extracellular matrix that lies beneath the epithelium and is believed to inhibit cell migration. The term is usually associated with electron microscopy, whereas the term *basement membrane* is usually associated with light microscopy.

basal layer, *n* See stratum basale.

basal metabolic rate (BMR) (bā'zəl met'əbol'ik), *n* a type of basal rate, or energy exchange, determined by means of a clinical test of oxygen consumption in a subject who has had a good night's rest, has fasted for 12 to 14 hours, and has been physically, mentally, and emotionally at rest for 30 minutes; usually indicated as a percentage of the normal calorie production per surface area, the normal values ranging between plus and minus 20%.

basal metabolism, *n* See basal metabolic rate.

basal seat, *n* the oral tissues and structures that support a denture.

basal seat area, *n* See area, basal seat.

basal seat outline, *n* an outline on the mucous membrane or on a cast of the entire area that is to be covered by a denture.

basal surface, *n* See surface, basal.

base, *n* **1.** the foundation or support on which something rests; the point of attachment of a part; the principal ingredient of a material. *n* **2.** a compound that yields hydroxyl ions in water solution and causes neutralization of acid to form a salt and water. **3.** the part of a denture that supports the prosthetic teeth and receives support from the oral mucosa, anchoring teeth, or alveolar ridge. See also basic. Opposite: acid.

base, acrylic resin, *n* a denture base made of an acrylic resin.

base, apical, *n* the portion of the jawbone that gives support to the denture base or alveolar process.

base, cement, *n* a layer of insulated, sometimes medicated dental cement placed in the deep portions of a cavity preparation to protect the pulp, reduce the bulk of the metallic restoration, or eliminate undercuts in a tapered preparation.

base, denture, *n* **1.** the part of a denture that fits the oral mucosa of the basal seat, restores the normal contours of the soft tissues of the dentulous oral cavity, and supports the artificial teeth. *n* **2.** the portion of a denture that overlies the soft tissue, usually fabricated of resin or combinations of resins and metal. *n* **3.** used in dentofacial orthopedics to describe the alveolar bone and the teeth contained in it.

base, extension (free-end), *n* a unit of a removable prosthesis that extends anteriorly or posteriorly, terminating without end support by a natural tooth.

base, film, *n* a thin, flexible, transparent sheet of cellulose acetate or similar material used to support the emulsion.

base, mandibular, *n* the body of the mandible, on which the teeth and alveolar tissues are situated.

base, material, *n* a substance from which a denture base may be made (e.g., acrylic resin, vulcanite, polystyrene resin, and metal).

base, metal, *n* the basal surface of a denture constructed of metal (e.g., aluminum, gold, and cobalt-chromium) to which the teeth are attached.

base, plastic, *n* a denture base, baseplate, or record base made of a plastic material.

base, record, *n* See baseplate.

base, shellac, *n* a resinous material adapted to maxillary or mandibular casts to form baseplates.

base, sprue, *n* See crucible former.

base, temporary, *n* See baseplate.

base, tinted denture, *n* a denture base that simulates the coloring and shading of natural oral tissues.

base, tongue, *n* the most posterior portion of the tongue.

base, trial, *n* See baseplate.

Basedow's disease (baz'ədōz), *n.pr* See goiter, exophthalmic.

baseline, *n* a reference point used to indicate the initial condition against which future measurements are compared.

basement lamina (lam'ənə), *n* the thin layer of noncellular material beneath epithelial cells that is composed primarily of collagen. Also known as the *basal lamina.*

basement membrane, *n* the extracellular material consisting of a basal and reticular lamina produced by the epithelium and connective tissue, respectively.

baseplate, *n* a temporary form representing the base of a denture and used for making maxillomandibular (jaw) relation records, arranging artificial teeth, or facilitating trial placement in the oral cavity.

baseplate, stabilized, *n* a baseplate lined with plastic or other material to improve its adaptation and stability.

baseplate wax, *n* See wax, baseplate.

basic, *adj* having the ability to neutralize acids.

basic life support (BLS), *n* fundamental emergency treatment consisting of cardiopulmonary resuscitation (CPR) or emergency cardiac care (ECC) that is provided until more precise medical treatment can begin.

basic metabolic rate, *n* See basal metabolic rate.

basic services, *n.pl* frequently insurance companies split dental procedures into basic and major categories. Basic services usually consist of diagnostic, preventive, and routine restorative dental services. The plan may provide different deductibles, coinsurance, and maximums for basic versus major services as incentives to good dental care.

basion (bā'sēon), *n* the midline point at the anterior margin of the occipital foramen.

basis, *n* the principal active ingredient in a prescription.

basophil (bā'səfil), *n* See leukocyte.

basophilia (bā'sōfil'ēə), *n* an aggregate of blue-staining granules found in erythrocytes; seen in lead poisoning, leukemia, malaria, severe anemias, and certain toxemias.

basophilic line (bā'sōfil'ik), *n* See line, basophilic.

bass wood interdental cleaner, *n* a triangular strip of wood that can be softened and used to clean a tooth that has little or no interdental papilla.

batch processing, *n* **1.** data processing in which a number of similar input data items are grouped together and processed during a single machine run with the same program. *n* **2.** the processing of a group of instruments through sterilization or disinfection.

Battle's sign, *n* See sign, Battle's.

bayonet (bā'ənet), *n* a binangled instrument, the nib or blade of which is generally parallel to the shaft; resembles a bayonet. See also angle former, bayonet and condenser, bayonet.

beading, *n* the scribing of a shallow groove (less than 0.5 mm in width or depth) on a cast that outlines the major connector. It is used to transfer the design to the investment cast and ensure tissue contact of the major connector.

beam, *n* a stream or approximately unidirectional emission of electromagnetic radiation or particles.

beam, central, *n* the center of the beam of roentgen rays emitted from the tube.

beam, useful, *n* the part of the primary radiation that passes through the aperture, cone, or other collimator.

beam alignment device, *n* a device used in intraoral radiography to align the position-indicating device in proper relation with the tooth and receptor.

beanbag dental chair, *n* a large self-adjusting form-fitting pad placed on top of a dental chair, filled with beans or small pellets, to more comfortably accommodate hypotonic and spastic patients who need more support but less restrictive stabilization in the dental environment.

beclomethasone dipropionate (bek'ləmeth'əsōn dī'prō'pēənāt'), *n brand names:* oral—Beclovent, Vanceril; nasal—Vancenase AQ Nasal, Beconase AQ Nasal; *drug class:* corticosteroid, synthetic; *action:* prevents inflammation by glucocorticoid receptors leading to inhibition of phospholipase A_2 and by depression of migration of polymorphonuclear leukocytes and fibroblasts and reversal of increased capillary permeability; *uses:* chronic asthma and rhinitis.

beeswax, *n* a wax that melts at low heat and is an ingredient of many dental waxes.

Begg's appliance, *n.pr* See appliance, Begg's.

behavior, *n* the manner in which a person acts or performs; any or all of the activities of a person, including physical action learned and unlearned, deliberate or habitual.

behavior guidance, *n* a continuum of techniques ranging from simple suggestion to conscious sedation employed to achieve the desired behavior of patients during dental treatment. Having expertise in behavior guidance is a very important aspect of practicing pediatric dentistry.

behavior management, *n* the techniques used to control or modify an action or performance of a subject. In dentistry, usually associated with the management of oral hygiene behavior, dietary behavior, or patient behavior under stress.

behavior modification, *n* alterations, changes, or transfers from a socially unacceptable and destructive act to a socially acceptable, nondestructive one. In dentistry, usually associated with oral habits such as finger or thumb sucking, oral cavity breathing, nail biting, and smoking.

behavior therapy, *n* psychotherapy that attempts to modify observable, maladjusted patterns of behavior by the substitution of a new response or set of responses to a given stimulus.

behavioral medicine, *n* a branch of clinical psychology that deals with behavior modification and may involve assertiveness training, aversion therapy, contingency management, operant conditioning, and systemic desensitization.

behavioral sciences, *n.pl* those sciences devoted to the study of human and animal behavior.

Behçet's syndrome (bechets´), *n* See syndrome, Behçet's.

bell stage, *n* the developmental stage of tooth development during which the cup-shaped enamel organ is transformed into a bell-shaped structure.

Fourth stage of odontogenesis, in which differentiation occurs to its furthest extent.

Bell's palsy, sign, palsy test, *n.pr* See palsy, Bell's; sign, Bell's; and palsy test, Bell's.

belladonna alkaloids, *n brand name:* Bellafoline; *drug class:* gastrointestinal anticholinergic; *action:* inhibits muscarinic actions of acetylcholine at postganglionic parasympathetic neuroeffector sites; *uses:* treatment of peptic ulcer disease and irritable bowel syndrome in combination with other drugs.

Benadryl, *n.pr* brand name for diphenhydramine hydrochloride, an antihistamine with anticholinergic (drying) and sedative side effects.

benazepril (bənă´zəpril´), *n brand name:* Lotensin; *drug class:* angiotensin-converting enzyme (ACE) inhibitor; *action:* selectively suppresses renin-angiotensin-aldosterone system; *uses:* treatment of hypertension.

Bence Jones protein, *n.pr* See protein, Bence Jones.

Benedict's test, *n.pr* See test, Benedict's.

beneficence (bənĕf´ĭsəns). *n* 1. the act of doing good; kindness. *n* 2. of benefit to the patient.

beneficiary, *n* 1. a person eligible for benefits under a dental plan. *n* 2. a person who receives benefits under a dental benefit contract. See also covered person; insured; member; and subscriber.

benefit booklet, *n* a booklet or pamphlet provided to the subscriber that contains a general explanation of the benefits and related provisions of the dental benefits program. Also known as a *summary plan description.*

benefit plan summary, *n* the description or synopsis of employee benefits required by the Employee Retirement Income Security Act (ERISA) to be distributed to employees.

benefits, *n.pl* 1. the monies paid and discounts applied for various procedures performed. *n.pl* 2. the dental services or procedures covered by the insurance policy, also known as the *schedule of benefits.*

benign (bēnīn´), *adj* a condition that, untreated or with symptomatic therapy, will not become life threatening. It is used particularly in relation to tumors, which may be benign or malignant. They do not invade surrounding tissues and do not metastasize to other parts of the body. The word is slightly imprecise, because some can, owing to mass effect, cause life-threatening complications.

Bennett angle, movement, *n* See angle, Bennett and movement, Bennett.

benzathine penicillin G (ben′zə then′), *n* a benzathine salt of natural penicillin that forms a slowly absorbable injectable antibiotic effective against penicillin-susceptible organisms.

benzene, abuse of, *n* an improper, recreational inhaling of the chemical hydrocarbon C6H6. It is found in gasoline and adhesives.

benzocaine (topical), *n brand names:* 20% liquid—Anbesol Maximum Strength, Orajel Mouth Aid; 20% gel—Anbesol Maximum Strength, Hurricaine, Orajel Brace-Aid; 10% gel—Denture Orajel, Baby Orajel Nighttime; *drug class:* topical ester local anesthetic; *action:* inhibits conduction of nerve impulses from sensory nerves and is derived from aminobenzoic acid; *uses:* treatment of oral irritation or sores, and pain caused by dental prostheses, orthodontic appliances, or teething. Mainly used for preanesthetic anesthesia of the oral mucosa. May cause localized allergic reactions and gag reflex if not used properly.

benzodiazepines (ben′zōdīaz′ə pēn), *n.pl* drugs used to decrease emotional stress, lessen anxiety, and bring about sleep. Sometimes used as sedatives during dental treatment.

benzol-arginine naphthylamide (ben′zol-ar′gənēn nafthil′əmīd), *n* a bacterial enzyme that mimics the activity of trypsin. It is used as a marker of bacterial growth in dental plaque or in the diagnosis of periodontal disease involving *Bacteroides gingivalis, B. forsythus,* and *Treponema denticola.*

benzonatate (benzon′ətāt′), *n brand name:* Tessalon; *drug class:* antitussive, nonnarcotic; *action:* inhibits cough reflex by anesthetizing

stretch receptors in respiratory system; *use:* nonproductive cough relief.

benzoyl peroxide, *n* **1.** a chemical incorporated into the polymer of resins to aid in the initiation of polymerization. *n* **2.** an antibacterial, keratolytic drying agent prescribed in the treatment of acne.

benztropine mesylate (benz′trō′ pēn mes′ilāt′), *n brand names:* Apo-benzotropin, benztropine mesylate; *drug class:* anticholinergic, antidyskinetic; *action:* blocks central acetylcholine receptors; *use:* treatment of Parkinson's disease symptoms.

bepridil HCl (bep′ridil), *n brand names:* Vascor, Bepadin; *drug class:* calcium channel blocker; *action:* inhibits calcium ion influx across cell membranes of cardiac muscle and blood vessels smooth muscle; *use:* treatment of stable angina, alone or in combination with propranolol or nitrates.

beriberi (asjike, athiaminosis, endemic multiple neuritis, endemic polyneuritis, hinchazon, inchacao, kakke, loempe, panneuritis endemica, perneiras) (ber′ēber′ē), *n* a nutritional disease resulting from a deficiency of thiamine. Classically it is characterized by multiple neuritis, muscular atrophy, weakness, cardiovascular changes, and progressive edema.

beryllium *(Be)* **(bəril′ēəm),** *n* a steel-gray, lightweight metallic element with an atomic number of 4 and an atomic weight of 9.01218. Alloys are used in fluorescent powders. Inhalation of beryllium fumes or particles may cause the formation of granulomas in the lungs, skin, and subcutaneous tissues.

beta cells, *n* See cells, beta.

beta receptors, *n* See receptors, beta.

beta-blocker, non-selective, *n* drug that targets both of the two β-adrenergic receptors, β_1 or β_2, of the effector organs, which in turn block the sympathetic autonomic nervous system action.

beta-blocker, selective, *n* a drug that specifically blocks either β_1 or β_2 adrenergic receptors of the effector organs, which in turn block the sympathetic autonomic nervous system action.

betamethasone (valerate, betamethasone benzoate, betamethasone dipropionate) (bā'təmeth'əsōn), *n* *brand names:* Uticort, Beben, and others; *drug class:* topical corticosteroid; *action:* binds to glucocorticoid receptors leading to inhibition of phospholipase A_2 and induces antiinflammatory effects; possesses antipruritic, antiinflammatory actions; *uses:* treatment of psoriasis, eczema, contact dermatitis, pruritus, and oral ulcerative inflammatory lesions.

betatron (bā'tətron), *n* a machine that produces high-speed electrons through magnetic induction.

betaxolol HCl (batak'səlol), *n* *brand name:* Kerlone; *drug class:* antihypertensive, selective β_1 –adrenergic receptor blocker; *action:* produces fall in blood pressure and reduction in heart rate; *use:* treatment of hypertension.

bethanechol chloride (bəthan'əkol), *n* *brand names:* Duvoid, Urecholine, Urebeth; *drug class:* cholinergic stimulant; *actions:* stimulates muscarinic acetylcholine receptors directly; stimulates gastric motility; *uses:* treatment of postoperative or postpartum urinary retention and neurogenic atony of bladder with retention.

bevel, *n* the inclination that one surface makes with another when not at right angles; in cavity preparation, a cut that produces an angle of more than 90° with a cavity wall.

bevel, cavosurface, *n* the incline or slant of the cavosurface angle of a prepared cavity wall in relation to the plane of the enamel wall.

bevel, contra, *n* blade placement toward the base of the periodontal pocket to separate the sulcular from the external epithelium. Also known as a *reverse,* or *internal bevel.*

bevel, incisal, *n* the angle of an incisor; it can be less than or greater than 90°.

bevel, instrument, *n* the sloping keen edge of a cutting instrument.

bevel, reverse, *n* See bevel, contra.

BHN, *n.pr* See number, Brinell hardness and test, Brinell hardness.

bias, *n* in statistics, the systematic distortion of a statistic caused by a particular sampling process.

bibulous (bib'yōōlus), *adj* pertaining to absorption; a material's ability to absorb fluids.

bibulous pad (saliva absorber), *n* a permeable cotton pad placed inside the cheek during the application of a sealant to staunch the flow of saliva and keep the treatment field dry.

bicarbonate, *n* a salt resulting from the incomplete neutralization of carbonic acid such as from passing excess carbon dioxide into a base solution.

Bicillin, *n.pr* the brand name for penicillin G benzathine.

bicuspid (bīkus'pid), *n* See premolar.

b.i.d., *adv* a Latin phrase meaning "twice a day"; abbreviation used in writing prescriptions.

bidi, *adj* an abbreviation for *bidirectional*; moving or occurring in two, usually opposite, directions.

bidigital palpation (bīdij'itəl), *n* a tactile method of oral examination in which the examiner uses the thumb and forefinger of one hand to rule out abnormalities.

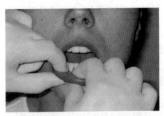

Bidigital palpation. (Fehrenbach/Herring, 2012)

Biermer's anemia (bir'murz), *n.pr* See anemia, pernicious.

bifid (bī'fid), *adj* divided in two.

bifid tongue, *n* See tongue, bifid.

bifid uvula, *n* See uvula, bifid.

Bifidobacterium **(bif'idōbakter'ē əm),** *n* a genus of anaerobic bacteria containing gram-positive rods of highly variable appearance. Pathogenicity for human beings or for animals has not been reported, although these bacteria have been isolated from the feces of infants and older people.

B

bifurcation (bī'furkā'shǝn), *n* the point of separation or division of a tooth's root structure into two parts or branches.

biguanides (bīgwan'īdz), *n.pl* orally administered agents used in the treatment of type 2 diabetes. They prevent the liver from breaking down glycogen into glucose and increases the sensitivity body tissues have to insulin, as well as other actions. See metformin HCl.

bilaminar embryonic disc, *n* the circular plate of bilayered cells developed from the blastocyst.

bilateral (bīlat'ǝrǝl), *adj* pertaining to both sides.

bilateral symmetry, *n* the configuration of an irregularly shaped body (as the human body or that of higher animals) that can be divided by a longitudinal plane into halves that are mirror images of each other.

bile, *n* an alkaline fluid secreted by the liver that breaks down fat and aids in its absorption in the small intestine. It has a yellow, green, or brown color and a bitter taste. Interference with its flow can result in jaundice.

bilharziasis (bil'härzī'ǝsis), *n* See also schistosomiasis.

biliary atresia (bil'ēǝrē'ǝtrē'zhǝ), *n* a congenital absence or underdevelopment of one or more of the biliary structures, causing jaundice and early liver damage.

bilirubinemia (bil'irōōbinē'mēǝ), *n* the presence of bilirubin in the blood. It may result from obstruction inside or outside the liver or from increased hemolysis. The total serum bilirubin in an adult is 0.2 to 0.7 mg/100 mL.

bilirubinuria (bil'irōōbinyōō'rēǝ), *n* the presence of bilirubin in the urine. More often, an excess of bilirubin in the urine resulting from excessive hemolysis.

billing, *n* the procedure of preparing a financial statement.

bimanual palpation, *n* a tactile method of oral examination in which the examiner uses both hands to examine the patient's oral cavity from both the inside and outside at the same time.

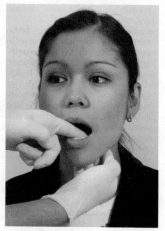

Bimanual palpation. (Hupp/Ellis/Tucker, 2008)

bimaxillary (bīmak'silerē), *adj* pertaining to the right and left maxillae; sometimes incorrectly used to refer to the maxillae and mandible.

bimaxillary protrusion, *n* See protrusion, bimaxillary.

bimeter (bīmē'tur), *n* a gnathodynamometer with a central bearing point adjustable to varying heights. See also gnathodynamometer.

Bimler's appliance, *n.pr* See appliance, Bimler's.

binangle (bin'anggǝl), *n* an instrument having two offsetting angles in its shank. The angles keep the cutting edge or the face of the nib within 3 mm of the axis of the shaft.

binder, *n* a substance, usually sticky, that holds the solid particles in a mixture together, thus aiding in the preservation of the physical form of the mixture.

binding, *n* a reversible combination of various drugs with body constituents such as plasma proteins.

binding site, *n* the location on the surface of a cell or molecule where other cell fragments or molecules attach to initiate a chemical or physiologic action.

binge-eating and purging, *n* a type of anorexia nervosa in which an individual consumes a large amount of food and then forces vomiting or uses enemas, laxatives, or diuretics to avoid additional weight gain.

binocular loupe, *n* See loupe, binocular.

bioburden, *n* the number of bacteria living on a surface before it is sterilized.

biochemistry, *n* the chemistry of living organisms and life processes.

biocidal (bī′ōsī′dəl), *adj* capable of destroying microorganisms.

biocompatible, *adj* compatible with living cells, tissues, organs, or systems, and posing no risk of injury, toxicity, or rejection by the immune system.

biocompatible material, *n* a substance that does not threaten, impede, or adversely affect living tissue.

biodegradability, *n* the natural ability of a chemical substance to be broken down into less complex compounds with fewer carbon atoms by bacteria or other microorganisms.

biodegradable (bī′ōdigrā′dəbəl), *adj* the ability to be broken down into smaller, harmless products by way of the action of living organisms.

bioelectrical impedance (bīōelek′trikəl impē′dəns), *n* a method of measuring total body fat that uses electrical current and is based on the premise that lean body mass is a better conductor of electricity than fat. See also body mass index calculation.

bioethics, *n* the study of social and moral issues raised in the field of biology, including medicine and dentistry.

biofeedback, *n* the instrumented process or technique of learning voluntary control over automatically regulated body functions; useful in the treatment of bruxism, temporomandibular joint dysfunction, and pain, and in facilitating anxiety control in the dental setting.

biofeedback, electromyographic (EMG) (əlek′trōmī′ōgraf′ik), *n* an instrumented process that helps patients learn control over muscle tension levels previously under automatic control; especially useful in treatment of dental disorders such as bruxism, temporomandibular joint dysfunction, tension headaches, and other disorders involving the muscles of mastication. In addition to

neuromuscular education, electromyographic type is useful in treating dental phobias and anxiety and facilitating pain control by helping patients learn deep-muscle relaxation techniques.

biofeedback, temperature, *n* an instrumented learning process whereby a patient learns to control temperature of body parts. Training in selfcontrolled vasodilation (hand-warming) technique has been found useful in treating migraine headaches and anxiety in dental patients.

biofilm (bi′ofilm′), *n* a very thin layer of microorganisms within an acellular matrix that covers the surfaces of an object.

biofilm, bacterial plaque, *n* a thick grouping of microorganisms that are very resistant to antibiotics and antimicrobial agents and that live on gingival tissues, teeth, and restorations, causing caries and periodontal disease; also known as *bacterial plaque biofilm.*

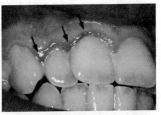

Accumulation of bacterial plaque biofilm (and the first symptoms of gingival inflammation). (Newman/Takei/Klokkevold, 2012)

biofilm, dental, *n* See biofilm, bacterial plaque.

biofilm, plaque, *n* See plaque.

biofilm, waterline, *n* a microbial growth that adheres to the waterlines used in dental procedures. Poses a serious risk for immunocompromised individuals.

bioflavonoids (bī′ōflav′ənoidz′), *n.pl* a broad category of plant-derived pigments that possess antioxidant and other properties.

bioglass, *n* a fused silica-containing aluminum oxide that presents a surface-reactive glass film compatible with connective and epithelial tissues.

Bioglass is used as a surface coating in blade and endosteal implants.

biointegration, *n* a condition that occurs when ceramic implant materials are used and there is no space located between the bone and dental implant.

biologic, *adj* pertaining to biology.

biologic death, n the permanent cessation of electrical activity in the central nervous system. Also called *brain death.*

biologic factors, n.pl the variables that influence life and living tissues.

biologic indicators, n.pl vials or strips that contain harmless bacterial spores and are used to determine whether sterilization has occurred. Also called *spore tests.*

biologic (permucosal) seal, n the health-protecting zone between the living soft tissue and the post or implant in patients with full replacement dental work. Works to prevent bacteria and any other health threatening organisms from breaching healthy tissue.

biologic science, n the science that deals with life processes.

biologic value (BV), n a number reached by comparing the amount of nitrogen retained with the amount absorbed to aid in determining protein quality.

biologic vector, n the live carrier, usually an arthropod, in which an infectious organism matures prior to infecting a receiver.

biologic age, *n* See age, biologic.

biologic width, *n* the combined height of the suprabony soft tissue attachment around a tooth that isolates the bone from the oral cavity; it is comprised of healthy connective tissue and junctional epithelium attachment to the root surface and crown.

biology, *n* the science of life or living matter in all its forms and phenomena.

biomarker, *n* a substance, usually a protein, whose concentration reflects the severity or presence of a particular disease state, or some other physiological state of an organism.

biomass, *n* the total quantity of living organisms in a particular volume of matter.

biomechanics (bī′ōməkan′iks), *n* See biophysics.

biomedical engineering, *n* a system of techniques in which knowledge of biologic processes is applied to solve practical medical problems and answer questions in biomedical research.

biometrics (bī′ōmet′riks), *n* the science of the application of statistical methods to biologic facts.

bionator (bī′ōnā′tər), *n* a removable orthodontic appliance designed to correct functional and skeletal anteroposterior discrepancies between the maxilla and mandible.

biophysics (bīōfiz′iks), *n* the science dealing with the forces that act on living cells of the body, the relationship between the biologic behavior of living structures and the physical influences to which they are subjected, and the physics of vital processes. Also known as *biomechanics.*

biophysics, dental, n the branch of biophysics that deals with the biologic behavior of oral structures as influenced by dental restorations.

biopsy (bī′opsē), *n* the removal of a tissue specimen or other material from the living body for microscopic examination to aid in establishing a diagnosis.

biopsy, aspiration, n See aspiration, fine needle (FNA).

biopsy, excisional (eksizh′ənəl), n the removal of an entire lesion, usually including a margin of contiguous normal tissue, for microscopic examination and diagnosis.

biopsy, exploratory, n an exploration combined with biopsy to determine method and degree of local extension, usually of bone or deep soft tissue lesions.

biopsy, incisional (insizh′ənəl), n the surgical removal of a selected mass of a lesion and adjacent normal tissue for microscopic examination and diagnosis.

biopsy, needle, n See aspiration, fine needle (FNA).

biopsy, oral brush, n a noninvasive procedure used to detect early oral cancer during which a sterile brush is rotated against the suspected lesion to obtain a tissue sample. Brand name: *OralCDx.*

biopsy, punch, n biopsy material obtained by use of a punch.

biopsy, shave, n a biopsy of skin or mucosal tissue made by removing part or all of a lesion with a scalpel held parallel to the base of the lesion.

bioresorbable, n the materials that can be broken down by the body and that do not require mechanical removal, such as sutures or the chlorhexidine chip.

biosynthesis, n the formation of a chemical compound by enzymes.

biotechnology, n **1.** the study of the relationships between humans or other living organisms and machinery. n **2.** the industrial application of the results of biologic research such as recombinant deoxyribonucleic acid (DNA) and gene splicing that permit the production of synthetic hormones or enzymes.

biotin (bī′ətin), n See vitamin, biotin.

biotransformation, n the chemical and physical changes produced in drugs after they enter the body (e.g., hydrolysis, conjugation).

biperiden lactate, n brand name: Akineton; *drug class:* anticholinergic; *action:* centrally acting competitive anticholinergic; *use:* treatment of Parkinson's disease symptoms.

bird face, n See brachygnathia; retrognathism.

birth control, n **1.** a regimen of one or more actions, devices, or medications followed in order to deliberately prevent or reduce the likelihood of a woman becoming pregnant or giving birth. n **2.** oral contraceptives, usually a mixture of a steroid having progestational activity and an estrogen.

birth, premature, n a birth in which the child is delivered before it has reached the full period of gestation (37 weeks).

birth weight, n the measured heaviness of a baby when born.

bis-, *pref* a prefix meaning that two like or mirror-image moieties are joined together to form a chemical compound.

bisacodyl (bisak′ədil), n brand names: Dulcolax, Fleet Bisacodyl, Bisacodyl Uniserts, Fleet Laxative; *drug class:* laxative, stimulant; *action:* acts directly on intestine by increasing motor activity; *uses:* short-term treatment of constipation, bowel

or rectal preparation for surgery or examination.

biscuit, n the firing bakes, or stages (referred to as *low, medium,* and *high*), during the fusing of dental porcelain preceding the final, or glaze, bake.

bisecting-angle technique, n See angulation, bisecting-angle technique.

bisecting-the-angle error, n an error in the bisecting angle technique in which the vertical angulation is incorrectly placed, resulting in either very long or short images. See also distortion; elongation; foreshortening.

Bismarck brown (Easlick's disclosing agent), *n.pr* one of a variety of dental applications, reveals deposits on the teeth by temporarily coloring them. Characterized by its brown color and licorice flavor.

bismuth (biz′məth), n a reddish, crystalline, trivalent metallic element that in combination with other elements forms salts that are used in the production of many pharmaceutical compounds.

bismuth poisoning, n See bismuthosis.

bismuth subsalicylate, n brand names: Bisamatrol, Pepto-Bismol; *drug class:* antidiarrheal; *action:* mechanism of action unknown; *uses:* treatment of diarrhea, prevention of diarrhea when traveling.

bismuthia (bizmyōō′thēə), n the discoloration of mucous membranes and skin from bismuth poisoning.

bismuthism, n See bismuthosis.

bismuthosis (biz′məthō′sis), n an acute or chronic bismuth intoxication resulting from the ingestion or injection of bismuth salts. Possible manifestations include albuminuria, exfoliative dermatitis, gastrointestinal disturbances, and stomatitis. Also known as *bismuth poisoning* or *bismuthism.* See also stomatitis, bismuth.

bisoprolol fumarate (bis′ōprō′lol fyōō′mərāt′), n brand name: Zebeta; *drug class:* antihypertensive, selective β_1 blocker; *action:* produces fall in blood pressure without reflex tachycardia or significant reduction in heart rate; *uses:* treatment of hypertension as a single agent or in combination.

bisphosphonate (bisfos′fənōt), n brand names: Fosamax, Boniva, Didronel; *drug class:* two classes: the

N-containing (alendronate) and non-N-containing (Etidronate); *action:* inhibits oseoclasts and bone resorption; *uses:* prevention and treatment of osteoporosis, osteitis deformans ("Paget's disease of bone"), bone metastasis (with or without hypercalcemia), multiple myeloma and other conditions that feature bone fragility. Can rarely cause osteonecrosis of the jaw; this may be reason to postpone drug treatment until after dental treatment, as they remain bound to the bone for a prolonged period. Most cases occur in high-dose intravenous types used in cancer patients, but a small proportion happens in patients on oral types. Also called *diphosphonate.* See also osteonecrosis, bisphosphonate-associated (BON).

bisphosphonate-related osteonecrosis of the jaw *(BONJ)*, *n* See osteonecrosis, bisphosphonate associated (BON).

bisulfite, allergy to (bĭsul'fāt), *n* a hypersensitive reaction to certain antioxidant substances, such as the preservatives sodium metabisulfite, acetone sodium bisulfite, and sodium or potassium bisulfite, which are used in local anesthetics containing vasoconstrictors.

bite, *n* **1.** the part of an artificial tooth on the lingual side between the shoulder and the incisal edge of the tooth. *n* **2.** an interocclusal record or relationship. See also denture space; distance, interarch; record, interocclusal; and record, maxilloman.

bite, balanced, n See occlusion, balanced.

bite block, n **1.** in intraoral radiography, a disposable or sterilized holder that the patient bites to provide stable retention of the receptor packet. *n* **2.** an occlusion rim. *n* **3.** a commercially available device, usually made of rubber, which can be used to prop open a patient's oral cavity during a prolonged treatment session.

bite, close, n See distance, small interarch.

bite, closed, n **1.** an abnormal overbite. *n* **2.** a decrease in the occlusal vertical dimension produced by factors such as tooth abrasion and loss or failure of eruption of supportive posterior teeth. See also distance, reduced interarch.

bite closing, n See dimension, vertical decrease.

bite, convenience, n See occlusion, acquired, eccentric.

bite, deep, n See overbite.

bite, edge-to-edge, n an occlusion in which the incisal edge of the maxillary incisors meets the incisal edge of the mandibular incisors. See also occlusion, edge-to-edge.

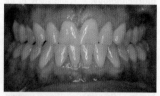

Edge-to-edge bite. (Courtesy Dr. Flavio Uribe)

bite force, n the interocclusal force produced in jaw closure, usually measured in grams or pounds.

bite fork, n See fork, face-bow.

bite guard, n See guard, bite.

bite guard splint, n See splint, acrylic resin bite-guard.

bite, human, n a puncture or laceration of tissue caused by human teeth. The markings may be distinctive and useful in forensic pathology to determine the person responsible. Human bite wounds may become infected, requiring antibiotic treatment and tetanus toxoid injection.

bite, locked, n See occlusion, locked.

bite marks, n.pl the distinctive tooth patterns in a wound that may have forensic or legal implications.

bite, normal, n See occlusion, normal.

bite, open, n See apertognathia.

bite opening bends, n.pl the bends made in maxillary and mandibular light round wires mesial to the molar tubes in orthodontics.

bite plate, n See plate, bite.

bite, power, n the strength of the closing motion of the mandible.

bite pressure, n the pressure produced by jaw closure per unit of area, usually measured in grams per square millimeter. See also pressure, occlusal.

bite raising, n See dimension, vertical, increasing occlusal.

bite record, *n* See path, generated occlusal.

bite rest, *n* See position, rest, physiologic.

bite rim, *n* See rim, occlusion.

bite, working, *n* See occlusion, working.

bite mark analysis, *n* See analysis, bite mark.

biteplane (bīt′plān), *n* a removable appliance that covers the occlusal surfaces of the teeth to prevent their articulation.

bite-wing film, *n* See film, bite-wing.

bite-wing radiograph, *n* See radiograph, bite-wing.

biting, cheek, *n* See habit.

biting, lip, *n* See habit.

biting, nail, *n* See habit.

biting pressure, *n* See pressure, occlusal.

biting strength, *n* See strength, biting.

bitolterol mesylate (bitol′ərol mes′ilāt′), *n brand name:* Tornalate; *drug class:* beta$_2$ adrenergic receptor agonist; *action:* causes bronchodilation; *uses:* treatment or prophylaxis of asthma, bronchitis, bronchospasm.

Black's Classification of Dental Caries and Restorations, *n.pr* a standard classification system used to indicate the location of caries and various methods to restore the tooth. G. V. Black developed this system in the early 1900s.

blackout, *n* the brief impairment of short- and long-term memory occurring during episodes of excessive alcohol consumption or of other substance abuse; consciousness is retained.

blade, *n* See specific instrument parts.

blanching, gingival, *n* See gingival blanching.

Blandin and Nuhn's gland, *n.pr* See gland, Blandin and Nuhn's.

blanket stitch, *n* See suture, blanket.

blastocyst, *n* the structure during prenatal development consisting of trophoblast cells and an inner mass of cells that develop into the embryo.

blastomatoid lesion (blastō′mə toid), *n* an overzealous reactive process that because of tumescence has some features of neoplasia. Specific tissue elements, such as fibroblasts, endothelial cells, osteoblasts, osteoclastic giant cells, or nerves, predominate in a specific lesion to form granuloma pyogenicum, giant cell reparative granuloma, traumatic fibroma, tori, or traumatic neuroma.

Blastomyces dermatitidis (blastōmī ′sēz dur′mətit′ədis), *n* a species of fungus causing North American blastomycosis.

blastomycosis (blastōmīkō′sis), *n* an infection resulting from the fungus *B. dermatitidis* (North American blastomycosis) or *B. brasiliensis* (South American blastomycosis); characterized by chronic suppurative lesions. The disseminated form is usually fatal.

blastomycosis, South American, *n* a fungal infection that often begins when organisms enter the body through the oral mucosa, producing local ulcers, or through an extraction site, producing papillary lesions. Dissemination leads to granulomatous lesions of the lymph nodes, gastrointestinal tract, liver, and lungs and to microabscesses of the skin. The causative agent is *B. brasiliensis.*

bleaching, *n* the use of a chemical oxidizing agent to lighten tooth discolorations. Preferred term is *whitening.* See also agent, whitening.

bleeding, *n* the flowing of blood.

bleeding disorders, *n.pl* hemorrhagic disorders including capillary abnormalities, platelet deficiencies, and blood clotting defects characterized by spontaneous and sometimes uncontrollable bleeding. Consideration before most invasive dental procedures.

bleeding, gingival, *n* See gingival bleeding.

bleeding, occult (əkult′), *n* a hemorrhage of such small proportions that the blood can be detected only by chemical test, microscope, or spectroscope.

bleeding points, *n.pl* a series of puncture points made through the gingival tissue; used as a guide for making the gingivectomy or internal bevel incisions.

bleeding time, *n* the time required for blood to stop flowing from a tiny wound. Normal bleeding time is from 2 to 6 minutes. Bleeding time is increased in disorders of platelet count, uremia, and ingestion of aspirin and other antiinflammatory medications.

bleomycin *n brand name:* Blenoxane; *drug class:* antibiotic antineoplastic; *action:* causes breaks in DNA; *uses:* testicular and head and neck cancer, Hodgkin's disease, GI tumors, sarcomas.

blepharophimosis (blef´ərō´fəmō´ sis), *n* a decrease in the size of the palpebral opening without a fusion of the eyelid margins.

blepharoptosis (blef´əroptō´sis), *n* a drooping of the upper eyelid.

blindness, color, *n* defective color vision characterized by decreased ability to detect differences in color. See also achromatopsia.

blindness, color, blue-yellow, *n* a color disability in which the spectrum is seen in reds and greens; a form of protanopia.

blindness, color, red-green, *n* the more common form of color disability, in which the entire spectrum is constituted by yellows and blues; a form of protanopia.

blindness, legal, *n* a condition distinguished by having less than 20/200 vision with the use of eyeglasses to correct vision.

blister, *n* See vesicle or bulla.

blisterform oral lesions, *n* well-defined, fluid-filled lesions in the oral cavity; may appear as pustules, vesicles, or bullae; characterized by elevation above the level of the surface where they are found, blisterform oral lesions are typically seethrough and soft. Color varies according to content of blister, which may include blood, serum, mucin, or suppuration; ranges in size from less than 1 cm in diameter to larger than 1 cm in diameter.

Bloch-Sulzberger syndrome (bloksulz´bergər), *n.pr* See syndrome, Bloch-Sulzberger.

block, *n* **1.** a mental obstacle that prohibits a patient from having favorable responses to the dental professional and suggested treatment plans. *n* **2.** the blocking of sensation like pain to an area. *n* **3.** a large amount of information.

block, data, *n* a physical unit of data that can be conveniently stored by a computer on an input or output device. The block is normally composed of one or more logical records or a portion of a logical record. Synonymous with *physical record.*

block, nerve, *n* See nerve block.

blocking, *n* the process of obstructing or deadening, as a nerve.

blocking agent, *n* See agent, blocking.

blockout, *n* the elimination of undesirable undercut areas on a cast to be used in the fabrication of a removable denture. Also known as *waxout.*

blood, *n* the fluid circulating through the heart, arteries, capillaries, and veins; carries nutrients and oxygen to body tissues.

blood alcohol concentration (BAC), *n* the amount of ingested alcohol absorbed into the body's cells and intercellular fluid; measured by a percentage based on milligrams of alcohol per deciliter of blood. The higher the BAC, the greater the physical and mental impairment. Most states have a legal limit of 0.10% (100 mg/dL) or lower for intoxication.

blood, arterial, *n* oxygen-rich blood taken away from the heart through the arteries and used as nourishment for the tissues of the body.

blood-borne diseases, *n.pl* disease-causing organisms transferred through contact with blood or other body fluids.

blood-borne pathogens, *n.pl* pathogenic microorganisms that are present in human blood and cause disease in humans.

blood-borne pathogens exposure control plan, *n* a plan that is compliant with Occupational Safety and Health Administration (OSHA) regulations and that explains ways to minimize or eliminate exposure of humans to blood-borne pathogens.

blood-brain barrier, *n* an anatomic-physiologic feature of the brain thought to consist of walls of capillaries in the central nervous system and surrounding glial membranes. It prevents or slows the passage of some drugs, other chemical compounds, radioactive ions, and disease-causing organisms such as viruses from the blood into the nerve tissues of the central nervous system.

blood calcium, *n* the level of calcium in the blood plasma, generally regulated by parathyroid gland activity in conjunction with the degree of calcium ingestion, absorption, use, and excretion. Normal value is 8.5 to 11.5 mg/100 mL of blood serum.

blood cell count, *n* an estimation of the number and types of circulating blood cells (e.g., red blood cells [erythrocytic series], white blood cells, differential).

blood cells, *n.pl* the formed elements of the blood, including red cells (erythrocytes), white cells (leukocytes), and platelets (thrombocytes).

blood chemistry, *n* the determination of the chemical constituents of blood by assay in a clinical laboratory as part of a diagnostic protocol.

blood circulation, *n* the circuit of blood through the body from the heart through the arteries, arterioles, capillaries, venules, and veins and back to the heart.

blood clot, *n* See clot, blood.

blood clotting, *n* the conversion of blood from a free-flowing liquid to a semisolid gel. Within seconds of injury to a blood vessel wall, platelets clump at the site. If normal amounts of calcium, platelets, and tissue factors are present, prothrombin will be converted to thrombin. Thrombin acts as a catalyst for the conversion of fibrinogen to a mesh of insoluble fibrin in which all the formed elements of blood are immobilized. Also called *blood coagulation.*

blood coagulation disorder, *n* a disturbance in the normal clotting mechanism of the blood.

blood, color index of, *n* a figure gained by dividing the hemoglobin percentage by the red blood cell percentage. In most anemias the result is lower than 1, but in pernicious anemia it is characteristically higher than 1.

blood, components of, *n.pl* a cellular fraction consisting of erythrocytes, leukocytes, and platelets, and a noncellular fraction made up of plasma.

blood component transfusion, *n* the administration of one or more elements of blood rather than the whole blood. May include red blood cells, platelets, and other elements.

blood disorders, *n.pl* hematologic dyscrasias that affect the component cells and plasma elements of the blood. They are generally divided into two broad groups: those in which an increase in bulk occurs (e.g., plethora, hydremia, polycythemia) and those in which a decrease in bulk occurs (e.g., anhydremia, dehydration, anemia).

blood dyscrasias (diskrā′zhēəz), *n* the pathologic conditions or disorders such as leukemia or hemophilia in which the constituents of the blood are abnormal or are present in abnormal quantity.

blood gas analysis, *n* the study of gas dissolved in the liquid part of the blood. Blood gases include oxygen, carbon dioxide, and nitrogen, all components of inspired air.

blood glucose level(s), *n/n.pl* the concentration of sugar (chiefly glucose—"true blood sugar") in the blood. It is usually kept within a narrow range by an interplay of many factors: glycogenolysis, glyconeogenesis, intestinal absorption, insulin, insulin antagonists, and other hormones. In the testing of total reducing substances, the normal range of concentration of fasting blood sugar is 80 to 120 mg/mL; in the testing of true blood sugar, the normal range of concentration is 70 to 100 mg/mL. An unusually low level results in hypoglycemia, whereas an abnormally high level causes hyperglycemia; an important level to monitor in diabetic patients, because changes in insulin levels can adversely affect glucose levels. Many methods of measurement are available, both invasive (finger prick) and noninvasive methods (must be used with traditional blood sampling). See also diabetes mellitus.

blood groups, *n.pl* the division of blood into types on the basis of the compatibility of the erythrocytes and serum of one individual with the erythrocytes and serum of another individual. The groups are immunologically and genetically distinct.

blood pressure (BP), *n* the pressure exerted on the arterial walls by the blood when the heart is in systole (systolic pressure), and the pressure maintained by the elasticity of the arteries when the heart is in diastole (diastolic pressure). A consistent arterial pressure greater than 120 over 80 is considered high and suggestive of hypertensive vascular disease. See also hypertension, systole, diastole.

blood pressure classification, n the rating system for blood pressure levels in millimeters of mercury (mm Hg), given as the systolic over the diastolic pressure. Both the systolic and diastolic pressure, if at increased levels, are indicators of concern for cardiovascular problems. Normal is less than 120 over 80; prehypertension is 120-139 over 80-89, stage 1 hypertension is 140-159 over 90-99; stage 2 hypertension is 159 or higher over 99 or higher. See also hypertension.

blood pressure, diastolic, n the pressure in the bloodstream when the heart relaxes and dilates, filling with blood. See also blood pressure; blood, pressure, stages; and diastole.

blood pressure, systolic, n the pressure exerted on the bloodstream by the heart when it contracts, forcing blood from the ventricles of the heart into the pulmonary artery and the aorta. See also blood pressure; blood, pressure, stages; and systole.

blood pressure cuff, n a part of a sphygmomanometer that fits over the patient's arm. It comes in four sizes, for children up to obese adults. It should be made of a nonelastic material, and the cuff used should be about 20% bigger than the arm it fits over— an undersized cuff will cause the blood pressure reading to appear higher than it is in reality, whereas an oversized cuff will cause the reading to appear too low.

blood pressure stages, n any of the three stages of hypertension marked by elevated blood pressure. Stage I is 140-159 over 90-99; Stage II is 160-179 over 100-109; Stage III is 180-209 over 110-119.

blood products, n the constituents of whole blood such as plasma or platelets that are used in replacement therapy.

blood transfusion, n the administration of whole blood or a component such as packed red cells to replace blood lost through trauma, surgery, or disease.

blood urea nitrogen *(BUN),* n the nitrogen in the form of urea in whole blood or serum. Its concentration is a gross measure of renal function. The upper limit of the normal range is 25 mg/100 mL.

blood, venous, n the deoxygenated blood that is returned from tissues throughout the body to the heart, then pumped into the lungs for reoxygenation.

blood vessel(s), n/n.pl the network of muscular tubes that carry blood. The kinds of blood vessels are arteries, arterioles, capillaries, venules, and veins.

blood vessels, periodontal ligament, n.pl a well-developed vascular system that enters the periodontal ligament and supplies blood to all the regions surrounding the tooth.

blood vessels, pulp, n.pl a well-developed vascular system that enters the apical foramen of the tooth and supplies blood to the pulp tissue.

blood, volume index of, n the volume of red blood cells divided by the total volume of blood times 100 times the volume percent of packed red blood cells (hematocrit index). A value greater than 1 indicates an abnormally large number or size of erythrocytes.

blower, chip, n See syringe, air, hand.

blowpipe, n a torch that employs gas-oxygen, or oxygen and acetylene, to melt metal in dental casting and soldering procedures.

blue, methylene (meth′əlēn), n **1.** a dye used to color bacteria for microscopic examination. n **2.** an aniline dye sometimes used as an antiseptic in the treatment of periodontal disease by photodisinfection.

blue nevus, n See nevus, blue.

BMR, n See basal metabolic rate.

board certification, n the examination program that establishes the clinical proficiency of a dental specialist according to the procedures established by the individual specialty certification board under the rules and authority of the Council on Dental Education of the American Dental Association.

board certified, adj the status of a dental specialist (such as an orthodontist) who has become a board diplomate by successfully completing the certification program of the recognized certification board in that area of practice.

board diplomate, *n* a dental specialist who has achieved certification by the recognized certifying board in that specialty, as attested by a diploma from the board.

board eligible, *adj* the status of a dental specialist whose educational qualifications have been verified by acceptance of an application for certification by the recognized certifying board. Board eligibility depends on advanced education in the specialty and timely progress toward completion of the certification procedure. Regular renewal is required to maintain eligibility until the examination is completed.

board qualified, *adj* an unrecognized term used variously and inaccurately to identify any of the stages from educational qualification to certification.

bodily movement, *n* See movement, body.

body, *n* any mass or collection of material.

body burden, *n* the activity of a radiopharmaceutical retained by the body at a specified time after administration.

body dysmorphic disorder (BDD), *n* See disorder, body dysmorphic.

body fluid, *n* a liquid portion of the body such as plasma, lymph, tears, saliva, and urine.

body, foreign, *n* an object or material that is not normal for the area in which it is located.

body height, *n* the overall length of the body from the crown to the bottom of the feet, usually taken in the standing position. Body length refers to the overall length taken in the supine position.

body image, *n* a person's subjective concept of personal physical appearance. The loss of a limb, breast, or tooth may cause psychologic trauma because of unresolved conflict in the change of body image. A distorted body image may be a causal factor in anorexia nervosa and bulimia. See also disorder, body dysmorphic (BDD).

body, ketone, *n* any of the compounds acetoacetic acid, betahydroxybutyric acid, and acetone that are formed in the liver and released in the blood. Elevated levels occur during excessive fat use such as in diabetes or starvation. See also ketoacidosis.

body mass index (BMI) calculation, *n* a method for assessing obesity and determining optimal weight, which involves dividing body weight in kilograms by height in square meters.

body mechanics, *n* the field of physiology that investigates actions and functions of the muscular system relating to body posture maintenance.

body, Schaumann's **(shou′mänz),** *n.pr* a round to oval cytoplasmic inclusion composed of concentric deposits of an amorphous material. Present in the giant cells of sarcoidosis, in beryllium lesions, and sometimes in other giant cells.

body shields, *n.pl* protective coverings patients are sometimes legally required to wear during radiographic examinations; usually a leaded apron containing lead 0.25 mm thick. The protective surface covers the torso and gonads.

body temperature, *n* the level of heat produced and sustained by body processes. Variations and changes in body temperature are major indicators of disease and other abnormalities.

Boeck's disease (boeks), *n.pr* See sarcoidosis.

Boeck's sarcoid, *n.pr* See sarcoidosis.

Bogarad's syndrome, *n.pr* See syndrome, Frey.

Bohn's nodules, *n* See cysts, palatal, of the newborn.

boil (furuncle), *n* a painful skin lesion caused by infection of a hair follicle, characterized by a central core surrounded by inflamed tissue.

boil, gum, *n* See parulis.

Boley gauge, *n.pr* See gauge, Boley.

Bolton analysis, *n.pr* a computation developed by Wayne Bolton for the evaluation of tooth size discrepancies between maxillary and mandibular arches.

Bolton-nasion plane, *n.pr* See plane, Bolton-nasion.

Bolton plane, *n.pr* See plane, Bolton-nasion.

Bolton point, triangle, *n.pr* See point, Bolton and triangle, Bolton.

bolus (bō′ləs), *n* a mass of food ready to be swallowed or a mass passing through the intestines.

bond, *n* the force that holds two or more units of matter together.

bond, peptide **(pep′tīd),** *n.pl* the linking mechanisms that bind together the amino acid building blocks of proteins.

bond, primary, *n* a chemical bond that requires some change in structure of matter. Primary bonds are ionic, covalent, or metallic.

bond, secondary, *n* a physical bond (sometimes called *van der Waals forces*) that involves weak interatomic attractions such as variations in physical mass or location of electrical charge.

bond strength, *n* the force with which a sealant holds fast to the surface of a tooth.

bonding, *n* an adhesion of orthodontic attachments to the teeth without use of an interposed band.

bonding agent, *n* See agent, bonding.

bonding, chemical, *n* the process of using a chemical in order to form a bond to the structure of the tooth. It is facilitated by the sharing and exchanging of electrons in order to form an arranged structure.

bonding, dentin, *n* the attachment of dental material to the dentin of tooth through various means, and the strength of that attachment.

bonding, direct, *n* direct placement of orthodontic brackets to the etched enamel surface using self cure or light cure adhesive.

bonding, enamel, *v* the process of adhering a coating, or liquid enamel, to the surface of a tooth. It is utilized for various aesthetic and functional reasons, including the repair of caries and chipped or cracked surfaces or to cover exposed roots caused by gingival recession. See also sealant, enamel.

bonding, indirect, *n* the positioning of orthodontic brackets on a dental cast and transfer of them to the teeth en masse for adhesion by means of a molded plastic matrix.

bone, *n* **I.** the material of the skeletons of the tissue composing bones. *n* **2.** dense, hard, and slightly elastic connective tissue in which the fibers are impregnated with a form of calcium phosphate similar to hydroxyapatite. *n* **3.** the bones of the human skeleton. *n* **4.** a single element of the skeleton such as a rib or femur.

bone, alveolar **(alvē′ələr),** *n* the specialized bone structure that contains the alveoli or sockets of the teeth and supports the teeth.

bone, alveolar, architecture, *n* the structural pattern of the alveolar bone and its subjacent latticework of supporting bone. The alveolar bone is thin and compact adjacent to the periodontal ligament. The trabecular bone connects and reinforces the individual alveoli. The architecture of a bone is the result of functional stimuli to that bone; the stimuli vary according to type, intensity, and duration.

bone, alveolar, metabolism, *n* the metabolic activity occurring within alveolar bone, which is generally slower than that occurring within metaphyseal bone but more rapid than that of diaphyseal bone.

bone apposition, *n* See bone deposition.

bone augmentation, *n* a term used to describe a variety of bone grafting procedures to build or enhance a deficient area of bone, usually in preparation for a dental implant site. Bone augmentation materials can be autogenous, allogenous, xenogenous, or allopastic sources.

bone, basal, *n* the part of the mandible and maxilla from which the alveolar process develops.

bone, bundle, *n* a histologic term for the portion of the bone of the alveolar process that surrounds teeth and into which the collagen fibers of the periodontal ligament are embedded. Bundle bone is functionally dependent in that it resorbs following tooth extraction or loss.

bone bur, *n* a drill designed to cut into bone.

bone, cadaver, *n* bone that has been donated for medical purposes from one person to another; used especially in bone grafting procedures. See also allogenic and allografts.

bone calcium content, *n* the amount of calcium stored in bone tissue. Plasma calcium is in constant exchange with the calcium of the extracellular fluid and bones. The parathyroid gland maintains the constancy of the calcium concentration in the plasma. The bones serve as a reservoir of calcium and phosphate to provide for the other needs of the

bone, cancellous (spongy bone, supporting bone, trabecular bone), *n* the bone that forms a trabecular network, surrounds marrow spaces that may contain either fatty or hematopoietic tissue, lies subjacent to the cortical bone, and makes up the main portion of a bone.

bone, cancellous, atrophy of disuse **(kan′seləs),** *n* the wasting of bone tissue occurring with loss of function of a part (e.g., a tooth). The supporting bone assumes an osteoporotic nature, and the marrow remains fatty or hematopoietic.

bone cells, *n.pl* the group includes osteoblasts, osteocytes, osteoclasts, and osteoprogenitor cells.

bone changes, mechanical factors, *n.pl* the pressure and tension forces that play an important role in determining bone structure. Improperly controlled appliances can resorb bone faster than deposition can occur, causing mobile teeth and traumatic occlusion. Poor vascularity as a concomitant cause of undue pressure and tension and may inhibit repair and cause necrosis.

bone chips, *n.pl* the small pieces of cancellous bone generally used to fill in bony defects and precipitate recalcification.

bone, compact, *n* the hard, dense bone composing the outer cortical layer and consisting of periosteal bone, endosteal bone, and haversian systems. Also known as *cortical bone.*

bone conduction, *n* See conduction, bone.

bone crest, *n* the most coronal portion of alveolar bone.

bone cyst, *n* **1.** a vascular cyst eccentrically placed within a bone. *n* **2.** ostitis fibrosa cystica, a parathyroid disorder characterized by cyst formation and the replacement of bone tissue with fibrous connective tissue.

bone defects, angular, *n.pl* a vertical defect in crestal bone adjacent to a tooth that results from inflammatory periodontal disease and/or occlusal trauma.

bone density, *n* the compactness of bone tissue. The demonstration of bone density by means of radiographs directly depends on the quantity of

inorganic salts contained in the bone tissue.

bone deposition, *n* the apposition or formation of new bone as a normal physiologic process.

bone development, *n* See bone, endochondral, formation; bone formation; and bone, intramembranous, formation.

bone, effect of external radiation to, *n* damage to the bones of adults is most often seen after heavy and localized radiation treatment.

bone, endochondral **(en′dōkon′drəl),** *n* a bone that is developed in relation to antecedent cartilages (e.g., long bones, mandible). See also bone, intramembranous.

bone, endochondral, formation, *n* a replacement of previously formed embryonic cartilage with an adult bony structure. The actual replacement of cartilage by bone is only part of the process, however; much of the bone is laid down directly external to the embryonic cartilage. See also bone, membrane, formation.

bone formation, *n* the deposition of an organic mucopolysaccharide matrix (osteoid) that is subsequently mineralized with calcium salts. See also bone apposition and bone deposition.

bone graft, autogenous **(ôtoj′ənəs),** *n* See graft, autogenous bone.

bone graft, donor site, *n* See donor site.

bone graft, onlay, *n* See graft, onlay bone.

bone graft, recipient site, *n* See recipient site.

bone groove, *n* an osteotomy into or near the crest of the alveolar ridge for placement of an endosteal blade type of implant.

bone groove, canted, *n* an osteotomy sloped to avoid the mandibular canal or keep the implant infrastructure within the medullary confines.

bone, horizontal loss of, *n* a resorption of bone caused by periodontal inflammation in which the bone crest remains even with the cementoenamel junctions of two adjoining teeth. The condition may be localized or generalized.

bone, internal reconstruction of, *n* the formation of bone on the tensional side of the periodontal ligament with concurrent resorption from the marrow space; contralaterally, resorption of alveolar bone with apposition from the endosteum in the marrow space.

bone, interproximal, *n* the bone that forms the septa between the teeth; consists primarily of a spongy supporting bone covered by a layer of cortical bone. See also septum, interdental.

bone, intramembranous, *n* a bone developed within a membrane but having no associated cartilage (e.g., parietal, frontal, bones of upper face). See also bone, endochondral.

bone, intramembranous, formation, *n* membrane bone forms directly from the mesenchyme, first as a thin, flattened, irregular bony plate or membrane in the dermis and gradually expanding at its margins and becoming thickened by the deposition of successive layers of additional bone on the inner and outer surfaces. See also bone, endochondral, formation.

bone involvement, *n* changes in the alveolar and supporting bone occurring as a sequel to or accompanying inflammatory or dystrophic disease; usually of a resorptive nature.

bone, lacrimal (lak′riməl), *n* the small, fragile, paired facial bone that helps form a part of the orbital wall and also a small part of the nasal cavity. The bone has four borders and two surfaces that articulate with four other facial bones.

bone lamella, *n* bone having the appearance of layers of thin leaves or plates. This appearance is produced by lines representing periods of inactivity of bone formation.

bone, malar (zygomatic bone), frontal process of, *n* a prominence on the zygomatic bone (cheekbone) that forms the anterior lateral orbital wall.

bone, malar (zygomatic bone), maxillary process of (zī′gəmat′ik mā′lər mak′sələr′ē), *n* a prominence on the zygomatic bone (cheekbone) that forms part of the inferior rim of the orbit and a small part of the orbital wall.

bone, malar (zygomatic bone), temporal process of, *n* a prominence on the inferior aspect of the zygomatic bone (cheekbone) that articulates with the zygomatic process of temporal bone to form the zygomatic arch.

bone, marble, *n* See osteopetrosis.

bone marrow, *n* the soft vascular tissue that fills bone cavities and cancellous bone spaces and consists primarily of fat cells, hematopoietic cells, and osteogenetic reticular cells.

bone marrow transplant, *n* the transplantation of bone marrow from healthy donors to stimulate production of formed blood cells. It is used in treatment of hematopoietic or lymphoreticular diseases such as aplastic anemia, leukemia, immune deficiency syndromes, and acute radiation syndrome.

bone membranes, *n.pl* the membrane structures associated with the growth, development, and repair of bone. They include the periosteum, a connective tissue layer adjacent to bone surfaces; periodontal ligament, a modified periosteum associated with tooth structure; and endosteum, a thin layer of connective tissue lining the walls of the bone marrow spaces.

bone, microscopic appearance of, *n* the composition of bone tissue as viewed under a microscope. Microscopically, bone is composed of osteocytes embedded within lacunae in a calcified intercellular matrix. Extending from the lacunae are small canals called canaliculi, which communicate with canaliculi of adjacent lacunae. Through this system of canals, nutrient material reaches the osteocytes and provides avenues for the removal of waste products of metabolism. It is deposited in incremental layers (lamellae) around haversian canals, the lamellae toward the surface of the bone being more or less parallel to it.

bone mineral content, chemistry of, *n* the hardness of bone results from its mineral content in the organic matrix. The minerals (commonly designated as bone salts) and the organic matrix make up the interstitial substance of bone. The bone salts consist essentially of hydroxyapatite $(Ca_{10}[PO_4]_6[OH_2])$, carbon dioxide, and water, with small amounts of other ions.

bone morphogenetic protein (BMP), *n* See protein, bone morphogenetic (BMP).

bone, normal level of, *n* the distance from the interdental bone crest to the cementoenamel junction in healthy teeth, usually 1 to 1.5 mm.

bone, occipital (əksip'itəl), *n* the saucer-shaped cranial bone that forms the most posterior part of the skull; the spinal cord passes through the foramen magnum, an opening at its base.

bone onlay, *n* See graft, onlay bone.

bone, perichondrial (perikon'drēəl), *n* bone that is deposited in concentric layers around the long shaft of the bone in a manner similar to that of the growth of endochondral bone.

bone, physical properties of, *n* a compact bone has the following physical characteristics: specific gravity, 1.92 to 1.99; tensile strength, 13,000 to 17,000 psi; compressive strength, 18,000 to 24,000 psi; compressive strength parallel to the long axis, 7150 psi; compressive strength at right angles to the long axis, 10,800 psi. These physical characteristics make bone particularly suitable for carrying out its functions of weight bearing, leverage, and protection of vulnerable viscera.

bone rarefaction (rar'əfak'shən), *n* a decreased density of bone such as a decrease in weight per unit of volume.

bone recession, *n* See recession, bone.

bone, resorption and repair of, *n* an adaptive physiologic mechanism occurring as long as the individual retains the natural dentition. See also resorption of bone.

bone, resting lines in, *n.pl* the regular lines created by alternating periods of bone formation and rest, giving a tierlike appearance to lamellar bone.

bone, reversal lines in, *n.pl* the irregular lines containing concavities directed away from the bundle bone and serving as histologic indications that resorption has taken place up to that line from the marrow side.

bone sequestrum, *n* See sequestrum.

bone, spongy, *n* See bone, cancellous.

bone support, *n* the amount of alveolar and trabecular bone adjacent to a tooth that can provide attachment, investment, and support for the tooth.

bone, supporting, *n* See bone, cancellous.

bone, supporting, atrophy of disuse, *n* See bone, cancellous, atrophy of disuse.

bone surgery, *n* See surgery, osseous.

bone, thickened margin of, *n* the widening of the crest of the alveolus, primarily on the buccal and lingual aspects, varying from a thick ledge to a "beading" of the bone margin; results in a more or less bulbous contour of the gingival tissue overlying it.

bone, trabecular (trəbek'yələr), *n* See bone, cancellous.

bone, vertical loss of, *n* apically directed resorption of bone caused by periodontal disease with or without occlusal trauma, in which the bone crest in one location (e.g. adjacent to a tooth) has moved apically more than the surrounding area resulting in an angular pattern. It can be localized (mainly) or generalized.

bone, vertical plates of the palatine, *n* the thin, oblong-shaped bone with two surfaces and four borders. It helps to form the floor of the orbit, the outer wall of the nasal cavity, and several adjoining structures.

bone volume (mass), age-affecting, *n* decreases that occur in human body bone mass after age 40. Diet and exercise may be contributing factors.

bone wax, *n* See wax, bone.

bone, woven, *n* a character and pattern of bone resulting from the interweaving of broad bands of skull.

bone(s), cranial, *n/n.pl* the eight bones that make up the cranium and protect the brain and include the ethmoid, frontal, occipital, sphenoid, two parietal, and two temporal bones.

bone(s), facial, *n/n.pl* the 14 bones that include the mandible, maxilla, frontal bones, nasal bones, and zygoma. With the exception of the mandible, maxilla, and vomer bones, the bones of the face occur in pairs, thus accounting for facial symmetry. They provide the framework for the face, serve as entry points for the digestive and respiratory systems, and provide the attachments for the muscles controlling facial expression.

bone(s), horizontal plates of pala-tine, *n/n.pl* the bones that form the posterior part of the hard palate and consist of four borders and two surfaces.

Bonwill-Hawley chart, *n.pr* See chart, Hawley.

Bonwill's triangle, *n* See triangle, Bonwill's.

bony crater, *n* a concave resorptive defect in the alveolar crest, often occurring interdentally but may also be observed at other surfaces and possibly completely surrounding a tooth.

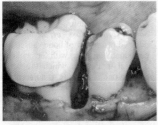

Bony crater. (Courtesy Dr. Perry Klokkevold)

bony crepitus, *n* See crepitus, bony.

borax, *n* a principal ingredient in casting fluxes. Used in gypsum products as a retardant for the setting reaction and a strengthener for hydrocolloids.

border, *n* a circumferential margin or edge.

border, denture (denture edge, denture periphery), *n* the limit, boundary, or circumferential margin of a denture base.

border, mandibular (mandibular plane), *n* a tangent to the inferior border of the mandible. A line joining point gonion to point gnathion.

border molding, *n* the shaping of an impression material by the manipulation or action of the tissues to determine the denture border position.

border movement, *n* See movement, border.

border seal, *n* the contact of the denture border with the underlying or adjacent tissues to prevent the passage of air or other substances.

border structures, *n.pl* the oral structures that bound the borders of a denture.

border tissues, movement, *n* the action of the muscles and other structures adjacent to the borders of a denture.

Bordetella pertussis (bor'dətel'ə pertus'is), *n.pl* the infectious bacteria responsible for whooping cough (pertussis), which is spread from person to person by direct contact with mucosal discharges.

Botulinum toxin (type A and type B) *n brand names:* Botox (type A), Myobloc (type B); *drug class:* inhibitor of acetylcholine from nerve endings; *action:* blocks the influx of calcium into the nerve terminal; *uses:* strabismus, ocular deviations, blepharospasms, skeletal muscle dystonias, relax facial muscle to prevent wrinkling.

boutons terminaux (bööt'ons ter'minō), *n.pl* See end-feet.

Bowen's disease, *n.pr* See carcinoma in situ.

box, light, *n* See illuminator.

boxing, *n* the building up of vertical walls, usually in wax, around an impression to produce the desired size and form of the base of the cast.

boxing strip, *n* See strip, boxing.

brace, *n* an orthotic device to support and hold part of the body in the correct position to allow function, such as a leg brace that permits walking and standing. Sometimes used to describe orthodontic appliances.

brachycephalic (brak'isəfal'ik), *adj* descriptive term applied to a broad, round head having a cephalic index of more than 80.

brachydactyly (brā'kēdak'təlē), *n* an abnormal shortness of the fingers, usually associated with some congenital syndrome.

brachygnathia (bird-face, micrognathia) (brak'ignā'thēə), *n* marked underdevelopment of the mandible; *adj* brachygnathous. See also retrognathism.

bracing, *n* a resistance to the horizontal components of masticatory force.

bracket, *n* a small slotted metal attachment bonded to a tooth that serves as a means of fastening an arch wire to the tooth. Brackets may also be welded to a band that is cemented to the tooth to receive the arch wire.

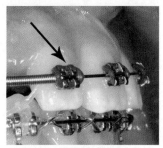

Bracket. (Courtesy Dr. Flavio Uribe)

▶ **bradycardia (brad′ikär′dēə),** *n* an abnormal slowness of the heart as evidenced by a slowing of the pulse rate (less than 50 beats per minute).

bradydiastole (brad′idīas′tōle), *n* an abnormal prolongation of diastole.

bradykinesia (brad′ikinē′zhə), *n* an irregular slowness in motions and reflexes.

bradykinin (brā′dəkī′nin), *n* one of a number of plasma kinins, a potent vasodilator; physiologic mediators of an anaphylactic reaction.

bradypnea (brad′ipnē′ə), *n* an abnormal slowness of breathing.

Braille (brāl), *n.pr* a printing and writing system using elevated dots to represent letters. The system allows those individuals with limited or no visual ability to read via touch.

brain, *n* the portion of the central nervous system that is enclosed within the cranium, continuous with the spinal cord, and composed of gray matter and white matter. It is the primary center for the regulation and control of bodily activities, receiving and interpreting sensory impulses, and transmitting information to the muscles and body organs. It is also the seat of consciousness, thought, memory, and emotion. Also called *encephalon.*

brain death, *n* an irreversible form of unconsciousness characterized by a complete loss of brain function while the heart continues to beat.

brain, electrical activity of, *n* the electrical energy that can be observed as waves with electroencephalographic equipment. These rhythms and patterns have been organized into a system that imputes values for the state of health and disease. Electrical evidence of it in the cerebral cortex reveals that different potential patterns are produced by different states of mental activity (e.g., tension, mental work, sleep).

brainstem, *n* the portion of the brain comprising the medulla oblongata, pons, and mesencephalon. It performs motor, sensory, and reflex functions.

branchial apparatus, *n* the group of structures that includes the branchial arches, branchial grooves and membranes, and the pharyngeal pouches.

branchial arches, *n.pl* the six stacked bilateral swellings of tissue that appear inferior to the stomodeum and include the mandibular arch.

branchial grooves, *n.pl* the grooves between neighboring branchial arches on each side of the embryo.

branchial nerve, *n* See nerve, branchial.

brand name, *n* a name given to a product by its manufacturer that becomes part of the product's identity.

Branemark technique, *n.pr* See osseointegration.

breach of contract, *n* See contract, breach of.

break-even point, *n* the level of patient visits or net revenues at which the revenues for a period are equal to the expenses incurred in that period.

breath, *n* the air inhaled and exhaled in respiration.

breath, bad (offensive), *n* See halitosis.

breathing check, *n* a series of steps, based on the pneumonic ABCD (*Airway, Breathing, Circulation, Disability*), used to determine the respiratory status of a patient in respiratory distress.

breathing, Kussmaul (kōōs′môl), *n. pr* a deep, slow breathing that requires great effort, which often occurs during a diabetic coma.

breathing, oral cavity, *n* the process of inspiration and expiration of air primarily through the oral cavity. It is commonly seen in nasal conditions such as deviated septum, hypertrophied adenoids, and allergies and may produce excessive drying of the oral mucosa with a tendency to gingival hyperplasia and inflammation of mainly the maxillary anterior teeth.

breathing, rescue, *n* an emergency treatment aimed at restoring natural respiration in a person who has stopped breathing in which the rescuer inflates the victim's lungs by breathing air into his or her oral cavity or nose directly or through a ventilation device. The technique may be combined with cardiac compressions if the victim has no pulse.

bregma (breg′mə), *n* the point at which the sagittal and coronary sutures meet.

Breuer's reflex, *n.pr* See reflex, Hering-Breuer.

▣ **bridge,** *n* a colloquial expression for a fixed partial denture. See also denture, partial, fixed.

bridge, cantilever, *n* See denture, partial, fixed, cantilever.

bridge, fixed, *n* See denture, partial, fixed.

bridge, removable, *n* a colloquial expression for a removable partial denture. See also denture, partial, removable.

bridge splint, *n* See splint, fixed.

Brill-Symmers disease, *n.pr* See lymphoma, giant follicular.

Brinell hardness number, *n.pr* See number, Brinell hardness.

Brinell hardness test, *n.pr* See test, Brinell hardness.

brittle, friable, *adj* technically a brittle material is one in which the proportional limit and ultimate strength are close together in value. See also ductility.

broach, *n* an instrument with numerous barbs protruding from a metal shaft. It is generally used to engage the dental pulp for extirpation.

broach, barbed, *n* See broach.

broach holder, *n* an instrument similar to a pin vise used to hold a broach.

broach, pathfinder, *n* See broach, smooth.

broach, smooth (pathfinder, pathfinder broach), *n* an instrument used for locating the opening of a root canal and exploring the canal to determine the accessibility of the root end.

broad spectrum, *adj* indicates that a chemical can be used for its intended function with a wide variety of microbes.

Broders' classification, *n.pr* See index, Broders'.

bromide (brō′mīd), *n* a broad-acting chemical agent used to disinfect surfaces in the dental environment; comes in tablet form and is for use on hard surfaces only.

bromine (brō′mēən), *n* a toxic, red-brown, liquid element of the halogen group. Bromine is widely used in industry, photography, the manufacture of organic chemicals, and pharmaceuticals.

bromism (brō′mizəm), *n* the toxic state induced by excessive exposure to or ingestion of bromine or bromine-containing compounds.

bromocriptine mesylate (brō′mō krip′tēn mes′ilāt′), *n brand name:* Parlodel; *drug class:* dopamine receptor agonist; *action:* inhibits prolactin release by activating postsynaptic dopamine receptors; *uses:* hyperprolactinemia, acromegaly, Parkinson's disease.

bromopnea (brəmop′nēə), *n* See halitosis.

brompheniramine maleate (brom ′fənē′rəmēn mā′lēāt), *n brand names:* Bromphen, Dehist, Veltane; *drug class:* antihistamine, histamine H1- receptor antagonist; *action:* acts on blood vessels and gastrointestinal and respiratory systems by competing with histamine for H1-receptor sites; *uses:* treatment of allergy symptoms, rhinitis.

bronchia (brong′kēə), *n.pl* the bronchial tubes smaller than bronchi and larger than bronchioles.

bronchiarctia (brong′kēärk′shēə), *n* the stenosis of a bronchial tube.

bronchiectasis (brong′kēek′təsis), *n* a chronic disease characterized by dilation of the bronchi and bronchioles, clinically recognizable by fetid breath and purulent matter; dilation of the bronchi, either local or general.

bronchiocele (brong′kēō sēl), *n* a dilation or swelling of a branch smaller than a bronchus.

▣ **bronchiole (brong′kēōl),** *n* a terminal division of a bronchium.

▣ **bronchitis (brongkī′tis),** *n* an acute or chronic inflammation of the mucous membranes of the tracheobronchial tree.

bronchium (brong′kēəm), *n* one of the subdivisions of a bronchus.

bronchoalveolar, *adj* referring to both the bronchia and alveoli of the lungs.

bronchoconstriction (brong'kōkən strik'shən), *n* the reduction of the caliber of the bronchi.

bronchodilation (brong'kōdīlā'sh ən), *n* the dilation of a bronchus; the operation of dilating a stenosed bronchus.

bronchodilator (brong'kōdīlā'tur), *n* a drug that dilates, or expands, the size of the lumina of the air passages of the lungs by relaxing the muscular walls.

bronchopneumonia (bron'kōnəmō 'nyə), *n* an acute inflammation of the lungs and bronchioles characterized by chills, fever, high pulse and respiratory rates, bronchial breathing, cough with purulent bloody sputum, severe chest pain, and abdominal distension.

bronchoscope, *n* a curved flexible tube for visual examination of the bronchi.

bronchoscopy (bronkos'kəpē'), *n* the visual examination of the tracheobronchial tree using a standard rigid, tubular metal bronchoscope or a narrower, flexible, fiberoptic bronchoscope. Bronchoscopy is used to secure a biopsy, aspirate fluids, and diagnose such conditions as lung abscess, bronchial obstruction, and localized atelectasis.

bronchospasm (brong'kōspaz'əm), *n* a spasmodic contraction of the muscular coat of the bronchial tubes such as occurs in asthma.

bronchostenosis (brong'kōstənō' sis), *n* the stenosis of the bronchi; bronchiarctia.

bronchus, *n* the subdivisions of the trachea serving to convey air to and from the lungs.

Brooke's tumor, *n.pr* See epithelioma adenoides cysticum.

brow lift, *n* a plastic surgery procedure designed to rejuvenate the upper ⅓ of the face or the area above the brow.

brow lift, petrichial, *n* incision is made in the front of the hairline at the top of the forehead. Also called *hairline browlift.*

brow lift, transpalpbral, *n* the incisions are made only in the upper eyelid creases.

brow lift, trichophytic, *n* the incision is placed directly in the hairline in a wavy fashion, camouflaging the incision.

brown dental stains, *n* the dark, mottled spots on teeth that may indicate fluorosis; may be caused by a prolonged exposure to a high concentration of fluoride during a crucial time in tooth development.

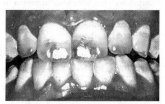

Brown dental stains. (Casamassimo, et al, 2013)

brown pellicle, *n* See pellicle, brown.

bruise, *n* a contusion or ecchymosis; injury, usually caused by blunt impact, in which the capillaries are damaged, allowing blood to seep into the surrounding tissue. Normally minor but painful. Can be serious, leading to hematoma, or can be associated with serious injuries, including fractures and internal bleeding. Minor ones are easily recognized by their characteristic blue or purple color in the days following the injury.

bruit (brōō'ē), *n* an extracardiac blowing sound heard at times over peripheral vessels; generally denotes cardiovascular disease.

brush, bristle polishing, *n* a polishing brush with natural or synthetic bristles.

brush, clasp, *n* a uniquely conceived tool, made to clean the clasps that connect a prosthesis to the natural teeth. Because the clasps are in a critical and difficult to reach position, the 2- to 3-inch tool features a twisted, tapered brush that removes plaque and other debris.

brush, Dixon bristle, *n* a soft brush used to polish the nonmetal parts of removable dentures.

brush, interdental, *n* a small dental brush designed to be used between teeth. It may be placed in a handle that enables enhanced interproximal maneuverability during oral care.

brush, interproximal, *n* See brush, interdental.

brush, polishing, *n* an instrument consisting of natural, synthetic, or wire bristles mounted on a mandrel or in a hub to fit on a lathe chuck; used to carry abrasive or polishing media to polish teeth, restorations, and prosthetic appliances.

brush, wheel polishing, *n* a polishing brush with bristles mounted similar to spokes of a wheel.

brush, wire polishing, *n* a polishing brush with bristles of wire, usually steel or brass.

brushing, *n* See abrasion, denture.

brushing plane, *n* See plane, brushing.

bruxism (bruk'sizəm), *n* the involuntary gnashing, grinding, or clenching of teeth. It is usually an unconscious activity, whether the individual is awake or asleep; often associated with fatigue, anxiety, emotional stress, or fear and frequently triggered by occlusal irregularities, usually resulting in abnormal wear patterns on the teeth, periodontal breakdown, and joint or neuromuscular problems.

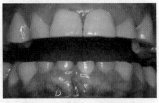

Bruxism. (Perry/Beemsterboer, 2007)

BSP test, *n* See test, Bromsulphalein.

bubo (byōō'bō), *n* a lymph node that is enlarged as a result of an infection. The process may lead to suppuration; seen in primary syphilis, chancroid, plague, malaria, and other infectious processes.

buccal (buk'əl), *adj* pertaining to or adjacent to the cheek.

buccal aspect, *n* See aspect, buccal.

buccal contour, *n* See contour, buccal.

▣ *buccal corridor width* **(buk'əl kor'idər),** *n* the negative space between the buccal surface of the maxillary first premolar and the inner point at which the lips join when the patient smiles. It is often stated as a ratio of the inner lip commissure width divided by the distance between the first maxillary premolars.

buccal flange, *n* See flange, buccal.

buccal lymph nodes, *n* See lymph nodes, buccal.

buccal mucosa, *n* See mucosa, oral.

buccal notch, *n* See notch, buccal.

buccal shelf, *n* See shelf, buccal.

buccal splint, *n* See splint, buccal.

buccal surface, *n* See surface, buccal.

buccal tube, *n* See tube, buccal.

buccal vestibule, *n* See vestibule, buccal.

▣ **buccinator muscle (buk'sinātər),** *n* the muscle consisting of three bands and composing the wall of the cheek between the mandible and the maxilla; it causes the cheek to stay tight to the teeth and the lip corners to pull inward. It is often known as the "cheek muscle."

buccoclusion (buk'ōklōō'zhən), *n* an occlusion in which the dental arch or group of teeth is buccal to the normal position.

buccolingual relationship (buk'ō ling'gwəl), *n* See relationship, buccolingual.

buccolingual stress, *n* See stress, buccolingual.

buccoversion (buk'ōvur'zhən), *n* a deviation from the normal line of occlusion toward the cheeks.

buck knife, *n* See knife, buck.

buckling, *n* the crowding of anterior teeth in the dental arch.

buclizine HCl (buk'lizēn), *n* brand name: Bucladin S; drug class: antihistamine, histamine H1-receptor antagonist; action: acts centrally by blocking chemoreceptor trigger zone; use: treatment for motion sickness.

▣ **bud stage,** *n* the second stage in the development of a tooth; it is the result of the proliferation of cells in the basal layer of the oral epithelium.

budesonide (byōōdes'ōnīd'), *n* brand names: Rhinocort Nasal Inhaler, Pulmicort; drug class: corticosteroid, synthetic; action: binds to steroid receptors to inhibit phospholipase A_2 and to induce antiinflammatory effects; uses: management of symptoms of allergic rhinitis in adults and children; perennial nonallergic rhinitis in adults.

budget plan, *n* a method of financing dental accounts in which arrangements are made for the patient to pay a series of small amounts on an account, usually over a period of 12 to 18 months.

buffer, *n* a substance in a fluid that tends to lessen the change in hydrogen ion concentration that otherwise would be produced by adding acids or alkalis.

buffer time, *n* time reserved on the schedule for emergency patients.

buffering capacity, *n* the body's ability to neutralize the acids that play a role in the demineralization of teeth; may be enhanced by eating firmly textured foods, which improve chewing and stimulate the flow of saliva.

bulb, speech, *n* See aid, speech, prosthetic, pharyngeal section.

bulimarexia (bōōlim′ərek′sēə), *n* an eating disorder distinguished by a combination of the symptoms prevalent in both anorexia nervosa and bulimia nervosa; develops primarily in teenage and young adult females.

bulimia (bəlē′mēə), *n* repeated secretive bouts of excessive eating followed by self-induced vomiting, purging, and anorexia, usually accompanied by feelings of guilt, depression, and self-disgust. Oral signs may include dental erosion of the lingual surface of the maxillary anterior teeth.

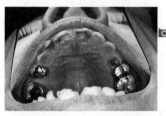

Lingual erosion caused by bulimia.
(Ibsen/Phelan, 2009)

bulla (bŏŏl′ə), *n* a circumscribed, elevated lesion of the skin containing fluid and measuring more than 5 mm in diameter.

bumetanide (byōōmet′ənīd′), *n* brand name: Bumex; *drug class:* loop diuretic; *action:* acts on the loop of Henle to decrease cotransport and reabsorption of chloride, sodium, and potassium with resultant diuresis;

uses: treatment of edema in chronic heart disease, renal disease, pulmonary edema, ascites, and hypertension.

BUN, *n* See blood urea nitrogen.

Bunnell test, *n.pr* See test, Paul-Bunnell.

Bunyaviridae **(bun′yəvir′idā),** *n* a grouping of enveloped, helix-shaped ribonucleic acid (RNA) viruses, implicated in certain forms of encephalitis and sandfly fever.

bupivacaine HCl (local) (byōōpiv′ə kān′), *n* brand names: Marcaine, Senorcaine; *drug class:* amide local anesthetic; *actions:* inhibits ion fluxes across membranes, particularly sodium transport across cell membranes; decreases rise of depolarization phase of action potential; blocks nerve action potential; *uses:* local dental anesthesia (which provides long duration of action), epidural anesthesia, peripheral nerve block, caudal anesthesia.

buprenorphine *n* brand name: Buprenex; *drug class:* opioid μ-receptor partial agonist, κ-receptor agonist; *action:* stimulates opioid receptors; *uses:* analgesia, treatment of opioid dependence.

bupropion (byōō′prō′pēon), *n brand names:* Wellbutrin, Zyban; *drug class:* antidepressant; *action:* weak uptake inhibitor of dopamine, serotonin, norepinephrine; mechanism unknown; *uses:* treatment of depression and anxiety disorders; tobacco cessation.

bur, *n* a rotary cutting instrument of steel or tungsten carbide, supplied with cutting heads of various shapes.

bur, carbide, *n* a bur made of tungsten carbide; used at high rotational speeds.

bur, crosscut, *n* a bur with blades slotted perpendicularly to the axis of the bur.

bur, end-cutting, *n* a bur that has cutting blades only on the end of its head.

bur, excavating, *n* a bur used to remove dentin and debris from a cavity.

bur, finishing, *n* a bur with numerous fine-cutting blades placed close together; used to contour metallic restorations.

bur, intramucosal insert basepreparing **(in′trəmyōōkō′səl),** *n* See insert, intramucosal.

bur, inverted cone, n a bur with a head shaped like a truncated cone, the larger diameter being at the terminal (distal) end.

bur, plug-finishing, n See bur, finishing.

bur, round, n a bur with a sphere-shaped head.

bur, straight fissure, n a bur without crosscuts that has a cylindrical head.

bur, tapered fissure, n a bur having a long head with sides that converge from the shank to a blunt end.

burden of proof, *n* in a legal proceeding, the duty to prove a fact or facts in dispute.

Burkitt tumor, *n.pr* See lymphoma, Burkitt.

Burlew wheel, *n.pr* a brand name for an abrasive-impregnated, knife-edged, rubber polishing wheel; used on a mandrel in the dental handpiece to smooth metallic restorations and tooth surfaces.

Burlew wheel, high luster, n a Burlew wheel in which jeweler's rouge or iron peroxide is used as the abrasive agent.

Burlew wheel, midget, n a miniature form of a Burlew wheel.

Burlew wheel, sulci, n See Burlew wheel, midget.

burn, *n* a lesion caused by contact of heat, radiation, friction, or chemicals with tissue. Thermal ones are classified as follows: first degree, by erythema; second degree, by formation of vesicles; third degree, by necrosis of the mucosa or dermis; and fourth degree, by charring into the submucous or subcutaneous layers of the body.

burn, aspirin, n an irregularly shaped, whitish area on the oral mucosa caused by the topical application of acetylsalicylic acid.

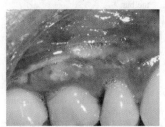

Aspirin burn. (Newman/Takei/Klokkevold, 2012)

burn, oral electrical, n. a severe burn to oral tissues, usually the labial commissure, due to intense heat created when a "live" electrical cord is placed in the mouth. This type of injury occurs most often in unattended children between six months and three three years of age.

burnisher, *n* an instrument shape with rounded edges used to burnish, polish, or work-harden metallic surfaces.

burnisher, ball, n a burnisher with a working point in the form of a ball.

burnisher, beaver-tail, n See burnisher, straight.

burnisher, fishtail, n a burnisher that slightly resembles a fish's tail in shape.

burnisher, straight, n a burnisher that resembles a beaver's tail in shape; the broad, flat blade is smoothly continuous with the shank, meeting it in a slight curve; the edges and the point are smoothly rounded.

burnishing, *n* a process related to polishing and abrading; the metal is moved by mechanically distorting the normal space lattice. Commonly accomplished during the polishing of soft golds.

burnout, *n* the elimination by heat of an invested pattern from a set investment to prepare the mold to receive casting metal.

burnout, high heat, n the use of temperatures higher than 1100°F (593.5°C) to effect wax elimination and prepare the mold to receive casting metal.

burnout, inlay (wax), n the elimination of wax from an invested inlay flask. See also wax elimination.

burnout, job, n the condition of having no energy left to care, resulting from chronic, unrelieved job-related stress and characterized by physical and emotional exhaustion and sometimes by physical illness.

burnout, radiographic, n the excessive penetration of the radiographic beam of an object or part of an object, producing a black, or overexposed, area on the image. Also known as *burnout, cervical.*

burnout, wax, n See burnout, inlay and wax elimination.

business area, *n* the area adjacent to the reception room in which the receptionist conducts the business affairs of the office and directly through which patients must pass to enter and leave the dental office.

business hours, *n.pl* the hours of the day during which professional, public, and other kinds of business are ordinarily conducted. Also called *office hours*

business office, *n* the room where the business of the dental practice is conducted.

buspirone HCl (byōōspī′rōn), *n brand name:* BuSpar; *drug class:* antianxiety agent; *action:* a partial agonist at serotonin 5HT-$_{1A}$ receptors; *use:* management and short-term relief of anxiety disorders.

busulfan (byōōsul′fən), *n brand name:* Myleran; *drug class:* antineoplastic; *action:* an alkylating agent, that interferes with biologic function of deoxyribonucleic acid; *use:* treatment of chronic myelocytic leukemia.

butoconazole nitrate (byōōtəkon′ə zōl′ nī′trāt), *n brand name:* Femstat; *drug class:* antifungal; *action:* binds sterols in fungal cell membrane, which increases permeability; *use:* treatment of vulvovaginal infections caused by *Candida.*

butamben, *n* an ester topical anesthetic; often combined with other topical anesthetics for use. It is an ester of 4-aminobenzoic acid and butanol.

butt, *v* to place directly against the tissues covering the residual alveolar ridge; to bring two square-ended surfaces into contact, as a butt joint.

button, *n* the excess metal remaining from the casting and sprue; located at the end of the sprue, opposite the casting.
   button, implant, n See insert, intramucosal.

buttonhole approach, *n* a method of surgical treatment of a periodontal abscess in which, after an incision is made in the fluctuant abscess, an additional attempt is made to curet the area adjoining the root and the fundus of the abscess through the destroyed portion of the alveolar plate or bone.

cachexia (kəkek′sēə), *n* the weakness, loss of weight, atrophy, and emaciation caused by severe or chronic disease, such as with AIDS.
   cachexia, hypophysial, n See disease, Simmonds'.
   cachexia hypopituitary, n See disease, Simmonds'.

CAD/CAM (computer aided design/computer aided manufacturing), *n* in dentistry, CAD/CAM can make crowns, bridges, or complete dentures by machining from metals or ceramics instead of last wax castings.

cadaver (kədav′ər), *n* a deceased body, most often used in reference to a body used for dissection and study.

cadaverine (kədav′ərēn′), *n* a foul-smelling diamine formed by bacterial decarboxylation of lysine. It is poisonous and irritating to the skin.

cadmium (Cd) (kad′mēəm), *n* a bluish-white metallic element that resembles tin. Cadmium bromide, used in engraving, lithography, and photography, can cause severe gastrointestinal symptoms if ingested.

café-au-lait spots, *n.pl* See spots, café-au-lait.

cafeteria plan, *n* an employee benefits plan in which employees select their medical insurance coverage and other nontaxable fringe benefits from a list of options provided by the employer.

caffeine (kafēn′, kaf′ēin), *n* a white, odorless, bitter compound isolated from tea and coffee that is used as a stimulant of the central nervous system.

CAGE questionnaire, *n.pr* a four question survey used to identify potential alcohol dependence. CAGE is an acronym for the four areas identified (felt need to *Cut back, Annoyance by critics, Guilt about drinking, and Eye-opening morning drinking*).

calcific metamorphosis (of dental pulp), *n* a frequently observed reaction to trauma, characterized by partial or complete obliteration of the pulp chamber and canal.

calcification (kal′sifikā′shən), *n* the process whereby calcium salts are deposited in an organic matrix. The condition may be normal, as in bone and tooth formation, or pathologic.

calcification, dystrophic, n the pathologic deposition of calcium salts in necrotic or degenerated tissues.

calcification, ectopic oral, n the displaced accumulation of hardened calcium salts in the oral cavity; stones found in pulp or saliva. See also salivary stone and denticle.

calcification, metastatic, n the pathologic deposition of calcium salts in previously undamaged tissues. This process is caused by an excessively high level of blood calcium, such as in the hyperparathyroid.

calcifying epithelial odontogenic tumor (Pindborg tumor), *n* an uncommon tumor arising from odontogenic epithelium characterized by focal areas of calcification. It has the same age, gender, and site distribution as the ameloblastoma.

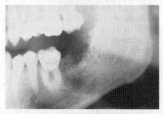

Calcifying epithelial odontogenic tumor. (Neville, et al, 2009)

calcination (kal′sinā′shən), *n* a process of removing water by heat; used in the manufacture of plaster and ▶ stone from gypsum.

calcinosis (kal′sənō′sis), *n* **1.** the deposition of calcium salts in various tissues because of hypercalcemia and tissue degeneration. *n* **2.** the presence of calcification in or under the skin. The condition may occur in a localized (calcinosis circumscripta) or generalized (calcinosis universalis) form.

calcipotriene (kal′sipōtri′ēn), *n brand name:* Dovonex; *drug class:* vitamin D3 derivative (synthetic); *action:* regulation of skin cell production and development; *use:* moderate plaque psoriasis.

calcite, *n* an abrasive agent made from crystallized natural calcium carbonate.

calcitonin (kal′sitō′nin), *n brand names:* Calcitonin, Calcimar, Miacalcin; *drug class:* synthetic polypeptide calcitonins; *actions:* inhibits bone resorption, reduces osteoclast function, reduces serum calcium levels in hypercalcemia; *uses:* Paget's disease, postmenopausal osteoporosis, hypercalcemia.

calcitriol (kal′sitri′ol), *n brand name:* Calcijex; *drug class:* vitamin D3 hormone; *action:* increases intestinal absorption of calcium and phosphorus; *uses:* hypocalcemia in chronic renal dialysis and rickets, nutritional supplement.

calcium *(Ca)* (kal′sēəm), *n* a basic element, with an atomic weight of 40.07, found in nearly all organized tissues. Essential for mineralization of bone and teeth. The normal level of it in the blood is 9 to 11.5 mg/ 100 mL. A deficiency of it in the diet or in use may lead to rickets or osteoporosis. Overexcretion in hyperparathyroidism leads to osteoporotic manifestations. See also factor IV.

calcium binding protein, n See calmodulin.

calcium, blood, n See blood calcium.

calcium carbonate, n brand names: Maalox Antacid, Rolaids Calcium Rich, Tums E-X; *drug class:* antacid; *actions:* neutralizes gastric acidity, supplies calcium; *uses:* antacid, calcium supplement.

calcium carbonate and magnesium hydroxide, n brand name: Rolaids; *drug class:* antacid; *action:* neutralizes gastric acidity; *use:* antacid.

calcium channel blocker, n a drug that inhibits the flow of calcium ions across the membranes of smooth muscle cells. The reduction of calcium flow relaxes smooth muscle tone and reduces the risk of muscle spasms. Calcium channel blockers are used in the prevention and treatment of coronary artery spasms.

calcium, dietary, n the amount of absorbable calcium ingested daily.

calcium fluoride, n a compound that is used as a flux in the manufacture of some silicate cements.

calcium hydroxide, n a white powder that is mixed with water or another medium and used as a base material in cavity liners and for pulp capping.

calcium hydroxyapatite, *n* the main inorganic crystal in enamel, bone, dentin, and cementum.

calcium oxalate, *n* an insoluble sediment in the urine and urinary calculi.

calcium phosphate, *n* an odorless, tasteless white powder, the various forms of which are sometimes used as abrasives in dentifrices.

calcium salts, *n.pl* the calcium present in salivary fluid as phosphates and carbonates. They are believed to form dental calculus on their precipitation from saliva.

calcium sulfate, *n* See alphahemihydrate, beta-hemihydrate, gypsum.

calcium tungstate, *n* a chemical substance used in crystal form to coat screens; the screens fluoresce when struck by roentgen rays.

calculogenesis (kal′kūlōjen′əsis), *n* the process during which calculus is formed.

calculogenic (kal′kūlōjen′ik), *adj* pertaining to the formation of calculus on tooth surfaces.

calculus (dental) (kal′kyələs), *n* a hard deposit on the exposed surfaces of the teeth and any oral prosthesis within the oral cavity. It is composed of calcium phosphate, calcium carbonate, magnesium phosphate, and other elements within an organic matrix composed of plaque, desquamated epithelium, mucin, microorganisms, and other debris. Factor in the initiation and continuation of periodontal disease. The colloquial term is *tartar.*

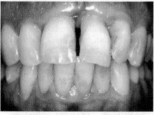

Calculus. (Perry/Beemsterboer, 2007)

calculus, identification of, by air application, *n* the use of compressed air to dry the periodontium and visualize minimal amounts of calculus, which are otherwise difficult to see, especially subgingivally.

calculus record, *n* a written accounting of the number and distribution of calculus deposits on tooth surfaces that becomes part of the patient's permanent chart and is used to monitor progress and plan treatment.

calculus, subgingival, *n* the calculus deposited on the tooth structure and found apical to the gingival margin within the periodontal pocket. Usually darker and denser than supragingival calculus. Older term is *serumal calculus.*

calculus, supragingival, *n* the calculus deposited on the teeth coronal to the gingival margin. Usually lighter in color (unless stained) and less dense than subgingival calculus. Older term is *salivary calculus.*

calibrated probe, *n* See probe, periodontal.

calibration (kal′əbrā′shən), *n* **1.** the process of comparing a measurement instrument against a verified standard instrument. The US Bureau of Standards maintains the national calibration instruments for weights and measures. *n* **2.** the comparison of procedures between clinicians to achieve a clinical standard.

calibration of radiography unit, *n* See unit, radiography calibration.

Caliciviridae **(kal′isēvir′idā),** *n* a grouping of nonenveloped, 20-sided RNA viruses, and includes the Norwalk gastroenteritis virus.

caliper, axis-orbital, *n* a caliper used to record facial measurements and transfer them to an adjustable articulator. It consists of the following: (1) a hinge-bow, (2) a bite fork covered with compound, (3) an indicator of the axis-orbital plane, (4) an upright rod to hold the orbital indicator in place, (5) a toggle to freeze the bow's base to the bite fork, and (6) a toggle to attach and allow adjustments for the support of the indicator. Also called *hinge-bow transfer recorder.*

Callahan's method, *n.pr* See method, chloropercha.

callus (kal′əs), *n* the tissue near and about the broken fragments of a bone that becomes involved in the repair of the fracture through various stages of exudate, fibrosis, and new bone formation.

calmodulin (kalmoj′əlin), *n* a calcium-binding protein that mediates a variety of biochemical and physiologic processes, including the contraction of muscles and the release of norepinephrine.

calorie (kal′ôrē), *n* the amount of heat required to raise 1 g of water 1° C at atmospheric pressure, also called gram calorie or small calorie. A great calorie, or kilocalorie, consists of 1000 small calories. The kilocalorie is the unit used to denote the heat expenditure of an organism and the fuel or energy value of food.

calorimetry (kal′ərim′ətrē), *n* the measurement of the amounts of heat radiated and absorbed.

Camper's line, *n.pr* See line, Camper's.

camphorated opium tincture (kam′fərā′təd), *n brand name:* Paregoric; *drug class:* antidiarrheal; *action:* antiperistaltic and analgesic with activity related to morphine content; *use:* diarrhea.

camphorated parachlorophenol (per′əklôr′ōfē′nol), *n* a mixture of 35% parachlorophenol and 65% camphor; used to treat root canals and periapical infections.

Campylobacter (kam′pəlōbak′tər), *n.pr* a microorganism associated with progressive periodontal destruction and refractory forms of periodontitis.

Campylobacter gastroenteritis, *n* a gastrointestinal tract infection with typical symptoms, caused by *C. jejuni* bacteria, the microaerophilic bacteria naturally occurring in humans.

Canadian Dental Hygienists' Association (CDHA), *n.pr* a nonprofit advocacy group established in 1964 representing Canadian dental hygienists nationwide. The CDHA promotes dental standards, releases position statements and safety alerts, and aims to educate the Canadian public on the importance of oral health.

canal (root), *n* **1.** the portion of the root that contains the pulp tissue and is surrounded by dentin. *n* **2.** an opening in bone that is long, narrow, and tubelike.

canal, accessory, *n* a lateral branching of the main root canal, usually occurring in the apical third of the root. Also called *lateral canal.*

canal, alimentary, *n* the entire digestive route, beginning at the oral cavity and ending at the anus, in which food enters, nourishment is extracted, and waste products are expelled.

canal, branching, *n* See canal, collateral pulp.

canal, calcified, *n* a root canal that has been subjected to calcification, the hardening of decaying of dead soft tissue.

canal, carotid, *n* he canal in the temporal bone that carries the internal carotid artery.

canal, collateral pulp (branching canal), *n* a pulp canal branch that emerges from the root at a place other than the apex.

canal, hypoglossal, *n* the canal in the occipital bone that carries the twelfth cranial nerve.

canal, infraorbital, *n* the canal off the infraorbital sulcus that terminates on the surface of the maxilla as the infraorbital foramen.

canal, interdental (nutrient canal), *n* the nutrient channels that pass upward through the body of the mandible. Present as radiolucent lines on radiographs.

canal, mandibular, *n* the canal in the mandible where the inferior alveolar nerve and blood vessels travel.

canal, optic, *n* the canal in the orbital apex between the roots of the lesser wing of the sphenoid bone.

canal, pterygoid, *n* the small canal at the superior border of each posterior nasal aperture.

canal, pulp, *n* the space in the radicular portion of the tooth occupied by the pulp.

canal, root, *n* the informal term for the endodontic procedure to remove infected root canal tissue and replace removed tissue with restorative material.

canal, root, measurements, *n.pl* a technique employing the use of radiographic images to determine the length of the root canal.

canaliculus (kan′əlik′yəlus), *n* a small channel that extends from or to the lacunae of bone and cementum and contains filamentous processes of the cells that occupy the lacunae; interconnects with canaliculi extending from neighboring lacunae.

cancellous (kan'seləs), *adj* possessing a permeable, porous structure. Frequently used in conjunction with *bone* to refer to the spongy, typically artery- and vein-rich section at the ends of long bones.

cancer (kan'sur), *n* a malignant neoplasm. The term is sometimes incorrectly used to include any neoplasm, whether benign or malignant. *Carcinoma* and *sarcoma* are more specific terms.

cancer, oral, *n* malignancies indicative of unchecked cell growth that are mainly found in and around the oropharynx, gingiva, floor of the oral cavity, lower lip, and base of the tongue.

cancrum oris (kang'krəm ôr'is), *n* See noma.

Candida albicans **(kan'didə al'bə kanz),** *n.pr* a budding, yeastlike fungus present in the normal flora of the mucous membrane of the female genital tract and respiratory and gastrointestinal tracts (including the oral cavity) that is capable of assuming a pathogenic role in the production of oral and systemic moniliasis, such as thrush and monilial infection.

candidiasis (kan'didĭəsis), *n* an infection by *C. albicans.* See also moniliasis; thrush.

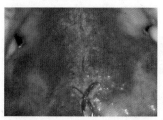

Candidiasis. (Courtesy Dr. James Scuibba)

candidiasis, angular cheilitis, *n* a condition that forms fissures or ulcers radiating from the corners of the oral cavity (commissures) often accompanied by white plaques. Usually observed in elderly patients, although when observed in a young person, it may be an indicator of HIV infection. Candidiasis of the esophagus, trachea, bronchi, or lungs is associated with group IV human immunodeficiency virus (HIV) infection. See also acquired immunodeficiency syndrome (AIDS).

candidiasis, erythematous (atrophic), *n* a condition that forms smooth red patches on the hard or soft palate, buccal mucosa, or dorsal surface of the tongue.

candidiasis, hyperplastic, *n* a condition that forms white plaques that cannot be removed by wiping or scraping.

candidiasis, pseudomembranous, *n* a condition that forms loosely adherent (wipeable), yellowish-white plaques on the oral mucosal surface.

canine (kā'nĭn), *n* one of the four pointed teeth situated one on each side of each jaw, distal to the lateral incisor; forms the keystone of the arch. Older term is *cuspid.*

canine eminence **(em'ənəns),** *n* a bony projection that covers the root of the canine tooth on the labial surface of the maxillary arch.

canine fossa, *n* See fossa, canine.

canine guidance, *n* a concept of occlusal function in which the canine teeth are assigned a major control role in the excursive movements of the mandible.

canine substitution, *n* orthodontic treatment in which the canine is moved mesially to assume the position of a congenitally missing lateral incisor. Usually it is performed in the maxilla.

canker (kang'kur), *n* See aphtha.

cannabis (kan'əbis), *n* a psychoactive herb derived from the flowering tops of a variety of hemp, *Cannabis sativa.* It is the active ingredient of marijuana. It has been used in the treatment of glaucoma and as an antiemetic in some cancer patients to counter the nausea and vomiting associated with chemotherapy. It is controlled under Schedule I of the Comprehensive Drug Abuse Prevention and Control Act of 1970.

cannula (kan'yələ), *n* a tube for insertion into the body; its caliber is usually occupied by a trocar during the act of insertion.

cannula, nasal, *n* a small, half-moon shaped plastic tube, the ends of which fit into the nostrils of an individual.

canthus, lateral (kan'thus), *n* a lateral angle between the upper and lower eyelids.

canthus, medial, *n* a medial angle between the upper and lower eyelids.

cantilever bridge (kan'tələ'vər), *n* See denture, partial, fixed, cantilever.

cantilever partial denture, *n* See denture, partial, cantilever fixed.

cap, *n* See crown.

🔲 **cap stage,** *n* the third period of development in a tooth bud. During this stage, the amorphous cellular structure of the bud takes shape, ultimately resulting in a caplike appearance.

capacity, *n* legal qualification, competency, power, or fitness.

capacity, functional residual, n (normal capacity), the volume of gas in the lungs at resting expiratory level.

capacity, iron-binding, n a measure of the binding capacity of iron in the serum; helps to differentiate the causes of hypoferremia. This capacity tends to increase in iron deficiency and diminishes in chronic diseases and during infection.

capacity, normal, n See capacity, functional residual.

capacity, total lung (TLC), n the volume of air in the lungs at the end of maximal inspiration.

capacity, vital (VC), n the maximum volume of air that can be expired after maximal inspiration.

capillarity (kap'iler'ĭtē), *n* the phenomenon by which a film of fluid is drawn and held between two closely approximating surfaces.

capillary (kap'ilerē), *n* the terminal vessels uniting the arterial with the venous systems of the body. They are organized into extensive branching reticular beds to provide a maximal surface for exchange of fluids, electrolytes, and metabolites between tissues and the vascular system.

capillary attraction, n the quality or state that, because of surface tension, causes elevation or depression of the surface of a liquid that is in contact with a solid. Considered to be one of the factors in retention of complete dentures.

capillary blood plexus, n.pl the groups of capillaries noted between the papillary layer and the deeper layers of the lamina propria.

capillary disorder, n a hemorrhagic disorder caused by increased fragility of the blood vessels that may cause hemorrhages in the skin and mucous membranes

capital budgeting, *n* the process of planning expenditures on assets, the returns of which are expected to extend beyond 1 year.

capitation (kap'ətā'shən), *n* **1.** the practice of dentistry financed by a set fee per person per given period of time. A form of contracted dental care, usually by a corporation, institution, or other group. *n* **2.** a system by which the contracting dental professional, assuming the financial risk, is compensated at a fixed per capita rate, usually on specific, predetermined dental services as appropriate and necessary to eligible subscribers. *n* **3.** a dental benefits program in which a dental professional or dental professionals contract with the program's sponsor or administrator to provide all or most of the dental services covered under the program to subscribers in return for payment on a per capita basis.

capitation fee, n a predetermined per-person charge made by the carrier for benefits available under an insurance plan.

capitulum (kəpich'əlum), *n* the European term for a small head, instead of *head* or *condyle.*

capitulum mandibulae, n See process, condyloid.

***Capnocytophaga* (kap'nositof'əgə),** *n* a species of gram-negative facultatively anaerobic bacteria belonging to the genus *Capnocytophaga.* It is present in both normal and diseased oral cavities. Possibly associated with periodontal disease.

capnography, *n* a method of monitoring the ventilation status of a patient. It uses an electronic device designed to determine the quality of the patient's respirations and it quickly alerts to any respiratory compromise. A useful patient monitoring device when a patient is sedated or undergoing general anesthesia.

capnophilic (kap'nōfil'ik), *adj* the ability to thrive in conjunction with carbon dioxide.

capping, direct pulp, *n* an application to the exposed pulp of a drug or material for the purpose of stimulating repair of the injured pulpal tissue.

capping, indirect pulp, *n* See indirect pulp treatment.

capping, pulp, *n* the covering of an exposed dental pulp with a material that protects it from external influences.

capsaicin (kapsā′isin), *n brand names:* Zostrix, Capzasin-P, Axsain; *drug class:* topical analgesic for selected pain syndromes; *action:* stimulates vanilloid or *TRPV1* receptors leading to depletion and preventing reaccumulation of substance P in peripheral sensory neurons; *uses:* neuralgia associated with herpes zoster, temporomandibular joint (TMJ) pain.

capsule, joint, *n* a fibrous sac or ligament that encloses a joint and limits its motion. It is lined with synovial membrane.

capsule, temporomandibular joint, *n* See articulation, temporomandibular, capsule.

captopril (kap′təpril), *n brand name:* Capoten; *drug class:* angiotensin-converting enzyme inhibitor; *action:* dilation of arterial and venous vessels; *uses:* hypertension, heart failure, diabetic nephropathy, useful after myocardial infarction.

carat, *n* a standard of fineness of gold, 24 carats being taken as expressing absolute purity.

carbamazepine (kär′bəmaz′əpēn), *n brand name:* Tegretol; *drug class:* anticonvulsant; *action:* inhibits nerve impulses by limiting influx of sodium ions across cell membrane; *uses:* tonic-clonic/complex/partial/mixed seizures, a specific analgesic for trigeminal neuralgia, sometimes used in the treatment of herpes zoster.

carbaminohemoglobin, *n* a hemoglobin compounded with CO_2.

carbenicillin indanyl (kärben′isil′in), *n* a semisynthetic penicillin that is acid resistant and rapidly absorbed from the small intestine and thus suitable for oral administration. Used for urinary tract infections.

carbide bur, *n* See bur, carbide.

carbides (kar′bīdz), *n.pl* **1.** in chemistry, carbon binary compounds with strong electron-releasing properties. *n.pl* **2.** mixtures of carbon with at least one heavy metal, e.g., the buror metal alloy bit of a dental drill has a composition of tungsten carbide.

carbidopa, *n brand names:* Lodosyn, Sinemet (when combined with levodopa); *drug class:* anti-Parkinson;

action: inhibits peripheral DOPA decarboxylase allowing levodopa to enter the brain before it is metabolized; *use:* adjunct in treating Parkinson's disease.

carbohemia (kär′bōhē′mēə), *n* an imperfect oxygenation of the blood.

carbohydrates, *n.pl* a group of organic compounds with the class name saccharides, which are the aldehydric or ketonic derivatives of polyhydric alcohols. Ones such as sugar, starch, cellulose, and gum are generally synthesized by green plants. They constitute the main energy source in the diet and are classified as mono-, di-, tri-, and polysaccharides.

carbohydrate tolerance, *n* See tolerance, carbohydrate.

carbon, *n* a nonmetallic tetravalent element that occurs in pure form in diamonds and graphite. It occurs as a component of all living tissue. Most of the study of organic chemistry focuses on the vast number of carbon compounds.

carbon coated, adj a vitreous carbon coating applied to either an endosteal or blade implant to improve tissue compatability.

carbon dioxide, n a colorless, odorless gas produced by the complete oxidation of carbon. It is a product of cell respiration and is carried by the blood to the lungs and exhaled. The acid-base balance of body fluids and tissues is affected by the level of it and its carbonate compounds.

carbon monoxide, n a colorless, odorless, poisonous gas produced by the combustion of carbon or organic fuels in a limited oxygen supply. It combines irreversibly with hemoglobin, preventing the formation of oxyhemoglobin and reducing the oxygen supply to the tissues.

carbonate, *n* a mineral salt of carbonic acid.

carbonate hydroxyapatite (kär′bənāt hīdrok′sēap′ətīt), n the composition and crystal structure of hard tissues.

carbonic acid, *n* an unstable acid formed by dissolving carbon dioxide in water. It is the basis of carbonated beverages and contributes the negative ion to carbonate salts.

carbonic anhydrase (kärbon′ik anhī′drās′), *n* an enzyme that plays a role in transferring carbon dioxide from tissue cells to the lungs by turning carbon dioxide into carbonic acid in red blood cells. Also called *carbonate dehydratase.*

Carborundum stone, *n.pr* See stone, Carborundum.

carboxylate, *n* a carboxylic acid salt, ester, or ion.

carboxylation (kärbok′səlā′shən), *n* the chemical process by which a carboxyl group (COOH) is added or displaces a hydrogen atom.

carboxypeptidase (kärbok′sēpep′ti dās), *n* an exopeptidase that stimulates the hydrolytic cleavage of the last or second to last peptide bond at the C-terminal end of a peptide or polypeptide.

carcinogen (kärsin′əjen), *n* a substance or agent that causes the development or increases the incidence of cancer.

carcinoma (kär′sinō′mə), *n* a malignant epithelial tumor. Also called *cancer.*

carcinoma, adenoid cystic, *n* a salivary gland malignancy of ductal and myoepithelial cells that may arise in both major and minor salivary glands. Although it grows slowly, perineural invasion and its relentless nature makes long-term survival poor.

carcinoma, basal cell (basal cell epithelioma, rodent ulcer, turban tumor), *n* an epithelial neoplasm with a basic structure resembling the basal cells of the epidermis. It develops from basal cells of the epidermis or from the outer cells of hair follicles or sebaceous glands, particularly the middle third of the face. It rarely, if ever, metastasizes but is locally invasive. It does not arise from oral mucosa. It develops as a plaque that then ulcerates in the center, becoming indurated.

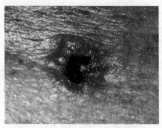

Basal cell carcinoma. (Regezi/Sciubba/Jordan, 2012)

carcinoma, basosquamous, *n* a carcinoma that histologically exhibits both basal and squamous elements. It may occasionally be seen in the oral cavity; considered to have a greater tendency to metastasize than does basal cell carcinoma.

carcinoma, epidermoid (ep′əder′moid), *n* a malignant epithelial neoplasm with cells resembling those of the epidermis. The term *squamous cell carcinoma* is used for intraoral lesions of this nature. See also carcinoma, squamous cell (SCC).

carcinoma, exophytic, *n* a malignant epithelial neoplasm with marked outward growth similar to a wart or papilloma.

carcinoma in situ, *n* a dysplastic epithelial disease involving the skin and mucous membranes and considered to be precancerous. Dysplasia is evident, but no invasion has yet occurred.

carcinoma, intraepithelial, *n* See carcinoma in situ.

carcinoma, mucoepidermoid (myōō′ kōep′əder′moid), *n* a malignant epithelial tumor of the salivary gland characterized by acini with mucus producing cells.

carcinoma, squamous cell (SCC), *n* the second most common skin cancer after basal cell carcinoma. It arises from the epidermis or oral mucosa and resembles the squamous cells that comprise most of the upper layers. It may occur on all areas of the body, including the mucous membranes, but is most common in areas exposed to the sun. Risk factors include actinic (sun) damage, alcohol use, and tobacco use.

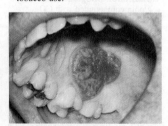

Squamous cell carcinoma. (Regezi/Sciubba/Jordan, 2012)

carcinoma, transitional cell, *n* a malignant tumor arising from a transitional type of stratified epithelium.

carcinoma, verrucous, n a squamous cell carcinoma, usually intraoral, that is exophytic and has a papillary appearance. Associated with spit tobacco.

cardia (kär′dēə), n the opening between the esophagus and the cardiac portion of the stomach; characterized by the absence of acid cells. Also an archaic term formerly used to describe the heart and the region surrounding it.

cardiac, *adj* relating to the heart.

cardiac arrest, n a stopping of heart action; a complete cessation of heart function.

cardiac dysrhythmia (disrith′mēə), n an irregular or abnormal heartbeat rhythm. Also known as *cardiac arrhythmia.*

cardiac massage, n See massage, cardiac.

cardiac output, n the volume of blood put out by the heart per minute; the product of the stroke volume and the heart rate per minute.

cardiac pacemaker, n See pacemaker.

cardiac surgery, n an operative procedure used to treat a disease of the heart or its blood vessels.

cardioinhibitory (kär′dēōinhib′itô rē), *adj* restraining or inhibiting the movements of the heart.

cardiokinetic (kär′dēōkinet′ik), *adj* exciting the heart; a remedy that excites the heart.

cardiology, n the scientific study of the anatomy, normal function, and disorders of the heart.

cardiomyopathy, hypertrophic, n a disease of the heart in which the heart is enlarged.

cardiopulmonary, *adj* pertaining to the heart and lungs.

cardiopulmonary resuscitation (CPR), n a basic emergency procedure for life support, consisting of mainly manual external cardiac massage and some artificial respiration.

cardiovascular disease (CVD), n any one of a number of abnormal conditions that involve dysfunction of the heart and blood vessels, including but not limited to systemic hypertension, atherosclerosis and coronary heart disease, and rheumatic heart disease.

cardiovascular system, n the network of structures, including the heart and blood vessels, that convey the blood throughout the body.

carditis, n an inflammation of the heart muscle tissue. Pericarditis, myocarditis, and endocarditis are types of carditis affecting specific regions of the heart.

care, n as a legal term, the opposite of negligence.

care, reasonable, n such care as an ordinarily prudent person would exercise under the conditions existing at the time that person is called on to act.

care plan, n strategies designed to guide health care professionals involved with patient care. Such plans are patient specific and are meant to address the total status of the patient. Care plans are intended to ensure optimal outcomes for patients during the course of their care.

caregiver, n a person providing treatment or support to a sick, disabled, or dependent individual.

caries (ker′ēz), n in dentistry, the decay of a tooth. Colloquial term is *cavity.*

caries, arrested, n the state existing when the progress of the decay process has halted. It is noted by its dark staining without any breakdown of tooth tissues.

Caries Assessment Tool (CAT), n.pr an analysis that examines the risk factors for the development of dental caries in infants and young children. Risk factors such as the environment, family history, and general health can be identified early, thereby reducing a patient's risk for developing dental caries and other diseases of the teeth and gingival tissues.

caries, baby bottle, n See caries, early childhood (EEC).

caries, cemental (root surface), n the decay of the cementum that occurs as a result of gingival recession and exposure of the root surface. See also caries, cervical (root surface).

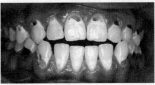

Cemental caries. (Bath Balogh/ Fehrenbach, 2011)

caries, cervical (root surface), *n* the decay that appears on the root at the cementoenamel junction or the neck as a result of gingival recession and exposure of the root surface. See also caries, cemental (root surface).

caries, chronic, *n* a form of caries that occurs over time and demands regular dental intervention.

caries, compound, *n* a type of caries that affects two or more surfaces of a tooth.

caries, early childhood (ECC), *n* a form of severe dental decay occurring in young children that is often caused by long and frequent exposure to liquids that are high in sugar, such as milk or juice. Because this form can damage the underlying bone structure, it may affect the development of permanent teeth.

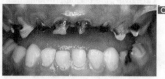

Early childhood caries. (Dean/Avery/McDonald, 2011)

caries, enamel, *n* the decay that occurs in the enamel of a tooth because of a fissure or the collection of bacterial plaque. It appears first as white spots, which later darken to brown.

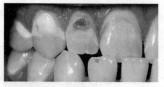

Enamel caries. (Sapp/Eversole/Wysocki, 2004)

caries, gross, *n* a form of caries with advanced dental decay that is easily seen clinically.

caries, healed, *n* See caries, arrested.

caries, incipient, *n* a decayed part of a tooth in which the lesion is just coming into existence.

caries management by risk assessment (CAMBRA), *n* a methodology in which the cause of a disease is identified through the assessment of risk factors for the individual patient and then the risk factors are managed through behavioral, chemical and minimally invasive procedures.

caries, nursing, *n* See caries, early childhood (EEC).

caries, pit-and-fissure, *n* See cavity, pit and fissure. See also sealant, enamel.

caries, plaque-related, *n* the caries associated with plaque formation. Most commonly located in the pits and fissures of the teeth, especially the molar and premolar teeth, and along the gingival tissue and also the margins associated with dental restorations.

caries, proximal, *n* decay occurring in the mesial or distal surface of a tooth.

caries, rampant, *n* a suddenly appearing, widespread, rapidly progressing type of caries.

caries, recurrent, *n* the extension of the carious process beyond the margin of a restoration. Also called *secondary caries.*

caries, residual, *n* (residual carious dentin), the decayed material left in a prepared cavity and over which a restoration is placed.

caries, risk assessment, *n* a procedure that considers a number of risk factors for a patient's caries development enabling the dentist to predict the patient's potential for the disease in the future.

caries, root, *n* tooth decay occurring on a portion of the root that is exposed.

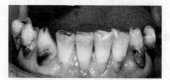

Root caries. (Sapp/Eversole/Wysocki, 2004)

caries, senile (senile decay), *n* older term for the decay noted particularly in the elderly when supporting tissues have receded; occurs in cementum, usually on proximal surfaces of the teeth.

caries, smooth surface, n the decay that occurs on the smooth surfaces of the tooth. See also caries, proximal dental and *S. mutans.*

caries, vaccine, n a vaccine currently under development to treat dental caries by inoculating against bacteria commonly known to contribute to their formation, particularly *S. mutans.*

cariogenesis (ker'ēōjen'əsis), n the process during which cavities develop in teeth.

cariogenic (kerēōjen'ik), adj contributing to the advancement of caries. Often used in the context of describing sugary foods.

cariogenic challenge, n an episode in which tooth enamel is exposed to acid, a byproduct of cariogenic foods and plaque bacteria.

cariogenicity (ker'ēōjənis'itē), n the ability of a substance to induce or potentiate the formation of dental caries.

cariostatic (ker'ēōstat'ik), adj tending to inhibit the development of dental caries, e.g., the cariostatic action of flouride. See also anticariogenic.

carious (ker'ēus), adj pertaining to caries or decay.

carious dentin, adj pertaining to caries or decay.

carisoprodol (ker'īsōprō'dol), n *brand names:* Soma, Vanasom; *drug class:* skeletal muscle relaxant, central acting; *action:* nonspecific central nervous system sedation; *use:* adjunct for relief of muscle spasm in musculoskeletal conditions.

carnauba wax, n See wax, carnauba.

carnitine (kar'nətēn'), n a compound found naturally in red meat and dairy, as well as in legumes and nuts, this quaternary ammonium compound assists in the movement of fatty acids through the membrane of the mitochondria.

Carnoy's solution, n.pr See solution, Carnoy's.

carotene (ker'ətēn), n an orange pigment found in carrots, leafy vegetables, and other foods that may be converted to vitamin A in the body.

carotenemia (ker'ətēnē'mēə), n excess carotene in the blood, producing a pigmentation of the skin and mucous membranes that resembles jaundice.

carotid (kərot'id), n either one of the two main right and left arteries of the neck.

carotid sheath, n the deep cervical fascia forming a tube which runs down the side of the neck.

carotid stenosis, n the narrowing and hardening of the carotid artery.

carotid triangle, n See triangle, carotid.

carpal tunnel syndrome, n an irritation and inflammation of the synovials surrounding the tendons controlling the fingers. It is a disabling condition for persons who work with their hands, particularly those engaging in keyboard activities, data management, and instrumentation such as those in the dental office.

carrier, n **1.** a person harboring a specific infectious agent without clinical evidence of disease and who serves as a potential source or reservoir of infection for others. May be a healthy or convalescent carrier. n **2.** the party of the dental plan contract who agrees to pay claims or provide service. Also called *insurer, underwriter,* and *administrative agent.* See also third party.

carrier, amalgam, n an instrument used to carry plastic amalgam to the prepared cavity or mold into which it is to be inserted.

carrier, foil, n See foil passer.

carteolol HCl (kär'teəlol), n *brand name:* Ocupress; *drug class:* β-adrenergic blocker; *action:* nonselective β-adrenergic receptor blocker, reduces production of aqueous humor by unknown mechanisms; *uses:* chronic open-angle glaucoma, ocular hypertension.

cartilage (kar'tlij), n a derivative of connective tissue arising from the mesenchyme. Typical hyaline type is a flexible, rather elastic material with a semitransparent, glasslike appearance. Its intercellular substance is a complex protein (chondromucoid) through which is distributed a large network of connective tissue fibers.

cartilage, articular, n a thin layer of hyaline cartilage located on the joint surfaces of some bones. Not usually found on articular surfaces of temporomandibular joints, which are covered with an avascular fibrous tissue.

cartilage, condylar **(kar′tlij kon′dələr),** *n* the cartilage containing a rounded articular protrusion, or condyle, present at bone joints. Condylar cartilage of the mandible is a common type.

cartilage, cricoid, *n* the most inferior cartilage of the larynx.

▣ *cartilage, Meckel's,* *n.pr* the cartilaginous process in the embryo derived from the mesenchymal tissue of the mandibular process.

cartilage, primary, *n* the cartilage formed during fetal development that is not replaced by bone.

cartilage, Reichert's **(rī′kherts),** *n. pr* the cartilaginous process located laterally in the embryonic tympanum; gives rise to styloid processes, stylohyoid ligaments, and lesser horns of hyoid bone.

cartridge, *n* in dentistry, a device of various configuration and composition used with a syringe for the application of anesthetic or other materials to a patient.

caruncle (ker′ungkəl), *n* a small, fleshy growth.

caruncle, sublingual **(subling′gwəl),** *n* See caruncle, submandibular.

caruncle, submandibular **(sub′man dib′yələr),** *n* the opening of the submandibular (Wharton's) duct that opens into the oral cavity on small papillae bilateral to the lingual frenum. The sublingual (Bartholin) duct opens here as well. See also gland, submandibular salivary, and gland, sublingual salivary.

carvedilol (kär′vədil′ol), *n brand name:* Coreg; *drug class:* nonselective β-adrenergic receptor blocking agent with α₁-adrenergic receptor blocking activity; *action:* produces fall in blood pressure without significant reflex tachycardia; *uses:* essential hypertension alone or with other antihypertensives, heart failure, after myocardial infarction.

▣ **carver (carving instrument),** *n* an instrument used to shape a plastic material such as wax or amalgam.

carver, amalgam, *n* an instrument used to shape plastic amalgam.

carving, *n* the shaping and forming with instruments.

case, *n* the term often incorrectly used instead of the appropriate noun (e.g., *patient, flask, denture, casting*). Case is not synonymous with patient because the latter is more than just the case of situations they present.

case charting, *n* the recording of a patient's status of health or disease.

case dismissal, *n* the technique of illustrating to the patient the results of treatment, usually done during the last appointment of a series.

case history, *n* See history, case.

case management, *n* the monitoring and coordination of treatment rendered to patients with specific diagnoses or requiring high cost or extensive services.

case presentation, *n* an explanation of dental needs to the patient.

case summary, *n* enumeration of all the services to be performed for an estimated amount of money.

case-control study, *n* an investigation employing an epidemiologic approach in which previously existing incidents of a medical condition are used in lieu of gathering new information from a randomized population. Control is obtained by comparing known cases of the medical condition with a group of persons who have not developed the medical problem.

cash budget, *n* a schedule showing cash flows (receipts, disbursements, net cash) for a firm over a specified period.

cash cycle, *n* the length of time between the purchase of raw materials and the collection of accounts receivable generated in the sale of the final product.

cash flow, *n* the reported net income of a corporation plus amounts charged off for depreciation, depletion, amortization, and extraordinary charges to reserves, which are bookkeeping deductions not paid out in actual dollars and cents. A measurement tool used in recent years to offer a better indication of the ability of a company to pay dividends and finance expansion from selfgenerated cash than the conventional reported net income figure.

Caspofungin acetate, *n brand name:* Cancidas; *drug class:* echinocandin antifungal; *action:* inhibits the synthesis of 1,3-β-D-glucan polymers, preventing cell wall synthesis on the fungal cell; *use:* systemic fungal infections, including candidiasis.

cassette (kəset′), *n* a light-tight container in which radiographic films are placed for exposure to radiation; usually backed with lead to eliminate the effect of backscattered radiation.

cassette, cardboard (cardboard film-holder), *n* a cardboard envelope of simple construction suitable for use in making radiographs on "direct exposure" or "no-screen" types of radiographic films.

cassette, screen-type, *n* a cassette usually made of metal, with the exposure side of low-atomic-number material, such as Bakelite, aluminum, or magnesium, and containing intensifying screens between which a "screen type" of film or films may be placed for exposure to radiation.

cast, *n* **1.** an object formed by pouring plastic or liquid material into a mold in which it hardens. *v* **2.** to throw metal into an impression to form the casting.

cast, bar splint, *n* See splint, cast bar.

cast, corrected master, *n* a dental cast that has been modified by the correction of the edentulous ridge areas as registered in a supplemental, correctable impression.

cast, dental, *n* a positive likeness of a part or parts of the oral cavity reproduced in a durable hard material.

cast, diagnostic, *n* a positive likeness of dental structures for the purpose of study and treatment planning.

cast, diagnostic, anatomic portion, *n* the section of a finished cast that contains the actual impression of the teeth and surrounding tissue. It should account for approximately 65% of the cast's total height.

cast, diagnostic, double-pour method, *n* a method of forming the base of a cast in which the inverted impression is held against the surface of prereadied stone while the sides and edges of the cast are shaped; eliminates the possibility of inverting the impression before the stone has set. Also called *two-step method.*

cast, diagnostic, implant, *n* a cast made from a conventional mucosal impression on which the wax trial denture and surgical impression trays are made or selected.

cast, gnathostatic **(nath′ostat′ik),** *n* a cast of the teeth trimmed so that the occlusal plane is in its normal position in the oral cavity when the cast is set on a plane surface. Such casts are used in the gnathostatic technique of orthodontic diagnosis.

cast, implant, *n* a positive reproduction of the exposed bony surfaces made in a surgical bone impression and on which subperiosteal implant frame is designed and fabricated.

cast, investment, *n* See cast, refractory.

cast, keying of, *n* the process of forming the base (or capital) of a cast so that it can be remounted accurately. Also referred to as the *split-cast method of returning a cast to an articulator.*

cast, master, *n* an accurate replica of the prepared tooth surfaces, residual ridge areas, or other parts of the dental arch reproduced from an impression from which a prosthesis is to be fabricated.

cast, mounted, *n* a reproduction of all or part of the oral cavity, which is then attached to a support for ease of display.

cast, preextraction, *n* a cast made before the extraction of teeth. See also cast, diagnostic.

cast, preoperative, *n* See cast, diagnostic.

cast, record, *n* a positive replica of the dentition and adjoining structures, used as a reference for conditions existing at a given time.

cast, refractory, *n* a cast made of materials that can withstand high temperatures without disintegrating and that, when used in partial denture casting techniques, expand to compensate for metal shrinkage.

cast, trimming diagnostic, *n* a set of finishing steps for a study cast in which the bases, posterior borders, sides, heels, and anterior surfaces are smoothed and shaped to ensure a finished product that is attractive, well proportioned, and useful as a diagnostic tool. The treatment is best accomplished using a mechanical model trimmer.

cast, working, *n* an accurate reproduction of a master cast; used in preliminary fitting of a casting to avoid injury to the master cast.

casting, *n* **1.** the process by which crowns, inlays, and other metallic restorations are produced. *v* **2.** to give a shape to (a substance) by pouring in liquid or plastic form into a mold.

casting flask, n See flask, refractory.

casting machine, n a mechanical device used for throwing or forcing a molten metal into a refractory mold.

casting machine, air pressure, n a casting machine that forces metal into the mold via compressed air.

casting machine, centrifugal, n a casting machine that forces the metal into the mold via centrifugal force.

casting machine, vacuum, n a casting machine in which the metal is cast by evacuation of gases from the mold. Atmospheric pressure actually forces metal into the mold.

casting model, n See cast, refractory.

casting ring, n See flask, refractory.

casting temperature, n See temperature, casting.

casting, vacuum, n the casting of a metal in the presence of a vacuum. See also casting machine, vacuum.

casting wax, n See wax, casting.

Castle's intrinsic factor, *n.pr* See factor, Castle's intrinsic.

castration anxiety (kastrā′shən), *n* **1.** the fantasized fear of injury to or loss of the genital organs. *n* **2.** a general threat to the body image of a person or the unrealistic fear of bodily injury or loss of power or control.

casualty insurance, *n* insurance against loss caused by accidents; usually applied to property but may apply to bodily injury or death from accident.

cat-scratch disease, *n* See disease, cat-scratch.

catabolism (kətab′ōlizəm), *n* the destructive processes (opposite of the anabolic-metabolic processes) by which complex substances are converted into more simple compounds. A proper relation between anabolism and catabolism is essential for the maintenance of bodily homeostasis and dynamic equilibrium.

catabolism of energy, n the dissipation of energy in living tissues as work or heat (one phase being metabolism, the other being anabolism).

catabolism of substance, n the destructive metabolism; the conversion of living tissues into a lower state of organization and ultimately into waste products.

catalase reaction (kat′əlās), *n* the response of bubbling in the presence of hydrogen peroxide given by blood exudates or transudates.

catalysis (kətal′əsis), *n* the increase in rate of a chemical reaction, induced by a substance called a *catalyst,* which takes no part in the reaction and remains unchanged.

catalyst (kat′əlist), *n* a substance that induces an increased rate of a chemical reaction without entering into the reaction or being changed by the reaction.

catamenia (kat′əmē′nēə), *n* menses. A term used frequently to designate age at onset of menses.

cataract (kat′ərakt), *n* an abnormal progressive condition of the lens of the eye, characterized by loss of transparency.

catatonia (kat′ətō′nēə), *n* a form of schizophrenia characterized by alternating stupor and excitement. A patient's arms often retain any position in which they are placed.

catecholamine (kat′əkō′ləmēn′), *n* any one of a group of sympathomimetic compounds composed of a catechol molecule linked to phenylethylamine. Some catecholamines (epinephrine and norepinephrine) are produced naturally by the body. Norepinephrine functions mainly as a neurotransmitter and to some extent a hormone, epinephrine functions primarily as a hormone.

catechol-o-methyl transferase (COMT), *n* an enzyme that deactivates epinephrine and norepinephrine.

catgut, *n* a sheep's intestine prepared as a suture and used for ligating vessels and closing soft tissue wounds.

catheter (kath′ətər), *n* a hollow, flexible tube that can be inserted into a vessel or cavity of the body to withdraw or instill fluids.

catheter, balloon-tip, n a tube with a balloon at its tip that can be inflated or deflated without removal after insertion.

catheter, indwelling, n a catheter left in place in the bladder; usually a type of balloon catheter.

catheterization (kath′ətərizā′sh ən), *n* the process of introducing a hollow, flexible tube into a blood vessel or body cavity to withdraw or instill fluids.

cathode (kath'ōd), *n* a negative electrode from which electrons are emitted and to which positive ions are attracted. In radiographic tubes, the cathode usually consists of a helical tungsten filament, behind which a molybdenum reflector cup is located to focus the electron emission toward the target of the anode.

cathode ray tube (CRT), *n* a vacuum tube in which a beam of electrons is focused to a small point on a luminescent screen and can be varied in position to form a pattern.

cathode-anode circuit, high-voltage, *n* one of the two electrical circuits required to expose radiographs, provides the power to accelerate electrons enough to create radiographic photons.

cation (kat'īon), *n* a positive ion carrying a charge of positive electricity, therefore attracted to the negatively charged cathode. In local anesthetics, the cation is the acid form which is water soluble and the active form of the molecule.

cationic detergent, See detergent, cationic.

causalgia (kō zal'jə), *n* a postextraction localized pain phenomenon usually characterized by a continuous burning sensation.

causality (kōsal'itē), *n* a relationship between one event or action that precedes and initiates a second action or influences the direction, nature, or force of a second action. In scientific study, causality must be observable, predictable, and reproducible and thus is difficult to prove.

cause of action, *n* a ground or reason for a legal action; a wrong that is subject to legal redress.

caustic (kôs'tik), *adj* destroying living tissue by chemical burning action.

cauterize (kô'tərīz), *v* to sear or burn living tissue in order to stop bleeding; a corrosive agent, hot metal, or electricity may be used.

cavernous sinus (kav'ərnəs), *n* one of a pair of irregularly shaped, bilateral venous channels located below the base of the brain between the sphenoid bone of the skull and the dura mater. Also called *cavernous venus sinus.*

cavernous sinus thrombosis, *n* an infection of the cavernous venous sinus. Increased risk with local anesthesia in the maxillary arch if infection is present ("needle track" infection).

cavitation (kav'itā'shun), *n* the formation and collapse of bubbles in the fluid spray released by a mechanized instrument used for debridement.

cavity (kav'itē), *n* a carious lesion or hole in a tooth.

cavity, access, *n* See access cavity.

cavity, amniotic, *n* the space between the developing fetus and the amnion, consisting of amniotic fluid.

cavity, axial surface, *n* a cavity occurring in a tooth surface in which the general plane is parallel to the long axis of the tooth.

cavity classification, *n* carious lesions are classified according to the surfaces of a tooth on which they occur (e.g., labial, buccal, occlusal), type of surface (i.e., pit, fissure, or smooth surface), and numerical grouping (G. V. Black's classification).

cavity classification, artificial (G. V. Black), *n* a classification of cavities.

cavity, complex, *n* a cavity that involves more than one surface of a tooth.

cavity, compound, *n* See cavity, complex.

cavity floor, *n* the base-enclosing side of a prepared cavity. See also cavity, prepared.

cavity, gingival (gingival third cavity), *n* a cavity occurring in the gingival third of the clinical crown of the tooth (G. V. Black's Class 5).

cavity lining, *n* the material applied to the prepared cavity before the restoration is inserted to seal the dentinal tubules for protection of the pulp.

cavity medication, *n* a drug used to clean or treat a cavity before inserting a dressing, base, or restoration.

cavity, nasal, *n* the two irregular spaces that are situated on either side of the midline of the face, extend from the cranial base to the palate, and are separated from each other by a thin vertical septum. In radiographs it appears over the roots of the maxillary incisors as a large, segmented, radio-lucent area. Also called *nasal fossa*.

cavity, pit and fissure, *n* a cavity that begins in microscopic faults in the enamel. Caused by imperfect closure of the enamel.

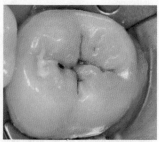

Pit and fissure cavity. (Heymann/Swift/Ritter, 2013)

cavity preparation, *n* the orderly operating procedure required to remove diseased tissue and establish in a tooth the biomechanically acceptable form necessary to receive and retain a restoration.

cavity, prepared, *n* the form developed in a tooth to receive and retain a restoration.

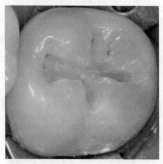

Prepared cavity. (Heymann/Swift/Ritter, 2013)

cavity, prepared, floor of, *n* the flat bottom or enclosing base wall of a prepared cavity; on an axial plane it is called the *axial wall,* and on the horizontal plane it is called the *pulpal wall.*

cavity, prepared, impression, *n* a negative likeness of a tapered type of prepared cavity.

cavity, proximal, *n* a cavity occurring on the mesial or distal surface of a tooth.

cavity, pulp, *n* the space in a tooth surrounded by the dentin; contains the dental pulp. The part of the pulp cavity within the coronal portion of the tooth is the pulp chamber, and the part found within the root is the pulp canal, or root canal.

cavity, simple, *n* a cavity that involves only one surface of a tooth.

cavity, smooth surface, *n* a cavity formed by decay beginning in surfaces of teeth that are without pits, fissures, or enamel faults.

cavity toilet, *n* G. V. Black's final step in cavity preparation. Consists of freeing all surfaces and angles of debris.

cavity varnish, *n* See varnish, cavity.

cavity wall, *n* See wall, cavity.

cavosurface angle (kā'vōsur'fəs), *n* See angle, cavosurface.

cavosurface bevel, *n* See bevel, cavosurface.

cavosurface margin, *n* See margin, cavosurface.

CBC, *n* the abbreviation for *complete blood cell count,* a procedure in which all the blood cells are counted per cubic millimeter, including a differential counting of the white blood cells (leukocytes).

CD-ROM, *n* the acronym for compact disk/read-only memory. These disks are used to store program information (software) for computer programs. Information and instructions can be retrieved from these disks, but information cannot be added or revised without destruction of the existing data.

CD4 (T4) lymphocyte, *n* an immunologically important white cell that is responsible for cell-mediated immunity. It is the cell invaded by the human immunodeficiency virus and in which the virus replicates itself.

CD8 (T8) lymphocyte, *n* a type of lymphocyte responsible for inducing the death of tumor cells or virally-infected somatic cells. Activation follows antigen presentation to surface T-cell antigen receptors; in turn there is a clonal expansion aided by cytokines (IL-2).

CDC, *n.pr* the acronym for the Centers for Disease Control and Prevention.

cecum (sē′kəm), *n* a cul-de-sac constituting the first part of the large intestine. It forms the junction between the ileum and the large intestine.

cefaclor (sef′əklor), *n brand names:* Ceclor, Ceclor CD; *drug class:* second-generation cephalosporin; *action:* inhibits bacterial cell wall synthesis; *uses:* eradication of gram negative bacilli from the upper and lower respiratory tract, treatment of urinary tracts, skin infections, and otitis media.

cefadroxil (sef′ədrok′səl), *n brand names:* Duricef, Ultracef; *drug class:* first-generation cephalosporin; *action:* inhibits bacterial cell wall synthesis, rendering cell wall osmotically unstable; *uses:* eradication of gram-negative bacilli from the upper and lower respiratory tracts, treatment of urinary tract, skin infections, otitis media.

cefazolin sodium (sifaz′ələn), *n brand names:* Ancef, Kefzol, Zolicef; *drug class:* first-generation cephalosporin; *action:* inhibits bacterial cell wall synthesis, rendering cell wall osmotically unstable; *uses:* eradication of gram-negative bacilli from the upper and lower respiratory tract, treatment of urinary tracts, skin, bone, joint, biliary, genital infections, endocarditis, surgical prophylaxis, septicemia.

cefepime (sef′əpēm), *n brand name:* Maxipime; *drug class:* fourth generation cephalosporin; *action:* inhibits cell wall synthesis in sensitive organisms; *uses:* respiratory tract, urinary tract, skin, other soft tissue infections associated with gram-negative organisms.

cefixime (sef′iksēm′), *n brand name:* Suprax; *drug class:* third generation cephalosporin; *action:* inhibits bacterial cell wall synthesis, rendering cell wall osmotically unstable; *uses:* uncomplicated urinary tract infections, pharyngitis and tonsillitis, otitis media, acute bronchitis, acute exacerbations of chronic bronchitis.

cefoxitin *n brand name:* Mefoxin; *drug class:* second generation cephalosporin antibiotic; *action:* inhibits cell wall synthesis; *uses:* respiratory, abdominal, urinary tract, and bone infections, septicemia, infections caused by one of several bacteria.

cefpodoxime proxetil (sef′podok′ sēm prok′sətil), *n brand name:* Vantin; *drug class:* third-generation cephalosporin; *action:* inhibits bacterial cell wall synthesis, rendering cell wall osmotically unstable; *uses:* upper and lower respiratory tract infections, pharyngitis, tonsillitis, gonorrhea, urinary tract infections, skin structure infections.

cefprozil monohydrate (sef′prōzil mon′ōhī′drāt), *n brand name:* Cefzil; *drug class:* second-generation cephalosporin; *action:* inhibits bacterial cell wall synthesis, which renders cell wall osmotically unstable; *uses:* pharyngitis, tonsillitis, otitis media, secondary bacterial infection of acute bronchitis, skin and skin structure infections.

ceftibuten (sef′tib′yōōtən), *n brand name:* Cedax; *drug class:* third generation cephalosporin; *action:* causes cell death by attaching to the bacterial membrane wall; *uses:* lower respiratory and urinary tract infections, gynecologic and enteric infections, pharyngitis, tonsillitis, otitis media caused by susceptible organisms.

cefuroxime axetil (sef′yōōrok′sēm ak′sətil), *n brand name:* Ceftin; *drug class:* second-generation cephalosporin; *action:* inhibits bacterial cell wall synthesis, rendering cell wall osmotically unstable; *uses:* eradication of gram-negative bacilli and gram-positive organisms, treatment of serious lower respiratory tract, urinary tract, skin, gonococcal infections, septicemia, meningitis.

celecoxib *n brand name:* Celebrex; *drug class:* non-steroidal antiinflammatory; *action:* selectively inhibits cyclooxygenase 2 (COX-2); *use:* pain.

celiac sprue (sē′lēak sprōō), *n* a genetic disorder in which the body cannot digest certain gluten proteins found in wheat, barley, rye, and oats. This leads to inflammation and flattening of the wall of the small intestine and a reduction in the body's ability to absorb nutrients. Also known as *celiac disease (CD).*

C

cell(s), *n/n.pl* the basic unit of vital tissue. One of a large variety of microscopic protoplasmic masses that make up organized tissues. Each cell has a cell membrane, protoplasm, nucleus, and a variety of inclusion bodies. Each type of cell is a living unit with its own metabolic requirements, functions, permeability, ability to differentiate into other cells, reproducibility, and life expectancy.

cell, beta, *n* any cell that produces insulin in the islets of Langerhans region of the pancreas.

cell, body, *n.pl* the part of the neuron containing the nucleus. It is responsible for protein synthesis and provides metabolic support for the neuron. Also called *soma.*

cell, bone-forming, *n.* See osteoblast.

cell, central, of the dental papillae, *n* the inner cells of the dental papilla within the concavity of the enamel organ that are the primordium of the pulp.

cell, centrioles of (sen′trēōls), *n.pl* cylinder-shaped organelles that contain microtubules. Function is to organize spindle fibers during cell division.

cell, connective tissue, *n* the fibroblast, which for purposes of clarity is characterized by such terms as *perivascular connective tissue cell* or *young connective tissue cell.*

cell count, *n* the number of cells contained in a unit volume; usually refers to red and/or white blood cells in a unit volume of blood.

cell culture, *n* living cells that are maintained in vitro in artificial media of serum and nutrients for the study and growth of certain strains, experiments in controlling diseases, or study of the reaction to certain drugs or agents.

cell cycle, *n* the sequence of events that occur during the growth and division of tissue cells.

cell, cytoplasm of (sī′tōplazəm), *n* the aqueous part of the cell in which are suspended all the organelles and inclusions. Site of all metabolic activities in the cell.

cell death, *n* the point in the process of dying at which vital functions have ceased at the cellular level. It precludes the use of tissue or organs as transplant donors.

cell, defense, *n* a cell, mobilized within inflamed, irritated, or otherwise diseased tissue, that acts as a protective element to neutralize or wall off the foreign irritant. Defense cells include plasma cells, polymorphonuclear leukocytes, and the cells of the reticuloendothelial system.

cell, dendritic (sel dendrit′ik), *n* the immune cells involved in the activation of T cells and B cells. They are primarily found in exposed tissue such as skin, the lungs, the stomach and intestines, and the membranes of the nose, but they are also found in blood. Not to be confused with dendrites.

cell differentiation, *n* the development of the cells into the various basic cell units of tissue: the epithelial cell and the nerve cell, which arise from the ectodermal tissue layer of the embryo; and the blood, muscle, bone, cartilage, and other connective tissue cells, which arise from the mesodermal tissue of the embryo. The mature tissue cell has many intermediary, transitional forms that are sequential in their development from the primitive, less differentiated anlage cell forms. These intermediary forms are evident clinically in disease in blood dyscrasias, tumors, and inflammation and in health in the normal processes of growth, development, healing, and repair.

cell, endoplasmic reticulum of, *n* See endoplasmic reticulum.

cell, endosteal, *n* a reticular cell that is modified and identified by its location; the endosteum is a condensation of the stroma of the bone marrow.

cell, filaments of, *n.pl* threadlike structures the function of which is to support the cytoskeleton; also integral parts of intercellular junctions.

cell, germ, *n* a cell of an organism the function of which is to reproduce an entity similar to the organism from which the germ cell originated. Germ cells are characteristically haploid.

cell, giant, *n* a large cell frequently having several nuclei.

cell, Golgi complex in, *n* See Golgi apparatus.

cell homeostasis, *n* See homeostasis, cell.

cell, homeostasis of (hŏ′mēōstā′sis), *n* See homeostasis, cell.

cell, inclusions of, *n.pl* nonliving bodies, by-products of cellular metabolism present in the cytoplasm.

cell, Langerhans, *n.pr* star-shaped cells of unknown function that appear to be permanent residents of the epithelium.

cell, lysosomes in (**lī'sōsōm**), *n.pl* membranous organelles produced from the Golgi complex; contain hydrolytic enzymes, which aid intracellular digestion.

cell membrane, *n* the outer covering of a cell. The membrane controls the exchange of materials between the cell and its environment.

cell, membrane of, transport through, *n* the movement of biomolecules into and out of cells. See diffusion, osmosis, active transport, phagocytosis.

cell, mesenchymal (**mezen'kəməl**), *n* an embryonic connective tissue cell with an outstanding capacity for proliferation and capable of further differentiation into reticular cells or osteoblasts. When persisting in the adult organism, the cells are usually arranged in loose connective tissue along the small blood vessels or in reticular fibers. They are identified by their location and capacity to differentiate into other cell types, such as smooth muscle cells in the formation of new arteries, phagocytes in inflammatory processes, and bone cells in the formation of new bone tissue.

cell, microtubules of, *n.pl* See microtubule.

cell, mitochondria of, *n.pl* See mitochondria.

cell, mucous, *n* a mucous-secreting cell.

cell, nucleus of, *n* See nucleus.

cell, outer, of the dental papillae, *n* an outer cell of the dental papilla within the concavity of the enamel organ that will differentiate into dentin-secreting cells or odontoblasts.

cell, plasma, *n* a cell of disputed origin (lymphatic versus undifferentiated mesenchymal cell) that is seen in chronic inflammation and certain disease states and tumors but not normally in the circulating blood. The cell is larger than a lymphocyte and has a cartwheel-like, eccentric nucleus with basophilic nuclear chromatin peripherally located. The cells synthesize antibodies (immunoglobulins).

cell, progenitor, *n* a cell that is able to transform into different types of cells through replication and differentiation.

cells, radiosensitivity of, *n* the amount of sensitivity of a particular cell to radiation, determined by three factors: cell metabolism—the higher the metabolic rate, the more sensitive; cell differentiation—less mature cells are more sensitive than specialized cells; and mitotic activity—cells are more sensitive when they are dividing or rapidly reproducing.

cell, replication, *n* See mitosis.

cell, reticular, *n* a cell of reticular connective tissue, such as in the stroma of the bone marrow, that retains both osteogenic and hematopoietic potencies; it is identified by its location, morphology, potency, and direct origin from mesenchymal cells.

cell, serous, *n* a specialized glandular epithelial cell that produces enzymatic secretions. These cells have a rounded nucleus and special secretory granules, or vesicles, in their cytoplasm. Serous cells include the acinar cells of the salivary glands and pancreas, gastric chief cells, and intestinal Paneth cells.

cell, somatic (**sōmat'ik**), *n* a cell that forms parts of the body, including the cells of the skin, bone, blood, connective tissue, and internal organs. From the Greek word *soma,* meaning "body."

cell, stem, *n.pl* the cells in the bone marrow from which all blood cells originate.

cell, typical, *n* See cell.

cell wall, *n* See cell membrane.

cell-surface marker, *n* an antigenic area on the surface of a cell that identifies that cell as a particular type.

cellulitis (**sel'yōōlī'tis**), *n* a diffuse inflammatory process occurring in response to an infection, that spreads along fascial planes and through tissue spaces without gross suppuration.

celluloid strip, *n* See strip, plastic.

cellulose (**sel'yōōlōs**), *n* the primary component of plant cell walls; provides the fiber and bulk necessary for optimal functioning of the digestive tract.

cellulose, oxidized, *n* cellulose, in the form of cotton, gauze, or paper, that has been made more or less completely oxidized.

cement, *n* a material that produces a mechanical interlocking effect on hardening.

cement, acrylic resin dental, *n* a dental cement, dispensed as a powder and a liquid, that is mixed as is any other cement. The powder contains polymethyl methacrylate, a filler, plasticizer, and polymerization initiator. The liquid monomer is methyl 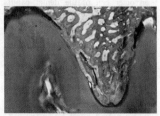 methacrylate with an inhibitor and an activator.

cement, copper dental, *n* a zinc phosphate cement to the powder of which has been added a copper oxide.

cement, dental, *n* the materials used in dentistry as luting agents, bases, and temporary restorations. See also cement, acrylic resin dental; cement, zinc.

cement, dental base, *n* an insulating layer of cement placed in the deeper portion of a prepared cavity to insulate the pulp.

cement dressing, *n* a postoperative dressing applied after periodontal surgery.

cement dressing, dental, Kirkland, *n. pr* See dressing, Kirkland cement.

cement, Kryptex dental, *n.pr* See cement, silicophosphate.

cement line, *n* See line, cement.

cement, polycarboxylate, *n* a dental cement used for cementation of cast restorations and orthodontic appliances and as bases. Prepared by mixing a zinc oxide powder with a liquid of polycarboxylic acid.

cement, resin, *n* See resin cement.

cement sealer, *n* a compound used in filling a root canal; it is inserted in a plastic condition, solidifies after placement, and fills any irregularities in the surface of the canal.

cement, silicate, *n* a relatively hard, translucent restorative material used primarily in anterior teeth. Prepared by mixing a liquid and a powder. The powder is an acid-soluble glass prepared by the fusion of CaO, SiO, Al_2O_3, and other ingredients with a fluoride flux. The liquid is a buffered phosphoric acid solution.

cement, silicious dental, *n* See cement, silicate.

cement, silicophosphate (sil′ikō fos′-fā t), *n* (Kryptex cement), a combination zinc phosphate and silicate cement. Less translucent, less irritating, and less soluble than silicate and stronger than zinc phosphate cement.

cement, zinc oxide–eugenol dental (ok′sīd-yōō′jənol), *n* the least irritating of the cements. The powder is essentially zinc oxide with strengtheners and accelerators. The liquid is basically eugenol.

cement, zinc phosphate, *n* a material used for cementation of inlays, crowns, bridges, and orthodontic appliances; occasionally used as a temporary restoration. Prepared by mixing a powder and a liquid. The powders are composed primarily of zinc oxide and magnesium oxides. The principal constituents of the liquid are phosphoric acid, water, and buffer agents.

cement-retained, *adj* referring to any of several methods for restoring lost or missing teeth by cementing them to a prosthetic attachment anchored in the jaw.

cemental, *adj* of or pertaining to the cementum of a tooth.

cemental repair, *n* See repair, cemental.

cemental spurs, *n.pl* the symmetrical spheres of cementum attached to the root surface.

cemental tear, *n* a small portion of cementum forcibly separated, either partially or completely, from the underlying dentin of the root. It often occurs as a result of occlusal force, and is most commonly seen on incisors; seen on the tension side in occlusal traumatism.

Cemental tear. (Newman/Takei/Klokkevold, 2012)

cementation (sē'mentā'shən), *n* attachment of an appliance or a restoration to natural teeth or attachment of parts by means of a cement.

◙ **cementicle** (səmen'tikəl), *n* a calcified body sometimes found in the periodontal ligament of older individuals. They may form from calcified epithelial rests, or from small spicules of cementum or alveolar bone traumatically displaced into the periodontal membrane. They may also be attached to or embedded in the cementum.

cementifying fibroma, *n* See fibroma, ossifying.

cementing line, *n* See line, cemental.

cementoblast (səmen'tōblast), *n* the cell that forms the organic matrix of cementum. Derived from the inner aspect of the dental sac during the initial formation of cementum or from the mesenchymal cell of the periodontal membrane after completion of primary cementogenesis. The cementoblast, trapped within cellular cementum, becomes a cementocyte.

cementoclasia (səmen'tōklā'zhə, -zēə), *n* the destruction of cementum by cementoclasts.

◙ **cementocyte** (səmen'tōsīt), *n* the cell found within lacunae of cellular cementum; possesses protoplasmic processes that course through the canaliculi of the cementum; derived from cementoblasts trapped within newly formed cementum.

cementoenamel junction *(CEJ),* *n* See junction, cementoenamel.

cementogenesis (sēmen'tōjen'ə sis), *n* the formation of cementum, the calcified connective tissue that covers the roots of teeth, from the epithelial root sheath. See also cementoblast.

cementoid (səmen'toid), *n* the cementum matrix produced by the cementoblasts, which forms the most recent uncalcified layer covering the surface of cementum.

cementoma (sēmentō'mə), *n* (traumatic osteoclasia), an apical lesion associated with the apices of teeth. It may be present as a mass of fibrous connective tissue, fibrous connective tissue with spicules of cementum, or a calcified mass resembling cementum and having few cellular elements.

cementoma, first-state, *n* See fibroma, periapical.

cementopathia (səmen'tōpath' ēə), *n* the concept wherein necrotic, diseased cementum and lack of productivity of cementum are implicated in the causation of periodontitis and periodontosis.

◙ **cementum** (səmen'tum), *n* a specialized, calcified connective tissue that covers the anatomic root of a tooth, giving attachment to the periodontal ligament.

cementum, abnormalities of, *n.pl* includes the reversal lines in the cementum, which represent bone tissue resorption or cementum resorption. Cementicles are calcified epithelial cells found in older persons. Hypercementosis is cementum overgrowth on the roots. See also reversal lines, cementicle, and hypercementosis.

cementum, acellular, *n* the cementum that contains no cementocytes.

cementum, cellular, *n* the portion of the calcified substance covering the root surfaces of the teeth. It is bonelike and contains cementocytes embedded within lacunae, with protoplasmic processes of the cementocytes coursing through canaliculi that anastomose with canaliculi of adjacent lacunae. The lacunae are dispersed through a calcified matrix arranged in lamellar form. It is localized primarily at the apical portion of the root but may deposit over the acellular cementum or serve to repair areas of cemental resorption.

cementum, collagen fibrils of, *n* the fibrils that penetrate the cementum surface and are continuous with the periodontal fibers necessary for tooth support.

cementum, lamellar, *n* the cementum in which layers of appositional cementum are arranged in a sheaflike pattern, the layers of cementum being more or less parallel to the cemental surface and demarcated by incremental lines that represent periods of inactivity of cementum formation.

cementum, necrotic, *n* nonvital cementum that is situated coronal to the bottom of the periodontal pocket.

cementum, properties of, *n.pl* the calcified, avascular connective tissue that is derived from the dental sac and functions in protecting the roots of teeth.

cementum, secondary, *n* the term used to describe all subsequent layers of cementum formed after the primary layer. It may be cellular or acellular.

center of rotation, *n* a point or line around which all other points in a body move.

Centers for Disease Control and Prevention (CDC), *n* the federal facility for disease eradication, epidemiology, and education, headquartered in Atlanta, Georgia.

central bearing, *n* the application of forces between the maxilla and mandible at a single point located as near as possible to the center of the supporting areas of the upper and lower jaws. The purpose is to distribute the closing forces of the jaws evenly throughout the areas of the supporting structures during the registration and recording of maxillomandibular (jaw) relations and the correction of occlusal errors.

central bearing device, *n* a device that provides a central point of bearing or support between upper and lower occlusion rims. It consists of a contracting point attached to one occlusion rim and a plate on the other rim that provides the surface on which the bearing point rests or moves.

central bearing point, *n* See point, central-bearing.

■ **central nervous system (CNS),** *n* that portion of the nervous system consisting of the brain and spinal cord. The portion of the nervous system beyond the brain and cord is known as the *peripheral nervous system.*

central occlusion, *n* See occlusion, centric.

central processing unit (CPU), *n* the primary processor of a computer, containing the internal memory unit (memory), arithmetic logic unit (ALU), and input/output control unit (I/O control).

central tendency, *n* the tendency of a group of scores to cluster around a central representative score. The statistics most frequently used for measures of central tendency are the mean, median, and mode.

centric (sen'trik), *adj* (objectionable as a noun) describing jaw and tooth relationships. See also position,

centric; relation, centric; occlusion, centric.

centric checkbite, *n* See record, occluding, centric relation.

centric occlusion, *n* See occlusion, centric.

centric position, *n* See position, centric.

centric relation, *n* See relation, centric.

■ **centric stops,** *n* the stable points of contact between occluded maxillary and mandibular teeth, located in the central pits, marginal ridges, and buccal and lingual cusps of posterior teeth and the incisals and linguals of anterior teeth.

centrifugal force (sentrif'əgəl), *n* See force, centrifugal.

cephalexin (sef'əlek'sin), *n* *brand names:* Ceporex, Keftab, Keflex; *drug class:* first-generation cephalosporin; *action:* inhibits bacterial cell wall synthesis, rendering cell wall osmotically unstable; *uses:* removal of gram-negative bacilli from the upper and lower respiratory tracts, urinary tract, skin; treatment of bone infections, otitis media.

cephalic index (sefal'ik), *n* an anthropometric value based on the ratio between the width and length of the head.

■ **cephalogram (sef'əlōgram),** *n* a cephalometric radiograph. On tracings of these films, anatomic points, planes, and angles are drawn that assist in the evaluation of the patient's facial growth and development.

cephalometer (sef'əlom'ətur), *n* See cephalostat.

cephalometer, radiographic, *n* See cephalostat.

cephalometric analysis (sef'əlōmet'rik), *n* See analysis, cephalometric.

cephalometric landmark, *n* See landmark, cephalometric.

cephalometric radiograph, *n* See radiograph, cephalometric.

cephalometric skeletal analysis, *n* an assessment of the facial type of a skeleton; the relationship of the parts to each other, to the skull, and to an estimated "normal."

cephalometric tracing, *n* a tracing of selected structures from a cephalometric radiograph made on translucent drafting paper or film for purposes of measurement and evaluation.

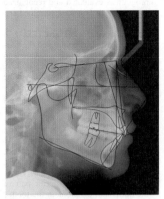

Cephalometric tracing. (Courtesy Dr. Flavio Uribe)

cephalometrics (sef´əlōmet´riks), *n* the scientific study of the measurements of the head.

cephalometry (sef´əlom´ətrē), *n* the measurement of the bony structure of the head using reproducible lateral and anteroposterior radiograms.

cephalophore (sef´əlō´fôr), *n* a cephalostat designed to take insequence-oriented facial photographs and gnathostatic models.

cephalosporins (sef´ələspor´ins), *n* semisynthetic derivatives of an antibiotic originally derived from the microorganism *Cephalosporium acremonium* (now *Acremonium chrysogenum*). They are similar in structure to penicillins.

cephalostat (sef´əlōstat), *n* a head-positioning device that ensures reproducibility of the relations between the x-ray beam, the head of a patient, and the radiographic receptor.

cephradine (sef´rədēn), *n brand name:* Velosef; *drug class:* first generation cephalosporin; *action:* inhibits bacterial cell wall synthesis, rendering cell wall osmotically unstable; *uses:* removal of gram negative bacilli and gram-positive organisms from respiratory tract, urinary tract, skin infections, otitis media.

ceramic coating, *n* a thin layer of ceramic material, commonly hydroxyapatite, used to cover dental implants.

This typically increases the hardness of the implant and can also make the implant bond more readily with bone.

ceramics, *n* the art of making dental restorations or parts of restorations from fused porcelain.

ceramics, orthoclase, *n* See feldspar.

cerebellum (ser´əbel´um), *n* a major division of the brain, behind the cerebrum and above the pons and fourth ventricle, consisting of a median lobe, two lateral lobes, and major connections through pairs of peduncles to the cerebrum, pons, and medulla oblongata. It is connected with the auditory vestibular apparatus and the proprioceptive system of the body and hence is involved in maintenance of body equilibrium, orientation in space, and muscular coordination and tonus.

cerebral arteries, *n.pl* the arteries to the brain that supply the cerebrum.

cerebral cortex, *n* a thin layer of gray matter on the surface of the cerebral hemisphere, folded into gyri with about two thirds of its area buried in fissures. It integrates higher mental functions, general movement, visceral functions, perception, and behavioral reactions.

cerebral hemorrhage, *n* an emergency condition indicated by the rupturing of a blood vessel in the brain and the subsequent bleeding into the tissues of the brain. Type of stroke or cerebrovascular accident (CVA).

cerebral infarction, *n* the blockage of the flow of blood to the cerebrum, causing or resulting in brain tissue death. Blockage may be caused by a thrombosis, an embolism, a vasospasm, or a rupture of a blood vessel. Type of stroke or cerebrovascular accident (CVA).

cerebral ischemia, *n* the reduction or loss of oxygen to the cerebrum; prolonged ischemia may lead to cerebral infarction.

cerebral palsy, *n* See palsy, cerebral.

cerebrospinal fluid, *n* the fluid that flows through and protects the four ventricles of the brain, subarachnoid space, and spinal canal.

cerebrovascular accident, signs and symptoms of, *n* a complete paralysis on one side of the body or various parts (e.g., face, arm, or leg), a diminished capacity to see, speak,

C

C

swallow, or control saliva, an increase or decrease in sensitivity to touch and pain, and an alteration in mental processes and personality; depends on the degree of involvement and the area of the brain damage.

cerebrum (ser'əbrum, sərē'brum), *n* the largest portion of the brain. Operating at the highest functional level and occupying the upper part of the cranium, it consists of two hemispheres united at the bottom by commissures of large bundles of nerve fibers. As with all parts of the nervous system, each part of it has highly specific functions (e.g., a specific outer cortical area controls voluntary mastication, whereas certain inner subcortical areas are involved in involuntary jaw posture).

cerium, *n* a ductile, gray rare-earth element. Cerium oxalate is used as a sedative, an antiemetic, and an antitussive. Cerium oxide is used in dental porcelains to stimulate the natural fluorescence found in human dental enamel.

Ceromer, *n.pr* an indirect filled resin material processed with combinations of heat/light/pressure to create semipermanent onlay or crown restorations.

certificate holder, *n* **1.** the person, usually the employee, who represents the family unit covered by the dental benefits program; other family members are referred to as *dependents*. *n* **2.** generally refers to a subscriber of a traditional indemnity program. *n* **3.** in reference to the program for dependents of active-duty military personnel, the certificate holder is called the *sponsor.* See also subscriber. Synonyms: subscriber, enrollee.

certificate of eligibility, *n* an official identification card or similar document issued to program beneficiaries as evidence of entitlement to services.

certificate of insurance, *n* a statement issued to a group member describing in general terms the policy provisions for eligibility, deductibles, coinsurance, allowances, and maximums. Used in lieu of issuing copies of the group or master contract to each individual employee member of an insured group.

certification, *n* a process by which an individual, institution, or educational program is evaluated and recognized as meeting certain predetermined criteria and standards.

certified dental assistant *(CDA),* *n* a person who has completed the Certification Board of the American Dental Assistant Association (ADAA).

cervical (sur'vikəl), *adj* relating to the neck, or cervical line, of a tooth.

cervical appliance, *n* See appliance, cervical.

cervical convergence, *n* See convergence, cervical.

cervical fibers, *n* See nerve fibers.

cervical line, *n* See junction, cementoenamel.

cervical ridge, *n* See ridge, cervical.

cervical third, *n* an inferior part of the horizontal divisions in the tooth's crown.

cervical triangle, posterior, *n* See triangle, cervical, posterior.

cervical vertebrae, *n* the first seven segments of the vertebral column that defines the neck.

cervical chain (lymph nodes), *n* one of three serially linked groups of lymph nodes located in the neck, including the superficial, deep, and posterior chains.

cervical collar, *n* flexible lead shield used to protect the thyroid gland from scatter radiation. Also known as *thyroid collar*. See also apron, lead.

cervical lymphadenectomy (limfad 'ənek'tōmē), *n* See neck dissection.

cesium (sē'zēəm), *n* an alkali metal element used in photoelectric cells and television cameras.

cestode (ses'tōd), *n* a tapeworm that resides in the small intestine or other vital organs (including the brain). It can be passed on to humans through contaminated or improperly cooked meats, including fish. Symptoms of infection, when they occur, are similar to mild food poisoning.

cetirizine HCl, *n brand names:* Reactine, Zyrtec; *drug class:* antihistamine; *action:* competitive antagonist at histamine H1 receptors; *uses:* treatment of symptoms of seasonal allergic rhinitis, perennial allergic rhinitis, chronic urticaria.

cetylpyridinium chloride (sē'tilpir'i din'ēum), *n* a quaternary amonium antiinfective agent used as a topical disinfectant and as a preservative in prepared pharmaceutical compounds.

cevimeline, *n brand name:* Evoxac; *drug class:* salivary stimulant; *action:* stimulates muscarinic cholinergic receptors; *use:* dry mouth (when salivary glands have retained some function).

Chagas' disease (chäg′əs), *n.pr* a parasitic disease caused by *Trypanosoma cruzi* transmitted to humans by the bite of bloodsucking insects.

chalazion forceps (kəlā′zēon), *n* See forceps, chalazion.

chalk, *n* an abrasive agent made from compact calcite.

chamber, *n* an enclosed area.

chamber, air-equivalent ionization, *n* a chamber in which the materials of the wall and electrodes produce ionization essentially similar to that produced in a free-air ionization chamber.

chamber, air-wall ionization, *n* an ionization chamber with walls of material of low atomic number, having the same effective atomic number as atmospheric air.

chamber, extrapolation ionization **(ekstrap′əlā′shən ĭ′ənīzā′shən),** *n* an ionization chamber with electrodes of which the spacing can be adjusted and accurately determined to permit extrapolation of its reading to zero chamber volume.

chamber, free-air ionization, *n* an ionization chamber in which a delimited beam of radiation passes between the electrodes without striking the walls or other internal parts of the equipment. The electric field is maintained perpendicular to the electrodes in the collecting region; as a result the ionized volume can be accurately determined from the dimensions of the collecting electrode and limiting diaphragm. This is the basic standard instrument for dosimetry within the range of 5 to 400 kV.

chamber, ionization **(ĭ′ənīzā′sh ən),** *n* an instrument for measuring the quantity of ionizing radiation, in terms of the charge of electricity associated with ions produced within a defined volume of air.

chamber, monitor ionization, *n* an ionization chamber used for checking the constancy of performance of the roentgen-ray apparatus.

chamber, pocket ionization, *n* a small, pocket-sized ionization chamber used for monitoring radiation exposure of personnel. Before use it is given a charge, and the amount of discharge is a measure of the quantity of radiation received.

chamber, pulp, (pulp cavity), *n* the space occupied by the pulp.

chamber, relief, *n* a recess in the impression surface of a denture created to reduce or eliminate pressure from the corresponding area of the oral cavity.

chamber, standard ionization, *n* See chamber, ionization, free-air.

chamber, suction, *n* See chamber, relief.

chamber, thimble ionization, *n* a small cylindrical or spherical chamber, usually with walls of organic material.

chamber, thin-wall ionization, *n* an ionization chamber having walls so thin that nearly all secondary corpuscular rays reaching them from external materials can penetrate them easily.

chamber, tissue-equivalent ionization, *n* a chamber in which the walls, electrodes, and gas are selected to produce ionization essentially equivalent to the characteristics of the tissue under consideration.

chamfer (autochthonous ulcer) (cham′fər), *n* in extracoronal cavity preparations, a marginal finish that produces a curve from an axial wall to the cavosurface.

chancre (shang′kur), *n* the primary lesion of syphilis, located at the site of entrance of the spirochete into the body, occurring about 3 weeks after contact. It begins as a papule and then develops into a clean-based shallow ulcer. Secondary infection may produce suppuration. Has the appearance of a buttonlike mass because of the contiguous induration and rolled border. Weeping characteristics also are present.

chancre of lip, *n* the primary lesion of syphilis that often appears as an ulcerated or crusted, indurated lesion with a brownish or copper-colored weeping base when located on the lip, which contains *T. pallidum.*

chancre, soft, *n* See chancroid.

chancroid (shang'kroid), *n* (soft chancre), a sexually transmitted disease caused by *H. ducreyi*. It is characterized by a soft chancre that is a necrotic draining ulcer similar to a chancre but without characteristic induration. A regional bubo may occur.

channel, *n* a definite furrow, groove, or tubelike passage.

channel, vascular, *n* a blood or lymph vessel through which inflammatory infiltrate and periodontitis proceed from a localized superficial area to involve the deeper structures of the periodontium.

change agent , *n* an event, organization, material thing or, more usually, a person that intentionally or unintentionally acts as a catalyst for social, cultural, or behavioral change.

Chantix (chan'tiks), *n* the brand name for the prescription drug verenicline, which is prescribed to aid in the cessation of smoking. Chantix provides minimal nicotine effects to ease symptoms of withdrawal and blocks the impact of nicotine if the user resumes smoking.

character, *n* one of a set of elementary symbols that may be arranged in groups to express information. They may include the decimal digits 0 to 9, the letters A to Z, punctuation marks, operation symbols, and any other single symbol that a computer may read, store, or write.

characteristics, acquired, *n.pl* environmentally influenced attributes that manifest after birth.

characteristics, sex, *n.pl* **1.** the primary sex characteristics are those organs concerned with reproduction such as the gonads and genitalia. *n.pl* **2.** secondary sex characteristics include differences in voice range and timbre, muscularity, and distribution of hair and adipose tissue.

charcoal, *n* a carbonized reduction of wood used as fuel and as an adsorptive substance to cleanse the air; it is used in some medical products.

Charcot's joint, *n.pr* See joint, Charcot's.

charges, *n.pl* the financial obligation made to a patient's account for services rendered, usually on a quoted fee for explicit services provided.

charlatan (shar'lətən), *n* a quack, a person who pretends to have skills or knowledge that he or she does not possess.

Charge-coupled device (CCD), *n* a solid-state detector found in the intraoral sensor used in digital imaging.

Charles' law, *n* See law, Charles'.

chart, *n* a sheet of paper or pasteboard that presents a graphic representation of a condition or state.

chart, Bonwill-Hawley, n.pr See chart, Hawley.

chart, dental, *n* a diagrammatic chart of the teeth on which the findings from the clinical and radiographic examinations are recorded.

chart, Hawley, n.pr (Bonwill-Hawley chart), graded outlines of dental arch sizes based on the mesiodistal diameters of the six anterior teeth.

chart, health, *n* See chart, history.

chart, history, *n* forms and records for obtaining a thorough medical and oral history combined with a complete record of findings that enable the practitioner to gather and have on hand the necessary records to render total patient care.

chart, periodontal, *n* a diagrammatic chart on which the findings from the periodontal examination are recorded. This includes pocket readings, furcations, tooth mobility, exudates and gingival recession.

chart, tooth, *n* See chart, dental.

Charters' method, *n.pr* See method, Charters'.

charting, *n* the tabulation of the progress of a disease; the compilation of a clinical record.

charting, computerized, *n* an automated method for documenting a patient's dental health, utilizing such computer innovations as voice activation and mouse-activated software to ensure accuracy and save time.

charting symbols, *n.pl* commonly accepted notations that are made to the patient's chart to indicate the condition, position, and restorative history of individual teeth.

Chayes' attachment (shāz), *n.pr* believed to be the first internal precision attachment. See also attachment, intracoronal.

Cheadle's disease (chēdls), See scurvy, infantile.

check key, *n* a device used to maintain accuracy while interchanging semiadjustable articulators.

checkbite, *n* See record, interocclusal.

   checkbite, centric, n See record, interocclusal, centric and record, maxillary.

   checkbite, eccentric, n See record, interocclusal, eccentric.

   checkbite, lateral, n See record, interocclusal.

   checkbite, protrusive, n See record, interocclusal, protrusive.

cheek, *n* the fleshy area on each side of the face below the eye and between the ear, nose, and oral cavity.

   cheek biting, n the chewing of one's cheek (buccal mucosa) because of malocclusion, oral habit, or lack of coordination in the chewing cycle. Can result in trauma to the area.

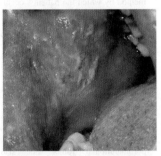

Cheek biting. (Sapp/Eversole/Wysocki, 2004)

cheilion (kīlē'ən), *n* the corner of the oral cavity.

cheilitis, actinic (solar cheilitis) (kīlī'tis aktin'ik), *n* crusting, desquamation, ulceration, atrophy, and inflammation of the lips, especially the lower lip, caused by chronic exposure to the elements and actinic rays of sunlight.

   cheilitis, cigarette paper, n focal areas of inflammation of the lips caused by cigarette paper sticking to the surface and injury produced by efforts to remove it.

   cheilitis, glandularis apostematosa (glan'jəlar'is apəstem'ətō'sə), n chronic diffuse nodular enlargement of the lower lip associated with purulent inflammatory hyperplasia of the mucous glands and ducts. Rare; unknown etiology.

   cheilitis, solar, n See cheilitis, actinic.

cheiloplasty (kī'əplastē), *n* corrective surgery or restoration of the lips.

cheilorraphy (kīlôr'əfē), *n* surgical repair of a congenital cleft lip.

cheilosis, actinic (kīlō'sis aktin'ik), *n* a diffuse degenerative change of the lower lip as a result of sun damage, which may result in cancer and present with white/red patches or non-healing ulcers, without a distinct border.

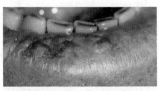

Actinic cheilosis. (Neville, et al, 2009)

cheilosis, angular, *n* See perleche.

cheilotomy (kīlôt'əmē), *n* incision into or excision of a part of the lip.

chelating agents, *n.pl* chemical compounds used to bind or inactivate metal poisons in the body.

chelation (kēlā'shən), *n* chemical reaction of a metallic ion (e.g., calcium ion) with a suitable reactive compound (e.g., ethylenediamine tetra-acetic acid) to form a compound in which the metal ion is tightly bound.

   chelation therapy, n the use of a chelating agent to bind firmly and sequester metallic poisons.

chemamnesia (kem'amnē'zhə, zēə), reversible amnesia produced by a chemical or drug.

Chemclave, *n.pr* the brand name for chemical vapor sterilizer that uses a mixture of alcohols, ketones, formaldehyde, and water heated to approximately 127°C under a pressure of at least 20 pounds per square inch. American Dental Association accepted. See also sterilization, chemical.

chemical cure, *n* a type of treatment in which a chemical process begins when the ingredients are completely mixed. The setting time depends on temperature and any added accelerator.

chemical dependence, *n* psychologic or physical reliance on any number of drugs, both legal and illegal, prescription and over the counter. The individual may experience withdrawal symptoms if the chemical is no longer taken into the body.

chemical inventory, *n* comprehensive list of every product used in the office that contains chemicals.

chemical solutions, darkroom, *n.pl* developer, fixer and distilled water use to mix the chemicals for processing radiographic films.

chemically induced, *adj* initiating biologic action or response by the introduction of a chemical.

chemistry, *n* the science dealing with the elements, their compounds, and the molecular structure and interactions of matter.

chemoreceptor (kē'mōrēsep'tər), *n* a specialized sensory end organ adapted for excitation by chemical substances (e.g., olfactory and gustatory receptors) or specialized sense organs of the carotid body that are sensitive to chemical changes in the bloodstream.

chemotaxis (kē'mōtak'sis), *n* a response involving movement that is positive (toward) or negative (away from) to a chemical stimulus.

chemotaxis, leukocyte, *n* the phagocytic activity of neutrophils and monocytes in response to chemical factors released by invading microorganisms.

chemotherapeutic agent, *n* See agent, chemotherapeutic.

chemotherapy, *n* a cancer treatment method that uses chemical agents to modify or destroy cancer cells; dental patients who are undergoing chemotherapy may have increased needs for certain nutrients and the treatment may affect the oral cavity. See also agent, chemotherapeutic.

chemotherapy, local, for gingivitis, *n* the treatment of gingivitis with a topical antibiotic agent.

chenodiol (kē'nōdī'ol), *n* *brand name:* Chenix; *drug class:* anticholelithic; *action:* increases amount of bile acids in relation to cholesterol; *use:* dissolving gallstones.

cherubism (familial intraosseous swelling) (cher'əbiz'əm), *n* 1. a fibroosseous disease of the jaws of genetic nature. The swollen jaws and raised eyes give a cherubic appearance; multiple radiolucencies are evident on radiographic examination. *n* 2. a familial form of fibrous dysplasia characterized by unilateral or, more often, bilateral swelling of the jaws in children. See also dysplasia, fibrous.

chest pain, *n* a physical complaint that requires immediate diagnosis and evaluation. It may be symptomatic of cardiac disease such as angina pectoris, myocardial infarction, or pericarditis or disease of the lungs and its linings. It also may be referred from the gastrointestinal tract or elsewhere. The differential diagnosis of chest pain is a crucial element of medical practice. See also angina pectoris.

chew-in record, functional, *n* the method by which the patient's occlusal paths in the wax patterns are recorded to be used in making restorations. In making the grooves and ridges in the wax patterns directly, the patient is asked to make right-and-left and fore-and-aft sliding occlusal strokes to generate the paths of the opposite prominences. See also path, generated occlusal.

chewing, *n* the movements of the mandible during mastication; controlled by neuromuscular action and limited by the anatomic structure of the temporomandibular joints. See also mastication.

chewing cycle, *n* See cycle, chewing.

chewing force, *n* See force, chewing.

chewing tobacco, *n* See smokeless tobacco.

Cheyne-Stokes reflex, *n.pr* See respiration, Cheyne-Stokes.

Cheyne-Stokes respiration, *n.pr* See respiration, Cheyne-Stokes.

chi square (kī), *n* a nonparametric statistic used with discrete data in the form of frequency count (nominal data) or percentages or proportions that can be reduced to frequencies. Used to determine differences between categories (e.g., yes-no; visits dental office every 6 months, 1 year, 2 years, 5 years); compares the observed results with the expected results to determine significant differences. May be used with many categories of response.

chickenpox, *n* See varicella.

child, *n* **1.** a person of either gender between the time of birth and adolescence, or puberty. **2.** in the law of negligence and in laws for the protection of children, a term used as the opposite of *adult* (generally under the age of puberty) without reference to parentage and distinction of gender.

child abuse, n the physical, sexual, or emotional maltreatment of a person under 18 years of age. Child abuse occurs predominantly with children under 3 years of age. Symptoms include bruises and contusions, medical record of repeated trauma, radiographic evidence of fractures, emotional distress, and failure to thrive.

child neglect, n a form of child abuse in which proper care is denied or withheld.

Child Protective Services, *n.pr* a governmental agency that responds to reports of child abuse or neglect. Dentists are mandated to report suspected child abuse or neglect to such service agencies.

Children's Health Insurance Program (CHIP), *n.pr* federal program created to cover medical care for children whose families have income too high to qualify for state medical assistance but cannot obtain private insurance. This may or may not include dental care.

chin, *n* the raised triangular extension of the anterior portion of the mandible below the lower lip. It is formed by the mental protuberance of the mandible.

chin cup, n See cup, chin.

chip, *n* a logic element containing electronic circuit components, both active and passive, embedded in a cohesive material of any shape.

chip blower, n See syringe, air, hand.

chiropractic, *n* a branch of the healing arts dealing with the nervous system and its relationship to the spinal column and interrelationship with other body systems in health and disease. The primary spinal and paraspinal structural derangements with which chiropractors are concerned are known as *chiropractic subluxations.*

Treatment is referred to as *chiropractic adjustment.*

chisel, *n* an instrument modeled after a carpenter's chisel intended for cutting or cleaving hard tissue. The cutting edge is beveled on one side only; the shank may be straight or angled.

chisel, contra-angle (binangle chisel), n a chisel-shaped, binangled, paired cutting instrument whose blade meets the shank at an angle greater than 12°.

chisel, posterior, n See chisel, contra-angle.

chisel, Wedelstaedt, n.pr a chisel with a blade that is continuous with the shank, has no constricting neck, curves rather than angles into the shank, and is available in varying widths.

Chlamydia (kləmid′ēə), *n.pr* a genus of microorganisms that live as intercellular parasites and have a number of properties in common with gramnegative bacteria. Two species have been identified; both are pathogenic.

C. psittaci (sit′əsē), *n.pr* an organism that infests birds and causes a type of pneumonia in humans (psittacosis).

C. trachomatis (trəkō′məetis′), *n.pr* an organism that lives in the conjunctivae of the eye and the epithelium of the urethra and cervix and is responsible for conjunctivitis, lymphogranuloma venereum, and trachoma.

chloral hydrate (klor′əl hī′drāt), *n* brand names: Aquachloral Supprettes, Novo-chlorhydrate; *drug class:* sedative-hypnotic chloral derivative; *action:* produces central nervous system depression; *uses:* sedation, treatment of insomnia, anesthesia adjunct.

chlorambucil (kloram′byəsil′), *n* brand name: Leukeran; *drug class:* antineoplastic alkylating agent; *action:* inhibits DNA function; *uses:* chronic lymphocytic leukemia, Hodgkin's disease, breast carcinoma, ovarian carcinoma.

chloramine solution, *n* See solution.

chloramphenicol, *n* a broadspectrum antibacterial and antirickettsial agent that should be reserved for serious infections in which other agents are ineffective.

chlordiazepoxide HCl, *n* brand names: Librium, Novopoxide; *drug* *class:* benzodiazepine antianxiety; *action:* produces central nervous system depression; *uses:* short-term management of anxiety, acute alcohol withdrawal, preoperatively for relaxation, treatment of convulsions.

chlorhexidine *(CHX)* gluconate, *n brand names:* Peridex, PerioGard; *drug class:* antiinfective oral rinse; *action:* absorbed by tooth surfaces, dental plaque, and oral mucosa; sustained reduction of plaque organisms; *uses:* as a rinse as a part of treatment of periodontal disease, irrigation during periodontal procedures, and possibly as an aseptic prerinse before dental procedures.

chloride shift (klôr′īd), *n* the exchange of a chloride ion for a bicarbonate ion across the enthrocyte membrane as part of the buffering system in the blood. It accounts for the greater chloride content of venous erythrocytes than arterial erythrocytes.

chlorine (klôr′ēn), *n* a yellowish-green gaseous element of the halogen group. It has a strong, distinctive odor that is irritating to the respiratory tract and is poisonous if ingested or inhaled. It occurs mainly as a compound of sodium chloride. It is used as a bleach and disinfectant. Chlorine compounds are used in solvents, cleaning fluids, and chloroform and formerly in general use as an anesthetic.

chlorine dioxide, *n* an oxidizing agent used in oral care to decrease amounts of volatile sulfur compounds that may cause halitosis.

chloroform, *n* a nonflammable, volatile liquid that was the first inhalation anesthetic to be discovered. It is no longer in general use because of its inherent risk factors and low margin of safety.

chloroformization (klôr′əfôrm′izā′shən), *n* the administration of chloroform.

Chloromycetin, *n.pr* the brand name for chloramphenicol. See also chloramphenicol.

chloropercha (klôr′ōpur′chə), *n* a solution obtained by mixing various amounts of chloroform with guttapercha.

chloropercha method, *n* See method, chloropercha.

chlorophyll (klôr′ōfil), *n* the pigment required for photosynthesis in plants.

chlorophyllin (klôr′əfilin), *n* any one of a number of products resulting from the reaction of certain decomposition products of chlorophyll with copper and other metallic ions.

chloroquine HCl/chloroquine phosphate, *n brand names:* Aralen HCl, Aralen Phosphate; *drug class:* antimalarial; *action:* inhibits parasite replication; *uses:* malaria, rheumatoid arthritis, amebiasis.

chlorothiazide (klor′əthī′əzīd′), *n brand name:* Diuril; *drug class:* thiazide diuretic; *action:* inhibits the sodium/chloride cotransporter in the distal tubule and increases the excretion of water, sodium chloride, and potassium; *uses:* edema, hypertension.

chlorpheniramine maleate (klor′fənir′əmēn′mā′lēāt), *n brand names:* Chlor-Trimeton, Novo-pheniram; *drug class:* antihistamine, blocks histamine H_1-receptors; *action:* acts on blood vessels, gastrointestinal system, respiratory system by competing with histamine for H_1-receptor site; *uses:* relief of allergy symptoms, rhinitis.

chlorphensin carbamate, *n brand name:* Maolate; *drug class:* skeletal muscle relaxant, central acting; *action:* unknown; may be related to sedative properties; does not directly relax muscle or depress nerve conduction; *use:* adjunct for relieving pain in acute, painful musculoskeletal conditions.

chlorpromazine HCl, *n brand name:* Thorazine; *drug class:* antipsychotic; *action:* blocks dopamine receptors in the cerebral cortex, hypothalamus, and limbic system; *uses:* psychotic disorders, mania, schizophrenia, nausea, vomiting, preoperatively for relaxation.

chlorpropamide, *n brand names:* Apo-Chlorpromide, Diabinese; *drug class:* antidiabetic, first generation sulfonylurea; *action:* causes functioning beta cells in pancreas to release insulin, leading to drop in blood glucose levels; *use:* stable type 2 diabetes mellitus.

chlortetracycline (klôr′tetrəsī′klēn), *n* (Aureomycin) a broad-spectrum antibiotic possessing bacteriostatic properties of some value in the treatment of disease produced by large viruses (the psittacosis and lymphogranuloma inguinale groups).

chlorthalidone, *n* *brand names:* Novothalidone, Apo-Chlorthalidone, Thalitone; *drug class:* diuretic; *action:* inhibits the sodium/chloride cotransporter in the distal tubule and increases the excretion of water, sodium chloride, and potassium; *uses:* edema, hypertension, chronic heart disease.

chlorzoxazone, *n* *brand names:* Paraflex, Parafon Forte DSC; *drug class:* skeletal muscle relaxant, central acting; *action:* depresses multisynaptic pathways in the spinal cord; *use:* adjunct for relief of muscle spasm in musculoskeletal conditions.

choice of path of placement, *n* See placement, choice of path of.

cholagogue (kŏ′ləgog), *n* a substance that stimulates emptying of the gallbladder and flow of bile.

cholera (kŏl′erə), *n* an acute bacterial infection of the small intestine characterized by severe diarrhea and vomiting, muscular cramps, dehydration, and depletion of electrolytes. The disease is spread by water and food that have been contaminated by feces of infected persons. The cholera vibrio produce an exotoxin, cholera toxin (choleragen), that stimulates the secretion of electrolytes and water into the small intestine, draining body fluids and weakening the patient. A vaccine is available.

choleretic (kŏ′ləret′ik), *n* a substance that stimulates production of bile by the liver.

cholestasis (kŏ′lstā′sis), *n* the interruption in the flow of bile through any part of the biliary system from the liver to duodenum.

cholesteatoma (kəles′tēətō′mə), *n* a cystic mass composed of epithelial cells and cholesterol that is found in the middle ear and occurs either as a congenital defect or as a serious complication of chronic otitis media.

cholesterol (kəles′tərôl), *n* a lipid common to all animal, but not plant, cells. As a sterol, it contains the cyclopentanophenanthrene nucleus. High levels are found in nerve tissue, atheromas, gallstones, and cysts.

cholestyramine, *n* *brand names:* Questran, Cholybar; *drug class:* antilipemic; *action:* absorbs, combines with bile acids to form insoluble complex that is excreted through the feces; lowers cholesterol levels; *uses:* primary hypercholesterolemia, pruritus associated with biliary obstruction, diarrhea caused by excess bile acid, xanthomas.

choline, *n* a nutrient essential for cardiovascular and brain function and for cellular membrane composition and repair. Classified as an essential nutrient by the Food and Nutrition Board of the Institute of Medicine (USA). Adequate intakes (AI) have been established.

choline salicylate, *n* *brand name:* Arthropan; *drug class:* salicylate analgesic; *action:* inhibits prostaglandin synthesis by interfering with cyclooxygenase need for biosynthesis; *uses:* relief of mild to moderate pain from fever, arthritis, juvenile rheumatoid arthritis.

cholinergic (parasympathomimetic) (kŏ′linur′jik), *adj* producing or simulating the effects of acetylcholine.

cholinergic blocking agent, n See agent, blocking, cholinergic.

cholinergic crisis, in myasthenia gravis, n a medical condition resulting from an administration of too much anticholinesterase, indicated by an immediate increase in muscle weakness, excessive pulmonarysecretions, excessive salivation, diarrhea, and cramps.

cholinesterase (kŏ′lines′tərās), *n* an esterase that hydrolyzes acetylcholine and other esters. Acetylcholinesterase is an esterase that is selective for acetylcholine. It is an enzyme that is widely distributed throughout the muscles, glands, and nerves of the body and that converts acetylcholine into choline and acetic acid.

cholinolytic (kŏ′linōlit′ik), *n/adj* See anticholinergic.

chondrodysplasia punctata (kon′ drŏdisplā′shə punkta′tə), *n* an inherited form of dwarfism characterized by skin lesions, radiographic epiphyseal stippling, and a pug nose. Two types are most often seen: a benign type marked by mild asymmetric limb shortening that is transmitted by an autosomal dominant gene and a lethal type with marked proximal limb shortening that is transmitted by an autosomal recessive gene.

chondroectodermal dysplasia (Ellis-van Creveld syndrome) (kon'drō ek'tōdur'məl displā'zhə), *n* a syndrome characterized by the following tetrad: (1) bilateral polydactyly; (2) chondrodysplasia of the long bones resulting in acromelic dwarfism; (3) anomalies of the teeth, nails, hair, and maxillary and mandibular region anteriorly; and (4) heart malformation.

chondroitin (kondroit'ən), *n* a mucopolysaccharide present in the intercellular substance or matrix of connective tissue, particularly cartilage.

chondroiton sulfate (kondrō'itin, kondroi'tin), *n* a mucopolysaccharide contained in skin, bones, teeth, and cartilage.

chondroma (kondrō'mə), *n* a benign tumor of cartilage. However, many chondrosarcomas arise in preexisting chondromas.

chondromyxosarcoma (kon'drō mik'sōsärkō'mə), *n* See chondrosarcoma.

chondrosarcoma (kon'drōsärkō' mə), *n* a malignant neoplasm composed of cartilage-like tissue.

chondrosarcoma, mesenchymal (mezen'kīməl), *n* a malignant cartilage tumor primarily found in younger adults, usually located in or near the jaw.

chorda tympani nerve (kor'də tim'pənē), *n* a nerve branch of the facial nerve that passes through the tympanic cavity to join the lingual branch of the mandibular nerve; it conveys taste sensation from the anterior two thirds of the tongue and carries parasympathetic preganglionic fibers to the submandibular and sublingual salivary glands.

chorea (St.Vitus' dance) (kôrē'ə), *n* a disorder of the central nervous system resulting in purposeless, involuntary athetoid (writhing) movements of the muscles of the face and extremities. It may be associated with or follow rheumatic fever (Sydenham's chorea), hysteria, senility, or infections, or it may be a hereditary disorder (Huntington's chorea).

choriamnionitis (kor'ēoam'nēōnī' tis), *n* an inflammatory reaction in the amniotic membranes caused by bacteria or viruses in the amniotic fluid.

Christian's disease, *n.pr* See disease, Hand-Schüller-Christian.

Christmas disease, *n.pr* See hemophilia B.

chroma, *n* a measurement of color saturation or the degree of color pureness. A color that is identified with a high chroma hue is almost completely free of white.

chromatin (krō'mətin), *n* the genetic material present in the nucleus, consisting of DNA and associated proteins, seen as irregular clumps in quiescent cells.

chromatography, *n* any one of several processes for separating and analyzing various gaseous or dissolved chemical materials according to differences in their absorbency with respect to a specific substance.

chromium (Cr), *n* a hard, brittle, metallic element with an atomic number of 24 and an atomic weight of 51.996. Chromium strongly resists corrosion and is used extensively to plate other metals and as an alloy to harden steel. Stainless steels are more than 10% chromium.

chromium-cobalt-molybdenum, *n* a stainless alloy used in interosseous implants for dental prostheses.

chromogenic (krō'mōjen'ik), *adj* pertaining to color production.

chromosomal, *adj* relating to chromosome, or a configuration within the cell's nucleus that contains a linear thread of DNA that conveys genetic data.

chromosomes (krō'məsōms), *n* the small, dark-staining, and more or less rod-shaped bodies situated in the nucleus of a cell. At the time of cell division, chromosomes divide and distribute equally to the daughter cells. They contain genes arranged along their length. The number of chromosomes in the somatic cells of an individual is constant (the diploid number), whereas just half this number (the haploid number) appears in germ cells.

chromosome aberration, n a rearrangement of chromosome parts as a result of breakage and reunion of broken ends.

chronic, *adj* characterized by a long, slow course, as opposed to *acute*.

chronic pulmonary emphysema, *n* a condition in which breathing is made difficult by an accumulation of mucus in the bronchioles and a loss of elasticity in the lungs.

chronology, *n* the arrangement of events in a time sequence, usually from the beginning to the end of an event.

chylomicrons (kī′lōmī′kronz), *n.pl* the tiny lipoproteins of approximately 2% protein that convey dietary fat throughout the body.

cicatricial pemphigoid (sikətrishəl pem′figoid′), *n* See pemphigoid, benign mucous membrane.

cicatrix (sik′ətriks) (scar), *n* the result of healing by secondary intention; characterized microscopically by excessive collagenation of the granulation tissue.

cicatrization (sikətrizā′shən), *n* the conversion of granulation tissue into scar tissue.

ciclopirox olamine (sik′lōpē′roks) (topical), *n brand name:* Loprox; *drug class:* topical antifungal; *action:* interferes with fungal cell membrane; *uses:* tinea cruris, tinea corporis, tinea pedis, tinea versicolor, cutaneous candidiasis.

Cidofovir, *n brand name:* Vistide; *drug class:* antiviral; *action:* inhibits DNA polymerase; *uses:* cytomegalovirus retinitis, herpes simplex skin and mucosal infections.

ciliophora protozoa (sil′ēof′ôrə), *n* the only human ciliate parasite *(Balantidium coli)* implicated in a type of dysentery and contracted from fecal contamination of water supplies.

cimetidine (simet′idēn′), *n brand names:* Tagamet, Apo-Cimetidine; *drug class:* H₂-histamine receptor antagonist; *action:* inhibits histamine at H₂-histamine receptor site in parietal cells, resulting in the inhibition of gastric acid secretion; *uses:* short-term treatment of duodenal and gastric ulcers by the control of hyperacidity, gastroesphogeal reflux disease.

cineradiography (sin′irā′dēog′rəfē), *n* the making of motion pictures by means of roentgen rays and image intensification. Studies are used for diagnosis and research purposes. Speech patterns can be studied during the process of phonation; the action of the tongue, jaws, and palate can be studied during mastication and deglutition.

cingulum (sing′gyū lum), *n* the portion of the incisor teeth and canines, occurring on the lingual surface, that forms a convex protuberance at the cervical third of the anatomic crown.

cingulum modification, *n* the alteration of the lingual form of an anterior tooth to provide a definite seat for the support of a rest unit of a removable partial denture.

ciprofloxacin, *n brand name:* Cipro; *drug class:* fluoroquinolone antibiotic; *action:* a broad-spectrum bactericidal agent that inhibits enzyme deoxyribonucleic acid (DNA) gyrase needed for replication of DNA; *uses:* adult urinary tract infection, uncomplicated gonorrhea, typhoid fever, diarrhea cause by sensitive bacteria, anthrax.

circuit voltmeter, *n* the device on the radiograph machine that records the line voltage on the circuit prior to the voltage being augmented by the transformer. Also may be used to measure the kilovoltage produced by the action of the transformer.

circuits, in radiograph machine, *n. pl* a radiograph machine contains two circuits, the low-voltage filament circuit and the high-voltage cathode-anode circuit. The low-voltage circuit uses a step-down transformer to form an electron cloud by heating up the filament. The high-voltage circuit uses a step-up transformer to increase the current enough to accelerate the electrons to the point that they create radiographic photons.

circular compression, *n* the compacting or pressing together of an object with equal circumventing force.

circulation, *n* the movement of blood through blood vessels.

circulation, peripheral, *n* the passage of fluids, electrolytes, and metabolites through the walls of terminal vessels of the vascular tree into and out of tissue spaces.

circulation, pulmonary, *n* the circulation of venous blood from the right ventricle of the heart to the lungs and back to the left atrium of the heart.

circulation, systemic, *n* the circulation of oxygenated blood from the left ventricle of the heart to the various tissues and of venous blood back to the right atrium of the heart.

circulatory system, *n* the system for the circulation of blood, consisting of the heart, arteries, arterioles, capillaries, venules, and veins.

circumferential fibers, *n.pl* See fibers, circular.

circumferential probing, *n* an examination technique in which the probe remains in the sulcus or periodontal pockets while it is "walked" around the oral cavity; prevents excessive trauma to the gingiva that can occur from repeated probe insertion and withdrawal.

circumferential wiring, *n* See wiring, circumferential.

cirrhosis (sirō'sis), *n* a chronic degenerative disease of the liver in which blood flow is restricted and metabolic and detoxification functions are impaired or destroyed. Cirrhosis is most commonly the result of chronic alcohol abuse.

cisplatin (sisplat'in), *n* an antineoplastic platinum-containing agent prescribed in the treatment of a wide variety of neoplasms such as metastatic testicular, prostatic, head and neck cancers, and ovarian tumors.

citalopram, *n* brand name: Celexa; *drug class:* antidepressant; *action:* selective serotonin re-uptake inhibitor; *use:* depression.

citric acid, *n* a white, crystalline, organic acid freely soluble in water and alcohol. It can be extracted from citrus fruits or through a fermentation of sugars. It is a key intermediary in metabolism. See also citric acid cycle.

citric acid cycle, *n* a sequence of enzymatic reactions involving the metabolism of carbon chains of sugars, fatty acids, and amino acids to yield carbon dioxide, water, and high-energy phosphate bonds. Also called *Krebs' citric acid cycle* or *tricarboxylic acid cycle.*

citrin (sit'rin), *n* See factor, platelet 1.

civil action, *n* a noncriminal legal action.

civil law, *n* a statutory law, as opposed to common law or judge-made law (such as case law). The Dental Practice Act in every state is a civil law.

claim, *n* **1.** in a juridic sense, a demand of some type made by one person or another. *n* **2.** a request for payment under a dental benefits plan. *n* **3.** a statement listing services rendered, the dates of services, and itemization of costs. Includes a statement signed by the beneficiary and treating dental professional that services have been rendered. The completed form serves as the basis for payment of benefit.

claim form, *n* the form used to file for benefits under a dental benefits program; includes sections for the patient and the dental professional to complete.

claimant, *n* a person who files a claim for benefits. May be the patient or the certificate holder.

claims payment fraud, *n* the intentional manipulation or alteration of facts submitted by a treating dental professional, resulting in a lower payment to the beneficiary or the treating dental professional than would have been paid if the manipulation had not occurred.

claims reporting fraud, *n* the intentional misrepresentation of material facts concerning treatment provided and charges made to cause a higher payment.

claims review, *n* **1.** in dental prepayment, the routine examination by a carrier or intermediary of the claim submitted to it for payment or predetermination of benefits; may include determination of eligibility, coverage of service, and plan liability. *n* **2.** in quality assurance, examination by organizations of claims as part of a quality review or use review process.

clamp, *n* a device used to effect compression or retention.

clamp, cervical, *n* See clamp, gingival.

clamp, Ferrier 212 gingival, *n.pr* a purposely unbalanced gingival rubber dam clamp for retracting gingival tissue from the field of operation. It must be stabilized to position with modeling compound.

clamp, gingival, *n* (cervical clamp), a rubber dam clamp intended to retract gingival tissues.

clamp, Hatch gingival, *n.pr* an adjustable gingival rubber dam clamp.

clamp, root rubber dam, *n* a clamp with jaws designed to fit on the root surfaces of a tooth; usually used for the retention of a rubber dam.

clamp, rubber dam, n (rubber dam retainer), a device made of spring metal and used to retain a rubber dam in place or improve the operating field by isolating it from the oral environment.

clarithromycin, *n brand name:* Biaxin; *drug class:* macrolide antibiotic; *action:* binds to 50S ribosomal subunits of susceptible bacteria and suppresses protein synthesis; *uses:* treatment of mild to moderate infections of the upper and lower respiratory tracts, otitis media, acute maxillary sinusitis, an alternative drug in dental prophylaxis.

Clark's rule, *n.pr* See rule, Clark's.

clasp, *n* an extracoronal direct retainer of a removable partial denture, usually consisting of two arms, a retentive arm and a reciprocal arm, joined by a body that may connect with an occlusal rest.

clasp, Adams', n.pr a formed wire clasp of modified arrowhead design using the buccomesial and distoproximal undercuts of a tooth for retention.

clasp, arm, n the clasp extensions, usually from minor connectors, that provide retention, reciprocation, or stabilization.

clasp, arm, fatigue of, n a situation in which the retentive arm of a clasp metal has undergone flexure at the same point repeatedly, and fracture has resulted. Tapering the clasp arm tends to distribute the flexure and reduce such tendency to fracture.

clasp, arm, reciprocal, n an arm of a clasp, usually at or occlusal to the height of contour, located in such a manner as to reciprocate any force arising from an opposing clasp arm on the same tooth.

clasp, arm, retentive (retention terminal), n a clasp arm that is flexible and engages the infrabulge area at the terminal end of the arm.

clasp, arrowhead, n a wire clasp, for retention of removable appliances, whose active elements are in the shape of an arrowhead and engage the mesioproximal and distoproximal undercuts on the buccal aspects of adjacent teeth.

clasp, back-action, n a clasp that originates on one surface of a tooth and traverses the suprabulge area to another surface, where it is supported by an occlusal rest; it then continues to encircle the tooth on the third surface, where it terminates in the infrabulge area beyond the opposite angle of the tooth surface where it originated.

clasp, bar, n a clasp with arms that are bar-type extensions from major connectors or from within the denture base; the arms pass adjacent to the soft tissues and approach the point of contact on the tooth in a cervicoocclusal direction.

clasp, bar, arm, n a clasp arm that originates from the denture base or from a major or minor connector. It consists of the arm, which traverses but does not contact the gingival structures, and a terminal end, which approaches its contact with the tooth in a cervicoocclusal direction.

clasp, cast, n a clasp made of an alloy that has been cast into the desired form and retains its crystalline structure.

clasp, circumferential (sərkum′fəre n′shəl), *n* a clasp that encircles more than 180° of a tooth, including opposite angles, and usually contacts the tooth throughout the extent of the clasp, at least one terminal being in the infrabulge area (cervical convergence).

clasp, circumferential arm, n a clasp arm that has its origin in a minor connector and follows the contour of the tooth approximately in a plane perpendicular to the path of placement of the removable partial denture.

clasp, combination, n a clasp that employs a wrought-wire retentive arm and a cast reciprocal or stabilizing arm. A clasp that employs a bar type of retentive arm and a cast reciprocal or stabilizing arm.

clasp, continuous, n a secondary lingual bar.

clasp design, n the determination of the shape and construction of a clasp with its position outlined on the cast.

clasp, embrasure (embrā′zhur), *n* a clasp used where no edentulous space exists. It passes through the embrasure, using two occlusal rests, and clasps the two teeth with circumferential clasps that have a common body.

clasp flexibility, n the property of a clasp that enables it to be bent without breaking and to return to its original form. Factors that affect the flexibility of a retentive clasp arm are its length, diameter, cross-section form, structure, and the alloy of which it is made.

clasp flexure, n See flexure, clasp.

clasp, formed, n See clasp, wrought.

clasp, mesiodistal **(mez′ēədis′təl),** n a type of clasp that embraces the distolingual and mesial surfaces of a tooth and takes its retention in either or both mesial and distal undercuts.

clasp, reciprocal, circumferential arm, n an arm of a clasp located in such a manner as to reciprocate any force arising from an opposing clasp arm on the same tooth.

clasp, retentive circumferential arm (retention terminal), n a circumferential clasp arm that is flexible and engages the infrabulge area at the terminal end of the arm.

clasp, Roach, n See clasp, bar.

clasp, stabilizing circumferential arm, n a circumferential clasp arm that is rigid and contacts the tooth at or occlusal to the surveyed height of contour.

clasp, stress-breaking action of, n the relief for the abutment teeth from all or part of torquing occlusal forces; partially achieved by having a retentive arm of maximum flexibility that will provide adequate retention.

clasp, wrought (formed clasp), n a clasp made of an alloy that has been drawn into various forms of wire.

classification, n the systematic arrangement according to characteristics of groups or classes.

classification, Angle's, n See Angle's classification of malocclusion (modified).

classification, Broders', n See index, Broders'.

classification, cavity, n See cavity, classification.

classification, Kennedy, n See Kennedy classification.

classification of habits, n a compilation of orofacial habits that may be a factor in the etiology of periodontal disease. Habit neuroses include lip biting, cheek biting, biting of foreign objects, and abnormal tongue pressure against the teeth. Occupational ones include thread biting, musician's habits, holding nails in the oral cavity, etc. Miscellaneous ones include thumb sucking, pipe smoking, incorrect toothbrushing habits, cracking nuts with the teeth, and oral cavity breathing.

classification of motion, n a classification system that identifies the extent of involvement of the body in completing a dental motor task.

classification of partial dentures, n grouping of partially edentulous situations based on various conditions (e.g., location of the edentulous space, location of remaining teeth, position of direct retainers, and ability of oral structures to support a partial denture).

classification of periodontal diseases, n the division of periodontal diseases into: (1) gingival disease; (2) chronic periodontitis; (3) aggressive periodontitis; (4) periodontitis as a manifestation of a systemic disease; (5) necrotizing periodontal diseases; (6) abscesses of the periodontium; (7) periodontitis associated with endodontic lesions; and (8) development of acquired deformities and conditions.

classification of pockets, n the division of periodontal pockets into two classes: (1) suprabony and (2) infrabony, according to the number of osseous walls (i.e., three osseous walls, two osseous walls, one osseous wall). See also pocket.

clavicle (klav′ikəl), n a long, curved, horizontal bone just above the first rib, forming the ventral portion of the shoulder girdle. It articulates medially with the sternum and laterally with the scapula.

cleansing, biomechanical, n the process of cleaning and shaping a root canal with endodontic instrumentation in conjunction with irrigating solutions.

cleansing solution, n See solution, cleansing.

clearance, *n* 1. a condition in which moving bodies may pass without hindrance. *n* 2. removal from the blood by the kidneys (e.g., urea or insulin) or by the liver (e.g., certain dyes).

clearance, interocclusal **(in'terəklō ō'səl),** *n* the difference in the height of the face when the mandible is at rest and when the teeth are in occlusion. This is determined by measuring the amount of space between the maxillary and mandibular teeth when the mandible is in the position of physiologic rest. The difference between the rest vertical dimension and the occlusal vertical dimension of the face, as measured in the incisal area. See also distance, interocclusal.

clearance, occlusal **(əklōō'səl),** *n* a condition in which the mandibular teeth may pass the maxillary teeth horizontally without contact or interference.

clearance time, *n* the time taken for a cariogenic exposure to pass from the oral cavity; depends largely upon type of food ingested, efficiency of the lips, teeth, and tongue, and the amount of saliva present in an individual's oral cavity.

cleat (klēt), *n* a fixed point of anchorage, usually in the form of a metal spur or loop embedded in the acrylic resin base of a Hawley retainer or soldered onto an arch wire, to which a rubber dam elastic or other device is attached during orthodontic tooth movement.

cleft (kleft), *n* a longitudinal fissure of opening.

cleft, facial, *n* the fissures along the embryonal lines of the junction of the maxillary and lateral nasal processes; usually extend obliquely from the nasal ala to the outer border of the eye (canthus).

cleft, gingival, *n* a cleft of the marginal gingiva; may be caused by many factors, such as incorrect toothbrushing, a breakthrough to the surface of pocket formation, or faulty tooth positions, and may resemble a V-shaped notch.

cleft lip, *n* a congenital anomaly of the face caused by the failure of fusion between embryonic maxillary and medial nasal processes.

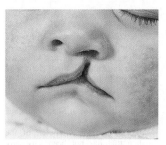
Cleft lip. (Swartz, 2010)

cleft, occult, *n* See submucous cleft.

cleft, operated, *n* (postoperative cleft), a cleft that has been surgically repaired.

cleft palate, *n* a congenital anomaly of the oral cavity caused by the failure of fusion between the embryonic palatal shelves.

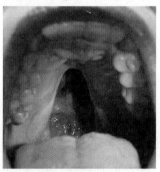
Cleft palate. (Swartz, 2010)

cleft palate, alveolar graft, *n* a bone graft placed at the site of a hard palate cleft before teeth have an opportunity to erupt through the gingiva tissue. It creates the architecture necessary for normal eruption of the maxillary teeth and provides support for adjacent teeth. It may also eliminate the need for prosthetic intervention in the future.

cleft palate, hard palate graft, *n* a bone graft used to block the oronasal passage in order to facilitate breathing in children with hard palate clefts.

cleft palate prosthesis, *n* See prosthesis, cleft palate.

cleft, postoperative, n See cleft, operated.

cleft, Stillman's, n the small fissures extending apically from the midline of the gingival margin in teeth subjected to trauma. Although these clefts may be found in traumatism, they are not necessarily diagnostic of occlusal trauma.

cleft, submucous, n See submucous cleft.

cleft, unoperated, n a cleft of the palate that has not been surgically repaired.

cleidocranial dysostosis, *n* See dysostosis, cleidocranial.

clemastine fumarate (klem′əstēn′ fyōō′mərāt′), *n brand names:* Tavist, Tavist-1; *drug class:* histamine H₁-receptor antagonist; *action:* acts on blood vessels and gastrointestinal and respiratory systems by competing with histamine for H₁-receptor sites; *uses:* allergy symptoms, rhinitis, angioedema, urticaria.

clenching (klen′ching), *n* the nonfunctional, forceful intermittent application of the mandibular teeth against the maxillary teeth. It can become habitual and cause damage to the periodontium.

cleoid (klē′oid), *n* a carving instrument having a blade shaped like a pointed spade or claw, with cutting edges on both sides and tip.

clicking, *n* a sound sometimes associated with the functioning of the temporomandibular joint; also the sound made by poorly fitting dentures.

clidinium bromide (klindin′ēəm brō′mid), *n brand name:* Quarzan; *drug class:* gastrointestinal anticholinergic; *action:* inhibits muscarinic actions of acetylcholine at postganglionic cholinergic neuroeffector sites; *use:* treatment of peptic ulcer disease in combination with other drugs.

climacteric (klīmak′tərik, klī′mak ter′ik), *n* the period during which women gradually lose their reproductive capabilities as a result of aging. Also used as an adjective to describe this period.

climate, occlusal, *n* the new occlusal relationship and environment produced by occlusal adjustment, orthodontic tooth movement, or a periodontal prosthesis.

clindamycin HCl/clindamycin palmitate HCl (klin′dəmī′sin pal′mətāt′), *n brand name:* Cleocin; *drug class:* lincomycin derivative antibiotic; *action:* binds to 50S subunit of bacterial ribosomes, suppresses protein synthesis; *uses:* infections caused by anaerobic bacteria, staphylococci, streptococci, pneumococci, topically for acne, bacterial vaginosis, an alternative drug for dental prophylaxis.

clinic, table, *n* a display or demonstration of a topic, limited in scope, for transmitting information to a small number of persons at a time.

clinical, *adj* pertaining to a clinic, direct patient care, or materials used in the direct care of patients.

clinical attachment level (CAL), n a measurement to determine periodontal health; consists of the distance in millimeters that exists between the edge of the enamel of a tooth to the gingival tissue that is adherent to its root, its epithelial attachment.

clinical crown, n See crown, clinical.

clinical crown : clinical root ratio, n See ratio, clinical crown : clinical root.

clinical contact surface, n surface touched by contaminated hands, instruments, or spatter during dental treatment.

clinical death, n a defined time at which bodily functions have ceased and are unable to be revived. In many instances, the definition of clinical death applies to circumstances where brain activity ceases despite the continuance of body functions.

clinical diagnosis, n See diagnosis, clinical.

clinical medicine, n the aspect of medicine that deals with direct patient care.

clinical protocol, n the detailed outline of the steps to be followed in the treatment of a patient.

clinical trials, n organized studies to provide large bodies of clinical data for statistically valid evaluation of treatment.

clinical trial, *n* a trial based upon the scientific method in which a control group and a test group are compared over time in order to study a single, differing factor.

clinician, *n* a licensed dental professional who provides preventative, therapeutic, and educational services that promote oral health.

clinoidale (klinoid'al), *n* the most superior point on the contour of the anterior clinoid.

clioquinol (klē'ōkwin'ol), *brand name:* Vioform; *drug class:* topical antifungal, antibacterial drug; *action:* topically to treat skin infections including angular cheilitis.

clobetasol propionate (klōbā'təsol' prō'pēənāt'), *n brand names:* Dermovate, Temovate, Temovate Emollient Cream; *drug class:* topical corticosteroid; *action:* possesses antipruritic and antiinflammatory properties; *uses:* psoriasis, exzema, contact dermatitis.

clock system, *n* **1.** system in which the dental instrument and the sharpening tool are held in such a way that the optimum angle required for sharpening is achieved. *n* **2.** the seating position for a clinician (and/or assistant) to facilitate instrumentation.

clocortolone pivalate (klōkor'təlōn piv'əlāt'), *n brand name:* Cloderm; *drug class:* topical corticosteroid; *action:* possesses antipruritic and antiinflammatory properties; *uses:* psoriasis, eczema, contact dermatitis, pruritus.

clofibrate (klōfī'brāt), *n brand names:* Abitrate, Atromid-S, Claripex, Novofibrate; *drug class:* an older antihyperlipidemic; *action:* inhibits DNA transcription and increases extrahepatic lipoprotein lipase and other effects leading to a decrease in VLDA and LDL; *uses:* hypertriglyceridemia, hypercholesterolemia.

clomiphene citrate (klō'məfēn' sit'rāt), *n brand names:* Clomid, Serophene, Milphene; *drug class:* nonsteroidal estrogen receptor antagonist and ovulatory stimulant; *action:* binds to estrogen receptors, resulting in increase of LH and FSH release from pituitary; *use:* female infertility.

clomipramine (klōmip'rəmēn'), *n brand name:* Anafranil; *drug class:* tricylic antidepressant; *action:* inhibits both norepinephrine and serotinin (5-HT) uptake in brain; *uses:* obsessive-compulsive disorder, panic disorder.

clonazepam (klōnaz'əpam'), *n brand names:* Klonopin, Rivotril; *drug class:* anticonvulsant, sedative benzodiazepine derivative; *action:* inhibits spike-wave formation; *uses:* akinetic myoclonic seizures, absence (petit mal) seizures, panic disorder.

clonic (klon'ik), *n* the alternating pattern of releasing and tightening a muscle.

clonidine HCl/clonidine transdermal, *n brand names:* Catpres, Dixarit, Catapres-TTS; *drug class:* antihypertensive, central α_2-adrenergic receptor agonist; *action:* inhibits sympathetic vasomotor center in central nervous system; *uses:* hypertension, opioid withdrawal, vascular headache.

clonus (klō'nəs), *n* an alternating muscular spasm and relaxation in rapid succession.

clopidogrel *n brand name:* Plavix; *drug class:* antiplatelet; *action:* blocks adenosine diphosphate (ADP) receptors preventing platelet aggregation; *uses:* adjunctive treatment of recent MI, ischemic stroke, peripheral vascular disease in patients with atherosclerosis, acute coronary syndrome.

clorazepate dipotassium (klor'əzepāt' dī'pətas'ēəm), *n brand names:* Tranxene, Gen-Xene, Apo-Chlorazepate, Tranxene-SD; *drug class:* benzodiazepine, sedative hypnotic; *action:* produces central nervous system depression; *uses:* anxiety, acute alcohol withdrawal.

closed bite, *n* See bite, closed. Synonymous to *deep bite*.

closed panel, *n* **1.** in a prepayment plan, a group of dental professionals sharing office facilities who provide stipulated services to an eligible group for a set premium. For beneficiaries of plans using closed panels, choice of dental professionals is limited to panel members. Dentists must accept any beneficiary as a patient. *n* **2.** a closed-panel dental benefits plan exists when patients eligible to receive benefits can receive them only if services are provided by dental professionals who have signed an agreement with the benefits plan to provide treatment to eligible patients. As a result of the dental professional reimbursement methods characteristic of a closed-panel plan, only a small percentage of practicing dental professionals in a given geographic area are typically contracted by the plan to provide dental services.

closed procedure, *n* the reduction of a fracture of the jaw or placement of an implant without surgical flap retraction.

closed reduction, for jaw fracture, *n* a process by which the broken portions of the jaw are approximated and stabilized without surgically opening the mucosal covering. The fixation of the reestablished approximation of the parts is accomplished with preformed bars attached to the teeth with ligatures or elastic bands.

Clostridium **(klostrid′ēəm),** *n* a genus of spore-forming anaerobic bacteria of the Bacillaceae family.

C. bifermentans **(bī′fermen′təns),** *n* causes gaseous gangrene.

C. botulinum **(boch′əli′nəm),** *n* causes botulism.

C. perfringens **(perfrin′jəns),** *n* the main cause of gas gangrene in humans; also causes food poisoning, cellulitis, and wound infections.

C. tetani **(tet′ənē′),** *n* causes tetanus.

closure, *n* the act or condition of being brought together or closed up.

closure, adjustive arcs of, n.pl the arcs of jaw closure found in deflective malocclusion caused by an intercusping of the teeth that does not coincide with a centrically related jaw closure.

closure, arcs of mandibular, n.pl the circular or elliptic arcs created by closure of the mandible.

closure, centric path of, n the path traversed by the mandible during closure when its associated neuromuscular mechanism is in a balanced state of tonus.

closure, open bite, n achieving anterior contact, either by orthodontic extrusion of anterior teeth or intrusion of posterior teeth.

closure, velopharyngeal **(vē′lōfərin′j ēəl),** *n* the closure of nasal air escape by the knee-action elevation of the soft palate and contraction of the posterior pharyngeal wall.

closure, voluntary arcs of, n.pl jaw closure directions consciously made by a patient.

clot, *n* coagulated blood, plasma, or fibrin.

clot, blood, n a coagulum formed of blood of a semisolidified nature. See also clotting factors.

clotrimazole **(klōtrim′əzōl′),** *n brand names:* Lotrimin, Canesten, Gyne-Lotrimin, Mycelex-7, Mycelex Troches; *drug class:* imidazole antifungal drug; *action:* interferes with fungal ergosterol synthesis; *uses:* tinea pedis, tinea cruris, tinea corporis, tinea vesicolor, and *C. albicans* infection of the oral cavity, pharynx, vulva, and vagina.

clotting factors, *n.pl* the chemical and cellular constituents of the blood responsible for the conversion of fibrinogen into a mesh of insoluble fibrin causing the blood to coagulate or clot.

cloxacillin sodium (klok′səsil′in), *brand names:* Apo Cloxi, Cloxapen, Novo-cloxin, Tegopen; *drug class:* penicillinase-resistant penicillin; *action:* interferes with cell-wall replication of susceptible organisms; *use:* penicillinase-producing staphylococcal infections.

clozapine **(klō′zəpēn′),** *n brand name:* Clozaril; *drug class:* antipsychotic, atypical; *action:* interferes with binding of dopamine at D_2 receptors; acts as a serotonergic 5-HT_{2A} receptor antagonist, also an antagonist at adrenergic, cholinergic, and histaminergic; *use:* management of psychotic symptoms in schizophrenic patients for whom other antipsychotics have failed.

clubbing (pulmonary osteoarthropathy), *n* a deforming enlargement of the terminal phalanges of the fingers. It is usually acquired and may be associated with certain cardiac and pulmonary diseases.

cluster, *n* in epidemiology, a composite of confirmed cases of a disease, defect, or disability that occur in close proximity to one another with regard to time or space.

cluster analysis, *n* a complex statistical technique of data analysis of numeric scale scores, producing clusters of variables related to one another.

cluster headache, *n* See histamine headache.

clutch, *n* a device made for gripping the teeth in a dental arch, to which face-bows or tracing devices may be attached rigidly enough to behave in space relations during the movements as if they were jaw outgrowths.

CMV, *n* the abbreviation for *cytomegalovirus.* See also cytomegalovirus.

coagulating current, *n* See current, coagulating.

coagulation (kōag′ūlā′shən), *n* causing a liquid to solidify; clotting.

coagulation time, *n* See time, coagulation.

coal tar, *n* an extract of coal used in combination with other compounds for the treatment of chronic skin diseases, such as eczema and psoriasis. Also a derivative of tobacco smoke that may act as an irritant and carcinogen.

coalescing (kōəles′ing), *n* a joining or fusing of parts.

coaptation (kō′aptā′shən), *n* the bringing together of two parts so as to create a seamless alignment.

coated tongue, *n* See tongue, coated.

coating, enteric (enter′ik), *n* a tablet covering that resists the action of the fluids and enzymes in the stomach but dissolves readily in the upper intestine.

coating material, *n* a biologically acceptable, usually porous nonmetal applied over the surface of a metallic implant with the expectation that tissue ingrowth will occur in the pores. Often a carbon polymer or ceramic substance.

cobalamin, *n* See vitamin, cobalamin.

cobalt-chromium alloy, *n* See alloy, cobalt-chromium.

cocaine (C, Cadillac, Charlie, coke, freebase, gold dust, joy powder, snow) abuse of, *n* the illegal recreational use of cocaine hydrochloride or one of its derivatives; *actions:* blocks re-uptake of catecholamines and serotonin, blocks sodium channels in nerves; *use:* medically prescribed for its anesthetic properties. Psychologic addiction may result from continued, compulsive use, typically by sniffing, injecting, applying topically, or smoking. Complications can occur with the concomitant use of it and epinephrine in the dental office. See also crack cocaine.

Coccidioides immitis (koksid′ēoid′ ēz im′itəs), *n* a dustborne fungus

endemic to the windblown desert dust of southwest United States. It is the chief culprit in coccidioidomycosis. Appears microscopically as uniformly scattered small ovals.

coccidioidomycosis (koksid′ēoid′ ōmīkō′sis), *n* an infectious fungal disease caused by the inhalation of spores of the bacterium *C. immitis,* which is carried on windborne dust particles. Although endemic in the southeastern United States, it is considered among the opportunistic infections that are indicators of AIDS.

code, *n* **1.** a system of recording information by symbols so that only selected people will know the meaning. Used also to conserve space. *n* **2.** a systematic statement.

code of ethics, n a series of principles used as a guide in assisting a dental professional to fulfill the moral obligations of professional dental practice.

codeine (kō′dēn), *n* a crystalline alkaloid, morphine methyl ether that stimulates opioid receptors and is used as an analgesic and antitussive. It is a controlled substance.

codeine sulfate/codeine phosphate, n generic codeine; *drug class:* narcotic analgesic, controlled substance schedule II, Canada N; *action:* depresses pain impulse transmission in central nervous system by interacting with opioid receptors; *uses:* mild-to-moderate pain, nonproductive cough.

coding, *n* writing instructions for a computer either in machine language or nonmachine language.

Coecal (kō′kôl), *n* the brand name for dental stone (hydrocal).

coefficient, absorption, *n* See absorption coefficient.

coefficient of thermal expansion, *n* See expansion, thermal coefficient.

coefficient, phenol, *n* the ratio of potency of a given germicide to that of phenol under standard conditions.

coenzyme (kōen′zīm), *n* a nonprotein substance, such as a B-complex vitamin, that combines with enzymes to assist in the catabolic process.

coenzyme A (CoA), *n* an important metabolite in the citric acid cycle. Although not a true enzyme, it plays a significant role in the transfer of

C

acetyl groups and the metabolism of acids and amino acids.

cofactor V, *n* See factor VII.

cognition (cognish′ən), *n* the higher mental processes, including understanding, reasoning, knowledge, and intellectual capacity.

cognitive (cog′nitiv), *adj/n* pertaining to the mental processes of knowing, perceiving, or being aware; an expression of intellectual capacity.

cognitive domain, *n* area of study that deals with the processes and measurable results of study, as well as the practical ability to apply intelligence.

cognovit note (kognō′vit), *n* a written authority of a debtor granting entry of a judgment against the debtor if the amount set forth in the note is not paid by the debtor when due. A cognovit note sets aside every defense that the maker of the note may otherwise have had.

cohere (kōhēr′), *v* to stick together, to unite, to form a solid mass.

coherent (Thompson/unmodified) scattering (kōhēr′ənt), *n* the dispersing of low-energy radiographs without losing photon energy, caused by elastic collision.

cohesion (kōhē′zhən), the ability of a material to adhere to itself.

cohesive, *n* the capability to cohere or stick together to form a mass.

cohort, *n* in statistics, a collection or sampling of individuals who share a common characteristic, such as the same age or sex.

cohort study, *n* a scientific study that focuses on a specific subpopulation, such as children born on a certain date in a specific environment.

coinsurance, *n* **1.** a means of sharing, dividing, or splitting the cost of dental services between the dental plan and the insured patient. A common division is 80/20. This means the insurance company will pay 80% of the cost of the dental service and that the patient will pay 20%. Percentages vary and may be applied to scheduled or usual, customary, and reasonable fee plans. *n* **2.** a provision of a dental benefits program by which the beneficiary shares in the cost of covered services, generally on a percentage basis. *n* **3.** the percentage of a covered dental expense that a beneficiary

must pay (after the deductible is paid). A typical coinsurance arrangement is one in which the third party pays 80% of the allowed benefit of the covered dental service and the beneficiary pays the remainder of the charged fee. Percentages vary and may apply to a table of allowance plans; usual, customary, and reasonable plans; and direct reimbursement programs.

coinsurance clause, *n* a provision in an insurance contract stipulating that the insurer will pay a specified share of dental expenses covered by the plan.

coitus (kō′itus), *n* the act of sexual intercourse.

col (kôl), *n* a depression in the gingival tissue of the interdental papilla apical to the contact.

colchicine (kol′chəsēn′), *n* generic colchicine; *drug class:* antigout agent; *action:* inhibits deposition of ureate crystals in soft tissues; *uses:* gout, gouty arthritis, pericarditis.

cold, clinical applications of, *n.pl* the clinical uses of cold to treat cold injury such as frostbite, relieve pain in burn injury, relieve pain in severe and acute inflammation (pulpitis), and relieve pain and swelling in contusions, abrasions, and sprains. See also heat, applied, and cold.

cold, physiologic effects of, *n* in reference to application of cold to a local area, marked vasoconstriction followed by vasodilation and edema. In extreme exposure the effects include a significant drop in temperature on the surface and a lesser drop in deeper tissue layers, depending on the degree of cold and duration of application; decreased phagocytosis; a decrease in local metabolism; and analgesia to varying degrees of anesthesia of the part exposed to cold.

cold sore, *n* See herpes labialis.

cold welding, *n* See welding, cold.

cold work, *n* a deformation of the space lattice of metals by mechanical manipulation at room temperature. The process alters certain properties (e.g., ductility).

cold-curing resin, *n* See resin, autopolymer.

colestipol HCl (kəles′təpol), *n* brand name: Colestid; *drug class:* antihyperlipidemic; *action:* absorbs, combines with bile acids to form insoluble complex that is excreted through feces; loss of bile acids lowers cholesterol levels; *uses:* primary hypercholesterolemia, xanthomas , pruritus caused by biliary obstruction.

colic (kŏl′ik), *n* a sharp visceral pain resulting from torsion, obstruction, or smooth muscle spasm of a hollow or tubular organ, such as a ureter or an intestine.

colitis (kəlī′tis), *n* an inflammatory condition of the large intestine. Most of the diseases of this group are of unknown origin.

collagen (kol′əjin), *n* an intercellular constituent of connective tissue and bone consisting of bundles of tiny reticular fibrils, most noticeable in the white, glistening, inelastic fibers of tendons, ligaments, and fascia.

collagenase (kol′əjənās′), *n* an enzyme capable of depolymerizing collagen, found in some microorganisms and believed to contribute to periodontal disease.

collapse, *n* a state of extreme prostration and depression with failure of circulation; abnormal falling in of the walls of any part or organ; with reference to a lung, an airless or fatal state of all or part of the lung.

collar, *n* the small part of the root of a tooth that is a part of an artificial tooth (denture).

collective bargaining, *n* the negotiations between organized labor and employers on matters such as wages, hours, working conditions, and health and welfare programs.

collimating film holder (kol′əmā′ting), *n* a stainless steel holder for radiographic film that provides rectangular lining-up (collimation) of the radiographic beam; useful when employing the paralleling technique for periapical survey. May also be called *precision film holder.*

collimation (kol′imā′shən), *n* in radiology, collimation refers to the elimination of the peripheral (more divergent) portion of a useful radiographic beam by means of metal tubes, cones, or diaphragms interposed in the path of the beam. See also diaphragm.

collimation, rectangular, *n* a method for minimizing patient exposure to unnecessary radiation during treatment by using a rectangular position-indicating device (PID) to reduce the size of the radiation beam.

collimator (kol′imātur), *n* a diaphragm or system of diaphragms made of an absorbent material (usually lead) and designed to define the dimensions and direction of a beam of radiation.

collision tumor, *n* See tumor, collision.

colloid (kol′oid), *n* **1.** a suspension of particles in a dispersion medium. The particles generally range in size from 1 to 100 mm. Hydrocolloids and silicate cements are examples of dental colloids. *n* **2.** material in the follicles of the thyroid reserved for production of thyroxine.

colon, *n* the body of the large intestine between the cecum and rectum.

color blindness, *n* See blindness, color.

color, temper, *n* the color produced by the thickening of the oxide coating on carbon steel as temperature is increased. Used as an indication of the degree of tempering.

coloring, extrinsic, coloring from without, as in the application of color to the external surface of a prosthesis.

coloring, intrinsic, *n* coloring from within. The incorporation of pigment within the material of a prosthesis.

Coloumb per kilogram *(C/kg)* (kōō′lōm pur kil′əgram), *n* the unit of measurement for radiation exposure from the French Système International d'Unités; can be converted to the traditional Roentgen (R) by the formula 1 R = 2.58×10^{-4} C/kg.

coma (kō′mə), *n* a state of unconsciousness from which the patient cannot be aroused, even by powerful stimulation. It is gradual in onset, prolonged, and not spontaneously reversible.

coma, diabetic, *n* the state of unconsciousness accompanying severe diabetic acidosis. It may develop from lack of insulin, surgical complications, or disregard of dietary restrictions. Premonitory symptoms include weakness, anorexia, dry skin and oral cavity, drowsiness, abdominal pain, and fruity breath odor. Late symptoms are coma, air hunger, low blood pressure, tachycardia, dehydration, soft and sunken eyeballs, glycosuria, hyperglycemia, and a high level of ecetoacetic acid. See also shock, insulin.

comatose (kō'mətōs), *adj* relating to the state of being unconscious and unable to wake.

combination clasp, *n* See clasp, combination.

command, *n* the portion of a computer-related instruction that specifies the operation to be performed. A term used with hardware operations.

comminution of food, *n* See food, comminution of.

Commission on Dental Accreditation *(CODA),* *n.pr* the body responsible for accrediting dental education programs. Sponsored by the American Dental Association and established in 1975, the Commission establishes quality standards and conducts program reviews to ensure that an educational program seeking accreditation meets these standards.

commissure (kəmish'ur), *n* the corners of the oral cavity.

common deductible, *n* a deductible amount that is common to the dental and another health insurance policy (usually a major medical policy). In a major medical policy with a $100 common deductible, once $100 of medical or dental expense has been incurred under either policy or both, no further deductible is required.

common law, *n* a judge-made law, as contrasted with statutory law. This body of law originated in England and was in force at the time of the American Revolution; modified since that time on a case-by-case basis in the courts.

communicable disease, *n* a disease transmitted from one person or animal to another directly or by vectors.

communicable period, *n* the period when the infectious agent that causes a communicable disease may be transmitted to a susceptible host, such as in diseases that initially involve the mucous membrane (e.g., diphtheria and scarlet fever). The period of communicability is from the time of exposure to the disease until termination of the carrier state, if one develops.

communication, *n* the technique of conveying thoughts or ideas between two people or groups of people.

communication, nonverbal, *n* the transmission of a message without the use of words. It may involve any or all of the five senses. Body language is used as a form of expression.

communication, privileged, *n* the class of communications between persons who stand in a confidential or fiduciary relationship to each other that the law will not permit to be divulged in court. Examples of confidential relationships are those of psychiatrist and patient and attorney and client. Confidentiality of communications depends on the law in each state.

community dentistry, *n* a branch, discipline, or specialty of dentistry that deals with the community and its aggregate dental or oral health rather than that of the individual patient. Formal recognition of dental professionals engaged in community dentistry is through the American Board of Public Health Dentistry. See dental public health.

community health aides, *n.pl* the paraprofessionals who assist in the treatment or support of patients (in their residential setting) within the patient's community environment.

Community Periodontal Index of Treatment Needs *(CPITN),* *n.pr* an assessment tool used to establish periodontal treatment priorities for individual children and adults or groups.

community water fluoridation, *n* the addition of fluoride to community water supplies.

compact, *v* to form by uniting or condensing particles with the application of pressure (e.g., the progressive insertion and welding of foil and the building up of plastic amalgam in a preparation).

compacter (kompak'tər), *n* a rotary instrument used in the McSpadden endodontic technique to condense the guttapercha cone into the root canal.

compaction (kompak'shən), *n* the act of compacting or the state of being compact.

compensating curve, *n* See curve, compensating.

compensation, *n* the monetary reward for rendering a service;

insurance providing financial return to employees in the event of an injury that occurs during the performance of their duties and that prohibits work. Compulsory in many states.

compensation, unemployment, n insurance covering the employee so that compensation may be provided for loss of income as a result of unemployment.

competence, *n* a measure of the degree of a person's ability to cope with all aspects of the environment.

competent, *adj* having legal capacity, ability, or authority.

compiler, *n* a computer program that translates a high-level language program into a corresponding machine instruction. The program that results from compiling is a translated and expanded version of the original program.

complaint, *n* an ailment, problem, or symptom disclosed by the patient.

complaint, chief (CC), n the main symptom or reason for which the patient seeks treatment. The most troublesome ailment, problem, or symptom.

complement (kom′pləmənt), *n* one of 11 complex, enzymatic serum proteins. In an antigen-antibody reaction, complement causes lysis. Complement is also involved in anaphylaxis and phagocytosis.

complement fixation, n an immunologic reaction in which an antigen combines with an antibody and its complement, causing the complement factor to become inactive, or "fixed."

complement-fixation test (C-F test), n a serologic test in which complement fixation is detected, indicating the presence of a particular antigen. The Wassermann test for syphilis is a C-F test, used to detect amebiasis, Rocky Mountain spotted fever, trypanosomiasis, and typhus.

complemental air, *n* See volume, inspiratory reserve.

complementary alternative medicine (CAM), *n* the use of herbs, natural products, and practices such as massage or yoga in health care.

complementary metal oxide semiconductor (CMOS), *n* a silicon-based detector used in digital imaging.

complete blood count, *n* See count, blood, complete.

complete denture, *n* See denture, complete.

complex, *n* a combination of a number of things; the sum or total of various things.

complex, craniofacial, n the bones and surrounding soft structure of the cranium and face.

complex odontoma, n See odontoma, complex.

complex, orofacial, n referring to the dentition and surrounding structures.

compliance (komplī′əns), *n* **1.** the fulfillment by the patient of the health care professional's recommended course of treatment. *n* **2.** the fulfillment of oversight criteria and/ or standards of care necessary for licensure, certification, and accreditation.

complication (kom′plikā′shən), *n* a disease or injury that develops during the treatment of an earlier disorder. An example is a bacterial infection acquired by a person weakened by a viral infection.

component(s), *n/n.pl* a part or element.

component, A, n See factor II.

component of force, n See force, component of.

component of partial denture, n See denture, partial, components of.

component, salivary, n See lysozyme.

component, thromboplastic cellular (TCC), n See factor, platelet, 3.

composite(s), *n* in dentistry, material made from mixture of resin and silica used in tooth-colored fillings and other restorative work. It was created as an alternative to metallic fillings, which were much more visible because of their dark coloring. Also known as a *resin matrix.*

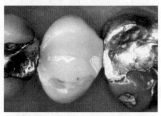

Composite restorations. (Torabinejad/ Walton, 2008)

composite cement, *n* a dental adhesive made of colloidal silica powder combined with the matrix monomer dimethacrylate.

composite odontoma, *n* See odontoma, compound.

composite resin, *n* See resin, composite.

composites, hybrid, *n.pl* resins made from a combination of macrofill and microfill particles that are generally considered easy to polish and highly resistant to fracture and wear. They may be used for either anterior or posterior applications. See also resin, composite and resin-filled.

composites, macrofilled, *n.pl* strong resins made from small particles filled with either glass or quartz. They may be difficult to polish. See also resin, composite and resin-filled.

composites, microfilled, *n.pl* filled resins made from finely ground silica used for anterior esthetic restorations because they polish well and retain their shine. See also resin, composite and resin-filled.

compound, *n* 1. a combination of elements held together in a welldefined pattern by chemical bonds. In pharmacy, a mixture of drugs. *n* 2. a thermoplastic substance used as a nonelastic impression material.

compound A, B, E, F, S, *n* See corticoid, adrenal.

compound cone, *n* a compound in the form of a cone or pyramid; used for impressions of individual preparations.

compound, impression (modeling compound), *n* See compound.

compound, intermetallic, *n* a compound of two metals in which the metals are only partially soluble in one another; exhibits a homogeneous grain structure, but the atoms do not intermingle randomly in all proportions.

compound, modeling, *n* See compound, impression.

compound, phenolic, *n* a mouthwash made from essential oils in combination with alcohol that is available over the counter and approved by the American Dental Association for use in controlling plaque and gingivitis. Also called *essential oils mouthrinses.*

compound tracing stick, *n* a compound dispensed in stick form.

compound, tray, *n* a compound similar to impression compound but with less flow and more viscosity when soft and more rigidity when chilled.

comprehensive dental care, *n* the coordinated delivery of the total dental care required or requested by the patient.

comprehensive health care, *n* the coordinated delivery of the total health care required or requested by the patient.

comprehensive orthodontic therapy, *n* a coordinated approach to improvement of the overall anatomic and functional relationships of the dentofacial complex, as opposed to partial correction with more limited objectives such as cosmetic improvement. Usually but not necessarily uses fixed orthodontic attachments as a part of the treatment appliance. Includes treatment and adjunctive procedures, such as extractions, maxillofacial surgery, other dental services, nasopharyngeal surgery, and speech therapy, directed at malrelationships within the entire dentofacial complex. Optimal care requires periodic evaluation of patient needs, especially during the growing years. Treatment is most effective when begun in the primary or mixed dentitions and accomplished in successive phases as the face matures. Active correction in the adult dentition can usually be accomplished in one phase.

compressed gas cylinders, *n.pl* the color-coded storage cylinders containing either nitrous oxide (light blue) or oxygen (green or white) under pressure; used in controlled combination to induce conscious sedation.

compression, *n* the act of pressing together or forcing into less space.

compression molding, *n* See molding, compression.

compression of tissue, *n* See tissue, displaceability.

compressive strength, *n* See strength, compressive.

compromise (käm′prəmīz′), *n* an arrangement arrived at, in or out of court, for settling a disagreement on terms considered by the parties to be fair.

Compton scatter radiation, *n.pr* the incidental radiation that is energized enough to break an electron bond, but instead strikes a weak bond. The leftover energy then continues in an altered direction.

compulsion (kəmpul′shən), *n* a repetitive, stereotyped, and often trivial motor action, the performance of which is compelled even though the person does not wish to perform the act. Oral habits such as bruxism and clenching may become compulsions.

computed tomography (CT) (tōmog′rəfē), *n* a radiographic body scanning technique in which thin or narrow layer sections of the body can be imaged for diagnostic purposes. The technique uses a computer-linked radiographic machine to focus the radiographs on a particular section of the body to be viewed.

computer, *n* a device capable of accepting data in the form of facts and figures, manipulating them in a prescribed way, and supplying the results of these processes as meaningful information. This device usually consists of input and output devices, storage, arithmetic and logic units, and a control unit. Usually an automatic, stored-program machine is implied.

computer, digital, *n* a computer that operates on discrete data by performing arithmetic and logic processes on them.

computer graphics, *n* the use of computers to create illustrations or designs.

computer imaging, *n* in general, a branch of computer science that works with digital images. In surgical terms, the production of hypothesized postprocedural images, e.g., to show a patient what his face will look like after cosmetic surgery; also called 🔲 *digital imaging.*

computer language, *n* the vocabulary and syntax of a set of symbols that are used to instruct a computer on what to do (e.g., Java, Ada, or C++).

computer literacy, *n* a functional knowledge of the use and application of computers, from word processing to data management.

computer output microfilm (COM), *n* 🔲 a system that allows a computer user to produce microfilm copies of computer output. The COM unit operates independently of the CPU and is therefore called an *off-line* device. Output from computer processing is recorded on generic media and later recorded on microfilm.

computer simulation, *n* the use of computers to replicate a mechanical or biologic function.

computer-controlled local anesthetic delivery system (CCLAD), *n* a computer-driven arrangement of software, hardware, and dental implements used to administer anesthetic injections in which the amount of drug and injection speed are predetermined by a software-driven motor. The injection itself is manually applied.

concavity, *n* **1.** the condition of being concave. *n* **2.** a concave surface, such as a depression on the surface of an organ or tissue.

concavity, facial, *n* the angle between the bridge of the nose, base of the upper lip and the chin. This angle is concave in a skeletal Class III jaw relationship.

conceal, *v* to hide; secrete; withhold from the knowledge of others.

concentration gradient, *n* a ratio of different substances (ions); extracelluar versus intracellular in relation to nerve conduction.

conchae, inferior nasal (kong′kē infē′rēr nā′zəl), *n* the most inferior of the three concha, or scroll-shaped bones, that protrude from the lateral wall of the nasal cavity.

concise, *n.pr* the brand name for diacrylate resin adhesives used in composite restorations and for bonding orthodontic appliances to the enamel.

concomitant drugs, *n.pl* two or more drugs in the systemic circulation at the same time.

🔲 **concrescence (känkres′əns),** *n* the union of two teeth after eruption, by the fusion of their cementum surfaces.

condensation (kän′densā′shən), *n* a commonly used term for the insertion and compression or compaction of dental materials into a prepared cavity. *Compaction* is a more accurate term than condensation. See also compaction.

🔲 **condenser (kənden′sur),** *n* an instrument or device used to compact or condense a restorative material into a prepared cavity. Its working end is called the *nib*, or *point;* the end of the nib is termed the *face.* The face may be smooth or serrated. Formerly called *plugger*.

condenser, amalgam (amalgam plugger), *n* an instrument used to condense plastic amalgam.

condenser, automatic, *n* See condenser, mechanical.

condenser, back-action, *n* a condenser with the shank bent into a U shape so that the condensing force is a pulling motion rather than the usual pushing force.

condenser, bayonet, *n* a condenser in which the offset of the nib and the approximately right-angled bends in the shank permit a better line of force for condensation of direct filling gold. There are many variations in angles, length, and diameter of the nib.

condenser, electromallet (McShirley's electromallet), *n* an electromechanical device for compacting direct filling gold. Frequency of blows may be varied from 200 to 3600 strokes/min; the intensity of the blow is controlled electronically.

condenser, foil, *n* a condenser used to compact direct-filling gold.

condenser, foot, *n* a foil condenser with the nib shaped like a foot.

condenser, hand, *n* an instrument that compacts material, the force being applied by the muscular effort of the clinician with or without supplementary force from a mallet in the hand of the assistant.

condenser, Hollenback, *n.pr* See condenser, pneumatic.

condenser, long-handled foil, *n* a hand condenser of varied design for compacting gold foil.

condenser, mechanical, (automatic mallet), *n* a device to supply an automatically controlled blow for condensing restorative material. It may be spring activated, pneumatic, or electronically controlled.

condenser, parallelogram (par′əlel′ə gram′), *n* a condenser the face of which is shaped like a rectangle or parallelogram.

condenser, pneumatic (Hollenback condenser) (nōō′mat′ik), *n* a pneumatic mechanical device developed by George M. Hollenback to supply a compacting force. The force is delivered by controlled pneumatic pressure. Blows are variable in intensity, with speed variable up to 300 strokes/min.

condenser point, *n* See point, condenser.

condenser, round, *n* a condenser the face of which has a circular outline.

condenser, stepping, *n* the orderly movement of a condenser point over the surface of gold foil or amalgam during its placement and compaction.

condensing force, *n* See force, condensing.

condensing osteitis, *n* See osteitis, condensing.

condensor (spreader), *n* an instrument used in filling a root canal to compress the filling material in a lateral direction.

conditioner, *n* **1.** an additive substance used to increase the effectiveness of another substance. *n* **2.** a substance added to enamel that improves a sealant's ability to adhere.

conditioning, *n* a form of learning based on the development of a response or set of responses to a stimulus or series of stimuli.

conduct, dishonorable, *n* conduct that mars the character and lessens the reputation; conduct that is shameful, disgraceful, base.

conduction, *n* the carrying of sound waves, heat, light, nerve impulses, and electricity.

conduction, air, *n* the process of transmitting sound waves to the cochlea by way of the outer and middle ear. In normal hearing, practically all sounds are transmitted in this way, except those of the hearer's own voice, which are transmitted partly by bone conduction.

conduction, bone, *n* the transmission of sound waves or vibrations to the cochlea by way of the bones of the cranium.

conduction, impulse, *n* the conduction of an impulse along the nerve fiber, accompanied by an alteration of the electrical potential of the fiber tissue and an exchange of electrolytes across the nerve fiber membrane.

conductivity, *n* the capacity for conduction; ability to convey.

conductivity, electrical, *n* the ability of a material to conduct electricity. Metals are usually good conductors, and nonmetals are poor conductors.

conductivity, thermal, *n* the ability of a material to transfer heat. Thermal conductivity is of great importance in dentistry, where a low thermal conductivity is desirable in restorative material and a high thermal conductivity is desirable when soft tissue is covered.

condylar (kän'dilur), *adj* pertaining to the mandibular condyle.

condylar axis, n See axis, condylar.

condylar cartilage, n See cartilage, condylar.

condylar guide, n See guide, condylar.

condylar guide inclination, n See guide, condylar, inclination.

condyle (kän'dīl), *n* the rounded surface at the articular end of a bone. Also called *capitulum.*

condyle head, n a redundant term— the word *condyle* means *head.* See also condyle.

condyle, lateral path, n the path of the condyle in the glenoid fossa when a lateral mandibular movement is made.

condyle, mandibular, n the articular process of the mandible; the condyloid process of the mandible.

condyle, neck of, n See process, condyloid, neck of.

condyle, occipital **(kän'dīl oksip'itl),** *n* the rounded projection that joins with the bones of the vertebrae located at the base of the occipital bone. It permits the head to rotate and flex.

condyle, orbiting, n See orbiting condyle.

condyle path, n the path traveled by the mandibular condyle in the temporomandibular joint during the various mandibular movements.

condyle, protrusive path, n the path of the condyle when the mandible is moved forward from its centric position.

condyle, rod, n See rod, condyle.

condyle, rotating, n the condyle on the side of the bolus formation, or the one that is braced and placed and rotated while the bolus is being chewed.

condylectomy (kän'dilek'tōmē), *n* the surgical removal of a condyle.

condyloid process (kon'dloid'), *n* See process, condyloid.

condyloplasty (kon'dəlōplas'tē), *n* a surgical procedure to alter the shape of the condyle to remove the effects of degenerative disease.

condylotomy (kän'dilot'ōmē), *n* a surgical division through, without removal of, a condyle; or removal of a portion, usually the articular surface, of a condyle.

cone, *n* **1.** a geometric shape with a circular base tapering evenly to an apex. *n* **2.** a solid substance, usually guttapercha or silver, having a tapered form similar in length and diameter to a root canal; used to fill the space once occupied by the pulp in the root of the tooth. *n* **3.** an accessory device on a dental x-ray tubehead, designed to indicate the direction of the central axis of its radiographic beam and to serve as a guide in establishing a desired source-to-receptor distance.

cone beam computed tomography (CBCT), n three-dimensional digital imaging method that uses a cone-shaped x-ray beam that rotates around the patient and acquires digital information.

cone distance, n the distance between the focal spot and the outer end of the cone; usually expressed in inches or centimeters. Modern dental roentgen-ray units usually have cone distances of from 5 to 20 inches (12.5 to 50 cm).

cone, long, n a tubular "cone" designed to establish an extended anode-to-skin distance, usually within a range of from 12 to 20 inches (30 to 50 cm).

cone, sharpening, n a tapered or straight cylindrical stone that is used primarily to sharpen the curvature of dental instruments. See also stone, Arkansas and stone, Carborundum.

cone, short, n a conical or tubular "cone" having as one of its functions the establishment of an anode-to-skin distance of up to 9 inches (22.5 cm).

cone socket handles, *n.pl* the hand-held parts of instruments that may be separated from the working ends in order to replace or exchange individual parts by screwing them together.

cone-cut, *n* a clear, unexposed area on a radiograph that occurs when the position-indicating device and x-ray beam are not centered over the receptor.

confidence interval, *n* a statistical device used to determine the range within which an acceptable datum would fall. Confidence intervals are usually expressed in percentages, typically 95% or 99%.

confidential, *adj* pertaining to information that is only shared with those directly responsible for patient care.

confidentiality, *n* the nondisclosure of certain information except to another authorized person.

confusion, *n* a mental state characterized by disorientation regarding time, place, or person that causes bewilderment, perplexity, lack of orderly thought, and inability to act decisively or perform the activities associated with daily living.

congenital, *adj* present at birth and usually developed in utero.

congestion, *n* See hyperemia.

congestive heart failure (kənjes'tiv), *n* an abnormal condition characterized by a reduction in cardiac contractility and cardiac output resulting in circulatory congestion with retention of fluids). The acute form may result from myocardial infarction of the left ventricle.

conjugate (kon'jəgāt'), *v* **1.** to unite. *n* **2.** the product of conjugation.

conjugation (kon'jəgā'shən), *n* in drug metabolism, the covalent linking of a drug or toxic substance with a normal constituent of the body, such as glucuronic acid, almost always forming an inactive product that is then eliminated.

conjunctiva (kon'junktī'və), *n* the mucous membrane lining the inner surfaces of the eyelids and anterior part of the sclera.

◎ conjunctivitis (kon'junktivī'təs), *n* an inflammation of the conjunctiva, caused by bacterial or viral infection, allergy, or environmental factors. Also called *pinkeye.*

connective tissue, *n* See tissue, connective.

connector, *n* the part of a partial denture that unites its components.

connector, anterior palatal major, n a major connector uniting bilateral units of a maxillary removable partial denture. It is a thin metal plate that is located in the anterior palatal region.

connector bar, n See bar, connector.

connector, cross-arch bar splint, n a removable cross-arch connector used to stabilize weakened abutments that support a fixed prosthesis by attachment to teeth on the opposite side of the dental arch. It can be removed by the dental professional but not by the patient.

connector, lingual bar major, n a type of connector used to unite the right and left components of a mandibular removable partial denture and occupy a position lingual to the alveolar ridge.

connector, linguoplate major **(ling'wōplāt'),** *n* a major connector formed by the extension of a metal plate from the superior border of the regular lingual bar, across gingivae, and onto the cingulum of each anterior tooth.

connector, major, n a metal plate or bar (e.g., lingual bar, linguoplate, palatal bar) used to join the units of one side of a removable partial denture to those located on the opposite side of the dental arch.

connector, minor, n the connecting link between the major connector or base of a removable partial denture and other units of the restoration, such as direct and indirect retainers and rests.

connector, nonrigid, n a connector used where retainers or pontics are united by a joint permitting limited movement. It may be a precision or a nonprecision type of connector.

connector, posterior palatal major, n (posterior palatal bar), a major transpalatal connector located in the posterior palatal region. It is used when the anterior palatal bar alone is insufficient to provide the necessary rigidity.

connector, rigid, n a connector used where retainers or pontics are united by a soldered, cast, or welded joint.

connector, saddle, n See connector, major.

connector, secondary lingual bar major (Kennedy bar), n often called a *continuous clasp* or *Kennedy bar.* It rests on the cingulum area of the lower anterior teeth and serves principally as an indirect retainer and/or stabilizer for weakened anterior lower teeth.

connector, subocclusal, n a nonrigid connector positioned gingival to the occlusal plane.

consanguinity (kon'sangwin'itē), n a hereditary or "blood" relationship between persons, by virtue of having a common parent or ancestor.

conscious, *adj* pertaining to the state of mind in which an individual is able to breathe on his or her own and to respond to verbal commands and physical prompts.

conscious sedation, n a state of sedation in which the patient remains aware of his or her person, surroundings, and conditions but without experiencing pain or anxiety.

consciousness, n a state in which the individual is capable of rational response to questioning and has all protective reflexes intact, including the ability to maintain a patent airway.

consent, n the concurrence of wills; permission.

consent, express, n consent directly given by voice or in writing.

consent, implied, n consent made evident by signs, actions, or facts, or by inaction or silence.

consideration, n inducement to make a contract. It may be a benefit to the promisor or a loss or detriment to the promisee. Consideration must be regarded as such by both parties.

Consolidated Omnibus Budget Reconciliation Act (COBRA), *n.pr* legislation relative to mandated benefits for all types of employee benefits plans. The most significant aspects within this context are the requirements for continued coverage for employees and their dependents for 18 months who would otherwise lose coverage (30 months for dependents in the event of an employee's death).

consonant, n a conventional speech sound produced, with or without laryngeal vibration, by certain successive contractions of the articulatory muscles that modify, interrupt, or obstruct the expired airstream to the extent that its pressure is raised.

consonant, semivowel, n consonants that are like vowels both perceptually and physiologically.

consonant, smile, n the curvature of the maxillary incisal edge is parallel to the lower lip when smiling.

constipation (kon'stipā'shən), n a difficulty passing stools or incomplete or infrequent passage of hard stools.

constituent (kənstich'ūənt), n a part of the whole; component.

constitution, n the general makeup of the body as determined by genetic, physiologic, and biochemical factors. An individual's constitution may be markedly influenced by environment.

constriction (kənstrik'shən), n an abnormal closing or reduction in the size of an opening or passage of the body.

construction, single denture, n the making of one maxillary or mandibular denture as distinguished from a set of two complete dentures.

consultant, n a professional or non-professional person who, by virtue of special knowledge of professional or nonprofessional aspects of a dental practice, is sought out for advice and training.

consultation (kon'səltā'shən), n a meeting of persons to discuss or decide an issue.

consultation, patient, n a meeting among a dental professional, patient, and other interested persons for the purpose of discussing the patient's dental needs, proposing treatment, making business arrangements, making appointments, and giving referrals.

consultation, professional, n a joint deliberation by two or more dental professionals and/or health care professionals to determine the diagnosis, treatment, or prognosis for a particular dental patient.

consumer, n one who may receive or is receiving dental service; the term is also used in health care legislation and programs as a reference to someone who is never a practitioner or is not associated in any direct or indirect way with the supplying or provision of dental services.

contact, n the act of touching or meeting, such as with the contact area, the portion of a tooth where adjacent tooth crowns in the same arch physically touch on each proximal surface.

contact, balancing, n the contact established between the maxillary and mandibular dentures at the side opposite the working side (anteroposteriorly or laterally) for the purpose of stabilizing the dentures.

contact, deflective occlusal, *n* (cuspal interference), a condition of tooth contacts that diverts the mandible from a normal path of closure to centric jaw relation or causes a denture to slide or rotate on its basal seat. See also contact, interceptive occlusal.

contact, faulty, *n* imperfections in the contact between adjacent teeth. Often leads to food impaction between the teeth, with subsequent initiation or perpetuation of periodontal lesions.

contact, indirect, *n* touching or in contact with a contaminated surface or instrument.

contact, initial, *n* the first meeting of opposing teeth on elevation of the mandible toward the maxillae.

contact, interceptive occlusal, *n* an initial contact of teeth that interferes with the normal movement of the mandible. See also contact, deflective occlusal.

contact, premature, *n* See deflective occlusal and contact, interceptive.

contact, working, *n* a contact of the teeth made on the side of the dental arch toward which the mandible has been moved.

contagious (kəntā′jus), *adj* capable of being transmitted from one person to another by direct or indirect contact.

contaminated (kəntam′inātid), *v* **1.** made radioactive by the addition of small quantities of radioactive material. *v* **2.** made contaminated by adding infective or radiographic materials. *n* **3.** an infective surface or object.

contamination, radioactive, *n* the deposition of radioactive material in any place where it is not desired, and particularly where its presence may be harmful or may constitute a radiation hazard.

contingent (kəntin′jənt), *adj* dependent for effect on something that may or may not occur.

continuant (kəntin′yōōənt), *n* a speech sound in which the speech organs are held relatively fixed during the period of production.

continuing education, *n* postgraduate study offered either in an institution of higher learning by groups with an organized dental program or by individuals who are especially qualified in certain areas. Required by most state licensing boards for license renewal for dental professionals. Credit accumulates for special qualifications to join special interest groups.

continuing education unit *(CEU),* *n* educational classes or experiences for licensed dental professionals that extend, update, or renew their knowledge of practices in their field. Some classes may be required for relicensing. Usually, one CEU equals 1 clock hour of instruction.

continuous bar retainer, *n* See retainer, continuous bar.

continuous clasp, *n* See retainer, continuous bar.

continuous loop wiring, *n* See wiring, continuous loop.

continuous variable, *n* variable that can be expressed by a large and infinite number of measure along a continuum and in a fraction; also considered quantitiative.

contour (kon′tōōr), *n* the external shape, form, or surface configuration of an object.

contour, anatomic height of **(an′ətom′ik),** *n* a line encircling a tooth to designate its greatest convexity.

contour, buccal, *n* the shape of the buccal aspect of a posterior tooth. It normally has occlusocervical convexity, with its greatest prominence at the gingival third of the clinical buccal surface.

contour, gingival, *n* the shape of the natural or artificial gingiva as it approximates the natural or artificial tooth.

contour, height of, *n* the greatest convexity of a tooth viewed from a predetermined position.

contour, proximal **(prok′səməl),** *n* the form of the mesial or distal surface of a tooth.

contour, restoration, *n* the restoration of a proper contour where surfaces of teeth have been destroyed by disease processes or excessive wear.

contour, tooth, *n* a shape of a tooth that is essential to a healthy gingival unit because it enables the bolus of food to be deflected from gingival margins during mastication.

contouring, occlusal, *n* the correction, by grinding, of gross disharmonies of the occlusal tooth form (e.g., uneven marginal ridges, plunger cusps, extruded teeth, malpositioned teeth) to establish a harmonious occlusion and protect the periodontium of the tooth.

contouring pliers, *n* See pliers, contouring.

contra-angle   (kän′trə-ang′gəl), *n* more than one angle. An instrument having two or more offsetting angles such that the end of the instrument is kept within 3 mm of the axis of the shaft.

contraception (kon′trəsep′shən), *n* a process or technique for the prevention of pregnancy by means of a medication, device, or method that blocks or alters one or more of the processes of reproduction in such a way that sexual union can occur without impregnation.

contract, *n* **1.** an agreement based on sufficient consideration between two or more competent parties to do or not to do something that is legal. *n* **2.** a legally enforceable agreement between two or more individuals or entities that confers rights and duties on the parties. Common types of contracts include (1) those contracts between a dental benefits organization and an individual dental provider to provide dental treatment to members of an alternative benefits plan. These contracts define the dental provider's duties both to beneficiaries of the dental benefits plan and the dental benefits organization, and usually define the manner in which the dental provider will be reimbursed; and (2) contracts between a dental benefits organization and a group plan sponsor. These contracts typically describe the benefits of the group plan and the rates to be charged for those benefits.

contract, breach of, n the failure, without legal excuse, to perform an obligation or duty in a contract.

contract   dentist/dental   professional, n a practitioner who contractually agrees to provide services under special terms, conditions, and financial reimbursement arrangements.

contract dentistry, n **1.** the providing of dental care under a specific set of

guidelines and for a specific set of individuals under an accepted written agreement by the patient, dental professional, and employer. *n* **2.** the practice of dentistry whereby the dentist/ dental professional enters into a written agreement with either patients or an employer to provide dental care for a set group of people.

contract, express, n a contract that is an actual agreement between the parties, with the terms declared at the time of making, being stated in explicit language either orally or in writing.

contract fee schedule plan, n a dental benefits plan in which participating dental professionals agree to accept a list of specific fees as the total fees for dental treatment provided.

contract, implied, n a contract not evidenced by explicit agreement of the parties but inferred by the law from the acts and circumstances surrounding the transactions.

contract, open-end, n **1.** a contract that permits periodic reevaluation of the dental plan during the contract year. If indicated by the reevaluation, dental services may be deleted or added to achieve a balance between the premium and cost of service provided. *n* **2.** a contract that sets no dollar limits on the total services to be provided to beneficiaries but does list the particular services that will be included in the plan.

contract practice, n a type of dental practice in which an employer or third-party administrator contracts directly with a dental professional or group of dental professionals to provide dental services for beneficiaries of a plan. See also closed panel.

contract term, n the period, usually 12 months, for which a contract is written.

contraction (kəntrak′shən), *n* **1.** a shortening, shrinkage, or reduction in length or size. **2.** a condition in which teeth or other maxillary and mandibular structures, such as the dental arch, are nearer than normal to the median plane.

contraction, concentric muscle, n an unresisted ordinary shortening of muscle.

contraction, eccentric muscle, n an increase in muscle tonus during lengthening of the muscle. Eccentric contraction occurs when muscles are used to oppose movement but not to stop it (e.g., the action of the biceps in lowering the forearm gradually and in a controlled manner). Eccentric contractions are called *isotonic,* because the muscle changes length.

contraction, isometric muscle (ī′sōmet′rik), *n* an increase in muscular tension without a change in muscle length, as in clenching the teeth.

contraction, isotonic muscle (ī′sōton′ik), *n* an increase in muscular tension during movement without resistance (either lengthening or shortening), as in free opening and closing of the jaws.

contraction, metal, *n* the shrinkage associated with the congealing of a metal from its molten state to a solid after having been cast. See also expansion, thermal.

contraction, muscle, *n* the development of tension in a muscle in response to a nerve stimulus.

contraction, muscle, changes in striation bands, *n.pl* alterations in bands of striated muscle during contraction. Striated muscle is composed of a darker A band and a lighter I band. Both these alternating bands develop tension during contraction but not to the same degree. In isometric contraction (clenched teeth), the sarcomere muscle unit remains unchanged in length, whereas the A band (the darker band) actually shortens and the I band (the lighter band) lengthens. When a muscle is passively stretched, such as when the mandible is opened by gravity, the A band lengthens relatively more than the I band, and during isotonic contraction, almost all the shortening is in the A segment. It is thus concluded that the contractile properties are not the same throughout the sarcomere, which is the unit of contractility. It is suggested that the darker A band has a greater concentration of contractile substance than the I band and that, in addition to contractile elements, the I band contains elastic noncontractile elements that constitute a series of elastic components throughout the fibril. Thus there is, throughout a fiber, an arrangement of dark, contractile components

alternating with lighter, elastic components.

contraction, muscle, chemical factors in, *n.pl* the chemical constituents and action involved in the contraction of muscle fibers. Muscle is a structure with working units built up largely from two proteins, actin and myosin, which appear to be organized into separate filaments running longitudinally through the muscle fibers. Neither type of filament runs continuously along the length of the fiber, although the effect is that of a continuous structure. The filaments are organized into a succession of groupings of one type of fiber. Each group is arranged in a regular palisade to overlap the next group of fibers, which are similarly arranged in palisades. This gives a banded appearance to the fiber. The thicker filaments contain myosin and are restricted to the A bands, where they give rise to a higher density and double refraction. The thinner filaments contain actin and extend to either side of the Z band, which is at the center of the I band. When the muscle contracts or is stretched, the two groups of filaments slide past each other like the alternating units of a sliding gate. The controlled sliding motion is presumably brought about through the mediation of oblique cross-links between the filaments. These cross-links are the structural expression of the biochemical interaction between actin and myosin. The chemical substance that initiates the interaction between these fibrils is adenosine triphosphate (ATP). The final effect of the interaction between ATP, myosin, and actin is to enable the two types of filaments to crawl past each other to create the shortened state of the muscle.

contraction, postural muscle (pos′churəl), *n* the maintenance of muscular tension (usually isometric muscular contraction) sufficient to maintain posture.

contraction, premature ventricular (PVC), *n* an extra heartbeat caused by premature contractions of the heart's ventricles resulting in palpitations, or a skipped beat, followed by a more pronounced beat.

contraction, smooth muscle, mechanism of, *n* the mechanisms that regulate the functions of smooth muscle fibers. These regulatory mechanisms vary and are affected principally by two methods. First, the parasympathetic and sympathetic nerve fiber endings of the autonomic nervous system form a reticulum around the muscle cells before entering them. The action of these fibers is antagonistic; they act directly on the muscle cell, not on each other. Examples of the structures principally under the control of the autonomic nerve mechanism are the blood vessels and the pilomotor fibers. Second, the selection response to rhythmic activity associated with the automaticity of a viscus or other organ depends on local or hormonal factors. An example of this mechanism is the function of the uterus under the control of the estrogenic hormone.

contraction, static muscle, n the contraction in which opposing muscles contract against each other and prevent movement. Fixation action of a muscle in a static contraction is termed *isometric,* because it develops tension without changing length.

contractor, independent, n one who, exercising an independent employment, contracts to do a piece of work according to the conditions of the contract and without being subject to control except as to the result of the work.

contracture (kǝntrak´chǝr), n a permanent shortening, or contraction, of a muscle.

contraindication (kon´trǝin´dikā´sh ǝn), n any symptom or circumstance indicating the inappropriateness of a form of treatment otherwise advisable. This is further divided into the concepts of absolutes and relative contraindications.

contralateral (kon´trǝlat´ǝrǝl), adj originating from or affecting the opposite side of the body.

contrast, radiographic (radiographic image), n the differences in photographic or film density produced on a radiograph by structural composition of the object radiographed or by varying amounts of radiation.

contrast, radiographic, long-scale, n an increased number of gradations of gray between the blacks and whites on a radiographic image. Higher

kilovoltages increase the scale of contrast.

contrast, radiographic, media, n See radiograph, contrast media.

contrast, radiographic, short-scale, n a minimum number of gradations of gray between the blacks and whites on a radiographic image. Lower kilovoltages decrease the scale of contrast.

contrast, subject, n See contrast, radiographic.

contributory negligence, n See negligence, contributory.

contributory plan, n a method of payment for group insurance coverage in which part of the premium is paid by the employee and part is paid by the employer or union.

contributory program, n a dental benefits program in which the enrollee shares in the monthly premium of the program with the program sponsor (usually the employer). Generally done through payroll deduction.

control group, n the group of participants in a clinical study who do not receive the drug or treatment being studied against which the reactions of individuals in the experimental group may be compared. See also controlled clinical trial.

control, stress, n a method used to diminish or remove the stress load generated by occlusal contact, whether the contact is functional in origin or the result of a habit cycle.

controlled clinical trial, n a research strategy that calls for two samples: an experimental sample of patients receiving a pharmaceutical, and a second sample of control patients receiving a placebo. Neither the patient nor the researcher knows which is receiving the pharmaceutical and which the placebo.

controlled substance, a drug as defined in the five categories of the federal Controlled Substances Act of 1970. The categories, or schedules, cover opium and its derivatives, hallucinogens, depressants, and stimulants.

controlled-release therapeutic systems, n a drug or hormone delivery system that releases predetermined amounts of drug or hormone into the body over a specified period.

contusion (kəntōō′zhən), *n* a bruise that is usually produced by impact from a blunt object and that does not cause a break in the skin.

convenience form, *n* See form, convenience.

convergence (kənvur′jəns), *n* the movement of two objects toward a common point , such as turning of the eyes inward to see an object close to the face.

convergence, cervical, *n* the angle formed between the cervicoaxial inclination of a tooth surface on one side and a diagnostic stylus of a dental cast surveyor in contact with the tooth at its height of contour.

conversion privilege, *n* the right of an individual covered by a group dental insurance policy to continue having coverage on a direct payment basis when association with the insured group is terminated.

converter, rotary, *n* a motor generator set or unit that, when operated by one type of current, produces another (e.g., the conversion of alternating to direct current).

convertin, *n* See thromboplastin, extrinsic.

convex (konveks′), *adj* having a surface that curves outward.

convexity, facial, *n* the angle between the bridge of nose, base of the upper lip and the chin. This angle is convex in a skeletal Class II jaw relationship.

convulsion (kənvul′shən), *n* an intense seizure.

coolant (kōō′lənt), *n* air or liquid directed onto a tooth, tissue, or restoration to neutralize the heating effect of a rotary instrument.

Cooley's anemia, *n.pr* See thalassemia major.

Cooley's trait, *n.pr* See thalassemia minor.

Coolidge filament transformer, tube, *n.pr* See transformer, Coolidge.

coordination, *n* the harmonious functioning of body systems.

coordination of benefits clause, *n* **1.** a provision in an insurance contract that when a patient is covered under more than one group dental plan, benefits paid by all plans will be limited to 100% of the actual charges after each deductible has been satisfied. *n* **2.** COB: a method of integrating benefits payable under more than one plan. Benefits from all sources should not exceed 100% of the total charges.

Copal resin (kōpəl), *n.pr* brand name for a mixed resin of diverse plant origin used in cavity varnishes. Its effectiveness in protecting the pulp from the phosphoric acid in dental cements is questioned.

copayment, *n* the beneficiary's share of the dental professional's fee after the benefits plan has paid.

cope, *n* the upper half of a flask in the casting art; hence also the upper, or cavity, side of a denture flask.

coping (thimble) (kō′ping), *n* a thin metal covering or cap over a prepared tooth.

coping, parallel, *n* a casting placed over an implant abutment to make it parallel to other natural or implant abutments.

coping, transfer, *n* a covering or cap, made of metal, acrylic resin, or other material used to position a die in an impression.

copolymer (kōpäl′imur), *n* a polymerization of two or more monomers that have slightly different chemical formulas. Used in dentistry to impart certain desirable physical properties such as flow.

copolymerization (kōpäl′imərizā′s hən), *n* the formation of a copolymer.

copper, *n* a malleable, reddish-brown metallic element. It is a component of several important enzymes in the body and is essential to good health. A deficiency is rare, because only 2 to 5 mg daily are necessary, and that amount is easily obtained in a normal diet.

coprolalia (kop′rōlā′lēə), *n* the uncontrollable vocalization of obscene or offensive words.

coproporphyria (kop′rōpôr′fir′ēə), *n* the presence of an abnormal concentration of coproporphyrin in the urine. Normal values range from 70 mg to 250 mg/day. An increased amount of coproporphyrin III occurs in the urine in clinical lead poisoning, exposure to lead without clinically apparent symptoms, infections, malignant disease, alcoholic cirrhosis, after ingestion of small amounts of ethanol, and normally in some individuals.

coproporphyrin (kop′rəpor′firin), *n* a nitrogenous organic substance normally excreted in the feces as a breakdown of bilirubin.

cord(s), *n/n.pl* a long, rounded organ or body.

cord, spinal, *n* the central nervous system cord contained in the vertebral column. It is essential to the regulation and administration of various motor, sensory, and autonomic nerve activities of the body. Through its pathways it conducts impulses from the extremities, trunk, and neck to and from the higher centers and to consciousness. It thus provides for simple reflexes, has control over visceral activities, and participates in the conscious activities of the body.

cord, vocal, *n* the membranous structures in the throat that produce sound; the thyroarytenoid ligaments of the larynx. The inferior cords are called the *true vocal cords,* and the superior cords are called the *false vocal cords.*

core, *n* the central part. A section of a mold, usually of plaster, made over assembled parts of a dental restoration or construction to record and maintain the relationships of the parts so that the parts can be reassembled in their original positions. Also called a *laboratory core.*

core, amalgam, *n* the foundational replacement of the badly mutilated crown of a tooth whose purpose is to provide a rigid base for retention of a cast crown restoration. The core may be retained by undercuts, slots, pins, or the pulp chamber of an endodontically treated tooth.

core, cast, *n* a metal casting, usually with a post in the canal or a root, designed to retain an artificial crown.

core, composite, *n* a composite resin buildup to provide retention for a cast crown restoration.

core, laboratory, *n* a section of a mold, usually of plaster, made over assembled parts of a dental restoration or construction to record and maintain the relationships of the parts so that the parts can be reassembled in their original positions.

cornea (kor′nēə), *n* the transparent anterior part of the eye.

cornification (kor′nifikā′shən), *n* the conversion of epithelium to a hornlike substance. *Keratinization* is a more specific term. See also keratin.

cornu (kôr′nōō), *n* a bony projection.

coronal, *adj* pertaining to the crown portion of teeth.

coronal, plane, *n* a plane dividing the body into anterior and posterior halves.

coronary angioplasty, percutaneous transluminal, *n* a surgical technique designed to improve circulation. It involves the insertion of a balloon-carrying catheter into a blood vessel of the heart that is clogged with plaque, then alternately inflating and deflating the balloon several times to flatten the plaque against the arterial walls and reestablish the free flow of blood. Also called *balloon angioplasty* or *coronary dilation.*

coronary artery bypass, *n* an open-heart surgery in which a section of a blood vessel is grafted onto one or more of the coronary arteries to improve the blood supply to the muscles of the heart.

Coronaviridae **(kôrō′nəvir′idā),** *n.pl* a family of enveloped, helical, airborne RNA viruses responsible for some respiratory and gastrointestinal diseases. It can also be contracted from unsanitary equipment or from human carriers.

coronoid notch, *n* See notch, coronoid.

coronoid process, *n* See process, coronoid.

coronoidectomy (kor′ōnoidek′tō mē), *n* the surgical removal of the coronoid process of the mandible.

corporate dentistry, *n* **1.** the dental care provided for a specific group of employees within a single business under a contract arrangement or on a salaried basis, with costs borne by the corporation. *n* **2.** a company owned-and-operated dental care facility that provides services to employees and sometimes dependents.

corpus callosum (kor′pəs kəlō′səm), *n* the largest commissure of the brain connecting the cerebral hemispheres.

corpuscle(s) (kor′pusəl), *n/n.pl* a small body, mass, or organ.

corpuscle, blood, *n* a formed element in the blood. See also erythrocyte, leukocyte, lymphocyte, monocyte.

corpuscle, Golgi's, n.pr a small, spindle-shaped proprioceptive endorgan located in tendons and activated by stretch.

corpuscle, Krause's, n.pr the bulboid encapsulated nerve endings located in mucous membranes and activated by cold.

corpuscle, Meissner's, n.pr the medium encapsulated nerve endings found in the skin and activated by light touch.

corpuscle, Merkel's, n.pr the specialized sensory nerve endings located in the submucosa of the oral cavity and activated by light touch.

corpuscle, Pacini's, n.pr the large sensory nerve endings, scattered widely in subcutaneous tissues, joints, and tendons and activated by deep pressure.

corpuscle, Ruffini's, n.pr the specialized sensory nerve organs in the skin and mucous membranes for perceiving heat. Temperature variations of less than 5°C are not readily received by these end organs.

corrected master cast, *n* See cast, master, corrected.

correction, occlusal, *n* the fixing of malocclusion, by whatever means is employed, including the elimination of disharmony of occlusal contacts.

corrective, *n* a prescription ingredient designed to compensate for or nullify specific undesirable effects of the principal pharmaceutical agent and the adjuvant.

correlation, *n* a statistical procedure used to determine the degree to which two (or more) variables vary together. Correlation does not suggest a cause-effect relationship but only the degree of parallelism or concomitance between the variables, the cause of which may be unknown. The *Pearson product-moment correlation (r)* is the most frequently used, and this coefficient is used unless another is specified.

correlation, coefficient number **(kŏ′əfish′ənt),** *n* the result of statistical computation that indicates the strength of the tendency of two or more variables to vary concomitantly. The coefficient is expressed in fractions (that is, r = 80), ranging from 21 to 11, and indicates the magnitude of the relationship between the variables.

Perfect direct correspondence is expressed by 11; perfect inverse correspondence by 21; complete lack of correspondence by 0. Fractional values are not read as percents.

correlation, linear, n a correlation in which the regression line, the line that best describes the relationship between the two variables, is a straight line, so that for any increase in the magnitude of one variable there will be a proportional change in the magnitude of the other variable.

correlation, multiple, n a complex correlation procedure in which scores on two or more variables are combined to predict scores on another variable, called the *dependent variable.*

correspondence, *n* written or typed communication between two individuals or groups of individuals.

corrosion, *n* an electrolytic or chemical attack of a surface. Usually refers to the attack of a metal surface.

cortex (kôr′těks′), *n* the outer layer of an organ or other structure.

cortex, adrenal, n the outer layer of the adrenal gland, the site of secretion of the adrenocortical hormones.

cortex, cerebral, n the outer gray matter of cerebrum, where many of the higher functions (such asvolition, consciousness, conceptualization) are carried out.

cortical, *adj* pertaining to or consisting of a cortex.

corticalosteotomy (kôr′tikəlos′tēot′ōmē), *n* an osteotomy through the cortex at the base of the dentoalveolar segment, which serves to weaken the resistance of the bone to the application of orthodontic forces.

corticoid, adrenal (kôr′tikoid), *n* an adrenal corticosteroid hormone (e.g., 11-dehydrocorticosterone, corticosterone, 11-deoxycorticosterone [cortexone, DOC], cortisone cortisol, 11-desoxycortisol aldosterone, androgen, progesterone, estradiol, and others). See also aldosterone, androgen, corticosterone, cortisone, estrogens, hydrocortisone, and progesterone.

corticosteroid (kôr′tikōstir′oid), *n* See steroid, adrenocortical.

corticosterone (Kendall's compound B) (kôr'tikōstir'ōn, kôr' tikos'tərōn), *n* an adrenal corticosteroid hormone necessary for the maintenance of life in adrenalectomized animals; protects against stress, influences muscular efficiency, and influences carbohydrate and electrolyte metabolism.

corticotropin (kôr'tikōtrō'pin), *n* a purified preparation of adrenocorticotropic hormone derived from the pituitary gland of animals. See also ACTH.

cortisol, *n* See hydrocortisone.

cortisone (17-hydroxy-11-dehydrocorticosterone, Kendall's compound E) (kor'tisōn'), *n* a hormone produced by the adrenal cortex; a glucocorticoid, 17-hydroxy-11-dehydrocorticosterone; useful in the treatment of rheumatoid arthritis, lupus erythematosus, and some allergic conditions. Has marked antiinflammatory properties. Excess production or administration produces signs of hyperadrenocorticalism (Cushing's syndrome) with hyperlipemia and obesity, hyperglycemia and edema.

cortisone acetate, n brand name: Cortone; *drug class:* gluocorticoid, short acting; *action:* decreases inflammation by binding to intracellular receptors resulting in inhibition of phospholipase A2 resulting in suppression of macrophage and leukocyte migration, reduction in capillary permeability and other effects; *uses:* inflammation, severe allergy, adrenal insufficiency, collagen, and respiratory and dermatologic disorders.

corundum, *n* See emery.

Corynebacterium (kor'ənēbakter' ēəm), *n* a common genus of rod-shaped, curved bacilli. The most common pathogenic species are *C. acnes,* commonly found in acne lesions, and *C. diphtheriae,* the cause of diphtheria.

cosmetic orthodontics, *n* limited orthodontic therapy for the purpose of improving appearance, such as the closing of an unsightly diastema between maxillary incisors that presents no other handicap.

cost containment, *n* the features of a dental benefits program or of the administration of the program designed to reduce or eliminate certain charges to the plan.

cost share, *n* the share of health expenses that a beneficiary must pay, including the deductibles, copayments, coinsurance, and charges over the amount reimbursed by the dental benefits plan.

cost-benefit analysis, *n* the comparative study of the service or production costs of a service or item and its value to the subject.

cost-effective, *n* the minimal expenditure of dollars, time, and other elements necessary to achieve the health care result deemed necessary and appropriate.

Costen's syndrome, *n.pr* See syndrome, Costen's.

cotherapist, *n* in oral health care, a designation for the relationships among patient, dental hygienist, and dental professional in securing the patient's regular treatment.

cotinine (kō'tinēn), *n* a metabolite of nicotine. The presence of this chemical in body fluids is considered proof of recent nicotine use.

cotton, absorbent, *n* the fibers or hairs of the seed of cultivated varieties of *Gossypium herbaceum,* so prepared that the cotton readily absorbs liquid.

cotton pliers, *n* See pliers, cotton.

cough, *n* a sudden, noisy expulsion of air from the lungs. See also mechanism, cough.

cough, gander, n the characteristic clanging, brassy cough of tracheal obstruction.

Council on Dental Therapeutics, *n. pr* an appointed council within the Division of Scientific Affairs of the American Dental Association directed to study, evaluate, and disseminate information with regard to dental therapeutic agents, their adjuncts, and dental cosmetic agents that are offered to the public or profession.

counseling, *n* the act of providing advice and guidance to a patient or the patient's family.

count, blood, complete, *n* the determination of the number of red blood cells (erythrocytes), white blood cells, and platelets in an accurately measured volume of blood. It usually includes the quantity of hemoglobin per cubic millimeter of blood. A

when the fragments of a fractured bone are rubbed together.

crest, *n* a projecting ridge or structure.

crest, alveolar, *n* See bone crest.

crest, gingival, *n* the coronal margin of the gingival tissue.

crest module, *n* the portion of a two-piece metal dental implant designed to hold the prosthetic component in place and to create a transition zone to the load-bearing implant body.

CREST syndrome, *n* See syndrome, CREST.

crestal resorption (kres'təl rēsôrp'shən), *n* bone resorption at the border or crest of the dental alveolus. This bone loss follows tooth extraction and may result from periodontal infection or through the use of heavy orthodontic forces.

cretin (krē'tən), *n* a thyroid-deficient dwarfed individual with mental subnormality.

cretinism (congenital hypothyroidism) (krē'tənizəm), *n* See hypothyroidism.

crevice, gingival, *n* See gingival, crevice.

crevicular fluid (krevik'yōolur), *n* an older term for a clear, usually unnoticeable fluid that can serve as a defense mechanism against infection by carrying antibodies and other substances between the connective tissue and sulcus or pocket. Also called *gingival sulcus fluid* or *sulcular fluid.*

crib, Jackson, *n.pr* a removable orthodontic appliance retained in position by crib-shaped wires.

crib, lingual, *n* an orthodontic appliance consisting of a wire framework suspended lingually to the maxillary incisor teeth; used to obstruct thumb and tongue habits.

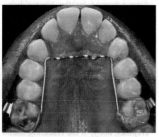

Lingual crib. (Courtesy Dr. Flavio Uribe)

crib splint, *n* See splint, crib.

cribriform plate (krib'rəform'), *n* **1.** the aveolar bone that forms the tooth socket and to which the periodontal ligament is attached (radiographically presents as the lamina dura). *n* **2.** the horizontal plate of the ethmoid bone that is perforated with foramina for the olfactory nerves.

cricoid cartilage (krī'koid), *n* See cartilage, cricoid.

cricoidynia (krī'koidi'nēə), *n* pain in the cricoid cartilage.

cricothyrotomy (krī'kōthirot'əmē), *n* an incision between the cricoid and thyroid cartilages for the purpose of maintaining a patent airway.

cri-du-chat syndrome (krē'- dōō -shä'), *n* See syndrome, cri-du-chat.

crisis, adrenal, an acute adrenocaortical insufficiency, with clinical manifestations of headache, nausea, vomiting, diarrhea, confusion, costovertebral angle pain, circulatory collapse, and coma. May occur in relation to stress of dental or medical procedures in patients with latent adrenal disease or in patients who have undergone prior ACTH or cortisone therapy, especially without control or termination of therapy.

crisis, thyroid, *n* a complication occurring after thyroidectomy, or before or during other surgical procedures where even mild hyperthyroidism is present. It is characterized by tachycardia, a high temperature, nervousness, and occasionally delirium.

crista galli, *n* the vertical midline continuation of the perpendicular plate of the ethmoid bone into the cranial cavity.

cristobalite (kristō'bəlīt), *n* a form of crystalline silica used in dental casting investments because of its relatively high capacity for thermal expansion and resistance to breaking down by heat.

criteria (krītēr'ēə), *n.pl* predetermined rules or guidelines for dental care, developed by dental professionals relying on professional expertise, prior experience, and the professional literature, with which aspects of actual instances of dental care may be compared. *Explicit* criteria are predetermined, specific, and measurable; *implicit* criteria are implied or understood but not directly expressed.

critical instrument, *n* item used to penetrate soft tissue or bone.

critical care, *n* See intensive care.

Crohn disease, *n* See disease, Crohn.

cromolyn sodium (krō′məlin′ sō′dēəm), *n brand names:* Intal, Nasalcrom, Rynacrom; *drug class:* antiasthmatic (prophylactic); *action:* stabilizes the membrane of the sensitized mast cell, preventing release of chemical mediators; *uses:* allergic rhinitis, severe perennial bronchial asthma, exercise induced bronchospasm.

cross-linkage, *n* See polymerization, cross.

cross-arch bar splint, *n* See connector.

cross-arch bar splint connector, *n* See connector, cross-arch bar splint.

cross-arch splinting, *n* See splinting, cross-arch.

crossbite, *n* an occlusion with the line of occlusion of the mandibular teeth anterior and/or buccal to the maxillary teeth. See also occlusion, crossbite.

crossbite, anterior, *n* the primary or permanent maxillary incisors locked lingual to mandibular incisors.

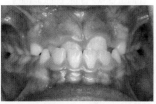

Anterior crossbite. (Courtesy Dr. Flavio Uribe)

crossbite, posterior, *n* the primary permanent maxillary posterior teeth in lingual position in relation to the man- 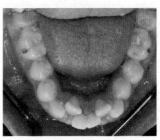 dibular teeth.

cross-contamination, *n* the transfer of an infection directly from one person to another or indirectly from one person to a second person via a fomite.

cross-examination, *n* the questioning of a witness by the party against whom he or she has been called and examined.

cross-infection, *n* the transmission of a communicable disease from one person to another because of a poor barrier protection.

cross-resistance, *n* See resistance, cross-.

cross-section form, *n* See clasp, flexibility of.

cross-sectional study, *n* the scientific method for the analysis of data gathered from two or more samples at one point in time.

cross-tolerance, *n* See tolerance, cross-.

crotch, furcation, *n* the point at which the root of a tooth forks into two or more branches.

Crouzon syndrome (krōōzonz′), *n. pr* See syndrome, Crouzon.

crowding, *n* **1.** in dentistry, when the dental arch length is less than the mesial distal width of the teeth intended to occupy it. *n* **2.** malocclusion characterized by inadequate arch circumference to accommodate the teeth in proper alignment.

Crowding. (Courtesy Dr. Flavio Uribe)

crown, *n* **1.** the natural portion of a tooth covered by enamel. *n* **2.** an artificial replacement for the natural crown of the tooth. Colloquial term is *cap.*

crown, anatomical, *n* the portion of dentin covered by enamel.

crown and bridge prosthodontics, *n* the division of prosthodontics that deals with crown restorations and the fixed type of tooth-borne partial denture prosthesis. See also prosthodontics, fixed.

crown, artificial, *n* a dental prosthesis restoring the anatomy, function, and esthetics of part or all of the coronal portion of the natural tooth.

crown, ceramic, *n* one of several materials that can make up a crown, which can be combined with other components such as porcelain or metal to improve long-term crown function.

crown, cervical aspect (ser′vikəl), *n* the clinical view of a crown from its most narrow angle of insertion into the gingival tissues.

crown, clinical, n **1.** the portion of enamel visibly present in the oral cavity. *n* **2.** the portion of a tooth that is occlusal to the deepest part of the gingival sulcus.

crown, complete, n a restoration that reproduces the entire surface anatomy of the clinical crown and fits over a prepared tooth stump.

crown, dowel, n a restoration that replaces the entire coronal portion of a tooth and derives its retention from a dowel extending into a treated (filled) root canal.

crown, extraalveolar clinical (ek′str əalvē′ələr), *n* the portion of a tooth that extends occlusally or incisally from the junction of the tooth root and the supporting bone.

crown, faced, n See crown, veneered metal.

crown, full, restoration, n an individual tooth prosthesis encompassing the entire prepared clinical crown. See also crown, complete veneer.

crown, gold, n a metal variety of crown using gold.

crown, jacket, n See crown, complete.

crown lengthening, n a surgical procedure to remove marginal gingival tissues to expose more of the crown of the tooth to facilitate a reconstructive or operative procedure.

crown, partial, n a restoration that covers three or more, but not all, surfaces of a tooth.

crown, porcelain-faced, n an artificial crown that makes use of porcelain inlayed in or veneered onto the labial or buccal surface.

crown, porcelain jacket, n a type of crown composed of porcelain mixed with metal, commonly used for its appearance and tooth-bonding properties.

crown remover, n one of a variety of clamps, hooks, levers, or adhesive blocks designed to remove crowns that have been cemented onto teeth.

crown, stainless steel, n a preformed steel crown used for the restoration of badly broken-down primary teeth and first permanent molars. Also used as a temporary restoration of fractured permanent incisors.

crown, temporary, n a short-term crown placed on a tooth while the final impression of the permanent crown is being cast.

crown, three-quarter, n a term frequently used to designate a partial veneer crown.

crown, veneer, n a restoration that reproduces the total clinical coronal surface contour of the tooth. Colloquial term is *veneers.*

crown, veneered metal, n a complete crown that has one or more surfaces prepared and covered by a tooth-colored substance such as porcelain or resin.

crown and loop, *n* an appliance consisting of a wire loop soldered to a stainless steel crown restoration and designed to prevent space loss in a dental arch when a tooth has been lost prematurely.

crown-implant ratio, *n* See ratio, crown-implant.

crown-root ratio, *n* the relation of the clinical crown to the clinical roots of the teeth—an important consideration in diagnosis, prognosis, and treatment planning.

crown-rump length, *n* the length of an embryo, fetus, or newborn as measured from the crown of the head to the prominence of the buttocks.

Crozat appliance, *n.pr* See appliance, Crozat.

CRT, *n* the abbreviation for cathode ray tube.

crucible (kroo′sibəl), *n* a vessel or container that will withstand high heat and is used for melting or holding material.

crucible crushing strength, n See strength, compressive.

crucible former (sprue base), n the stand or base into which a sprued pattern is placed. It establishes the shape or form of the hollowed-out end of the investment in the casting ring, which will receive the molten metal on its course through the sprue hole. See also sprue former.

crust, *n* a hard-coating surface layer composed of coagulated tissue fluid and blood products mixed with epithelial and inflammatory cells covering a lesion formed by the rupture of a bulla, vesicle, or pustule.

cryolite (krī′ōlīt), *n* a fluoride often used as a flux in the manufacture of silicate cements. Also called sodium aluminum fluoride (Na3AlF6).

cryosurgery (krī′ōsur′jərē), *n* the use of subfreezing temperature to destroy tissue. Cryosurgery is used to cause the edges of a detached retina to heal, to remove cataracts, and in the treatment of Parkinson's disease.

cryotherapy (krī′ōther′əpē), *n* a use of cryosurgery in the treatment of cutaneous tags, warts, actinic keratosis, and dermatofibromas. The agent is usually liquid nitrogen, applied briefly with a sterile cotton-tipped applicator.

cryptococcosis (krip′tōkäkō′sis), *n* a fungal infection from the organism *C. neoformans,* found primarily in pigeon feces. It often affects individuals with weakened or compromised immune systems.

cryptogenic (krip′tōəjen′ik), *n* a condition distinguished by an unknown cause.

crystal(s), *n/n.pl* a naturally produced solid. The ultimate units of the substance from which it was formed are arranged systematically.

crystal, fluorapatite **(flōōrap′ətīt),** *n* the crystalline structure that occurs after hydroxyapatite changes into fluorapatite as a result of the tooth being exposed to fluoride.

crystal gold, *n* See gold, mat.

crystal, silver halide **(hal′īd),** *n* the silver compounds, usually silver bromide and silver iodide, that are impregnated in the photographic emulsion of film. These compounds, when acted on by actinic rays, are disintegrated, with the formation of metallic silver in a finely divided state. The photographic image results when the film is subjected to processing.

crystallization (kris′təlīzā′shən), *n* the production or formation of crystals, either by cooling a liquid or gas to a solid state or by cooling a solution until the solute precipitates as a crystalline deposit.

cubital (kū′bitəl), *adj* pertaining to the forearm.

cubitus (kū′bitus), *n* the forearm.

cuboid (kū′boid), *adj* (cuboidal), resembling a cube in form.

cuboidal, *adj* See cuboid.

cue, *n* a stimulus that determines or may prompt the nature of a person's response.

cultural competency, *n* awareness and understanding of cultural difference.

cultural diversity, *n* a population consisting of two or more cultural groups.

cultural sensitivity, *n* awareness and understanding of cultures different from one's own.

culture, *n* **1.** the growth of microorganisms or other living cells on artificial media. *n* **2.** a set of learned values, beliefs, customs, and behavior that is shared by a group of interacting individuals.

culture, bacterial, *n* the bacterial growth on or in an artificial medium. The medium used may be selective for a given type or genus of organism (e.g., tomato juice agar for lactobacilli).

culture, endodontic, *n* the growth of microorganisms obtained from root canals or periapical tissues.

culture, endodontic medium, *n* a type used for endodontic cultures.

culture medium, *n* a type used for cultivating bacteria.

cumulative, *adj* increasing in effect.

cup, chin, *n* **1.** an orthopedic device that directs a posterior and/or vertical force to the mandible, through the attachment of a cup fitting over the chin to a headcap. *n* **2.** a drug used to cause muscle relaxation during anesthesia by blocking acetylcholine at the neuromuscular and synaptic junctions.

cure, *n* **1.** the successful treatment of a disease or wound. *n* **2.** a procedure or reaction that changes a plastic material to a hard material (e.g., vulcanization and polymerization). See also process.

curet, (curette) (kyōōret′), *n* a periodontal or hand instrument having a sharp, spoon-shaped working blade; used for debridement. It is available in many sizes and shapes; used for root planing and gingival curettage, both surgically and nonsurgically.

curet, area-specific, *n* any of a number of curets designed for use on specific tooth surfaces. It may feature an elongated shank or shortened blade.

curet, mini-bladed, n a small dental instrument employed in the surgical removal of unwanted materials, useful in getting at narrow or closed-off areas of the teeth and oral cavity.

curet, nonsurgical Gracey, n an instrument used for removal of subgingival deposits and root debridement.

curet, nonsurgical Langer, n an instrument that has combined features of the Gracey curet and universal curet.

curet, nonsurgical rigid, n an instrument made with a rigid shank that is stronger and aids in removal of tenacious deposits.

curet, nonsurgical universal, n an instrument designed to permit access to all surfaces of the tooth without the need to change instruments during deposit removal or root planing.

curet, universal, n an instrument used on subgingival sufaces. It has a blade with an unbroken cutting edge that curves around the toe and a flat face that is set at a 90° angle to the lower shank.

curettage (kyŏŏ′rətäzh′), n/v the scaling or removal of tissue with a curet.

curettage, angle for gingival, n an angle between 45° and 90° at which the curet should be held against the gingiva to clean out a pocket effectively. See also curettage, subgingival.

curettage, apical, n the curettement of diseased periapical tissue without excision of the root tip. See also curettage, subgingival.

curettage, gingival, n See curettage, subgingival.

curettage, gingival, closed, n See curettage, subgingival.

curettage, inadvertent **(kyŏŏ′rətazh′ in′ədver′tənt),** n the accidental removal of the gingival tissues with typical surgical instrument usage.

curettage, infrabony pocket, n the enucleation, by means of suitable instrumentation, of the inflammatory soft tissue elements lying within and surrounding the crest of an infrabony resorptive defect; also includes the

debridement and planing of the root surface of the pocket.

curettage, root (root planing), n the debridement and planing to smoothness of the root surface of a tooth to eliminate deposits on the root.

curettage, subgingival, n the process of debridement of the epithelial attachment, the ulcerated and entire (pocket) epithelium, and subjacent inflamed and altered gingival tissues. The procedure is no longer recommended for the health of the periodontium.

curette, n See curet.

curie (kyŏŏ′rē), a measurement of radioactivity produced by the disintegration of unstable elements. The curie is that quantity of a radioactive nuclide in which the number of disintegrations per second is 3.700 times 10^{10}. Because the curie is a relatively large unit, the millicurie (0.001 curie) and the microcurie (one millionth of a curie) are more often used. The curie is based on the number of nuclear disintegrations and not on the number or amount of radiations emitted.

curing, n the act of polymerization.

curing, denture, n See denture curing.

curing light, n a blue light held by the dental professional to harden photopolymerized sealants of tooth-colored restorations, the process of which takes approximately 20 to 60 seconds; special protective glasses or shields must be used by the dental professional and patient to protect against retinal damage from the light.

current, n a measure of the number of electrons per second that pass a given point on a conductor.

current, alternating, n a current that alternately changes its direction of flow. It usually consists of 60 complete cycles/sec.

current, coagulating, n an electrical current, delivered by a needle, ball, or other variously shaped points, that coagulates tissue.

current dental terminology (CDT), n a listing of descriptive terms and identifying codes developed by the American Dental Association (ADA) for reporting dental services and procedures to dental benefits plans.

current, direct, n an electrical current in which the electron flow is in only one direction.

current, galvanic, *n* a direct current created by a battery.

current procedural terminology (CPT), *n* a listing of descriptive terms and identifying codes developed by the American Medical Association (AMA) for reporting practitioner services and procedures to medical plans and medicare.

current, saturation, *n* the maximum current in a roentgen-ray tube that fully uses all electrons that are available at the cathode for the production of roentgen rays.

curriculum, *n* a course of study; the linked series of academic courses leading to mastery of a discipline.

cursor, *n* the pointer on a PC monitor or other display that indicates where the next character will be entered.

curvature, occlusal, *n* See curve of occlusion.

curve, *n* a nonangular deviation from a straight line or surface.

curve, alignment, *n* See alignment.

curve, anti-Monson, *n.pr* See curve, reverse.

curve, compensating, *n* the curvature of alignment of the occlusal surfaces of the teeth that is developed to compensate for the paths of the condyles as the mandible moves from centric to eccentric positions. A means of maintaining posterior tooth contacts on the molar teeth and providing balancing contacts on dentures when the mandible is protruded. Corresponds to the curve of Spee of natural teeth.

curve, dose-effect, *n* a curve relating the dose of radiation with the effect produced.

curve, dose-response, *n* a graphical representation of the relationship between dosage (x-axis) and degree of response (y-axis); used to determine the effective dose of any given drug.

curve, milled-in, *n* See path, milledin.

curve, Monson **(mon'sən),** *n.pr* the curve of occlusion, described by Monson, in which each cusp and incisal edge touch or conform to a segment of the surface of a sphere 8 inches (20 cm) in diameter, with its center in the region of the glabella. See also curve, compensating.

curve of occlusion (occlusal curvature), *n* **1.** a curved occlusal surface that makes simultaneous contact with the major portion of the incisal and occlusal prominences of the existing teeth. *n* **2.** the curve of a dentition on which the occlusal surfaces of the teeth lie. See also curve, reverse.

curve of Spee, *n.pr* **1.** an anatomic curvature of the occlusal alignment of teeth, beginning at the tip of the mandibular canine, following the buccal cusps of the natural premolars and molars, and continuing to the anterior border of the ramus, as described by von Spee. *n.pr* **2.** the curve of the occlusal surfaces of the arches in vertical dimension, brought about by a dipping downward of the mandibular premolars, with a corresponding adjustment of the maxillary premolars.

curve of Wilson, *n.pr* the curvature of the cusps, as seen from the front view. The curve in the mandibular arch is concave, whereas the one in the maxillary arch is convex.

curve, reverse, *n* a curve of occlusion that is convex upward when viewed in the frontal plane.

curve, sine, *n* the wave form of an alternating current, characterized by a rise from zero to maximum positive potential, then descending below zero to its maximum negative value, and then rising to its maximum positive potential, to fall to zero again.

curve, survival, *n* a curve obtained by plotting the number or percentage of organisms surviving at a given time against a given dose of radiation. A curve showing the percentage of individuals surviving at different intervals after a particular dosage of radiation.

Cushing's syndrome, *n.pr* See syndrome, Cushing's.

cusp (kusp), *n* a notably pointed or rounded eminence on or near the masticating surface of a tooth.

cusp, angle, *n* See angle, cusp.

cusp of Carabelli, *n* the small cusp usually seen on a permanent maxillary first molar.

cusp-fossa relations **(kusp fos'ə),** *n. pl* the organic relations between a stamp cusp and its fossa.

cusp height, *n* the shortest distance between the deepest part of the central fossa of a posterior tooth and a line connecting the points of the cusps of the tooth.

cusp ridges, n.pl ridges that descend from each cusp tip on posterior teeth.

cusp, shoeing, n See restoration of cusps.

cusp slopes, n.pl two ridges on the incisal edge of canines, which are divided by the cusp tip.

cusp, talon, n an extra well-defined cusp that may be found on the lingual surfaces of the anterior teeth.

cusp tips, n the points on the occlusal surface of the molars, premolars, or canines that are used for tearing or chewing.

cuspal interference, n See contact, deflective occlusal.

cuspid (kus′pid), n See canine.

cuspidor (kus′pədor), n a fixture provided on some dental operating units into which patients can expectorate. In current practice, most operating fields are kept clear of saliva by high-volume suction saliva ejectors.

customary fee, n the fee level determined by the administrator of a dental benefits plan from actual submitted fees for a specific dental procedure to establish the maximum benefit payable under a given plan for that specific procedure. See also fee, usual and fee, reasonable.

cutaneous (kūtā′nēus), adj relating to the skin. Tests of cutaneous hypersensitivity may be indicators of malnutrition and are useful in determining a patient's readiness for surgery.

cuticle (kyōō′tikəl), n the outer layer of the skin. Also, a layer that covers the free surface of an epithelial cell.

cuticle, primary, n **1.** the transitory remnants of the enamel organ and oral epithelium covering the enamel of a tooth after eruption. *Synonym:* Nasmyth's membrane. n **2.** is believed to be the last substance formed by ameloblasts, mediating the attachment of ameloblasts to the enamel.

cuticle, secondary, n **1.** the second cuticle formed when the ameloblasts are replaced by the oral epithelium. It then covers the primary cuticle on the enamel and is the only cuticle on the cementum. n **2.** a keratinized pedicle found between the gingival epithelium and the surface of a tooth.

cuticula dentis (kūtik′ūlə den′tis), n See cuticle, primary.

cutting edge, n the edge of a periodontal instrument formed where the lateral side and face of the instrument meet.

cutting instrument, n See instrument, cutting.

CVA, n See accident, cerebrovascular.

cyanocobalamin (sī′ənō′kōbal′ə min), n (vitamin B$_{12}$), *brand names* (some): Alpha Redisol, Betalin-12, Cobex; *drug class:* Vitamin B$_{12}$ water-soluble vitamin; *action:* needed for adequate nerve functioning, protein and carbohydrate metabolism, normal growth, red blood cell development, and cell reproduction; *uses:* vitamin B$_{12}$ deficiency, pernicious anemia, hemolytic anemia, hemorrhage, and renal and hepatic diseases.

cyanosis (sī′ənō′sis), n a characteristic bluish tinge or color of the skin and mucous membranes associated with reduction in hemoglobin brought about by inadequate respiratory change (5 gm/100 mL are necessary for color to be perceptible).

cyclamate (sī′kləmāt′), n a noncaloric artificial sweetening agent used in conjunction with saccharin; presently banned by the FDA because of its carcinogenic potential.

cycle, chewing, n a complete course of movement of the mandible during a single masticatory stroke.

cycle, masticating, n the three-dimensional patterns of mandibular movements formed during the chewing of food.

cyclic AMP (cyclic adenosine monophosphate) n a cyclic nucleotide formed from adenosine triphosphate by the action of adenylyl cyclase. Known as a "second messenger," ' that participates in the action of catecholamines, vasopressin, adrenocorticotropic hormone, and many other hormones.

cyclic neutropenia (nōō′trəpē′nēə), n a hereditary disease primarily afflicting young children and infants; characterized by flulike symptoms (weakness, tenderness in the pharynx, aching head, and fever) as well as stomatitis, periodontitis, and gingivitis; cycles every 3 to 4 weeks with painful lesions and damage to the alveolar bone; should be medicated with antibiotics prior to any oral surgery.

cyclizine HCl/cyclizine lactate, trade (sīklǝzēn lak´tāt), *n brand name:* Marezine; *drug class:* antihistaminic, antiemetic, anticholinergic; *action:* blocks histamine H₁ receptors peripherally and centrally; *uses:* motion sickness, prevention of postoperative vomiting.

cyclobenzaprine HCl (sīklōben´zǝp rēn´), *n brand names:* Cycoflex, Flexeril; *drug class:* skeletal muscle relaxant, centrally acting tricyclic; *action:* has actions similar to those of tricyclic antidepressants; *uses:* adjunct for relief of muscle spasm and pain in musculoskeletal conditions.

cyclophosphamide (sīklŏfos´fǝm īd´), *n brand names:* Cytoxan, Neosar, Procytox; *drug class:* antineoplastic alkylating agent; *action:* alkylates DNA, RNA; inhibits enzymes that allow synthesis of amino acids in proteins; *uses:* Hodgkin's disease; lymphomas; leukemia; cancer of female reproductive tract, lung, prostate; multiple myeloma; neuroblastoma; retinoblastoma; Ewing's sarcoma.

cycloserine (sī´klōserēn), *n brand name:* Seromycin Pulvules; *drug class:* antitubercular; *action:* inhibits cell wall synthesis, analog of D-alanine; *use:* pulmonary tuberculosis.

cyclosporine (sī´klōspor´ēn), *n brand name:* Sandimmune; *drug class:* immunosuppressant; *action:* produces immunosuppression by inhibiting lymphocytes; *uses:* to prevent rejection of tissues and/or organ transplants.

cyclothymia (sī´klōthī´mēǝ), *n* See psychosis, manic-depressive.

cyclotron (sī´klǝträn), *n* a device for accelerating charged particles to high energies by means of an alternating electrical field between electrodes placed in a constant magnetic field.

cylinder, glass, *n* one of several components forming the cartridge, a fundamental component of the anesthesiologist's kit; its cylindrical body contains the volume and content of the anesthesia.

cylindroma (sil´indrō´mǝ), *n* **1.** an obsolete term for an adenoid cystic carcinoma. See carcinoma, adenoid cystic. **2.** a benign adnexal neoplasm of skin that most often occurs on the scalp.

cyproheptadine HCl (sī´prōhep´tǝd ēn´), *n brand name:* Periactin; *drug class:* histamine H1 receptor antagonist, also blocks serotonin 5-HT₂ₐ receptors; *action:* acts on blood vessels, gastrointestinal and respiratory systems by competing with histamine for H1 receptor site; *uses:* allergy symptoms, rhinitis, pruritus, cold urticaria.

cyst (sist), *n* a pathologic space in bone or soft tissue containing fluid or semifluid material and, in the oral regions, almost always lined by epithelium.

cyst, aneurysmal bone **(an´yǝriz´mǝl),** *n* a benign osteolytic lesion expanding a long bone jaws or within a vertebra in which the space, filled with blood, is networked with fibrous tissue containing multinucleated giant cells.

cyst, apical periodontal, n See cyst, periapical.

cyst, branchial, n (branchial cleft cyst), a soft-tissue cyst usually seen on the lateral side of the neck, arising from epithelial illusions within the cervical lymph nodes. Microscopic examination shows the epithelial lining of stratified squamous epithelium surrounded by lymphoid tissue.

cyst, calcifying odontogenic (Gorlin cyst), n a cyst arising from odontogenic epithelium, with abundant production of keratin-containing ghost cells and areas of dystrophic calcification. This lesion has a predilection for young adults.

cyst, cervical, n a developmental cyst formed when branchial grooves do not become obliterated.

cyst, dental, n See cyst, periodontal.

cyst, dental lamina **(lam´ǝnǝ),** *n* See cyst, eruption.

cyst, dentigerous **(dentij´ǝrǝs),** *n* an epithelium-lined sac filled with fluid or semifluid material that surrounds the crown of an unerupted tooth or odontoma.

cyst, dentoalveolar, n See cyst, periodontal.

cyst, dermoid **(der´moid),** *n* an epithelium-lined sac with one or more skin appendages (hair follicles, sweat glands, sebaceous glands) in its wall. It may be found in the floor of the oral cavity. This lesion should not be confused with the teratomatous dermoid cyst of the ovary.

cyst, developmental, *n* a pathologic fluid sac that may be caused by infection or disease. See also cyst, dentigerous and cyst, odontogenic.

cyst, epidermoid (ep′əder′moid), *n* a fluid or keratin-filled epithelial-lined sac.

cyst, eruption, *n* a dentigerous cyst that causes a clinically evident bulging of the overlying alveolar ridge.

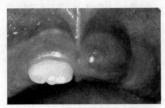

Eruption cyst. (Neville, et al, 2009)

cyst, extravasation, *n* See cyst, traumatic.

cyst, fissural, *n* a cyst that arises from the entrapped epithelium in maxillary suture lines caused by fusion of the embryonic processes of the facial bones.

cyst, follicular (fəlik′yələr), *n* See cyst, dentigerous.

cyst, gingival, of the adult, *n* a rare gingival cyst, usually painless, that originates on dental laminar rests. It is usually categorized as an extraosseous instance of a lateral periodontal cyst.

cyst, gingival, of the newborn, *n* a keratin-filled benign cyst on the alveolar mucosa that is common among newborn infants. Similar to palatal cysts of the newborn.

cyst, globulomaxillary (globyəlōma k′səler′ē), *n* thought to have been a developmental fissural cyst arising in the area between the nasal process and maxillary process. It is now believed that all these lesions are actually other odontogenic cysts, such as odontogenic keratocysts or lateral periodontal cysts.

cyst, Gorlin, *n* See cyst, calcifying odontogenic (Gorlin cyst).

cyst, hemorrhagic (hem′əraj′ik), *n* an extravasation cyst or lesion; traumatic bone cyst or lesion. This is not a true cyst but is probably a defect in the bone produced by trauma and repair. It appears as a definite radiolucent area with a sharply marked radiopaque border. It contains air and is lined by a thin endosteum. See also cyst, solitary bone.

cyst, incisive canal, *n* See cyst, nasopalatine.

cyst, indefinite bone, *n* See cyst, traumatic.

cyst, lateral, *n* See cyst, periodontal.

cyst, lateral periodontal (botryoid odontogenic cyst), *n* a developmental cyst found in the tooth-generating tissue on the lateral surface of the root of a tooth.

cyst, median palatal, *n* an epithelium-lined sac containing fluid; appears as a radiolucency in the midline of the palate. It is of developmental origin.

cyst, multilocular (mul′tilok′yələr), *n* a follicular cyst containing many loculi, or spaces, and not associated with a tooth.

cyst, nasoalveolar (nā′zōalvē′əl ər), *n* a fluid-containing sac lined by epithelium and located at the ala of the nose. A developmental cyst, it may simulate a nasal or periapical abscess.

cyst, nasopalatine duct (nā′zōpal′ə tīn), *n* a cyst arising within the nasopalatine canal. Radiographically it may appear as a heartshaped or round radiolucency between the maxillary central incisors. Histologically it may show mucous cells and nerve bundles in addition to a lining of stratified squamous or respiratory epithelium. The incisive canal cyst and the cyst of the papilla incisiva are the recognized subtypes.

cyst, nonodontogenic, *n* a soft tissue abnormality that may develop in any number of locations within the oral cavity but is not directly associated with a tooth.

cyst, odontogenic, *n* an epithelium-lined sac produced from the tooth-forming tissues (e.g., primordial, dentigerous, and periodontal cysts).

cyst, palatal, of the newborn, *n* a common developmental cyst found on the hard palates of most infants. It is small, white, and filled with keratin. Called Epstein's pearls when found on the midline of the palate, and Bohn's nodules when found elsewhere on the palate, though both types are the same.

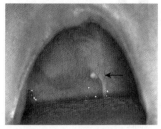

Palatal cyst of the newborn. (Casamassimo, et al, 2013)

cyst, periapical, n a cyst that has a fibrous connective tissue wall and a lining of stratified squamous epithelium and that is attached to the apex of the root of a tooth with a nonvital pulp or a defective root canal filling.

cyst, periodontal (dental root cyst, dentoalveolar cyst, lateral cyst, periapical cyst), n an epithelium lined sac containing fluid usually found at the apex of a pulp-involved tooth. Lateral types occur less frequently along the side of the root.

cyst, primordial (prīmor′dēəl), n an epithelium-lined sac containing fluid and appearing as a radiolucency in the jaws. It is derived from an enamel organ before any hard tissue is formed.

cyst, radicular (periapical cyst, root end cyst) (rədik′yələr), n See cyst, periapical.

cyst, residual, n an odontogenic cyst that remains within the jaw after the removal of the tooth with which it was associated. May be radicular or follicular.

cyst, root end, n See cyst, periapical.

cyst, simple bone, n a bone cavity that forms around the roots of teeth, easily identifiable during radiologic exam. Of uncertain origin. Previously

known as *traumatic bone cyst* and *solitary bone cyst.*

cyst, soft tissue, n a broad classification of oral abnormalities that may include blisterlike obstructions of salivary glands and growths in the thyroglossal tract, lymph nodes, and epithelial cells on the floor of the oral cavity.

cyst, soft tissue developmental, n a pathologic fluid sac that occurs in mucous membranes or other soft tissue of the body, as opposed to those occurring in bone or teeth. See also cyst, thyroglossal duct and cyst, lateral cervical.

cyst, solitary bone, n See cyst, simple bone.

cyst, thyroglossal duct (thī′rōglos′əl), n an epithelium-lined sac containing fluid formed in portions of the incompletely involuted thyroglossal duct, which connects the primitive pharynx with the tongue in embryonic life. These cysts may appear in the midline at any region from the subhyoid to the base of the tongue.

cyst, traumatic bone, n See cyst, simple bone.

cystadenoma (sist′adənō′mə), n an adenoma with the development of cystic spaces caused by dilation of acinar or ductal structures.

cystadenoma, papillary, lymphomatosum (Warthin's tumor), n a benign salivary gland tumor that consists of numerous cystic spaces lined by a double layer of epithelium. A dense aggregate of lymphocytes containing germinal centers surrounds the cystic spaces.

cysteine (sis′təēn′), n a nonessential amino acid found in many proteins in the body.

cystic fibrosis (sis′tik fībrō′sis), n an inherited disorder of the exocrine glands, causing those glands to produce abnormally thick secretions of mucus, elevation of sweat electrolytes, increased organic and enzymatic constituents of saliva, and overactivity of the autonomic nervous system.

cystinuria (sis′tinyŏŏ′rēə), n a hereditary defect caused by the dysfunctional reabsorption of the amino acid cystine into the kidneys; it results in regular, abnormally high levels of cystine in urine.

cystostomy (sistos'təmē), *n* creating a surgical opening into the urinary bladder or gallbladder.

cytochrome (sī'təkrōm'), *n* one of a class of hemoproteins that act in electron transport. Cytochromes are classified as *a, b, c, d,* and P450

cytodifferentiation, *n* the development of different cell types.

cytokine (sī'təkīn'), *n* a nonantibody protein, such as lymphokine. Cytokines are released by a cell population on contact with a specific antigen. Cytokines act as intercellular mediators in the generation of immune response.

cytologic smear (sī'təloj'ik), *n* the product of a diagnostic technique where cells are scraped off the surface of a lesion found in the oral cavity. The gleaned cells are then examined under a microscope for indications of a variety of diseases. Considered a preliminary diagnostic test, it is not used to detect more serious conditions that require deeper tissue samples.

cytology (sītol'əjē), *n* the study of the anatomy, physiology, pathology, and chemistry of a cell.

cytology, exfoliative, *n* the study of desquamated cells.

cytomegalic inclusion disease, *n* See disease, salivary gland.

Cytomegalovirus (CMV), *n* a visceral disease virus, a member of the group of herpesviruses having special affinity for the salivary glands. Considered one of the indicator infections of AIDS.

cytoplasm, *n* the fluid portion contained within the cell membrane.

cytoskeleton, *n* the intracellular filaments that serve to support or stiffen cells.

cytosol, *n* the totality of the intracellular substance exclusive of mitochondria and endoplasmic reticulum components.

cytotoxicity (sī'tōtoksis'itē), *n* a description of the extent of the destructive or killing capacity of an agent. Most often used to describe the character of immune activity or toxicity of certain drugs that limit the development of cancer cells.

cytozyme (sī'tōzīm), *n* See thromboplastin.

DAQT System, *n.pr* a system to designate teeth: *D* for dentition, *A* for arch, *Q* for quadrant, and *T* for tooth type.

Dacarbazine, *n* brand name: DTIC; *drug class:* triazine alkylating drug; *action:* covalently binds to and inhibits DNA; *uses:* Hodgkin's disease, melanoma, sarcomas.

dactinomycin (actinomycin D), *n* brand name: Cosmegen; *drug class:* antibiotic antineoplastic; *action:* intercalates into DNA, inhibits RNA synthesis; *uses:* Wilm's tumor, Ewing's sarcoma, rhabdomyosarcoma, choriocarcinoma, testicular cancer.

d-lysergic acid diethylamide (LSD) (lisur'jik as'id dīeth'əlam'id), *n* a hallucinogenic street drug taken to induce a perceived state of euphoria, freedom, and control.

daily food requirements, *n* actively teaching patients proper nutrition, personal diet analysis, reasonable portion sizes, and how to choose foods to enjoy overall good health.

Dalton's law, *n* See law, Dalton's.

dam, a barrier to the passage of moisture or saliva.

dam, post-, *n* See seal, posterior palatal.

dam, rubber, *n* a thin sheet of latex rubber used to isolate a tooth or teeth and keep them dry during a dental procedure.

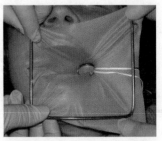

Rubber dam. (Dean/Avery/McDonald, 2011)

dam, rubber, punch, n a hand-punch instrument with progressively larger openings, used to make a hole(s) in the rubber dam.

damages, n.pl compensation or indemnity that may be recovered in the courts by any person who has suffered loss, detriment, or injury to person, property, or rights through the unlawful act or negligence of another.

damages, compensatory, n.pl a sum that compensates the injured party for injury only.

damages, exemplary (punitive damages) (**igzem'plərē**), n.pl damages awarded to the plaintiff over those that will barely compensate for property loss. Such compensation may be awarded when the wrong done to the plaintiff involves violence, malice, or fraud by the defendant. The object is to provide compensation for mental suffering or loss of pride. It may be employed as punishment of the defendant.

damages, nominal, n.pl a small sum awarded to a plaintiff in an action in which there is no substantial loss or injury to be compensated but in which the law still recognizes a technical invasion of rights or a breach of the defendant's duty. Also awarded in cases in which, although there has been a real injury, the plaintiff's evidence is not sufficient to show its amount.

damages, punitive, n.pl See damages, exemplary.

danazol (**dan'əzol'**), n brand name: Danocrine; drug class: androgen, α-ethinyl testosterone derivative; action: decreases FSH and LH output; uses: endometriosis, prevention of hereditary angioedema, fibrocystic breast disease.

dantrolene sodium (**dantrōlēn**), n brand name: Dantrium; drug class: skeletal muscle relaxant, direct acting; action: interferes with intracellular release of calcium necessary to initiate contraction; uses: spasticity in multiple sclerosis, stroke, spinal cord injury, cerebral palsy, malignant hyperthermia.

dapsone *(DDS)* (**dap'sōn**), n brand name: Avlosulfon; drug class: leprostatic, antibacterial; action: bactericidal and bacteriostatic against M.

leprae; may also be immunosuppressant; uses: leprosy, dermatitis herpetiformis.

Darier's disease, n.pr See disease, Darier's.

darkroom, n a completely lightproof room or cubicle where photographic, medical, and dental films are handled and processed. See also safe light.

darkroom, features of, n a darkroom for developing radiographic films, should be absolutely devoid of white light, as well as chemicals or dust that could damage the film while it is being processed; a filtered safe light of less than 15 watts should be the only light in the room.

Darvon, n.pr the brand name for propoxyphene hydrochloride, a weak opioid receptor agonist used to treat pain but with little justification for its use because of weak analgesic effects and yet with substantial toxicity.

data, n.pl facts and figures; data are processed and interpreted to yield information.

data aggregation (**ag'grəgā'shən**), n a collection of protected health information used to conduct data analysis relating to the health care operations of the entity.

database, n an organized collection of data. A medical database is all the information that exists in the practice at any time.

data processing, n the collection of data, processing of the data to obtain usable information, and communication of this usable information.

data set, n a hardware device that converts digital pulses (square waveform) into modulated frequencies (sinusoidal wave) for transmission, a process called modulation. It also converts modulated frequencies into voltage pulses, a process called demodulation. Also called *modem.*

daughter (decay product), n **1.** a nuclide formed from the radioactive decay of another nuclide called the parent. n **2.** after meiosis, one parent cell produces four daughter cells. These cells have half the number of chromosomes found in the original parent cell and, with crossing over, are genetically different.

day sheet, n a form that permits systematic record keeping of treatment of patients and of monies received and spent.

Day's syndrome, *n.pr* See syndrome, Riley-Day.

daylight loader method, *n* method for developing radiographic films without a darkroom, using a flexible apparatus that allows hands to be inserted into a dark space without admitting any light. Insert the exposed radiographic film in the daylight loader compartment and remove the protective packets. With ungloved hands, process the film, touching only the edges.

DDC, *n* the abbreviation for dideoxycytidine. See dideoxycytidine.

DDI, *n* the abbreviation for dideoxyinosine. See dideoxyinosine.

dead space, *n* See space, physiologic dead space, and anatomic dead space.

deaf, *adj* without usable hearing.

deafen, *v* to make deaf; to cause the loss of all usable hearing.

deafness (def'nes), *n* a condition characterized by a partial or complete loss of hearing.

deafness, central, *n* impaired hearing caused by interference with cerebral auditory pathways or in the auditory centers in the brain (e.g., cerebrovascular accidents and other degenerative brain diseases). Hearing aids are of little benefit.

deafness,   conduction **(kənduk′shən),** *n* See deafness, transmission.

deafness, nerve, *n* impaired hearing caused by pathologic conditions in the auditory nerve or the hair cells of the organ of Corti in the inner ear (e.g., high-tone deafness, which comes with age; damage to the organ of Corti by noise; or a tumor of an auditory nerve). Hearing aids are usually of little benefit.

deafness, transmission (conduction deafness), *n* impaired hearing caused by interference with passage of sound waves through the external ear (e.g., interference caused by wax) or middle ear (e.g., interference caused by otitis media, aerotitis media, or otosclerosis). May be characterized by greater interference with hearing of low tones. Hearing aids that amplify may be helpful.

deaminated   (dēam′inātəd), *adj* pertaining to α-amino acids that have

undergone the chemical alteration that removes ammonia (NH_3) from glutamate.

deamination   (dēam′inā′shun), *n* the removal of an amino group form a chemical compound.

deanesthesiant (dē′anəsthē′zēənt), *n* anything that will arouse a patient from a state of anesthesia.

death (deth), *n* **1.** the cessation of life; the stoppage of life beyond the possibility of resuscitation. *n* **2.** the cause or occasion of loss of life. *n* **3.** the total absence of activity in the brain and central nervous system, the cardiovascular system, and the respiratory system as observed and declared by a physician or other legally authorized agent.

death, brain, *n* in addition to the generally accepted definition of death, some states, either by statute or court decision, have added a "brain death" definition to the law, applicable when there has been an irreversible cessation of brain function.

death certificate, *n* the signed affidavit that life has ceased, giving the time, place, and cause of death. It is required by law to be filed in the proper local or regional geopolitical office.

debility (debil′itē), *n* weakness; lack of strength; asthenia.

debonding, *n* a procedure by which brackets and bonding resin are removed and the surface of the tooth is restored to its previous condition.

debridement (dabrēd′mənt), *n* the removal of foreign material and/or devitalized tissue from the vicinity of a wound.

debridement, epithelial (deepitheliazation), *n* See curettage, subgingival.

debridement, nonsurgical periodontal, *n* the removal of deposits on the tooth surface. See also scaling.

debris (debrē′), *n* foreign material or particles loosely attached to a surface. In dentistry, food deposits (Materia alba) or cellular matter on a surface, such as a tooth or its roots.

debt, *n* a sum of money due by agreement; the contract may or may not be express and does not necessarily set the precise amount to be paid.

debug, *v* to locate and correct any errors (bugs) in a computer program.

decalcification (dēkal'sifikā'shən), *n* an older term for the loss or removal of calcium salts from calcified tissues. Newer term is *demineralization.*

decarboxylation (dē'karbok'səlā' shən), *n* a chemical reaction involving the removal of a molecule of carbon dioxide from a carboxylic acid.

decay, *v* to decompose.

decay, dental, *n* See caries.

decay product, *n* See daughter.

decay, radioactive, *n* the disintegration of the nucleus of an unstable nuclide by the spontaneous emission of charged particles and/or photons.

decay, senile, *n* See caries, senile dental.

decayed teeth, indices and scoring methods for, *n.pl* See index, DEF and index, DMF.

deceleration (dēsel'ərā'shən), *n* a decrease in the speed or velocity of an object or reaction.

decibel (des'ibel), *n* a logarithmic ratio unit that indicates by what proportion one intensity level differs from another.

deciduous (dēsid'ūəs), *adj* that which will be shed (exfoliated). Older term pertaining specifically to the first dentition. Preferred term is *primary.*

deciduous dentition, *n* See dentition, primary.

deciduous teeth, *n* See teeth, primary.

decision-making, *n* the process of coming to a conclusion or making a judgment.

decision-making, evidence-based, *n* a type of informal decision-making that combines clinical expertise, patient concerns, and evidence gathered from scientific literature to arrive at a diagnosis and treatment recommendations. See also evidence-based care.

decision-making, statistical, *n* a type of formal decision-making that proceeds from a hypothesis to a conclusion by incorporating such techniques as statistical inference and significance, probability analysis, literature review, sampling, and discussion.

decision tree, *n* an algorithm or a formal stepwise process used in coming to a conclusion or making a judgment. Published decision trees are helpful to dentists in treating complex conditions with many variables.

declaration and provision for affairs, *n* a systematic statement of the affairs and estate of a person, in which all assets and property are listed.

decompensate, *n* to improve the angulation of teeth to the basal bone with orthodontics so that they are positioned normally in relation to their apical base. Decompensation is usually undertaken prior to orthognathic surgery.

decompression, *n* **1.** a technique used to readapt an individual to normal atmospheric pressure after exposure to higher pressures, as in diving. *n* **2.** the removal of pressure caused by gas or fluid in a body cavity such as the stomach or intestinal tract.

decompression, nerve, *n* the release of pressure on a nerve trunk by surgical widening of the bony canal.

decontamination, *n* the process of making a person, object, or environment free of microorganisms, radioactivity, or other contaminants.

deductible (diduk'təbəl), *n* **1.** a stipulated sum the covered person must pay toward the cost of dental treatment before the benefits of the program go into effect. The deductible may be annual or payable only once and may vary in amount from program to program. *n* **2.** the amount of dental expense for which the beneficiary is responsible before a third party will assume any liability for payment of benefits. Deductible may be an annual or one-time charge and may vary in amount from program to program. See also family deductible.

deductible amount, *n* the portion of dental care expense the insured must pay before the plan's benefits begin.

deductible clause, *n* a provision in an insurance contract stipulating that the insurer will pay only that amount that is in excess of a specified amount.

deductive reasoning, *n* the ability to distill the pertinent facts and details of a situation from a wider body of evidence and generalizations.

deep, *n* the structure(s) that are located inward, away from the body surface.

deep bite, *n* See overbite.

deepithelization (dēep'ithē'lizā' shən), *n* See debridement, epithelial.

D

deep sedation, *n* an intentional drug-induced state of a patient who cannot be easily aroused but responds purposefully after repeated verbal or painful stimulation.

DEF rate, See rate, DEF.

defamation (def'əmā'shən), *n* the act of detracting from the reputation of another. The offense of injuring a person's reputation by false and malicious statements.

default, *n* **1.** an omission of that which should be done. *v* **2.** to fail to fulfill an obligation or a promise.

defecation, *n* the elimination of feces from the digestive tract through the rectum.

defect, *n* **1.** the absence of some legal requisite. *n* **2.** an imperfection.

defect, atrial septal, *n* a congenital defect in the heart that is often present from birth. It is sometimes referred to as a "hole" in the heart and is caused by the unsuccessful closure of the septum between the atria of the heart. The failure of the septum to close properly leaves a hole between the right and left atria.

defect, operative, *n* the incomplete repair of bone after root resection or periapical curettage.

defect, osseous, *n* a concavity in the bone surrounding one or more teeth, resulting from periodontal disease.

defect, speech, *n* deviation of speech that is outside the range of acceptable variation in a given environment.

defective, mentally, *adj* a mentally subnormal individual. A person in whom a basic nervous system defect may be assumed because of social and intellectual deficiencies (e.g., persons afflicted with microcephaly, hydrocephalus, or mongolism).

defendant, *n* the party against whom relief or recovery is sought in a lawsuit.

defense, *n* the reasons, in law or fact, offered by the defendant in a legal proceeding as to why the plaintiff should not prevail.

defense cell, *n* See cell, defense.

defense mechanism, *n* an unconscious, intrapsychic reaction that offers protection to the self from threatening or stressful situations. Defense mechanisms may be useful to diminish anxiety and facilitate coping behaviors, or may be harmful because of denying, displacing, isolating, or repressing anxiety and preventing useful coping responses.

Deferoxamine, *n brand name:* Desferal; *drug class:* metal chelator; *action:* binds (chelates) iron and aids in its removal; *use:* acute and chronic iron toxicity.

defibrillation (dēfib'rilāshən), *n* the arrest of fibrillation, usually that of the cardiac ventricles. An intense alternating current is briefly passed through the heart muscle, throwing it into a refractory state.

defibrillator (dēfib'rilā'tur), *n* a device for defibrillating the ventricles of the heart.

defibrillator, automatic external (AED), *n* a mobile electric device attached to the abdomen or chest that terminates erratic heartbeat by shock, thereby restoring the normal cardiac rhythm.

deficiency, *n* a lack or defect.

deficiency, ac-globulin, *n* See parahemophilia.

deficiency, dietary, *n* an inadequate amount of food intake or an insufficiency of any of the food elements necessary for proper nutrition.

deficiency, mineral, *n* a form of nutritional deficiency produced by the inadequate ingestion, absorption, use, and/or overexcretion of essential inorganic elements such as calcium, magnesium, and phosphorus.

deficiency, nicotinic acid (nik'ətin 'ik), *n* a deficiency of nicotinic acid in the diet, resulting in acute erythematous stomatitis, papillary atrophy of the tongue, and ulcerative gingivitis.

deficiency, nutritional, *n* See deficiency, dietary.

deficiency, plasma thromboplastic antecedent (throm'bōplas'tik), *n* See hemophilia C.

deficiency, protein, *n* a malnutritive state produced by inadequate ingestion, absorption, use, or overexcretion of essential protein elements. Degenerative lesions produced in the periodontium include osteoporosis of the alveolar and supporting bone and disappearance of fibroblasts and connective tissue fibers of the periodontal membrane.

deficiency, PTA, *n* See hemophilia C.

deficiency, salivary (sal'əvar'ē), *n* an insufficiency in the amount of saliva produced by the salivary glands. The lack of saliva production can result in dry mouth (xerostomia), caries, and infection of the oral cavity.

deficiency, vitamin A, gingival hyperplasia in, n the hyperplastic and hyperkeratotic gingival changes occurring with decreased ingestion, diminished absorption, faulty use, or overexcretion of vitamin A. In diabetes mellitus, the liver often cannot effectively convert carotene to vitamin A.

definition (image), n the property of projected radiographic images relating to their sharpness, distinctness, or clarity of outline. Penumbra width is a measure of definition. See also resolution.

definitive care, n the completion of recommended treatment.

deflective occlusal contact, n See contact, deflective occlusal.

defluoridation, n the process of removing excessive natural fluorine from water supply.

deformation (dē'fôrmā'shən), n a distortion; a disfigurement.

deformation, elastic, n the change in shape of an object under an applied load from which the object can recover or return to its original unloaded state when the load is removed.

deformation, inelastic, n a deformation occurring when a material is stressed beyond its elastic limit.

deformation, permanent, n a deformation occurring beyond the yield point so that the structure will not return to its original dimensions after removal of the applied force.

deformity, n a distortion or disfigurement of a portion of the body; may be congenital, familial, hereditary, acquired, pathologic, or surgical.

deformity, gingival, n a deviation from the normal gingival topographic and architectural pattern.

degassing (dēgas'ing), *adj* related to degasification, the process by which dissolved gas is removed from water or other liquid solutions.

degeneration, ballooning (dijen'ərā'shən), n a condition seen in vesicles of viral origin in which epithelial cells are washed from the vesicle wall. The cells swell and their nuclei undergo amitotic division, resulting in multinucleated giant cells that may be seen floating in vesicular fluid.

degeneration, basophilic granular, See basophilia.

degenerative joint disease, n See osteoarthritis.

degloving (dēgluv'ing), n an intra-oral surgical exposure of the bony mandibular anterior region. This procedure can be performed in the posterior region if necessary.

deglutition (dē'glootish'ən), n (swallowing), a succession of muscular contractions from above downward or from the front backward; propels food from the oral cavity toward the stomach. The action is generally initiated at the lips; it proceeds back through the oral cavity, and the food is moved automatically along the dorsum of the tongue. When the food is ready for swallowing, it is passed back through the fauces. Once the food is beyond the fauces and in the pharynx, the soft palate closes off the nasopharynx, and the hyoid bone and larynx are elevated upward and forward. This action keeps food out of the larynx and dilates the esophageal opening so that the food may be passed quickly toward the stomach by peristaltic contractions. The separation between the voluntary and involuntary characteristics of this wave of contractions is not sharply defined. At birth the process is already well established as a highly coordinated activity, (i.e., the swallowing reflex.)

degradation (deg'rədā'shən), n the reduction of a chemical compound to a less complex compound.

degrees of freedom *(df),* *n.pl* a statistic, based on the number of observations and groups in a study, that is necessary to determine statistical significance. One looks up the degrees of freedom and the significance level in a table of significance values to determine if the magnitude of the value obtained is significant. Used with the t-test, chi square, analysis of variance, and correlation.

dehiscence (dēhis'əns), n a fissural defect in the facial alveolar bony plate extending from the gingival margin apically that results in incomplete coverage of the root (or implant) by bone.

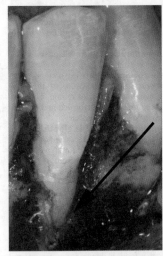

Dehiscence. (Rose/Mealey/Genco, 2004)

dehiscent mandibular canal, n a condition caused by bone resorption that leaves the mandibular canal without a covering or roof of bone.

dehydration (dē'hīdrā'shən), n **1.** the removal of water (e.g., from the body or tissue). n **2.** a decrease in serum fluid coupled with the loss of interstitial fluid from the body. It is associated with disturbances in fluid and electrolyte balance.

dehydration of gingivae, n the drying of gingival tissue, leading to a lowered tissue resistance, which can result in gingival inflammation; seen in mouth breathing. See also breathing, mouth and oral cavity.

dehydrogenase (dē'hīdroj'ənās'), n an oxidoreductase class (EC 1) enzyme that induces the transportation of electrons or hydrogen from a donor, which usually indicates the dehydrogenase, to an acceptor compound.

delayed expansion, n See expansion, delayed.

delict (dilikt'), n a wrong or an injury; an offense; a violation of public or private obligation.

delinquent (deling'kwent), n pertaining to a debt or claim that is due and unpaid at the time due.

delirium (delir'ēəm), n a condition of mental excitement, confusion, and clouded sensorium, usually accompanied by hallucinations, illusions, and delusions; precipitated by toxic factors in diseases or drugs.

DELPHI method, n.pr a structured method of gathering groups of experts together to develop a consensus and forecasts. At least two rounds of information are collected, with feedback in between, so that a group can receive and modify their response after receiving the anonymous responses of others.

delirium tremens (DT), n See alcohol withdrawal delirium.

Delta Dental Plan, n.pr an active member organization of the Delta Dental Plans Association (a not-for-profit organization), formed and guided by state dental societies to provide prepaid dental care to the public on a group basis.

delusion, n a persistent, aberrant belief or perception held inviolable by a person despite evidence to the contrary.

demand, n in economics, refers to the buying of services or goods; in dental care, generally denotes the active request for and purchase of dental care services.

demeclocycline HCl (dem'əklōsi'klēn), n brand name: Declomycin; drug class: tetracycline antibiotic; action: inhibits protein synthesis, in microorganisms; uses: uncommon gram-positive or gram-negative bacteria or both, diseases caused by rickettsiae.

dementia (dimen'shə), n a progressive, organic mental disorder characterized by chronic personality disintegration, confusion, disorientation, stupor, deterioration of intellectual capacity and function, and impairment or control of memory, judgment, and impulses (e.g., senile psychosis, also associated with AIDS).

Demerol (dem'ərôl), n.pr the brand name for meperidine hydrochloride.

demilune, serous (dem'ēloon sēr'əs), n a half-moon–shaped body of serous cells located on the surface of some mucoserous acini in salivary glands.

demineralization (dēmin′əral′īzā′shən), *n* a measurable decrease in the level of inorganic salts or minerals such as bone or enamel. Older term is *decalcification.*

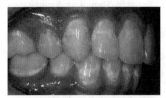

Demineralization. (Cobourne/DiBiase, 2010)

demography (dimog′rəfē), *n* the study of populations, particularly the size, distribution, and characteristics of members of population groups. Demographic techniques are employed in the long-term continuing study of the residents of Framingham, Massachusetts, by the National Institutes of Health.

demurrer (dēmur′ər), *n* an admission of the facts charged by the opponent while maintaining that those facts are legally insufficient to establish liability.

demyelinate (dēmī′əlināt), *n* the process of removing or damaging the myelin sheath surrounding a nerve.

denasality (dēnəzal′itē), *n* the quality of the voice when the nasal passages are obstructed, preventing adequate nasal resonance during speech.

dendrite (den′drīt), *n* **1.** the finger-like projections formed during the solidification of crystalline materials. *n* **2.** a branched, treelike protoplasmic process of a neuron that carries nerve impulses toward the cell body. See also axon.

denervation (de′nurvā′shən), *n* the sectioning or removal of a nerve to interrupt the nerve supply to a part.

dens, *n* the odontoid process of the second cervical vertebra.

dens evaginatus (denz ivaj′ənātəs), *n* See dens in dente.

dens in dente (denz in den′tā), *n* (older terms: *dens invaginatus, gestant odontoma),* an anomaly of the tooth found mainly in maxillary lateral incisors; characterized by invagination of the enamel, giving a radiographic appearance that suggests a "tooth within a tooth."

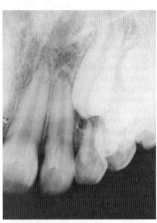

Dens in dente. (Dean/Avery/McDonald, 2011)

dens invaginatus (denz invajinā′təs), *n* See dens in dente.

Densite (den′sīt), *n.pr* the brand name for a form of α-hemihydrate with a low setting expansion and greater hardness; used for dies, models, and casts; sometimes referred to as a Class II stone.

densitometer (den′sitom′ətur), *n* an instrument for determining the degree of darkening of developed photographic or radiographic film, based on the use of a photoelectric cell to measure the light transmission through a given area of the film.

density (den′sitē), *n* the concentration of matter, measured by mass per unit volume.

density, radiographic, n the degree of darkening of exposed and processed photographic or radiographic film, expressed as the logarithm of the opacity of a given area of the film.

dental, *adj* relating to the teeth.

dental abutment, n See abutment.

dental alloy, n See alloy.

dental amalgam, n See amalgam.

dental ankylosis (ang′kəlō′sis), n See tooth, ankylosed.

dental anxiety, n See anxiety.

dental app, n a software program or application which allows dental information to be accessed on a mobile device, such as a mobile phone or tablet.

dental arch, *n* See arch, dental.

dental articulator, *n* See articulator.

dental assistant, *n* See assistant, dental.

dental auxiliary, *n* See auxiliary personnel.

dental benefits organization, *n* an organization offering a dental benefits plan. Also known as dental plan organization.

dental benefits plan, *n* the plan entitles covered individuals to specified dental services in return for a fixed, periodic payment made in advance of treatment. Such plans often include the use of deductibles, coinsurance, or maximums to control the cost of the program to the purchaser.

dental benefits program, *n* the specific dental benefits plan being offered to enrollees by the sponsor.

dental biofilm, *n* **l.** in dentistry, a biofilm noted in the oral cavity. It consists of salivary proteins, microorganisms, and other byproducts of the microorganism. A type of intercellular matrix is also present. It forms on the oral cavity surface after the formation of the salivary pellicle using selective attachment factors. It is a factor in initiation and continuation of dental caries and periodontal disease. Older terms: *mucin plaque, bacterial plaque.* See also biofilm, bacterial plaque.

dental bonding, *n* See bonding.

dental calculus, *n* See calculus.

dental care, *n* the treatment of the teeth and their supporting structures.

dental care delivery, *n* the way that dental care is provided to the public.

dental care for children, *n* See pediatric dentistry.

dental caries, *n* See caries.

dental caries susceptible, *n* See susceptible.

dental cavity lining, *n* See cavity lining.

dental cement, *n* See cement, dental.

dental cementum, *n* See cementum.

dental chart, *n* See chart, dental.

dental claim, *n* patient's formal request for insurance payment for a dental procedure that was rendered.

dental claim form, *n* standard dental document used to file a claim

or request authorization for a procedure.

dental clinic, *n* See clinic.

dental cooperative, *n* a dental facility organized to provide dental services for the benefit of subscribers and not for profit. There is no discrimination as to who may subscribe, and each subscriber has equal rights and voice in the control of the cooperative. The operation of the cooperative usually rests with a lay board of directors elected by subscribers.

dental deposit, *n* See calculus.

dental disability, *n* caries, periodontal disease, dentoalveolar trauma, and other oral conditions that, if ignored and untreated, can negatively impact a child's development and an individual's participation in life activities.

dental dysfunction, *n* See dysfunction, dental.

dental enamel, *n* See enamel.

dental enamel, hypoplastic, *n* See hypoplasia.

dental engine, *n* See engine, dental.

dental equipment, *n* See equipment.

dental fissure, *n* See fissure.

dental fistula, *n* See fistula.

dental floss, *n* a waxed or plain thread of nylon or silk used to clean the interdental areas; an aid in oral physiotherapy. Shredproof Teflon expanded polytetrafluoroethylene (ePTFE), ultra-high molecular weight polyethylene (UHMWPE), or nylon flosses are still believed to be the best materials for removing dental biofilm (dental plaque) from the teeth.

dental fluorosis, *n* See fluorosis, dental.

dental formula, *n* a formula for each dentition that is used when comparing human teeth with those of other mammals.

dental geriatrics, *n* See geriatrics.

dental granuloma, *n* See granuloma, dental.

dental handpiece, *n* See handpiece.

dental health services, *n* the sum of the diagnostic, preventive, consultative, supportive, and therapeutic dental care offered by the dental profession or that portion provided a member of a dental health plan.

dental health surveys, *n* the use of questionnaires and oral examinations of a target population to determine the need or demand for dental care or the opinions or attitudes of patients or consumers.

dental history, n See history.

dental home, n ongoing relationship between the dentist and the patient, includes all aspects of oral health care delivery in a comprehensive, accessible, and family-centered way. Establishment of a dental home should begin no later than one year of age and includes referrals to specialists when needed.

dental hygiene armamentarium, n See armamentarium.

dental hygiene diagnostic model, n one of four approaches to patient care. Its purpose is to arrive at a plan for recommended treatment by the systematic use of six steps that cover the major aspects of care, from initial inquiry to problem solving to patient education.

dental hygiene instrumentarium, n See instrumentarium.

dental hygiene movement, n inception and evolution of the use of the dental hygienist to provide dental care.

dental hygiene process model, n one of four approaches to patient care, characterized by the documentation of a patient's expressed needs as they relate to a range of possible causes. Patient is questioned about various areas of concern, including overall health care.

dental hygienist, n See hygienist, dental.

dental identification, n the process of establishing the unique characteristics of teeth and dental work of an individual, leading to the identification of an individual by comparison with the person's dental charts and records. Used in forensic dentistry.

dental implant, n See implant.

dental impression material, n See impression.

dental index, n standardized, quantitative method for measuring, scoring, and analyzing oral conditions in individuals and groups.

dental instrument, n See instruments.

dental insurance, n a policy that insures against the expense of treatment and care of dental disease and accident to teeth.

dental jurisprudence (jur′isprū′dəns), n the application of the principles of law as they relate to the practice of dentistry. See also jurisprudence, dental.

dental laboratory technician, n See technician, dental laboratory.

dental lamina, n See lamina, dental.

dental material, n See material, dental.

dental model, n See model.

dental neglect, n the purposeful denial of the minimum amount of oral health care or maintenance required to sustain properly functioning periodontium and teeth, free from pain and infection. The caretaker may exhibit a disregard for the patient's health and may focus primarily on pain relief for the patient. It is considered a warning sign of possible child or elder abuse.

dental nurse, n term used in New Zealand for a school dental staff member. See also dental therapist.

dental occlusion, n See occlusion.

dental papilla, n See papilla.

dental pathology, n that branch of dentistry that deals with all aspects of dental disease. See also pathology.

dental perioscopy (per′ēos′kəpē), n See endoscopy, periodontal.

dental phobia, n unfounded fear or morbid dread of dental treatment.

dental pin, n See pin.

dental plan, n an organized method for the financing of dental care.

dental plaque, biofilm, n See dental biofilm.

dental plexus, n a network or vessels of nerves.

dental porcelain, n See porcelain, dental.

dental prepayment, n a system for budgeting the cost of dental services in advance of their receipt.

dental prophylaxis, n See prophylaxis.

dental prosthesis, n See prosthesis.

dental prosthetic restoration, n See prosthesis, dental.

dental public health, n may also be called *public health dentistry.* The specialty of dentistry devoted to the science and art of preventing and controlling dental diseases and promoting dental health through organized community efforts. It is that form of dental practice that serves the community as a patient rather than the individual. It is concerned with the dental health education of the public, with applied dental research, and with the administration of group dental care programs as well as prevention and control of dental diseases on a community basis. This is one of the nine recognized specialties in dentistry. See also community dentistry.

dental pulp, n See pulp.

dental pulp capping, n See capping, pulp.

dental pulp cavity, n See cavity, pulp.

dental pulp exposure, n See exposure.

dental record, n a confidential document containing the clinical and financial data of the dental patient, including the patient's identity, pertinent history, medical and dental conditions, services rendered, and charges and payments made.

dental research, n the formal scientific study of issues related to dentistry.

dental review committee, n a group of dental professionals and administrative personnel that reviews questionable dental claims and can suggest policy decisions regarding dental care.

dental sac, n a portion of the tooth germ consisting of ectomesenchyme surrounding the outside of the enamel organ, which produces the periodontium of a tooth. Older term is *dental follicle.*

dental scaling, n See scaling.

dental sealant, n See sealant.

dental senescence, n See senescence, dental.

dental service corporation, n a legally constituted, not-for-profit organization that negotiates and administers contracts for dental care. Delta Dental and Blue Cross/Blue Shield corporations are two such organizations.

dental service, hospital, n **1.** the location of the dental facility within a hospital. n **2.** the array of dental procedures offered within a hospital setting.

dental spa, n a dental facility supervised by a licensed oral health care provider in which dental services are provided alongside spa treatments, such as massages, skin treatments, and body treatments.

dental splint, n See splint, dental.

dental staff, n the personnel employed or engaged by the dental professional to conduct the assignable professional and management functions of the dental clinic, office, or practice.

dental stone, n See stone, dental.

dental supply person, n a representative of a dental supply company who provides dental supplies, product information, services, and repairs.

dental tape, n See tape, dental.

dental technician, n See technician.

dental therapist, n provider of restorative care under the general supervision of dentists, found mostly in the United Kingdom and in former countries of the British Commonwealth, such as Australia, Canada, and Nigeria.

dental unit, n See unit, dental.

dental unit waterline (DUWL), n small-bore tubing usually made of plastic, used to deliver dental treatment water through a dental unit.

dentate (den′tāt), *adj* having teeth.

denticle (den′tikəl), n (endolith, pulp nodule, pulp stone), a calcified body found in the pulp chamber of a tooth; it may be composed either of irregular dentin (true denticle) or an ectopic calcification of pulp tissue (false denticle).

dentifrice (toothpaste) (den′tə fris′), n a pharmaceutical compound used in conjunction with the toothbrush to clean and polish the teeth. Contains a mild abrasive, a detergent, a flavoring agent, a binder, and occasionally deodorants and various medicaments designed as caries preventives (e.g., antiseptics).

dentifrice abrasion, n See abrasion, dentifrice.

dentifrice, anticalculus **(an′tōkal′ky ələs),** n a commercially available toothpaste, gel, or powder formulated to inhibit the development of new calculus and which contains, among other ingredients, either pyrophosphate or zinc. It has no effect on existing calculus.

dentifrice, calculus-control, n See dentifrice, anticalculus.

dentifrice, cosmetic, n a dentifrice, or solution, applied to a toothbrush or other cleaning device in order to remove tooth deposits such as stain and dental biofilm (dental plaque). It has an effect on teeth appearance over the short term.

dentifrice, flavoring agents, n an additive in liquid, powder, or paste oral hygiene products designed to enhance the product's taste. Flavors tend to be mint and are derived primarily from essential oils.

dentifrice, foaming agents in, n the detergents or surfactants that generate foam. These nontoxic, chemically compatible ingredients also serve to remove unwanted matter from dental surfaces, make teeth feel smoother, and break down stains and deposits.

dentifrice, therapeutic (den′təfris ther′əpū′tik), *n* a material or substance, such as mouthwash, prompting physical changes that positively influence dental health.

dentigerous cyst, *n* See cyst, dentigerous.

dentin (den′tin), *n* the portion of the tooth that lies subjacent to the enamel and cementum. Consists of an organic matrix on which mineral (calcific) salts are deposited; pierced by tubules containing the processes of the odontoblasts that line the pulpal chamber and canal. It is of mesodermal origin. Older term is *dentine.*

dentin bonding agent, n a tissue compatible adhesive that adheres to dentin.

dentin, carious, n the dentin that is involved in or affected by the carious process.

dentin, circumpulpal, n a layer of dentin around the outer pulpal wall.

dentin dysplasia, n See dysplasia, dentinal.

dentin eburnation (ē′burnā′shən), *n* a change in carious teeth in which the decayed dentin assumes a hard, brown, polished appearance and becomes arrested.

dentin, globular, n part of dentinal matrix consisting of completely fused and calcified globules of predentin.

dentin, hereditary opalescent (ō′p əles′ənt), *n* See dentinogenesis imperfecta.

dentin, hyperesthesia of (hī′pəristhē ′zhə), *n* an excessive sensibility of dentin.

dentin, interglobular, n the incompletely calcified dentinal matrix present between the calcified globules.

dentin, intertubular, n the dentin present between the dentinal tubules.

dentin irritation (tertiary dentin, reparative dentin), n the dentin formed in response to an injury or irritant.

dentin, mantle, n the outer portion of dentin bordering the enamel or cementum of the tooth.

dentin, peritubular, n a type of dentin that creates the wall of the dentinal tubule.

dentin, primary, n a type of dentin, made of straight dentinal tubules, that develops until the apical foramen of the root of the tooth is fully formed.

dentin, residual carious, n See caries, dental, residual.

dentin, sclerotic, n See dentin, transparent.

dentin, secondary, n the dentin formed or deposited on the walls of pulp chambers and canals subsequent to the complete formation of the tooth; caused by certain metabolic disturbances that result in irritation and stimulation of the odontoblasts to renewed activity.

dentin, tertiary, n the dentin formed in response to a localized injury to the exposed dentin.

dentin, transparent (sclerotic dentin) (sklərot′ik), *n* dentin formed as a defense mechanism in reaction to various stimuli. Dental tubules are obliterated by deposits of calcium salts that are harder and denser than normal dentin. This dentin appears transparent in ground sections.

dentin wall, n the portion of the wall of a prepared cavity that consists of dentin.

dentinal (den′tənəl), *adj* pertaining to the dentin.

dentinal dysplasia, n See dysplasia, dentinal.

dentinal fluid, n the tissue fluid in the dentinal tubule that surrounds the odontoblastic process.

dentinal hypersensitivity, n exposed dentin that is sensitive to various stimuli.

dentinal permeability, n the degree to which fluids can pass through intact dentin.

dentinal tubule, n a microscopic tube within dentin that spreads outward from the tooth's center. It carries dentinal fluid.

dentine, *n* See dentin.

dentinocemental junction (DCJ) (dentin'ōsēmen'təl), *n* See junction, dentinocemental.

dentinoenamel junction (DEJ) (den'tinōinam'əl), *n* See junction, dentinoenamel.

dentinogenesis, *n* the apposition of predentin by the odontoblasts.

dentinogenesis imperfecta (den'ti nōjen'əsis), *n* (hereditary opalescent dentin) **1.** a disturbance of the dentin of genetic origin; characterized by early calcification of the pulp chambers and root canals, marked attrition, and an opalescent hue to the teeth. 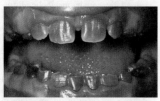 *n* **2.** a localized form of mesodermal dysplasia affecting the dentin of the tooth. It may be hereditary and may be associated with osteogenesis imperfecta. *n* **3.** a hereditary condition associated with a defect in dentin formation; the enamel remains normal.

Dentinogenesis imperfecta. (Dean/Avery/McDonald, 2011)

dentinoma (den'tinōmə), *n* an odontogenic tumor containing regular or irregular dentin.

dentist, *n* a person who is qualified by training and licensed by a state or region to diagnose and treat abnormalities of the teeth, gums, and underlying bone, including conditions caused by disease, trauma, and heredity. Required training consists of 2 to 4 years in an undergraduate college, a satisfactory score on a Dental Aptitude Test, and 4 years at an American Dental Association–accredited dental college. After completing dental college, a dentist is awarded a degree of either Doctor of Dental Surgery (D.D.S.) or Doctor of Dental Medicine (D.M.D.); the two degrees are equivalent.

dentistry, *n* the evaluation, diagnosis, and/or treatment (nonsurgical, surgical, or related procedures) of diseases, disorders, and/or conditions of the oral cavity, maxillofacial area, and/or the adjacent and associated structures and their impact on the body; provided by dental professionals, within the scope of his/her education, training, and experience, in accordance with the ethics of the profession and applicable law.

dentistry, forensic, *n* a branch of forensic science that applies dental science to the identification of unknown human remains and bite marks.

dentistry, four-handed, *n* the technique of chairside operating in which four hands are kept busy working in the oral cavity simultaneously.

dentistry, neuromuscular **(ner'ō mus'kyələr),** *n* a subdiscipline of dentistry concerned with correcting alignment problems at the temporomandibular joint. This branch of dentistry focuses primarily on caring for the muscles, nerves, and other tissue as opposed to teeth and bones.

dentistry, operative, *n* the branch of oral health service concerned with operations to restore or reform the hard dental tissue (e.g., operations necessitated by caries, trauma, and impaired function, and for improvement of appearance).

dentistry, preventive, *n* a subdiscipline of dentistry concerned with preventing cavities and other dental disorders and preserving healthy teeth and gingival tissue.

dentistry, prosthetic, *n* See prosthodontics.

dentistry, psychosomatic **(sī'kəsōma t'ik),** *n* a type of dentistry that concerns itself with the mind-body relationship.

dentistry, washed-field, *n* the constant flushing of the operative field with an irrigant (usually water) and the evacuation of the washing (debris) from the oral cavity by vacuum airstream. See also technique, hydroflow.

dentition (dentish'ən), *n* the natural teeth in position in the dental arches.

dentition, artificial, *n* the artificial substitutes for the natural dentition. See also denture.

dentition, deciduous, *n* See dentition, primary.

dentition, mixed, *n* the teeth in the jaws after the eruption of some of the permanent teeth but before all the primary teeth are exfoliated. This period usually begins with the eruption of the first permanent molars and ends with the exfoliation of the last primary tooth. Also called the *transitional dentition.* See also ugly duckling stage.

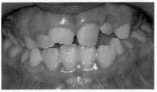

Mixed dentition. (Dean/Avery/McDonald, 2011)

dentition periods, *n* the three periods that occur throughout a lifetime: primary, mixed, and permanent dentition periods.

dentition, permanent (secondary dentition, permanent teeth), *n* the 32 teeth of adulthood that either replace or are added to with the shedding (exfoliation) of the primary teeth.

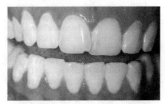

Permanent dentition. (Robinson/Bird, 2007)

dentition, primary, *n* the 20 teeth present that erupt first and are usually replaced by the permanent teeth. This term is currently preferred over *deciduous.*

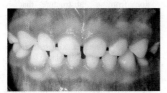

Primary dentition. (Robinson/Bird, 2007)

dentition, prognosis of, *n* an evaluation by the dental professional of the prospect of recovery from dental disease, combined with a forecast of the probability of maintaining the dentition and its associated structures in function and health.

dentition, secondary, *n* See dentition, permanent.

dentition, transitional, *n* See dentition, mixed.

dentoalveolar surgery (den'tōalvē' əlur), *n* the category of oral surgery concerned with the extraction of teeth and the repair or restructuring of supporting bone. See also exodontics.

dentoform (den'tōform'), *n* See typodont.

dentogenesis (den'tōjen'əsis), *n* formation of the connective tissue, dentin, from odontoblasts during the development of the tooth. See also dentin.

dentogingival junction (DGJ), *n* See junction, dentogingival.

dentogingival junctional tissue, *n* the tissue that includes the sulcular epithelium and junctional epithelium.

dentulous (dent'yoolǝs), *adj* (dentulism), having the natural teeth present in the oral cavity. Opposite term: *edentulous.*

denture (den'chǝr), *n* an artificial substitute for missing natural teeth and adjacent tissue.

denture, acrylic resin, *n* a denture made of acrylic resin.

denture adhesive, *n* a pliable, self-adjusting product used to hold a dental prosthesis in position. Also referred to as an *adherent.*

denture, artificial, *n* See denture.

denture, basal surface of (impression surface of denture, foundation surface of denture), *n* the part of a denture base that is shaped to conform to the basal seat for the denture.

denture-bearing area, *n* See area, basal seat.

denture, bilateral partial, *n* a dental prosthesis that supplies teeth and associated structures on both sides of a semiedentulous arch.

denture brush, *n* a brush designed especially for cleaning dentures.

denture characterization, *n* a modification of the form and color of the denture base and teeth to produce a more lifelike appearance.

denture cleanser, *n* a variety of products designed to safely remove stains, deposits, and debris from the surfaces of dental prostheses, by means of immersion or brushing with a denture brush and paste, toothpaste, or powder.

denture cleanser, alkaline hypochlorite, *n* a chemical ingredient used in some solutions to clean removable oral prostheses. The active ingredient is dilute sodium hypochlorite. It effectively removes food, stains, and dental biofilm (dental plaque), and is readily available in household bleach; it has a strong lingering scent and may damage prostheses.

denture cleanser, alkaline peroxide, *n* a light-duty denture cleaner; active ingredient is typically sodium perborate or sodium percarbonate. Comes in tablet or powder form; when combined with water, it creates bubbles. Does not effectively deal with calculus or darker staining.

denture cleanser, dilute acid, *n* a chemical containing inorganic acids as its active ingredient; used to clean prosthetic dental appliances in an immersion regimen. Solutions range includes 3% to 5% hydrochloric acid or a combination of phosphoric and hydrochloric acids. Regular use of dilute acids can damage any metal on the prosthetic device.

denture cleanser, enzyme, *n* an agent that is sometimes added to immersion cleaning solutions, which works by weakening polysaccharides and dental biofilm (dental plaque) proteins.

denture, complete (complete dental prosthesis), *n* a dental prosthesis that replaces all the natural dentition and associated structures of the maxillae or mandible. It may be supported solely by the mucosa or attached to implants in the alveolar process.

    denture, complete, lower, *n* a prosthetic replacement of all the teeth in the mandibular dental arch.

    denture, complete, upper, *n* a prosthetic replacement of all the teeth in the maxillary dental arch.

denture, coping, *n* See overdenture.

denture coverage, *n* the extent to which the oral tissue is covered by the denture base.

denture curing, *n* the process by which the denture base materials are hardened in a denture mold to the form of a denture. See also process.

denture delivery, *n* See denture placement.

denture deposits, *n* these deposits range in degree of severity and ease of removal. They first appear as easily dissolved food matter or mucin, can progress to dental biofilm (dental plaque) or yeast infection, and in severe cases can result in the formation of calculus, a deposit that requires professional intervention to remove.

denture design, *n* a planned visualization of the form and extent of a denture.

denture dislodging force, *n* See force, denture dislodging.

denture, duplicate, *n* a second denture intended to be a copy of the first denture.

denture edge, *n* See border, denture.

denture engraving tool, *n* a tool used to permanently inscribe the patient's name on the flange of his or her dental prosthesis for identification purposes.

denture esthetics, *n* See esthetics, denture.

denture, finish of, *n* the final perfection of the form of the polished surfaces of a denture.

denture flange, *n* See flange.

denture foundation, *n* the portion of the oral structures that supports the complete or partial denture base under occlusal load. See also area, basal seat.

    denture foundation, surface of, *n* See denture, basal surface of.

denture, full, *n* improper term. See denture, complete.

denture, heel of, *n* See distal end.

denture, immediate (immediate-insertion denture), *n* a removable dental prothesis constructed for placement immediately after removal of the remaining natural teeth.

denture, implant, *n* a denture that gains its support, stability, and retention from a substructure that is implanted under the soft tissue of the basal seat of the denture and is in contact with bone.

    denture, implant, substructure, *n* See substructure, implant.

    denture, implant, superstructure, *n* See superstructure, implant.

denture, impression surface of, *n* See denture, basal surface of.

denture, inclusion markers, n the temporary labels affixed to the impression surface of the denture for identification during processing.

denture, insertion, n See denture, placement.

denture, interim (in'terəm), n a dental prosthesis that is to be used for a short interval of time.

denture liner, n a resin used to coat the tissue surface of a dental prosthesis to restore or improve the conformation of the prosthesis to the tissue; generally used to improve the retention of the denture.

denture, maintenance of, n an important part of prosthodontic treatment and a major factor in the longevity of the service that the restoration can be expected to give.

denture, metal base, n a denture with a base of gold, chrome-cobalt alloy, aluminum, or other metal.

denture, model, wax, n See denture, trial.

denture overlay, n a complete denture that is supported by both tooth and mucosa. Remaining teeth are used to provide additional stability to the denture.

denture packing, n See packing, denture.

denture, partial (partial dental prosthesis), n a prosthesis that replaces one or more, but less than all, of the natural teeth and associated structures.

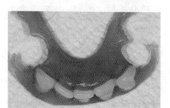

Partial denture. (Garg, 2010)

denture, partial, cantilever (kan'tə lē'vər), n See denture, partial, cantilever fixed.

denture, partial, cantilever fixed, n a fixed dental prosthesis that has one or more abutments at one end of the denture supporting pontic(s) at its other end.

denture, partial, components of, n the units that compose a removable partial denture (e.g., the base, the artificial teeth, direct and indirect retainers, major and minor connectors).

denture, partial, construction of, n the science and technique of designing and constructing partial dentures.

denture, partial, extension, n a removable partial denture that is retained by natural teeth at one end of the denture base segments only; a portion of the functional load is carried by the residual ridge.

denture, partial, fixed, n a tooth-borne partial denture that is intended to be permanently attached to the teeth or roots that furnish support to the restoration.

denture, partial, removable, n a partial denture that can be readily placed in the oral cavity and removed by the wearer.

denture, partial, temporary, n See denture, partial, treatment.

denture, partial, tissue-borne, n a removable partial denture that is not supported entirely by the natural teeth.

denture, partial, tooth-borne, n a partial denture that is supported entirely by the teeth that bound the edentulous area covered by the base.

denture, partial, tooth-borne/tissue-borne, n a partial denture that gains support from both an abutment tooth or teeth and from the structures of the edentulous area covered by the base.

denture, partial, treatment (temporary partial denture), n a dental prosthesis used for the purpose of treating or conditioning the tissue that are needed to support and retain a denture base.

denture, partial, unilateral (ū'nələ t'ərəl), n a dental prosthesis that restores lost or missing teeth on one side of the arch only.

denture periphery, n See border, denture.

denture placement, n the act of inserting a dental prosthesis into the place in a patient's oral cavity for which it was designed. Also called *denture delivery* or *denture insertion*.

denture, polished surface of, n the portion of the surface of a denture that extends in an occlusal direction from the border of the denture and includes the palatal surface. It is the part of the denture base that is usually polished and includes the buccal and lingual surfaces of the teeth.

denture processing, n See processing, denture.

denture, provisional (prōvizh'ənəl), n a prosthetic appliance to be used for a short period for reasons of esthetics, function, or occlusal support; more commonly referred to as a temporary, interim, or transitional denture. A provisional denture is usually an immediate denture and is most often employed in the maxillary arch.

denture repair, n the restoration of a broken or damaged dental prosthesis.

denture retention, n See retention, denture.

denture-sore oral cavity, n See oral cavity, denture-sore.

denture space, n the space between the residual ridges and the cheeks and tongue that is available for dentures. See also distance, interarch.

denture stability, n See stability, denture.

denture, stomatitis, n See oral cavity, denture-sore.

denture supporting area, n See area, basal seat.

denture supporting structure, n See structure, denture supporting.

denture, temporary, n a denture intended to serve for a very short time in a temporary or emergency situation.

denture, tooth-mucosa-supported, n See denture.

denture, transitional, n a removable partial denture that serves as a temporary prosthesis to which teeth will be added as more teeth are lost and that will be replaced after postextraction tissue changes have occurred. A transitional denture may become an interim denture when all the teeth have been removed from the dental arch.

denture, trial (wax model denture), n a temporary denture, usually made of wax on a baseplate, that is used for checking jaw relation records, occlusion, and the arrangement and observation of teeth for esthetics.

denturist (den'chərist), n a person other than a dental professional (usually a technician) who engages in the practice of dentistry that is usually limited to making and fitting complete or partial dentures. Dental practice acts vary in allowing this.

denudation (den'yoodā'shən), n stripping bare; the process of removing the outer (epithelial) layer by surgery or disease.

deoxyribonucleic acid *(DNA)* (dēo k'sērī'bōnooklā'ik), n See DNA.

deoxyribonucleic acid *(DNA)* **probes,** n a nucleic acid fragment labeled with a radioisotope that is complementary to a sequence in another nucleic acid fragment that will bind to it and thus identify it. It can be used as a diagnostic tool to identity the species of microbe involved in an infectious process such as refractory periodontal disease.

dependence, physical, n the level of substance abuse at which disagreeable or severe physiologic symptoms will occur if use of the substance is suddenly terminated.

dependency, n the state of being dependent.

dependency, drug, n a psychologic craving for, habituation to, or addiction to a chemical substance; the term is distinct from drug addiction, which emphasizes physiologic craving.

dependency, emotional, n an emotional need manifested by a marked and habitual inclination to rely on another for comfort, support, guidance, and decision making; the tendency to seek help from others in making decisions or in carrying out difficult actions; the need to be mothered, loved, taken care of, emotionally supported. In extreme cases such persons lose their ability to function independently.

dependents, n.pl the spouse and children of a subscriber, as defined in a contract. Under some contracts, arents or other members of the family may be beneficiaries.

dependent variable, n in a clinical study, the variable that is being tested.

deplaquing, n the removal of dental biofilm (dental plaque) from the tooth's surface or the gingival tissue.

depletion, salt (dēplē'shən), n a condition resulting from inadequate water intake, low intake of sodium and chlorides in the alimentary tract, and secretion of sweat and urine. The most significant of these losses are the gastrointestinal fluid losses resulting from vomiting, diarrhea, and fistulas.

depolarization (dēpō′lərizā′shən), *n* a neutralization of polarity; the breaking down of polarized semipermeable membranes, as in nerve or muscle cells in the induction of impulses.

deponent (dipō′nənt), *n* one who gives under oath testimony reduced to writing.

deposit, bismuth, *n* See stomatitis, bismuth.

deposit, calcareous, *n* See calculus.

deposition (dep′ōzish′ən), *n* the evidence given by a witness under interrogation, oral or written, and usually written down by an official person and intended to be used in the trial of an action in court.

deposits, assessment of, *n* the examination of the teeth for evidence of calculus and debris, which, if not removed, may lead to caries and/or periodontal infection.

deposits, nonmineralized (soft), *n.pl* the soft deposits, consisting of acquired pellicle, dental biofilm (dental plaque), and debris, that accumulate on tooth surfaces and within the gingival sulcus or periodontal pockets. If left unattended, will harden into calculus and may lead to caries and/or periodontal disease.

depot (dē′pō), *n* in physiology, the site of accumulation, deposit, or storage of body products not immediately or actively involved in metabolic processes (e.g., a fat depot).

depreciation, *n* the charges against earnings to write off the cost, less salvage value, of an asset over its estimated useful life. It is a bookkeeping entry and does not represent any cash outlay, nor are any funds earmarked for the purpose. There are three classic methods of applying depreciation: straight line, sum of the year's digits, and double declining balance.

depressant (dēpres′ənt), *n* a medicine that diminishes functional activity.

depressed oral lesions, *n.pl* lesions characterized by their subsurface appearance and nonuniform shape. They may be classified as either erosions, which are considered superficial (i.e., having a depth of less than 3 mm), or the more frequently occurring ulcers, which may be up to 3 mm in depth. Ulcers may be the result of elevated lesions that have burst, and vary in appearance, with centers being yellow to gray, while the borders are typically red.

depression (dēpresh′ən), *n* **1.** a decrease of functional activity. *n* **2.** a pitted area on a tooth or other anatomic surface.

depression, developmental, *n* depression seen in a defined region on a tooth.

depression, mandible, *n* the lowering of the mandible caused by rotational movement of the temporomandibular joint.

depression, postpartum, *n* a moderate to severe form of depression that occurs in women beginning approximately 2 to 3 weeks after childbirth as a result of physical and psychologic factors. Symptoms include fatigue, loss of appetite, and lack of enthusiasm for everyday activities.

depression, psychologic, *n* a clinical syndrome of neurotic or psychotic proportions, consisting of lowering of mood tone (feelings of painful dejection), difficulty in thinking, and psychomotor retardation. As commonly used, depression ordinarily refers only to the mood element, which would be more appropriately labeled dejection, sadness, gloominess, despair, or despondency. Many such patients lack motivation and concern for their oral health or dental needs.

derivative (dēriv′ətiv), *n* a chemical substance that is the result of a chemical reaction.

dermabrasion (dur′məbrā′zhən), *n* a treatment for the removal of superficial scars on the skin by the use of revolving wire brushes or sandpaper. An aerosol spray is used to freeze the skin for this procedure. Dermabrasion is performed to reduce facial scars of severe acne. See also microdermabrasion.

dermal undergloves, *n* an additional pair of protective hand coverings, worn to protect sensitive skin from the latex or nonlatex material of the outer glove.

dermatalgia (durmətal′jēə), *n* pain, burning, and other sensations of the skin unaccompanied by any structural change; probably caused by some nervous disease or reflex influence.

dermataneuria (dur′matənŏŏrēə), *n* a derangement of the nerve supply of the skin, causing disturbance of sensation.

dermatitis (durmətī′tis), *n* an inflammation of the skin.

dermatitis, allergic contact, n the reaction of the skin to direct contact with a specific antigen. Poison ivy rash is a common example of an allergic contact dermatitis.

dermatitis, atopic (ātō′pik), n an atopic eczema characterized by the distinctive phenomenon of atopy, a familial related allergic response associated with IgE antibody.

dermatitis, contact, n a delayed type of induced sensitivity (allergy) of the skin with varying degrees of erythema, edema, and vesiculation, resulting from cutaneous contact with a specific allergen. It is an occupational hazard in dentistry.

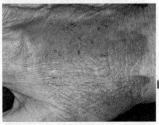

Contact dermatitis caused by latex glove. (Krouse, 2008)

dermatitis herpetiformis (hərpet′i formis), n dermatitis characterized by grouped, erythematous, papular, vesicular, pustular, or bullous lesions occurring in various combinations, often accompanied by vesicobullous and ulcerative lesions of the oral mucosa.

dermatitis infectiosa eczematoides (Engman's disease), n a pustular eczematous eruption that frequently follows or occurs coincidentally with some pyogenic process.

dermatitis, occupational, n a contact dermatitis associated with allergens found in the workplace.

dermatitis, radiation, n an inflammation of the skin resulting from a high dose of radiation. The reaction varies with the quality and quantity of radiation used and is usually transitory.

dermatitis, seborrheic (seb′ərē′ik), n a chronic inflammatory skin disease that can affect the scalp, face, ears, armpits, breasts, and groin. Its symptoms include moist, greasy, or dry scaling and patches of yellowish crust. Although the cause is unknown, it can be treated with selenium sulfide shampoos, topical antibiotics, and topical and oral corticosteroids.

dermatoglyphics (dur′mətöglif′iks), *n* the study of the skin ridge patterns on fingers, toes, palms of hands, and soles of feet. The patterns are used as a basis of identification (fingerprinting).

dermatology, *n* the study of the skin, including the anatomy, physiology, and pathology of the skin and the diagnosis and treatment of skin disorders.

dermatoma (dur′mətō′mə), *n* a circumscribed thickening or hypertrophy of the skin.

dermatome (dur′mətōm′), *n* **1.** an instrument for cutting thin slices or layers of skin for grafting or for sequentially removing small lesions. *n* **2.** dermatologic regions of sensory innervation supplied by particular posterior root spinal nerves.

dermatomyositis (dur′mətōmī′ōsī′tis), *n* (polymyositis, dermatomucosomyositis) a form of connective tissue disease related to scleroderma and lupus erythematosus. The skin lesions are diffuse erythematous desquamations or rashlike lesions. The skin symptoms are related to a variety of patterns of myositis.

dermatophyte (dərmat′əfit′), *n* fungi that cause parasitic skin disease.

dermatosclerosis (dur′mətōsklərō′sis), *n* See scleroderma.

dermatosis (dur′mətō′sis), *n* a disease of the skin.

dermis (dur′mis), *n* the layer of skin just below the epidermis consisting of vascular connective tissue.

dermoid cyst, *n* See cyst, dermoid.

desaturation (dēsat'yərā'shən), *n* the conversion of a saturated compound such as stearin into an unsaturated compound such as olein by the removal of hydrogen.

desensitization (dēsen'sitizā'shən), *n* **1.** a condition of insusceptibility to infection or an allergen; established in experimental animals by the injection of an antigen that produces sensitization or an anaphylactic reaction. After recovery, a second injection of the antigen is made, bringing about no reaction and thus producing desensitization. *n* **2.** a reduction in dentin hypersensitivity by the addition of medicaments to the exposed dentin surface.

desensitization, psychologic, *n* the deliberate exposure of an individual to imagined or actual emotionally stressful experiences to treat phobias and other related conditions.

descriptive approach, *n* a variety of methods (including surveys, case studies, developmental studies, documents or content analysis, trend studies, and correlational studies) used in research.

descriptive statistics, *n. pl* procedures that are used to summarize, organize, and describe quantitative data.

desflurane, *n brand name:* Suprane; *drug class:* inhalation, general anesthetic; *action:* inhibits nerve conduction by several potential mechanisms; *use:* general anesthesia.

desiccate (des'ikāt), *n* to dry by chemical or physical means; e.g., electrocoagulation can produce desiccation in tissue.

desiccation (des'ikā'shən), *n* an excessive loss of moisture; the process of drying up. See also electrocoagulation.

design, *v* **1.** to plan or delineate by drawing the outline of a proposed prosthesis. *n* **2.** the graphical and artistic representation of a plan.

designer drugs, *n.pl* the synthetic organic compounds that are designed as analogs of illicit drugs and have the same narcotic or other dangerous effects.

desipramine HCl (dəsip'rəmēn), *n brand names:* Norpramin, Petrofrane; *drug class:* antidepressant, tricyclic;

action: inhibits both norepinephrine and serotonin (5-HT) uptake in the brain; *use:* depression.

desmins (dez'minz), *n.pl* α-amino acids, usually lysine and norleucine, condensed through their side chains rather than through the α-amino and carboxyl groups. They copolymerize with vimentin to form constituents of connective tissue.

desmolysis (desmol'isis), *n* the destruction and disintegration of connective tissue. Some authorities associate this desmolytic process with the destruction of connective tissue lying between the enamel and oral epithelium, which thus permits proliferation of the oral epithelium and fusion of enamel and oral epithelium.

desmopressin acetate (des'mō pres'ən as'ətāt), *n brand names:* Stimate, DDAVP; *drug class:* synthetic antidiuretic hormone; *action:* promotes reabsorption of water by action on renal tubular epithelium; *uses:* primary nocturnal enuresis, hemophilia A with factor VIII levels of less than 5%, von Willebrand disease, neurogenic diabetes insipidus.

desmosomes, *n.pl* See epithelium, desmosomes of.

desonide (des'ənīd'), *n brand names:* DesOwen, Tridesilon; *drug class:* topical corticosteroid, group IV low potency; *actions:* possesses antipruritic, antiinflammatory actions; *uses:* psoriasis, eczema, contact dermatitis, pruritus.

desoximetasone (desok'sēmet'əs ōn), *n brand names:* Topicort, Topicort LP; *drug classes:* topical corticosteroid, group II potency (0.25%), group III potency (0.05%); *action:* interacts with steroid cytoplasmic receptors to induce antiinflammatory effects; *uses:* psoriasis, eczema, contact dermatitis, pruritus.

desquamation (des'kwəmā'shən), *n* a naturally occurring process in which the outer layer of skin or mucosa cells is sloughed off.

detector, radiation, *n* See radiation detector.

detention, *n* restraint; custody; confinement.

detergent (dētur'jənt), *n* a cleanser. Also applied in a more specific sense to chemicals that possess surface active properties in water and whose

D

solutions are therefore able to wet surfaces that are normally water repellent, thereby assisting in the mechanical dispersion and emulsification of fatty or oily material and other substances that soil the surface.

detergent, anionic, n a detergent in which the cleansing action resides in the anion. Soaps and many synthetic detergents are anionic.

detergent, cationic, n a detergent in which the cleansing action resides in the cation. Many are strong germicides (e.g., those that contain quaternary ammonium compounds).

detergent, nonionic, n a cleanser that acts by depressing the surface tension of water but does not ionize.

detergent, synthetic, n a cleanser, other than soap, that exerts its effect by lowering the surface tension of an aqueous cleansing mixture.

determinants of health, n. pl factors that interact to creat specific healh conditions, including physical, biological, behavioral, social, cultural, and spiritual.

detoxicate (dētok′sikāt), *v* See detoxify.

detoxify, *v* (detoxicate), to remove the toxic quality of a substance.

detritus (det′ritus), *n* the fragments or scraps that cling to teeth, gingival tissue or other oral surfaces.

deuterium (dootēr′ēəm), *n* a stable isotope of the hydrogen atom, used as a tracer. Also called *heavy hydrogen.* Deuterium oxide, or heavy water, is formed from an isotope of hydrogen, which has twice the weight of ordinary hydrogen (hence the name).

developed countries, *n.pl* the countries with an economic base built largely on manufacturing and technology rather than agriculture. Although the need for medical and dental care may not differ from undeveloped to developed countries, the effective demand does vary. They have the available health professionals, the economic base to support the purchase of health care, and an informed public.

developer, *n* a chemical solution used in film processing that converts the invisible (latent) image on a film into a visible one composed of minute grains of metallic silver.

developer stain,′ *n* See film fault, black spots.

developing countries, *n.pl* the countries in transition from an agrarian economy to a manufacturing- and technology-based economy.

developing, time-temperature method, *n* the procedure of developing dental films; a solution of fixed temperature is used, and the films are immersed in the solution for a specific length of time.

developing, visual method, *n* the procedure of developing dental films by placing the films in the developing solution and holding them from time to time before a safelight. Correct development has occurred when the film becomes so dark that it is difficult to distinguish between tooth and bone structure.

development, *n* the process by which an individual reaches maturity.

development hyperactivity, *n* a condition distinguished by continuous movement, restlessness, impetuosity, excitability, and a short span of attention. Also called *hyperkinesis.*

developmental biology, *n* the study of life processes occurring during growth and maturation.

developmental disabilities (DD), *n. pl* the pathologic conditions that have their origin in the embryology and growth and development of an individual. DDs usually appear clinically before 18 years of age. The limitations of physiologic or mental function usually persist throughout life.

deviation (dē′vēā′shən), *n* the turning from a regular course; deflection.

device, scavenging (skav′ənjing), *n* a device that collects and removes exhaled nitrous oxide during the administration of nitrous oxide and oxygen for sedation. The device is recommended by the American Dental Association to avoid occupational exposure to the gas.

devital tooth, See tooth, pulpless.

dexamethasone/dexamethasone acetate/dexamethasone sodium phosphate (dek′səmeth′əsōn), *n brand names:* Decadron, Hexadrol, Oradexan; *drug class:* glucocorticoid, long-acting; *action:* binds to intracellular receptors affecting RNA production leading to a decrease in inflammation due to inhibition of phospholipase A_2 and suppression of macrophage and leukocyte migration and reduction in capillary permeability; *uses:* inflammation, allergies, neoplasm, cerebral edema, shock, collagen disorders.

dexamethasone/dexamethasone sodium phosphate, *n brand name:* Decaderm; *drug class:* synthetic topical corticosteroid; *action:* binds to intracellular receptors affecting RNA production leading to a decrease in inflammation due to inhibition of phospholipase A_2 and suppression of macrophage and leukocyte migration and reduction in capillary permeability; *uses:* corticosteroid-responsive dermatoses, oral ulcerative inflammatory lesions.

dexchlorpheniramine maleate (deks′klorfənir′əmēn′ māleāt), *n brand name:* Polaramine; *drug class:* antihistamine; *actions:* acts on blood vessels, gastrointestinal system, respiratory system by competing with histamine for H_1 receptor sites; decreases allergic response by blocking histamine; *uses:* allergy symptoms, rhinitis, pruritus, contact dermatitis.

dexmedetomidine, *n brand name:* Precedex; *drug class:* alpha$_2$ adrenergic receptor agonist; *action:* stimulation of alpha$_2$ adrenergic receptors in the brainstem and the dorsal horn of the spinal cord causes sedation and analgesia, respectively; *uses:* sedation, pain relief in intensive care, certain procedures.

dextran (dek′stran), *n* ($C_6H_{10}O_5$) a water-soluble polymer of glucose of high molecular weight. A purified form, having an average molecular weight of 75,000, is used in a 6% concentration in isotonic sodium chloride solution to expand plasma volume and maintain blood pressure in emergency treatment of hemorrhagic and traumatic shock.

dextro-, *adj/comb* the prefix designating that an aqueous solution of a substance rotates the plane of polarized light to the right. See also isomers, optical.

dextroamphetamine sulfate (dek′s trōamfet′əmēn′ sul′fāt), *n brand names:* Dexedrine, Oxydess II; *drug class:* amphetamine, *action:* increases release of norepinephrine and

dopamine in the cerebral cortex, the reticular activating system and other areas; *uses:* narcolepsy, attention deficit disorder with hyperactivity.

dextromethorphan hydrobromide (dek′strōməthor′fan hī′drōbrō′ mīd), *n brand names:* Benylin DM, Robitussin Pediatric, Vicks Formula 44; *drug class:* antitussive, nonnarcotic; *action:* depresses cough center in medulla; *use:* nonproductive cough.

dextrorotatory (dek′strōrō′tətôrē), *adj* turning the plane of polarization, or rays of polarized light, to the right.

dextrose (dek′strōs), *n* dextrorotatory glucose, a monosaccharide occurring as a white, crystalline powder; colorless and sweet.

diabetes (dīəbē′tēz), *n* a deficiency condition involving carbohydrate metabolism and characterized by increased urination.

diabetes, bronzed, *n* the combination of hemochromatosis and diabetes mellitus. The skin takes on a bronzed appearance as a result of the deposition of an iron-containing pigment in the skin.

diabetes, gestational (jestāshənəl), *n* the term describing patients who acquire glucose intolerance when pregnant.

diabetes insipidus (insip′idəs), *n* **1.** a metabolic disturbance characterized by marked urinary excretion and great thirst but no elevation of sugar in the blood or urine. *n* **2.** a pituitary dysfunction characterized by an insufficient output of antidiuretic hormone, leading to polyuria and polydipsia.

diabetes, juvenile, *n* an older term for diabetes mellitus occurring in children and adolescents, usually of a more severe and rampant nature than diabetes mellitus in adults, with consequent difficulty of regulation. Now considered a form of type 1 diabetes mellitus.

diabetes mellitus (DM) (mel′ətəs), *n* a metabolic disorder caused primarily by a defect in the production of insulin by the islet cells of the pancreas, resulting in an inability to use carbohydrates. Characterized by hyperglycemia, glycosuria, polyuria, hyperlipemia (caused by imperfect catabolism of fats), acidosis, ketonuria, and a lowered resistance to infection. Periodontal manifestations if

D

blood sugar is not being controlled may include recurrent and multiple periodontal abscesses, osteoporotic changes in alveolar bone, fungating masses of granulation tissue protruding from periodontal pockets, a lowered resistance to infection, and delay in healing after periodontal therapy. See also blood glucose level(s).

diabetes mellitus, amputation, n a great number of limb amputations are caused by diabetes, especially amputations of the feet; blood infections in the feet can go unnoticed by the patient because of a lack of feeling caused by diabetic neuropathy.

diabetes mellitus, type 1, n diabetes that usually includes patients requiring the administration of insulin to prevent ketosis. Previously called *insulin-dependent diabetes mellitus (IDDM), juvenile-onset diabetes, brittle diabetes,* and *ketosis-prone diabetes.*

diabetes mellitus, type 2, n diabetes that includes patients who can maintain proper blood sugar levels without the administration of insulin. Previously called *non–insulin-dependent diabetes mellitus (NIDDM), maturity-onset diabetes, adult-onset diabetes, ketosis-resistant diabetes,* and *stable diabetes.*

diabetes, phlorizin (flor′əzin), n a condition of glycosuria caused by inhibition of phosphorylation of phlorizin. It is not related to an endocrine disturbance.

diabetic (dī′əbet′ik), adj of or pertaining to diabetes.

diabetic ketoacidosis (DKA) (kē′tōas ′idō′sis), n a diabetic coma; an acute, life-threatening complication of uncontrolled diabetes mellitus in which urinary loss of water, potassium, ammonium, and sodium results in hypovolemia, electrolyte imbalance, extremely high blood glucose levels, and the breakdown of free fatty acids causing acidosis. Causes "fruity" or acetone breath. See also acetone breath.

diabetic nephropathy (nəfro′pət hē′), n the negative effects on the kidneys or renal system caused by diabetes mellitus. The condition may necessitate dialysis or kidney transplant.

diabetic neuropathy, n the complications to the nervous system that can be caused by diabetes mellitus, some of which may necessitate amputation or result in oral or facial symptoms.

diabetic retinopathy (ret′inop′ət hē), n the complication to the eye that can be caused by diabetes mellitus, some of which may result in blindness.

diadochokinesia (dīad′əkōkīnē′zēə, -zhə), n the act or process of repeating at maximum speed a simple cyclical, reciprocating movement such as raising and lowering of the mandible or protrusion and retracting the tongue.

diagnose, v to distinguish irregularities and other issues of concern based upon a patient's examination and interview.

diagnosis, n the translation of data gathered by clinical and radiographic examination into an organized, classified definition of the conditions present.

diagnosis, clinical, n the determination of the specific disease or diseases involved in producing symptoms and signs by examination of the patient and use of analogy.

diagnosis, dental hygiene, n the professional determination of a dental hygienist, including evaluation and recommendation, regarding a patient's personal hygienic needs.

diagnosis, differential, n the process of identifying a condition by differentiating all pathologic processes that may produce similar lesions.

diagnosis, final, n the diagnosis arrived at after all the data have been collected, analyzed, and subjected to logical thought. Treatment may be necessary in some instances before the final diagnosis is made.

diagnosis, laboratory, n a diagnosis made from chemical, microscopic, microbiologic, immunologic, or pathologic study of secretions, discharges, blood, or tissue sections.

diagnosis, oral, n the identification of the cause of a dental disease or abnormality.

diagnosis, radiographic, n a limited term used to indicate those radiologic interpretations that cannot be verified or disproved by clinical examination.

diagnosis-related group (DRG), *n* a system of classifying hospital patients on the basis of diagnosis consisting of distinct groupings. A DRG assignment to a case is based on the patient's principal diagnosis, treatment procedures performed, age, gender, and discharge status.

diagnosis, surgical, *n* a surgical incision into a body part or the excision of a lesion for the purpose of determining the cause or nature of an illness.

diagnostic cast, *n* See cast, diagnostic.

diagnostic equilibration (ikwil′əbrā′shən), a measuring method of determining and recording on dentodes the amount and direction that interfering cusps deflect the closure direction of the mandible, as can be seen in mountings.

diagnostic error, *n* a mistake in judgment regarding the cause of an illness.

diagnostic imaging, *n* the use of radiographic, sonographic, and other technologies to create a graphic depiction of the body part(s) in question.

diagnostic services, *n.pl* the imaging and laboratory capabilities available for determining the cause of an illness.

diagnostic wax-up, *n* a process in which wax is applied to a model of the patient's teeth to simulate the procedure and results of planned reconstruction, repair, or enhancement.

dialysis (dīal′isis), *n* a type of filtration used to separate smaller molecules from larger ones contained in a solution. The molecular solution is placed on one side of a semipermeable membrane and water on the other side. The smaller molecules pass through the membrane into the water; the larger molecules are retained in the solution.

dialysis, kidney, artificial, *n* See kidney dialysis, artificial.

diamond, *n* a crystalline carbon substance, the hardest natural substance known, used industrially and in dentistry for cutting and grinding.

diamond particles, *n.pl* the elements of a diamond polishing paste that are used to bring out the natural luster of porcelain surfaces.

diaphoresis (dī′əfərē′sis), *n* excessive sweating.

diaphragm (dī′əfram), *n* **1.** a musculotendinous partition that separates the thorax and abdomen. *n* **2.** a metal barrier plate, often of lead, pierced with a central aperture so arranged as to limit the emerging, or useful, beam of roentgen rays to the smallest practical diameter for making radiographic exposures. See also collimation; collimator; distance, cone.

diaphragm, lead, *n* a collimating device with a small opening, designed to limit the size of the outgoing x-ray beam. It is usually made of lead one-eighth of an inch thick and located between the position-indicating device and the radiographic tube itself.

diaphragm, Potter-Bucky, See grid, Potter-Bucky.

diaphysis (diaf′isis), *n* the shaft of a long bone.

diarrhea (dī′ərē′ə), *n* a condition with the frequent passage of loose, watery stools. The stool may also contain mucus, suppuration, blood, or excessive amounts of fat. It is usually a symptom of some underlying disorder. See also antidiarrheals.

diarthrosis (dī′ärthrō′sis), *n* See synovial joint.

diastema (dī′əstē′mə), *n* an abnormal space between two adjacent teeth in the same dental arch. The gap between the maxillary central incisors is very noticeable.

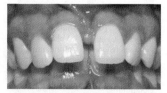

Diastema. (Proffit/Fields/Sarver, 2013)

diastole (dīas′təlē), *n* **1.** the rhythmic period of relaxation and dilation of a chamber of the heart during which it fills with blood. *n* **2.** the period after the contraction of the heart muscle, during which the aorta releases the potential energy stored in its elastic tissue. The energy is converted into kinetic energy and sustains the pressure necessary for steady flow of blood in the vessels. The pressure measured at this period is the lowest attained during the cardiac pumping cycle and is called the *diastolic pressure.* The normal pressure in the adult is approximately 120/80 mm Hg (systolic/diastolic) and increases with age from 128/85 at 45 years of age to 135/89 at 60 years of age. See also blood pressure classification.

diathermy (dī'əthur'mē), *n* a generalized rise in tissue temperature produced by a high-frequency alternating current between two electrodes. The temperature rise is produced without causing tissue damage.

diathesis (dīath'əsis), *n* a tendency, based on body makeup or constitutional, hereditary, or acquired states of the body, that causes a predisposition or susceptibility to disease.

diathesis, hemorrhagic **(hem'əraj'ik),** *n* a condition that may be caused by defects in the coagulation mechanism, blood vessel wall, or both.

diazepam (dīaz'əpam'), *n brand name:* Valium; *drug class:* benzodiazepine, anxiolytic; *action:* produces CNS depression by enhancing the effect of gamma aminobutyric acid (GABA) in parts of the limbic system and the thalamus and hypothalamus, inducing a calming effect; *uses:* management of short-term anxiety disorders, relief of symptoms of anxiety, short-term relief of skeletal muscle spasm, acute alcohol withdrawal, convulsions.

Dick's test, *n* See test, Dick's.

diclofenac (dīklō'fənak'), *n brand names:* Cataflam, Voltaren; *drug class:* nonsteroidal antiinflammatory; *action:* inhibits prostaglandin synthesis; *uses:* acute and chronic rheumatoid arthritis, osteoarthritis, ankylosing spondylitis.

dicloxacillin sodium (dīklok'səsil'ən), *n brand names:* Dycill, Dynapen, Pathocil; *drug class:* penicillinase-resistant penicillin; *action:* interferes with cell wall synthesis of susceptible organisms; *use:* infections caused by penicillinase-producing *Staphylococcus.*

dicyclomine HCl (dīsī'kləmēn'), *n brand names:* Antispas, Dibent; *drug class:* GI anticholinergic; *action:* inhibits muscarinic actions of

acetylcholine at postganglionic parasympathetic neuroeffector sites; *uses:* peptic ulcer disease in combination with other drugs; irritable bowel.

didanosine (dīdan'əsin'), *n brand name:* Videx; *drug class:* synthetic antiviral; *action:* inhibits reverse transcriptase in HIV; *use:* HIV infections in combination with other drugs.

dideoxycytidine (dī'dēok'sēsī'ti dēn'), *n* See zalcitabine.

dideoxyinosine (dī'dēok'sēin'əsēn'), *n* See didanosine.

die, *n* the positive reproduction of the form of a prepared tooth in any suitable hard substance, usually in metal or specially prepared (improved) artificial stone.

die, lubricant, *n* a material applied to a die to serve as a separating medium so that the wax pattern will not adhere to the die but may be withdrawn from it without sticking.

die, stone, *n* a positive likeness in artificial (dental) stone; used in the fabrication of a dental restoration.

die, waxing, *n* a mold into which wax is forced for the production of standardized wax patterns.

diencephalon (dīənsef'əlon), *n* the division of the brain that consists of the thalamus and hypothalamus.

dienestrol (dī'ənes'trol), *n brand name:* Ortho Dienestrol; *drug class:* nonsteroidal synthetic estrogen; *action:* stimulates estrogen receptors; *uses:* atrophic vaginitis, kraurosis vulvae.

diet, *n* **1.** the food and drink consumed by a given person from day to day. Not all the diet is necessarily used by the body. For this reason, diet and nutrition must be differentiated. *v* **2.** to eat according to a plan.

diet, alkaline, *n* a diet that is basic in reaction; produced by the addition of alkaline salts, including sodium bicarbonate.

diet, cariogenic, *n* the intake of food that is heavy in refined carbohydrates and other food stuffs that support the growth of caries-producing bacteria.

diet, lysine-poor, *n* a diet deficient in lysine, an essential amino acid. All the essential amino acids must be present in the diet; should one or more be absent, proper use of the others cannot occur. Periodontal changes described in experimental animals with lysine deficiency include osteoporosis of supporting bone and disintegration and failure of replacement of peri-odontal fibers.

dietary carbohydrates, *n* the amount of simple and complex sugars con-sumed; the physical character of the diet. It may tend to produce or modify periodontal disease.

dietary fiber, *n* a generic term for nondigestible chemical substances found in plant cell walls. Foods high in dietary fiber are fruits, green leafy vegetables, root vegetables, and whole-grain cereals and bread.

dietary history, *n* See analysis, dietary.

dietary reference intakes *(DRIs), n. pl* a set of nutritional guidelines concerning the intake of vitamins and minerals from food rather than supplements.

dietetics (dī′itet′iks), *n* the science of applying nutritional principles to the planning and preparation of foods and the regulation of the diet in rela-tion to both health and disease.

diethylpropion HCl (dīeth′əlprō′ pēən), *n brand names:* Tenuate, Ten-Tab; *drug class:* anorexant, amphetamine-like analog; *action:* releases norepinephrine and other catecholamines from nerve endings with an effect on the satiety center of the hypothalamus; *use:* exogenous obesity.

dietitian, registered *(RD)* **(dīətish′ ən),** *n* an individual who meets the requirements of the American Dietetic Association (ADA) including posses-sion of a bachelor's degree in dietetics or nutrition, a passing grade on the registration exam, and a demonstrated commitment to continuing education through updated courses taken annually.

difenoxin HCl with atropine sulfate (dif′ənok′sin at′rəpēn′ sul′fāt), *n brand name:* Motofen; *drug class:* antidiarrheal; *action:* inhibits gastric motility by acting on mucosal recep-tors responsible for peristalsis; *uses:* acute nonspecific diarrhea, acute exacerbations of chronic functional diarrhea.

differential force, *n* a term sometimes used to describe the design and appli-cation of an orthodontic appliance to distribute the reciprocal forces of the appliance over significantly different root areas with the objective of elicit-ing a differential response.

differentiation (dif′ərən′shēā′shən), *n* the change in the embryonic cells, which are genetically identical but become quite distinct structurally and functionally.

difficult eruption, See teething.

diffusibility (difūz′ibil′itē), *n* capable of being diffused.

diffusion (difū′zhən), *n* a property of ions or molecules of a solute that permits them to pass through a mem-brane or to intermingle by rapid or gradual permeation with the mole-cules of a solvent.

diffusion barrier, n a thin layer of material placed between two other materials to prevent one from corrupt-ing the other.

diffusion, facilitated, n an absorption process during which only certain rec-ognized molecules are allowed to pass into the receiving area.

diflorasone diacetate (dif′lorəsōn dīas′ətāt), *n brand names:* Florone, Maxiflor, Psorcon, Apexicon E; *drug class:* topical corticosteroid; *action:* binds to glucocorticoid recep-tors and reduces itching; *uses:* pso-riasis, eczema, contact dermatitis, pruritus.

diflunisal (dīfloo′nəsal′), *n brand name:* Dolobid; *drug class:* salicylate derivative, nonsteroidal antiinflam-matory; *action:* inhibits cyclooxygen-ase thereby inhibiting prostaglandin synthesis; *uses:* mild to moderate pain, symptoms of rheumatoid arthri-tis and osteoarthritis.

digestion, *n* the conversion of food into absorbable substances in the GI tract.

digit, *n* **1.** a single symbol or character representing a quantity. *n* **2.** a finger or toe.

digit sucking, n an oral habit, usually referred to as *finger* or *thumb sucking,* that is not unusual in preschool children. Prolonged, persistent, or vigorous sucking into the transition dentition period can cause tooth dis-placement malocclusions.

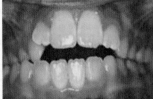

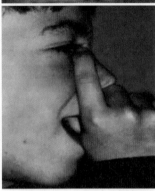

Digit Sucking. (Dean/Avery/McDonald, 2011)

digital, *adj* **1.** involving the use of the fingers. *adj* **2.** a means of data storage in which information is converted to numeric strings. *adj* **3.** using alphanumeric characters to display data, as opposed to analog, which uses the relative position of needles or "hands" (as with a clock) against a background scale.

digital imaging, *n* a method of capturing a radiographic image using a sensor, breaking it into electronic pieces, and presenting and storing the image using a computer, a film-less imaging system.

digital image, *n* electronic signals captured by sensors and displayed on computer monitors.

Digital Imaging and Communications in Medicine *(DICOM),* *n* the universal format for handling, storing and transmitting three-dimensional digital images; information exchanged is referred to as DICOM data.

digital massage, *n* a manual technique developed to increase blood flow to the area of the oral cavity where dentures are worn. The technique involves a moderate, pulse/squeeze movement with the index finger and the thumb over the affected region.

digitalization (dij'italiza'shən), *n* the administration of digitalis in sufficient amount by any of several types of dosage schedules to build up the concentration of digitalis glycosides in the body of a patient.

digitize, *v* convert (data or an image) to digital form.

digoxin (dijok'sin), *n brand names:* Lanoxicaps, Lanoxin, Novadigoxin, Digitek; *drug class:* cardiac glycoside; *action:* acts by inhibiting the sodium-potassium ATPase, which indirectly makes more calcium available for contractile proteins; *uses:* congestive heart failure, atrial fibrillation, atrial flutter.

dihydrocodeine, *n brand name:* Synalgos-DC (in combination with aspirin and caffeine); *drug class:* opioid narcotic analgesic; *action:* binds to opioid receptors leading to pain relief; *use:* pain.

dihydrotachysterol (DHT) (dīhī' drōtəkis'tərol), *n brand names:* DHT Intensol, Hytakerol; *drug class:* vitamin D analog; *actions:* increases intestinal absorption of calcium, increases renal tubular absorption of calcium; *uses:* nutritional supplement, rickets, hypoparathyroidism, postoperative tetany.

dihydroxyaluminum sodium carbonate (dīhī'drok'sēaloo'mənəm), *n brand name:* Rolaids; *drug class:* antacid; *action:* neutralizes gastric acidity; *use:* antacid.

dilaceration (dīlas'ərā'shən), *n* a severe angular distortion in the root of a tooth or at the junction of the root and crown. It results from trauma during tooth development.

Dilantin enlargement, *n.pr* See hyperplasia, gingival, Dilantin.

Dilantin gingival hyperplasia, *n.pr* See hyperplasia, gingival, Dilantin.

Dilantin sodium (dīlan'tin sō' dēəm), *n.pr* the brand name for phenytoin sodium.

dilation (dīlā'shən), *n* the act of stretching or dilating.

diltiazem HCl (dīltī'əzem), *n brand names:* Cardizem, Cardizem SR, Cardizem CD; *drug class:* calcium channel blocker; *actions:* inhibits calcium ion influx across cell membranes in cardiac muscle and smooth muscles of blood vessels, produces relaxation of coronary vascular smooth muscle, dilates coronary arteries, reduces SA node automaticity, slows AV node conduction; *uses:* chronic stable angina pectoris, coronary artery spasm, hypertension.

diluent (dil′ūənt), *n* an agent that dilutes the strength of a solution or mixture; medication that dilutes any of the body fluids.

dilute (diloot′, dīloot′), *v* to make weaker the strength of a solution or mixture.

dimenhydrinate (dī′menhī′drināt), *n brand names:* Calm-X, Dimentabs, Dinate, Dramamine; *drug class:* antihistamine, histamine H_1 receptor antagonist; *actions:* acts on blood vessels and gastrointestinal and respiratory systems by competing with histamine for H_1 receptor sites; decreases allergic response by blocking histamine; *uses:* motion sickness, nausea, vomiting.

dimension, vertical, *n* **1.** a vertical measurement of the face between any two arbitrarily selected points that are conveniently located one above and one below the oral cavity, usually in the midline. *n* **2.** the vertical height of the face with the teeth in occlusion or acting as stops. See also relation, vertical.

dimension, vertical, decrease (loss), *n* a decrease of the vertical distance between the mandible and the maxillae by modifications of teeth or the positions of teeth or occlusion rims, or through alveolar or residual ridge resorption. Also accomplished with orthodontics by using skeletal anchorage to intrude the posterior teeth.

dimension, vertical, increase, *n* an increase of the vertical distance between the mandible and the maxillae by modifications of teeth or the positions of teeth or occlusion rims.

dimension, vertical, occlusal, *n* the vertical dimension of the face when the teeth or occlusion rims are in contact in centric occlusion.

dimension, vertical, rest, *n* the vertical dimension of the face with the jaws in the rest relation.

dimension, vertical, rest, decrease, *n* may or may not accompany

a decrease in occlusal vertical dimension. It may occur without a decrease in occlusal vertical dimension in patients with a preponderant activity of the jaw-closing musculature, as in chronic gum chewers or patients with muscular hypertension.

dimension, vertical, rest, increase, *n* may or may not accompany an increase in occlusal dimension. It sometimes occurs after the removal of remaining occlusal contacts, perhaps as a result of the removal of noxious reflex stimuli.

dimensional stability, *n* See stability, dimensional.

dimercaprol *(BAL), n drug class:* metal chelator; *action:* selectively binds (chelates) certain heavy metals; *uses:* poisoning due to mercury, gold or arsenic, acute lead poisoning in combination with Ethylenediaminetetraacetic acid (EDTA).

dimethyl sulfoxide (dīmeth′əl sulfok′sīd), *n* an organic solvent.

dimethylbenzene (dīmeth′ilben′z ēn), *n* See xylene.

diopter magnification (dīop′tər mag′nifikā′shən), *n* an optical feature that allows an enlarged, focused view of a small area.

diphenhydramine HCl (dīfenhī′dr əmēn), *n brand names:* Benadryl, Sominex Formula 3; *drug class:* antihistamine, histamine H_1 receptor antagonist; *actions:* acts on blood vessels and gastrointestinal and respiratory systems by competing with histamine for H_1-receptor sites; decreases allergic response by blocking histamine; *uses:* allergy symptoms, rhinitis, motion sickness, Parkinsonism, insomnia, infant colic.

diphenoxylate HCl with atropine sulfate (dī′fenok′səlät′ at′rəpēn sul′fāt), *n brand names:* Lofrol, Logene, Lomotil, Lonox; *drug class:* antidiarrheal (opioid with atropine); *action:* inhibits gastric motility by acting on mucosal receptors responsible for peristalsis; *use:* simple diarrhea.

diphtheria (difthir′ēə), *n* an acute, sometimes fatal disease caused by *C. diphtheriae* resulting in swelling of the pharynx and larynx with fever. Vaccination is available.

dipivefrin HCl (dīpiv′əfrin), *n brand name:* Propine; *drug class:* adrenergic agonist; *action:* converted in the eye to epinephrine resulting in decreased production and increased outflow of aqueous humor; *use:* open-angle glaucoma.

diplococci, morphologic form of (dip′lōkôk′ē môr′fəloj′ik), *n.pl* the uniformly scattered pairs of half ovals, resembling shoeprints, which are characteristic of the diplococci bacteria.

diplomate (dip′ləmāt′), *n* a dental specialist who has achieved certification by the recognized certification board in that specialty, as attested by a diploma from the board.

diplopia (diplō′pēə), *n* seeing a single object as two images. May occur after fracture of the bony orbital cavity as a result of displacement of the globe of the eye inferiorly.

dipyridamole (dīpir′idəmol′), *n brand name:* Persantine; *drug class:* platelet aggregation inhibitor; *actions:* inhibits phosphodiesterase increasing the level of cyclic AMP in platelets, inhibits tissue uptake of adenosine; these actions inhibit the ability of platelets to aggregate; *uses:* prevention of transient ischemic attacks (TIA), inhibition of platelet aggregation to prevent myocardial reinfarction, prevention of coronary bypass graft occlusion (given with aspirin).

direct (dīrekt′), *adj* relating to any restorative procedure performed directly on a tooth without the use of a die (e.g., composite or silver amalgam restorations, a wax pattern formed in the prepared cavity, or a gold foil restoration).

direct access storage device, *n* a device used for storage of direct access files. It could be a magnetic disk or diskette units.

direct billing, *n* a process whereby the dental professional bills a patient directly for his or her fees.

direct digital imaging, *n* technique in which the image is captured on an intraoral sensor and then is viewed on a computer monitor.

direct gold, *n* any of the forms of pure gold that may be compacted directly into a prepared cavity to form a restoration.

direct pulp capping, *n* See capping, pulp, direct.

direct reimbursement, *n* a self-funded program in which the individual is reimbursed based on a percentage of dollars spent for dental care provided, allowing the beneficiary to seek treatment from the dental professional of his or her choice.

direct retainer, *n* See retainer, direct.

direct retention, *n* See retention, direct.

direct supervision, *n* a circumstance of treatment in which the dental professional must be present on the premises to diagnose, authorize, and approve all work performed on the patient by the members of the dental staff.

director, *n* **1.** a person elected by shareholders at the annual meeting to establish company policies. The directors appoint the president, vice presidents, and all other operating officers. Directors decide, among other matters, if and when dividends shall be paid. *n* **2.** the manager of an institution, office, or clinic.

directory, *n* **1.** an organized list of names, organizations, or other data bases for ease of retrieval or reference. *n* **2.** the listing of files in a computer storage system.

dirithromycin (dīrith′rōmī′sin), *n brand name:* Dynabac; *drug class:* macrolide antibiotic; *action:* binds to 50S ribosomal subunits of susceptible bacteria to inhibit bacterial growth; *uses:* treatment of secondary bacterial infection of acute bronchitis, community-acquired pneumonia, streptococcal pharyngitis, uncomplicated skin and skin structure infections.

disability, *n* the inability to function in the normal or usual manner; examples of an outcome measure are days missing from work or lessened productivity.

disability, denial of, *n* a symptom in which patients deny the existence of a disease or disability. Denial by these patients is a nonrealistic attempt to maintain their predisease status. These patients regard ill health and disability as an imperfection, a weakness, and even a disgrace.

disaccharide (dīsak′ərīd), *n* a general term for simple carbohydrates (sugars) formed by the union of two monosaccharide molecules. Sucrose is the most common disaccharide sugar.

disarticulation (dis'ärtik'ūlā'shən), *n* the amputation or separation of joint parts, as in hemimandibulectomy, with inclusion of the condyloid process of the mandible.

disc of the temporomandibular joint, *n* a plate of fibrous tissue that divides the joint into an upper and lower synovial cavity. The disc is attached to the articular capsule and moves forward with the condyle in free opening and protrusion. Also called *meniscus.* See also articulation, temporomandibular.

discharge, *v* **I.** to release; liberate; annul; unburden. *v* **2.** To cancel a contract; to make an agreement or contract null and void. *n* **3.** a substance that exudes from an opening.

discharge, purulent, n See suppuration.

discharge summary, n the clinical notes written by the discharging physician or dental professional at the time of releasing a patient from the hospital or clinic, outlining the course of treatment, the status at release, and the postdischarge expectations and instructions.

disclosing solution, *n* a chewable tablet that forms a dye in the mouth or a solution of dye applied directly to teeth that stains plaque on the surfaces of teeth. It is used to help patients identify plaque in their own oral cavities. See also plaque.

disclosing solution, two-tone, n a type that stains older dental biofilm (dental plaque) blue and newer dental biofilm (dental plaque) red.

disclosure, *n* a release of information.

disclusion (diskloo'zhən), *n* a separation of the occlusal surfaces of the teeth directly and simply by opening the jaws, or indirectly in excursions by the anterior teeth.

discoid (dis'koid), *n* a carving instrument with a blade of circular form that has a cutting edge around the entire periphery.

discoloration, enamel, *n* See tetracycline.

discoloration, gingival, *n* See gingival discoloration.

discoplasty (dis'kōplas'tē), *n* the surgical shaping or contouring of the meniscus of the temporomandibular joint.

discount, *n* **I.** an allowance or deduction made from a gross sum. *v* **2.** to reduce the amount of a professional fee.

discrete (categorical) variable, *n* variable made up of distinct and separate units or categories and counted only in whole numbers; also referred to as *mutually exclusive.*

discrimination, legal, *n* a situation that leads one to treat unequally or unfairly on the basis of race, gender, national origin, religion, or handicap.

discrimination, tactile, *n* the ability to perceive two simultaneous touch stimuli; two-point discrimination. When the distance between the two stimuli is diminished to the point where only one stimulus is perceived, a value is determined for the two-point discrimination capacity of a special part. When patients are anesthetized by local agents, they have diminished tactile sense and frequently bite their lips rather severely without being aware of it. Thus patients should be instructed not to eat or chew until the "numbness" has completely gone and full tactile sense has returned.

disease(s) (dizēz'), *n/n.pl* a definite deviation from the normal state characterized by a series of symptoms. Disease may be caused by developmental disturbances, genetic factors, metabolic factors, living agents, or physical, chemical, or radiant energy, or the cause may be unknown.

disease, Adams-Stokes (Adams-Stokes syndrome), n.pr a disease characterized by a slow and perhaps irregular pulse, vertigo, syncope, occasional pseudoepileptic convulsions, and Cheyne-Stokes respirations.

disease, adaptation (adaptation syndrome), n the metabolic disorders occurring as a result of adaptation or resistance to severe physical or psychologic stress. See also syndrome, general adaptation.

disease, Addison's, n.pr a chronic adrenocortical insufficiency caused by bilateral tuberculosis, aplasia, atrophy, or degeneration of the adrenal glands. Symptoms include severe weakness, weight loss, low blood pressure, digestive disturbances, hypoglycemia, lowered resistance to infection, and abnormal pigmentation (bronze color of the skin, with associated melanotic pigmentation of the oral mucosa, especially of the gingival tissue).

disease, adrenocortical, n the disorders of adrenocortical function, giving rise to Addison's disease, Cushing's syndrome, adrenogenital syndrome, and primary aldosteronism.

disease, Albers-Schönberg, n.pr See osteopetrosis.

disease, autoallergic, n See disease, autoimmune.

disease, autoimmune (autoallergic disease, autoimmunization syndrome, chronic hypersensitivity), n a disease that is believed to be caused in part by reactions of hypersensitivity of the host tissue (antigens). Includes various hemolytic anemias, idiopathic thrombocytopenias, rheumatoid arthritis, systemic lupus erythematosus, glomerulonephritis, scleroderma, Hashimoto's thyroiditis, and Sjögren's syndrome.

disease, Barlow's, n.pr See scurvy, infantile.

disease, Basedow's, n.pr See goiter, exophthalmic.

disease, Behçet's, n.pr See syndrome, Behçet's.

disease, Besnier-Boeck-Schaumann, n.pr See sarcoidosis.

disease, bleeder's, n See hemophilia.

disease, blood, n a disease affecting the hematologic system (e.g., anemia, leukemia, agranulocytosis purpura, infectious mononucleosis). Such a disease often results in lesions of the oral structures, particularly the mucosal surfaces.

disease, Bowen's, n.pr See carcinoma in situ.

disease, Brill-Symmers, n.pr See lymphoblastoma, giant follicular.

disease, brittle bone, n See osteogenesis imperfecta.

disease, Caffey's, n.pr See hyperostosis, infantile cortical.

disease, Cannon's, n.pr See nevus, white sponge.

disease, cardiac, n a disease affecting the heart.

disease, cat-scratch, n a granulomatous disease caused by *B. henselae* that occurs at the site of a scratch or bite of a house cat. Local lesions occur at the site of injury with a regional adenitis that is out of proportion to the primary lesion occurring within 1 to 3 weeks. Systemic symptoms of infection may occur. Diagnosis is confirmed by serologic tests.

disease, celiac, n See celiac sprue.

disease, Cheadle's, n.pr See scurvy, infantile.

disease, Christmas, n.pr See hemophilia B.

disease, chronic hypersensitivity, n See disease, autoimmune.

disease, chronic obstructive pulmonary (COPD), n a disease marked by decreased expiratory flow rates resulting in increased total lung capacity. Patients with this condition are prone to acute respiratory failure from infections or general anesthesia.

disease, collagen (group disease, visceral angiitis) (kol'əjin), n a group of diseases affecting the collagenous connective tissue of several organs and systems. These diseases have similar biochemical structural alterations and include rheumatic fever, scleroderma, rheumatoid arthritis, systemic lupus erythematosus, periarteritis, and serum sickness.

diseases, communicable, n a disease that may be transmitted directly or indirectly to a well person or animal from an infected person or animal. A disease with the capacity for maintenance by natural modes of spread (e.g., by contact, by airborne routes, through drinking water or food, by arthropod vectors).

disease, congenital, n a disease present at birth, or, more specifically, one that is acquired in utero.

disease, Coxsackie A, n.pr See herpangina.

disease, Crohn, n a type of inflammatory bowel disease that may affect any part of the gastrointestinal tract, from mouth to anus. Oral aphthous ulcers (canker sores) are common in individuals with Crohn disease. Also known as regional enteritis.

disease, Crouzon, n.pr See syndrome, Crouzon.

disease, Cushing's, n.pr hypercortisolism that results from an adrenal or pituitary neoplasm. The term Cushing's syndrome refers to hypercortisolism that is not related to an endogenous process.

disease, cytomegalic inclusion, generalized, *n* See disease, salivary gland.

disease, Darier's (keratosis follicularis), *n.pr* an apparently genetic dermatologic disease that also involves mucous membranes. The oral lesions are whitish papules of the gingiva, tongue, or palate. It is characterized histologically by the presence of corps ronds.

disease, deficiency, *n* a disturbance produced by lack of nutritional or metabolic factors. Used mainly in reference to avitaminosis.

disease, degenerative joint, *n* See osteoarthritis.

disease, dermatologic, *n* a disease affecting the skin; often accompanied by pathologic manifestations of various mucosal surfaces (e.g., the oral mucosa, genital mucosa, conjunctiva).

disease, end-stage, *n* the last phase of an illness, at which point the patient's life is gravely endangered.

disease, Engman's, *n.pr* See dermatitis infectiosa eczematoides.

disease, exanthematous (**eg′zanthē′ mətəs**), *n* a group of diseases caused by a number of viruses but having as a prominent feature a skin rash (e.g., smallpox, chickenpox, cowpox, measles, rubella).

disease, familial, *n* a disease occurring in several members of the same family. Often used to mean members of the same generation and occasionally used synonymously with hereditary disease.

disease, Feer's, *n.pr* See erythredema polyneuropathy and acrodynia.

disease, fibrocystic (mucoviscidosis) (**fī′brōsis′tik mū′kōvis′idō′sis**), *n* a hereditary defect of most of the exocrine glands in the body, including the salivary glands. The secretion of the affected mucous glands is abnormally viscous.

disease, fifth, *n* a viral infection caused by the human parvovirus B19; spread via the upper respiratory tract, this virus impacts on children more strongly than adults. Also called erythema infectiosum.

disease, Fordyce's, *n.pr* See Fordyce granules.

disease, functional, *n* a disease that has no observable or demonstrable cause.

disease, Gaucher's (**gôshāz′**), *n.pr* a constitutional defect in the metabolism of the cerebroside kerasin. This glycoprotein accumulates in the reticuloendothelial system and leads to splenomegaly, hepatomegaly, lymph node enlargement, and bone defects.

disease, graft-versus-host (GVHD), *n* a potentially deadly condition resulting from allogenically transplanted hematopoietic cells that reject host cells in the transplant recipient. In early stages, this condition may result in lichenoid and erosive lesions on the oral mucosa.

disease, Graves', *n.pr* See goiter, exophthalmic.

disease, hand-foot-and-mouth (aphthous fever, epidemic stomatitis, epizootic stomatitis) (**af′thəs**), *n* primarily a disease of animals caused by a filterable virus that may be transmitted to humans and that occasionally produces symptoms. The human form is characterized by fever, nausea, vomiting, malaise, and ulcerative stomatitis. Skin lesions consisting of vesicles may appear, usually on the palms of the hands and soles of the feet. Ulcers may occur anywhere in the mouth. Spontaneous regression usually occurs within 2 weeks.

disease, Hand-Schüller-Christian (chronic disseminated histiocytosis X), *n.pr* a type of cholesterol lipoidosis characterized clinically by defects in membranous bones, exophthalmos, and diabetes insipidus.

disease, Hansen's, *n.pr* See leprosy.

disease, heart, *n* an abnormal condition of the heart (organic, mechanical, or functional) that causes difficulty.

disease, heart, arteriosclerotic, *n* a variety of functional changes of the myocardium that result from arteriosclerosis.

disease, heart, congenital, *n* a defective formation of the heart or of the major vessels of the heart.

disease, heart, ischemic (**iskē′mik**), *n* a heart condition in which an inadequate supply of oxygenated blood reaches the heart, resulting in damage to the heart muscle; it is usually caused by atherosclerosis, a buildup of fatty plaque deposits in the main coronary arteries that leads to narrowing or hardening of the arteries. Symptoms include chest pain or discomfort (angina pectoris), ventricular fibrillation, heart attack (myocardial infarction), or sudden death. Also known as *coronary artery disease* and *coronary heart disease*.

disease, heart, rheumatic, n a scarring of the endocardium resulting from involvement in acute rheumatic fever. The process most often involves the mitral valve.

disease, heart, thyrotoxic (thī'rōto k'sik), n cardiac failure occurring as the result of hyperthyroidism or its superimposition on existing organic heart disease. Thyrotoxicosis is an important cause of atrial fibrillation.

disease, hemoglobin C, n a disease resulting from an abnormal hemoglobin (hemoglobin C); occurs primarily in African Americans and causes a mild normochromic anemia, target cells, and vague, intermittent arthralgia.

disease, hemolytic, of newborn, n a hemolysis caused by isoimmune reactions associated with Rh incompatibility or with blood transfusions in which there is an incompatibility of the ABO blood system. Several forms of the disease occur: erythroblastosis fetalis, congenital hemolytic disease, icterus gravis neonatorum, and hydrops fetalis.

disease, hemophilioid (hēməfil'ē oid), n a hemophilic states (conditions) that clinically resemble hemophilia (e.g., parahemophila, hemophilia B [Christmas disease]).

disease, hemorrhagic, of newborn (hem'əraj'ik), n a hemorrhagic tendency in newborn infants occurring usually on the third or fourth day of life; believed to be caused by defects of prothrombin and factor VII, resulting from a deficiency of vitamin K.

disease, hereditary, n a disease transmitted from parent to offspring through genes. Three main types of mendelian heredity are recognized: dominant, recessive, and sexlinked.

disease, hidebound, n See scleroderma.

disease, Hodgkin, n.pr See lymphoma, Hodgkin.

disease, hypersensitivity, n See disease, autoimmune.

disease, iatrogenic (īat'rəjen'ik), n a disease arising as a result of the actions or words of a health care professional.

disease, idiopathic (id'ēōpath'ik), n a disease in which the etiology is not recognized or determined.

disease, infectious, n the pathologic alterations induced in the tissue by the action of microorganisms and/or their toxins. Some infectious diseases involving the oral tissue are herpes zoster, herpetic gingivostomatitis, moniliasis, syphilis, and tuberculosis.

disease, inflammatory neoplastic, n See granuloma; tumor, inflammatory.

disease, kissing, n See mononucleosis, infectious.

disease, Langerhans cell (Langerhans cell histiocytosis), n a group of three diseases identified by an abundance of Langerhans cells—eosinophils combined with histiocytic cells. See also disease, Letterer-Siwe; disease, Hand-Schüller-Christian; and granuloma, eosinophilic.

disease, Letterer-Siwe (sē'vä), n.pr (acute disseminated histiocytosis X, nonlipid histiocytosis, nonlipid reticuloendotheliosis), a fatal febrile disease of unknown cause occurring in infants and children; characterized by focal granulomatous lesions of the lymph nodes, spleen, and bone marrow. Results in enlargement of the lymph nodes, spleen, and liver, defects of the flat and long bones, anemia, and sometimes purpura.

disease, lipoid storage (lipoidosis, reticuloendothelial granuloma) (lip' oid ritik'yəlōen'dōthē'lēəl gran'yə lō'mə lipoidō'sis), n group of diseases in which lipid substances accumulate in the fixed cells of the reticuloendothelial system. Included are Gaucher's disease, Niemann-Pick disease, and the Hand-Schüller-Christian disease complex. Other storage diseases include lipochondrodystrophy (gargoylism) and cerebral sphingolipidosis.

disease, Lobstein's, n.pr See osteogenesis imperfecta.

disease, macrovascular, n a disease of the large blood vessels, including the aorta, and coronary arteries. Fatty plaque buildup and thrombosis formation in these vessels may lead to a myocardial infarction, cerebral infarction, and circulation problems in the limbs. It is often a complication of long-term diabetes.

disease, Marie's, *n.pr* See acromegaly.

disease, Mediterranean, *n.pr* See thalassemia major.

disease, metabolic bone, *n.pl* the diseases of the bone which may be attributed to cellular changes or to nutritional deficiencies/excesses brought on by dietary imbalances. These include hyperparathyroidism, osteoporosis, osteomalacia, rickets, and the many diseases associated with an abnormal abundance of Langerhans cells.

disease, Mikulicz' **(mik′ūlich′əz),** *n.pr* a benign hyperplasia of the lymph nodes of the parotid or other salivary glands and/or the lacrimal glands.

disease, Moeller's, *n.pr* See scurvy, infantile.

disease, molecule, *n* a disease associated with genetically determined abnormalities of protein synthesis at the molecular level.

disease, muscle, *n* the pathologic muscle tissue changes that can lead to disease. Such changes reveal few structural alterations, and the highly differentiated contents of muscle fibers tend to react as a whole. The pathologic features that distinguish one muscle disease from another are the age and character of changes within a muscle, distribution of those changes within one or several muscles, presence of inflammatory cells and parasites, and coexistence of pathologic changes in other organs. Muscles undergo a number of degenerative changes. There are alterations in the striation in certain pathologic states caused by cloudy swelling, granular degeneration, waxy or hyaline degeneration, and other cellular modifications such as multiplication of the sarcolemmic nuclei and phagocytosis of muscle fibers.

disease, neuromuscular, *n* a condition in which various areas of the central nervous system are affected; results in dysfunction or degeneration of the musculature and disabilities of the organ.

disease, Niemann-Pick **(nē′män),** *n.pr* a congenital, familial disorder occurring mainly in Jewish female infants that terminates fatally before the third year and is characterized by the accumulation of the phospholipid sphingomyelin in the cells of the reticuloendothelial system.

disease, oral, hereditary, *n* the heritable defects of oral and paraoral structures (excluding the dentition) without generalized defects; includes ankyloglossia, hereditary gingivofibromatosis, and possibly cleft lip and cleft palate. Many oral and paraoral defects are associated with generalized defects (e.g., Peutz-Jeghers, Franceschetti, Ehlers-Danlos, Pierre Robin, and Sturge-Weber syndromes; hemorrhagic telangiectasia; Crouzon's disease; sickle cell disease; acatalasemia; white spongy nevus; xeroderma pigmentosum; gargoylism; neurofibromatosis; familial amyloidosis; and achondroplasia).

disease, oral manifestations of systemic, *n* the lesions in association with systemic disease, often influenced by the local environmental factors within the oral cavity.

disease, organic, *n* a disease in which actual structural changes have occurred in the organs or tissue.

disease, Osler's, *n.pr* See erythremia.

disease, Owren's, *n.pr* See parahemophilia.

disease, Paget's, of bone (osteitis deformans), *n.pr* a bone disease characterized by thickening and bowing of the long bones and enlargement of the skull and maxillae. It is represented radiographically by a cotton-wool appearance of the bone and microscopically by a mosaic bone pattern with so-called reversal lines. Hypercementosis and loosening of the teeth may be significant manifestations. Increased serum alkaline phosphatase may be an early finding.

disease, Parkinson's, *n.pr* a progressive neurologic disorder for which there is no known cure that is thought to be the result of neuron degeneration in the section of the brain controlling spontaneous movement and balance. The disease causes postural changes, tremors, muscle rigidity, and weakness. Oral manifestations include difficulty in swallowing and excess salivation.

disease, periodic, n See disorder(s), periodic.

disease, periodontal **(per′ēōdon′əl),** *n* a disturbance of the periodontium. Diseases affecting the periodontium include aggressive and necrotizing types, as well as gingivitis. Etiologic factors may be local or systemic or may involve an interplay between the two. Periodontal diseases may be involved in increasing the risk and course of systemic diseases.

disease, periodontal, etiologic factors of, n.pl the local and systemic factors, singly or in combination, that initiate periodontal lesions.

disease, periodontal, local factors of, n.pl the environmental conditions within the oral cavity that initiate, enable, or alter the course of diseases of the periodontium (e.g., calculus, diastemata between teeth, food impaction, prematurities in the centric path of closure, and tongue habits).

disease, peripheral vascular, n a disease of arteries, veins, and/or lymphatic vessels.

disease, pink, n See acrodynia.

disease, Pott's, n.pr a spinal curvature (kyphosis) resulting from tuberculosis.

disease progression, n the course of the disease within a patient/host from onset to resolution.

disease, psychosomatic **(sī′kōsōmat′ik),** *n* a disease that appears to have been precipitated or prolonged by emotional stress; manifested largely through the autonomic nervous system. Various conditions may be included (e.g., certain forms of asthma, dermatosis, migraine headache, and hypertension). See also disorder, psychophysiologic, autonomic, and visceral.

disease, Quincke's, n.pr See edema, angioneurotic.

disease, Rendu-Osler-Weber **(ron′ doo),** *n.pr* See telangiectasia, hereditary hemorrhagic.

disease, rheumatic, n See rheumatism.

disease, rickettsial **(riket′sēəl),** *n* a disease caused by microorganisms of the order Rickettsiales (e.g., Rocky Mountain spotted fever, rickettsialpox, typhus, and Q fever).

disease, Riga-Fede **(rē′gə-fā′də),** an ulceration of the lingual frenum of infants caused by abrasion by natal or neonatal teeth.

disease, Sainton's, n.pr See dysplasia, cleidocranial.

disease, salivary gland (generalized cytomegalic inclusion), n a generalized infection in infants caused by intrauterine or postnatal infection with a cytomegalovirus of the group of herpesviruses. Manifestations include jaundice, purpura, hemolytic anemia, vomiting, diarrhea, chronic eczema, and failure to gain weight.

disease, Schüller's **(shü′lerz),** *n.pr* See osteoporosis.

disease, Selter's, n.pr See acrodynia.

disease, sex-linked, n a hereditary disorder transmitted by the gene that also determines sex (e.g., hemophilia).

disease, sickle cell, n a hematologic disorder caused by the presence of an abnormal hemoglobin (hemoglobin S) that permits the formation or results in the formation of sickle-shaped red blood cells. Two forms of the disease occur: sickle cell trait and sickle cell anemia. See also anemia, sickle cell; trait, sickle cell.

disease, Simmonds' (pituitary cachexia, hypophyseal cachexia, hypopituitary cachexia), n.pr a panhypopituitarism resulting from destruction of the pituitary gland, usually from hemorrhage or infarction.

disease, Sturge-Weber-Dimitri (encephalotrigeminal angiomatosis), n.pr See angiomatosis, Sturge-Weber.

disease susceptibility, n the degree to which a patient or host is vulnerable to a disease.

disease, Sutton's, n.pr See periadenitis mucosa necrotica recurrens.

disease, Swift's, n.pr See acrodynia.

disease, systemic, n a disease involving the whole body.

disease, Takahara's **(tä′kəhä′rəz),** *n.pr* a form of rare progressive oral gangrene occurring in childhood and seen only in Japan. Apparently related to a congenital lack of the enzyme catalase (acatalasemia). Characterized by a mild to severe form of a peculiar type of oral gangrene that may develop at the roots of the teeth or the tonsils. Loss of teeth occurs, with necrosis of the alveolar bone. Patients become symptom free after puberty.

disease, transmissible, *n* a disease capable of being transmitted from one individual to another; a disease capable of being maintained in successive passages through a susceptible host, usually under experimental conditions such as by injection. See also disease, communicable.

disease transmission, *n* the method by which a disease is passed from one patient or host to another. The three most common methods of transmission are direct contact, aerosols, and vectors, such as insects.

disease, Vaquez' (väkēz'), *n.pr* See erythremia.

disease vectors, *n.pl* the intermediary hosts that carry the disease from one species to another, such as mosquitoes, ticks, and rabid animals.

disease, von Recklinghausen's, *n.pr* See hyperparathyroidism; osteitis; generalized fibrosa cystica; and neurofibromatosis.

　disease, von Recklinghausen's, of bone (fōn rek'linghouzenz), See hyperparathyroidism; osteitis fibrosa cystica.

　disease, von Recklinghausen's, of skin, *n.pr* See neurofibromatosis.

disease, von Willebrand's (fōn vil'ebränts), *n.pr* an inherited blood coagulation disorder attributed to a deficiency or malfunction of factor VIII. It may cause prolonged or excessive gingival bleeding.

disease, Weil's (epidemic jaundice) (vīlz), *n.pr* an acute febrile disease caused by Leptospira icterohaemorrhagiae or L. canicola. Manifestations include fever, petechial hemorrhage, myalgia, renal insufficiency, hepatic failure, and jaundice.

disease, Werlhof's (verl'hofs), *n.pr* See purpura, thrombocytopenic.

diseases, demyelinating (dēmī'ələnā' ting), *n* the diseases that have in common a loss of myelin sheath, with preservation of the axis cylinders (e.g., multiple sclerosis, Schilder's disease).

diseases, dental, hereditary, *n.pl* the heritable defects of the dentition without generalized disease, which include amelogenesis imperfecta, dentinogenesis imperfecta, dentinal dysplasia, localized and generalized hypoplasia of enamel, peg-shaped lateral incisors, familial dentigerous cysts, missing teeth, giantism, and fused primary mandibular incisors. Dental defects occurring with generalized disease include dentinogenesis imperfecta with osteogenesis imperfecta, missing teeth with ectodermal dysplasia, enamel hypoplasia with epidermolysis bullosa dystrophica, retarded eruption with cleidocranial dysostosis, missing lateral incisors with ptosis of the eyelids, missing premolars with premature whitening of the hair, and enamel hypoplasia in vitamin D–resistant rickets.

diseases, group, *n* See disease, collagen.

disharmony, occlusal (əkloo'səl), *n* a phenomenon in which contacts of opposing occlusal surfaces of teeth are not in harmony with other tooth contacts and with the anatomic and physiologic controls of the mandible. See also contact, deflective occlusal; contact, interceptive occlusal; and malocclusion.

disinfect (dis'infekt'), *v* to destroy pathogenic microorganisms.

disinfectant (dis'infek'tənt), *n* a chemical intended to destroy most pathogenic microorganisms. Does not cause sterilization.

　disinfectant, alcohol, *n* an unaccepted method of sterilization. Although ethanol and isopropanol both have cleansing properties when used on the skin, they are insufficient as sterilizers.

　disinfectant, chlorine dioxide, *n* a chemical disinfectant that can be used for 24 hours once it is activated. It can corrode some steel tools.

　disinfectant holding solution, *n* an antimicrobial liquid into which an object can be temporarily placed while awaiting sterilization.

disinfection, *n* the process of destroying pathogenic organisms or rendering them inert.

　disinfection, full oral cavity, *n* a procedure used to reduce active periodontal disease, usually completed within a certain short time frame.

disintegration, induced nuclear, *n* the disintegration resulting from artificial bombardment of a material with high-energy particles such as alpha particles, deuterons, protons, neutrons, or gamma rays.

disintegration, nuclear, *n* a spontaneous nuclear transformation (radioactivity) characterized by the emission of energy or mass from the nucleus. When numbers of nuclei are involved, the process is characterized by a definite half-life.

disk, *n* **1.** a thin, flat, circular object. *n* **2.** another word for *disc.*

disk, abrasive, *n* a disk with abrasive particles attached to one or both of its surfaces or its edge.

disk, diamond, *n* a disk of steel with diamond chips bonded to its surface.

disk, garnet, *n* a disk with particles of garnet as the abrading medium.

disk, Joe Dandy, *n.pr* the brand name for a separating disk. See also disk, separating.

disk, lightning, *n* a steel separating disk.

disk, Merkel's, *n.pr* See corpuscle, Merkel's.

disk, pack, *n* a set of circular magnetic surfaces mounted coaxially on a shaft for computer storage of files. Can be used for storage of serial or direct access files.

disk, polishing, *n* a disk with an extremely fine abrasive; used to finish and polish a surface.

disk, safe-side, *n* a separating disk with abrasive on one side only; the other side is smooth.

disk, sandpaper, *n* an abrasive disk with sandpaper as the abrading medium.

disk, separating, *n* a disk of steel or hard rubber.

disk, storage, *n* a storage device that uses magnetic recording on flat, rotating disks.

disking, *v* the act of grinding or reducing the superficial surface of the tooth with an abrasive material.

dislocation, *n* the displacement of any part, especially a bone or bony articulation.

dislodgment, *n* the movement or removal of a prosthesis from its established position.

disopyramide **(dīsōpir′əmīd′),** *n* *brand name:* Norpace CR; *drug class:*

antidysrhythmic (Class IA); *actions:* reduces automaticity, prolongs action potential duration and effective refractory period; *uses:* ventricular tachycardia.

disorder(s), *n/n.pl* derangement of function.

disorder, bipolar (bīpō′lər), *n* a major mood disorder characterized by alternating periods of mania or elation and depression. Formerly called *manic-depressive disorder.*

  disorder, bipolar, type I, *n* symptoms consists of major depression and mania.

  disorder, bipolar, type II, *n* symptoms consists of major depression and hypomania (lesser form of mania).

disorder, body dysmorphic (BDD) (dismôr′fik), *n* a mental disorder in which an otherwise physiologically healthy person obsesses about an imaginary physical defect. It is considered a form of somatoform disorder.

disorder(s), coagulation, *n/n.pl* any one of the hemorrhagic diseases caused by a deficiency of plasma thromboplastin formation (deficiency of antihemophilic factor, plasma thromboplastic antecedent, Hageman factor, Stuart factor), deficiency of thrombin formation (deficiency of prothrombin, factor V, factor VII, Stuart factor), and deficiency of fibrin formation (afibrinogenemia, fibrinogenopenia).

disorder, conversion, *n* conversion disorder is a monosymptomatic somatoform disorder that affects the voluntary motor system or sensory functions. The patient may experience blindness, deafness, paralysis, or an inability to speak or to walk.

disorder, cumulative trauma, *n* a disorder of the musculature and skeleton after repetitive strain injuries to muscles, tendons, joints, bones, and nerves.

disorder, panic, *n* an anxiety disorder marked by repeated panic attacks and fear, which interrupts normal functioning.

disorder(s), periodic, *n/n.pl* a variety of disorders of unknown cause that have in common periodic recurrence of manifestations. Such disorders are usually benign, resist treatment, often begin in infancy, and occasionally have a hereditary pattern. Included are periodic sialorrhea, neutropenia, arthralgia, fever, purpura (anaphylactoid purpura), edema (angioneurotic edema), abdominalgia, and periodic parotitis (recurrent parotitis).

disorder, pervasive developmental, n a disorder of behavioral and sensory impairment that generally appears during infancy or early childhood and continues to affect the individual's ability to communicate and interact with others throughout his or her life. See also autism.

disorder(s), platelet, n/n.pl a hemorrhagic disease caused by an abnormality of the blood platelets (e.g., thrombocytopenia, thrombasthenia).

disorder(s), posttraumatic stress, n an anxiety disorder characterized by acute or recurring anxiety which has been brought about as the result of experiencing a traumatic event, such as a natural disaster, terrorist attack, military combat, rape, physical torture, or childhood sexual abuse. Symptoms may include flashbacks, nightmares, mild to severe depression, and panic attacks.

disorder(s), psychophysiologic, autonomic, and visceral, n/n.pl the standard psychiatric nomenclature for what are commonly known as psychomotor disorders. The disorders are disturbances of visceral function, secondary to chronic attitude and long-continued reaction to stress. These disorders may occur in any organ innervated by the autonomic nervous system, since overactivity or underactivity of that system as a result of stress appears to trigger the disorder. See also disease, psychosomatic.

disorder(s), visual, n/n.pl disorders that may result from injury or disease to the eyeball and its adnexa, the retina, or the cornea (e.g., contusions of the orbit and eyelids, opacities of the lens, corneal scars, vascular changes to the retina). These peripheral disorders are effective in causing partial or total loss of vision in one or both eyes. They are simple, concrete, and fundamental. One sees or one does not see, and gray visions are generally quantitative differences that affect the perception of light and shadow and color and form. They may

also result from injury or disease to the optic tract fibers, optic chiasma, cerebral pathways, and visual cortex in the occipital region of the cerebrum. These are qualitative deviations from normal, and the symptoms include visual field defects such as tubular vision found in hysteria, complete blindness in one or both eyes as a result of optic nerve injury, and hemianopsia, in which vision may be lost in one half of the visual field of one or both eyes. Others include night and day blindness, color blindness, and the serious visual agnosia that results from trauma, tumor, or vascular disorders in the visual cortex of the cerebrum.

disorder(s), cognitive impairment, n/n.pl the mental disorders distinguished by a limitation of mental functions (e.g., memory, comprehension, and judgment).

disorder(s), dissociative, n/n.pl the mental disorders distinguished by the psychologically induced, distinct partition of separate mental functions from normal behavior or consciousness (e.g., dissociative amnesia and depersonalization disorder).

disorder(s), factitious **(faktish′əs),** *n/n.pl* the mental disorders distinguished by the self-induced creation of artificial physical or mental symptoms to assume the role of a sick individual.

disorder(s), feeding, n/n.pl conditions distinguished by an inability to eat sufficiently, a continual need to consume abnormal items of food or substances lacking nutrients, or frequent vomiting episodes without any indications of a gastrointestinal infection.

disorder(s), impulse control, n/n.pl the mental disorders distinguished by an uncontrollable tendency to commit an unplanned behavior (e.g., pathologic gambling, kleptomania, and pyromania).

disorder(s), sexual, n/n.pl disorders of sexual performance or desire, which may include sexual dysfunction, feelings of discomfort about one's gender, and perverse sexual urges or activities. Also called paraphilia.

disorder(s), sleep, n/n.pl conditions characterized by a disruption in normal sleeping patterns, which may be the result of serious medical conditions, including breathing difficulties or thyroid disorders, or external factors such as stress or substance abuse. Manifestations include insomnia, sleep apnea, and narcolepsy.

disorder(s), somatoform (sō'matə form'), *n/n.pl* disorders characterized by symptoms that seem to suggest the presence of an illness, but for which there is no physical proof. Often may be attributed to unresolved emotional conflicts. Types include conversion disorder, hypochondriasis, body dysmorphic disorder, and pain disorder.

disorder(s), substance-related, *n/n.pl* conditions or illnesses that may be directly attributed to overuse of drugs, alcohol, nicotine, or caffeine and may also include nutritional deficiencies, cardiovascular disease, oral lesions, liver disease, and sleep disorders.

disorder(s), tic, *n/n.pl* conditions characterized by involuntary and sometimes violent muscle spasms, including Tourette's syndrome and chronic motor or vocal tic disorders.

disprove, *v* to refute or to prove false by affirmative evidence to the contrary.

dissection, neck, *n* the removal of the lymph nodes and contiguous tissue from a primary site in the mandibular or maxillofacial area as treatment of neoplastic cells that have involved the regional cervical lymphatic system.

disseminated intravascular coagulation (DIC) (disem'ənātəd in' trəvas'kyələr kōag'yəlā'shən), *n* a grave coagulopathy resulting from the overstimulation of clotting and anticlotting processes in response to disease or injury, such as septicemia, acute hypotension, poisonous snake bites, neoplasms, and severe trauma.

dissociation (disō'shēā'shən), *n* the psychologically induced, distinct partition of separate mental functions (e.g., identity, memory, and awareness) from normal behavior or consciousness.

dissociation constant (pKa), *n* the equilibrium constant for a reversible dissociation; the ratio of concentrations when equilibrium is reached in a reversible reaction (when the rate of the forward reaction equals the rate of the reverse reaction).

dissociative fugue (fūg), *n* a sudden departure from a home or workplace without any ability to recall personal history or identity.

dissolve, *v* to terminate, cancel, annul, disintegrate. To release the obligation of anything, as to dissolve a partnership.

distal (dis'təl), *adj* away from the median sagittal plane of the face and following the curvature of the dental arch.

distal contact, *n* a contact area on the distal surface of a tooth.

distal end, *adj* the most posterior part of a removable dental restoration or denture flange.

distal marginal ridge, *n* a marginal ridge on the distal portion of the lingual surface of anterior teeth or the distal portion of the occlusal table on posterior teeth.

distal step, *n* see step, distal.

distance, *n* the measure of space intervening between two objects or two points of reference.

distance, cone, *n* the distance between the focal spot and the outer end of the cone; usually expressed in inches or centimeters. Modern dental roentgen-ray units usually have cone distances of from 5 to 20 inches (12.5 to 50 cm).

distance, interarch (interridge distance), *n* the vertical distance between the maxillary and mandibular arches under conditions of vertical relations that must be specified.

distance, interocclusal (interocclusal gap, freeway space), *n* the distance between the occluding surfaces of the maxillary and mandibular teeth when the mandible is in its physiologic rest position. This can be determined by calculating the difference between the rest vertical dimension and the occlusal vertical dimension of the face.

distance, interridge, *n* See distance, interarch.

distance, large interarch, *n* a large distance between the maxillary and mandibular arches.

distance, long (extended) cone, *n* the distance is usually 14 to 20 inches (35 to 50 cm). See also cone, long.

distance, object-film, *n* the distance, usually expressed in centimeters or inches, between the object being radiographed and the cassette or film.

distance, operator, n See positions at the chair.

distance, short cone, n a focal-skin distance of 9 inches (22.5 cm) or less; usually refers to the distance as determined by the cone supplied by the manufacturer of the basic radiograph unit.

distance, small interarch, n a small distance between the maxillary and mandibular arches.

distance, target-receptor (anode-receptor distance, focal-receptor distance), n the distance between the focal spot of the tube and the receptor; usually expressed in inches or centimeters.

distention, n a state of dilation.

distoclusion   (dis'tŏkloo'zhən), n the mandibular teeth occluding distal to their normal relationship to the maxillary teeth, as in an Angle Class II malocclusion. It can present either bilaterally or unilaterally.

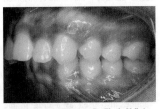
Distoclusion. (Courtesy Dr. Flavio Uribe)

distolingual marginal groove, n a developmental groove that crosses the distal marginal ridge on the lingual surface and extends onto the root on certain anterior teeth.

distomolar   (dis'tŏmŏ'lər), n a supernumerary (fourth) molar located posterior to the third molar.

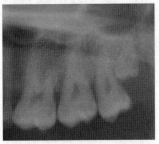
Distomolar. (Proffit/Fields/Sarver, 2013)

distortion, n **1.** a deviation from the normal shape or condition. n **2.** a modification of the speech sound in some way so that the acoustic result only approximates the standard sound and is not accurate. n **3.** a twisting or deformation. A loss of accuracy in reproduction of cavity form.

distortion, film-fault, n an imperfection in the size or shape of an image by either magnification, elongation, or foreshortening.

distortion, horizontal, n a disproportional change in size and shape of the image in the horizontal plane as a result of oblique horizontal angulation of the radiographic beam.

distortion, magnification, n a proportional enlargement of a radiographic image, a variation of the true size and shape of the object being radiographed. It is always present to some degree in oral radiography.

distortion, vertical, n a disproportional change in size, either elongation or foreshortening, caused by incorrect vertical angulation or improper receptor placement.

distoversion (dis'tōver'zhən), n the placement of a tooth farther than normal from the median plane or midline.

distraction, n the placement of teeth or other maxillary or mandibular structures farther than normal from the median plane.

distraction   osteogenesis   (DO) (distrak'shən os'tēəjen'isis), n a surgical process in which two bony segments are separated and gradually distracted so that bone will form between them. There are three periods to this process: latency, distraction, and consolidation.

disturbances,   occlusal, n.pl the derangements in the patterns of occlusion.

disulfiram (dīsul'fəram'), n *brand name:* Antabuse; *drug class:* aldehyde dehydrogenase inhibitor; *action:* blocks oxidation of alcohol at acetaldehyde stage; *use:* chronic alcoholism (as adjunct).

ditch (ditching), n the undesirable loss of tooth substance in the region of a restoration margin (usually gingival).

ditching, n the placement of a defining groove around a dental stone die just apical to the preparation margin.

diuretic (dī'yəret'ik), *n* **I.** a drug that increases the formation of urine. *adj* **2.** pertaining to the increased formation of urine. Used mainly in the initial treatment of hypertension (high blood pressure).

diuretic, loop, n a high-potency therapeutic agent used to control hypertension by exerting influence on the loop of Henle in order to facilitate the removal of surplus water and sodium from the body. See furosemide.

diurnal (dīur'nəl), *adj* relating to or happening in the daytime or portion of the day that is light.

diverticulitis (dī'vurtik'yŏŏlō'sis), *n* an inflammatory pouching of the intestinal wall.

dizziness, *n* a sensation of faintness or an inability to maintain normal balance in a standing or seated position. A patient who experiences it should be carefully lowered to a safe position on a bed, chair, or floor because of the danger of injury from falling. See also syncope.

DMF index rate, *n* See rate, DMF index.

DNA, *n* an acronym for deoxyribonucleic acid. A type of nucleic acid that contains genetic instructions for the development of cellular life forms. Capable of replicating itself and of producing another type of nucleic acid known as RNA.

DNA, bacterial, n the DNA specific to a bacterial strain.

DNA fingerprinting, n the use of DNA analysis to identify a subject from blood or other suitable tissue.

DNA probe, n See deoxyribonucleic acid probes.

DO cavity, *n* a cavity on the distal and occlusal surfaces of a tooth. See also cavity, Class 2.

double-blind study, *n* a type of experimental research in which neither the subjects nor the investigators know who is in the control (or placebo) group and who is in the other (independent variable) group that receives the experimental treatment.

docosanol *n brand name:* Abreva; *drug class:* topical antiviral; *action:* inhibits the fusion of the viral lipid envelope with the plasma membrane of the host; *use:* herpes labialis.

doctor, *n* a learned person; one qualified in a science or art; one who has received the highest academic degree in a particular field. See also dentist and physician.

documentation, *n* the permanent recording of information properly identified as to time, place, circumstances, and attribution.

docusate calcium/docusate potassium/docusate sodium (dok' usāt), *n brand names:* Colace, Correctol Extra Gentle, Sulfalax; *drug class:* laxative; *action:* increases water, fat penetration in intestine; allows for easier passage of stool; *use:* stool softener.

dolichocephalic (dol'ikōsəfal'ik), *adj* pertaining to a long and narrow head (with a cephalic index below 75).

dolor (dō'lôr), *n* any condition of physical pain, mental anguish, or suffering from heat.

donor site, *n* the portion of the body from which an organ or tissue is removed for transplant or grafting.

donor tissue, *n* the tissue contributed by a donor to be used in tissue or organ transplant.

dopa (dō'pə), *n* an amino acid derived from tyrosine that occurs naturally in plants and animals. It is a precursor of dopamine, epinephrine, and norepinephrine.

dopamine (dō'pəmēn'), *n* an endogenous sympathomimetic catecholamine, also used as a drug in the treatment of shock, hypotension, and low cardiac output.

dope, *n* a colloquial term denoting a drug taken temporarily or habitually without medical cause and that is intended to alter mood.

dornase alfa (dor'nās al'fə), *n brand name:* Pulmozyme; *drug class:* recombinant human deoxyribonuclease (DNase); *action:* reduces sputum viscosity; *uses:* cystic fibrosis, reduces incidence of pulmonary infection, improves pulmonary function.

dorsal (dôr'səl), *adj* pertaining to the back or to the posterior part of an organ.

dorsal surface of the tongue, n the top surface of the tongue.

dorsum sellae (dôr'səmsel'ē), *n* the most posterior point on the internal contour of the sella turcica.

dosage (dō'səj), *n* the amount of a medicine or other agent administered for a given case or condition.

dose, *n* **1.** the quantity of drug necessary to produce a desired effect. *n* **2.** the total radiation delivered to a specified area or volume or to the whole body. See also dose, radiation-absorbed.

dose, absorbed (D), n the amount of energy imparted by ionizing particles to unit mass of irradiated material at a place of interest. The unit of absorbed dose is the rad (100 ergs/Gm).

dose, air, n a radiographic dose delivered at a point in free air; expressed in roentgens. It consists only of the radiation of the primary beam and the radiation scattered from surrounding air; does not include backscatter from radiated matter (e.g., tissue).

dose, booster, n the portion of an immunizing agent given at a later time to stimulate the effects of a previous dose of the same agent.

dose, cumulative (kū′myələtiv), *n* the total accumulated dose resulting from a single or repeated exposure to radiation of the same region or of the whole body. If used in area monitoring, it represents the accumulated radiation exposure over a given period.

dose, depth, n the absorbed dose of radiation imparted to matter at a particular depth below the surface, usually expressed as "percentage depth dose." See also dose, percentage depth.

dose, distribution, n a representation of the variation of dose with position in any region of an irradiated object. The dose distribution may be measured using detectors small enough to avoid disturbing the distribution, or it may be calculated and expressed in mathematical form.

dose, doubling, n the amount of ionizing radiation, absorbed by the gonads of the average person in a population over a period of several generations, that will result in a doubling of the current rate of spontaneous mutations.

dose, effect curve, n See curve, dose effect.

dose, equivalent (DE), n the product of absorbed dose and modifying factors, namely the quality factor (QF), distribution factor (DF), and any other necessary factors. The unit of dose equivalent is the rem (rads times qualifying factors).

dose, erythema (erəthē′mə), *n* the dose of radiation necessary to produce a temporary redness of the skin. This dose varies with the quality of radiation.

dose, exit, n the absorbed dose delivered by a beam of radiation at the surface through which the beam emerges from a phantom or patient.

dose, exposure, n See exposure.

dose, fractionation, n a dose given by a number of shorter exposures over a longer period than would be required if the dose was given by a continuous exposure in one session at the same dose rate.

dose, gonadal, n the dose of radiation absorbed by the gonads.

dose, integral (integral absorbed dose, volume dose), n the total energy absorbed by a part or object during exposure to radiation. The unit of integral dose is the gram rad (100 ergs/gm).

dose, lethal, n **1.** the amount of a drug that would prove fatal to the majority of persons. *n* **2.** the amount of radiation that will be or may be sufficient to cause the death of an organism.

dose, maintenance, n the quantity of drug necessary to sustain a normal physiologic state or a desired blood or tissue level of drug.

dose, maximum permissible (MPD), n the maximum relative biologic effect dose that the body of a person or specific parts thereof shall be permitted to receive in a stated period. In most instances, for the roentgen rays used in dental radiography, it is satisfactory to consider the RBE dose in rems numerically equal to the absorbed dose in rads and the absorbed dose in rads numerically equal to the exposure dose in roentgens. See also dose, weekly permissible.

dose, median effective (ED50), n a dose that, under standard conditions, is effective in 50% of a randomly selected group of subjects.

dose, median lethal (LD50), n the amount of ionizing radiation or drug required to kill, within a specified period, 50% of the individuals in a large group or population of animals or organisms.

dose, minimum lethal (MLD), n the minimal amount of a drug that will kill an experimental animal.

dose, percentage depth, n the ratio (expressed as a percentage) of the absorbed dose at a given depth in an irradiated body, to the absorbed dose at a fixed reference point on the central ray, usually the surface-absorbed dose.

dose, priming, n a quantity several times larger than the maintenance dose; used at the initiation of therapy to rapidly establish the desired blood and tissue levels of the drug.

dose, protraction (prōtrak'shən), n a method of radiation administration delivered continuously over a relatively long period at a relatively low dosage rate.

dose, radiation, n the amount of energy absorbed per unit mass of tissue at a site of interest. Note: This definition limits the use of "dose" to conform with the 1962 recommendations of the International Commission on Radiological Units and Measurements (ICRUM). The following terms therefore become obsolete but will be found in this dictionary under the general heading of exposure: air dose, cumulative dose, exposure dose, and threshold dose.

dose, radiation-absorbed (rad), n the unit of absorbed dose, with a value of 100 ergs per gram.

dose, rate, n the time rate at which radiation dose is applied, expressed in either roentgens per unit time or rads per unit time.

dose, safely tolerated (STD), n the dose that can be safely tolerated without producing serious acute toxicity.

dose, skin, n See dose, surface-absorbed.

dose, subantimicrobial (sub'antē mīkrō'bēəl), n the quantity of medication to be taken at one time for purposes other than the elimination of disease-causing microorganisms.

dose, surface-absorbed, n the absorbed dose delivered by a radiation beam at the point where the central ray passes through the superficial layer of the phantom or patient.

dose, therapeutic, n a quantity several times larger than the maintenance dose; used in vitamin therapy in which a marked deficiency exists.

dose, threshold, n the minimum dose that will produce a detectable degree of any given effect.

dose, tissue, n the dose absorbed by a tissue or tissues in a region of interest.

dose, tolerance, n See dose, maximum permissible.

dose, toxic, n the amount of a drug that causes untoward symptoms in the majority of persons.

dose, transit, n a measure of the primary radiation transmitted through the patient and measured at a point on the central ray at some point beyond the patient.

dose, U.S.P, n See dose, median effective (ED50); dose, lethal.

dose, volume, n See dose, integral.

dose, weekly permissible, n a dose of ionizing radiation accumulated in 1 week and of such magnitude that, in view of present knowledge, exposure at this weekly rate for an indefinite period of time is not expected to cause appreciable bodily injury during a person's lifetime.

dosimetry (dōsim'etrē), n the accurate and systematic determination of the amount of radiation to which an animal or person has been exposed during a given period.

dosimeter, thermoluminescent (TLD), n measures ionizing radiation exposure by measuring the amount of visible light emitted from a crystal in the detector when the crystal is heated. The amount of light emitted is dependent upon the radiation exposure.

dovetail (dov'tāl), n a widened or fanned-out portion of a prepared cavity, usually established deliberately to increase the retention and resistance form.

dovetail, lingual, n a dovetail established as a step portion, with lingual approach, in some Class 3 and Class 4 preparations; used to supplement the retentions and resistance form.

dovetail, occlusal, n a dovetail established at the terminal of the occlusal step of a proximal cavity.

dowel, n a post or pin, usually made of metal, fitted into a prepared root canal of a natural tooth to improve retention of a restoration.

Down syndrome, n a congenital condition characterized by varying degrees of mental retardation and multiple developmental defects. It is most commonly caused by the presence of an extra chromosome 21. It is also called *trisomy 21* and *trisomy G syndrome.* The term *mongolism* is no longer used.

downcoding (doun′kō′ding), *n* a practice of third-party payers in which the benefits code has been changed to a less complex or lower cost procedure than was reported.

downtime, *n* the time interval during which a device is malfunctioning or inoperative.

doxazosin mesylate (doksā′zōsin mes′ilāt′), *n brand name:* Cardura; *drug class:* peripheral α-adrenergic receptor blocker; *action:* peripheral blood vessels are dilated, peripheral resistance lowered, sphincter and trigone muscles of the urinary bladder are relaxed; *uses:* hypertension, benign prostate hyperplasia.

doxepin HCl, *n brand name:* Sinequan; *drug class:* antidepressant, tricyclic; *action:* inhibits both norepinephrine and serotonin (5-HT) reuptake in synapses in brain; uses: major depression, anxiety.

doxepin (topical) (dok′səpin), *n* brand name: Zonalon; *drug class:* topical antipruritic (tricyclic antidepressant); *action:* antipruritic mechanism unknown; has antihistaminic activity; also produces drowsiness; *uses:* pruritus associated with eczema, atopic dermatitis, lichen simplex chronicus.

doxorubicin, *n* brand names: Adriamycin, Doxil; *drug class:* antibiotic antineoplastic; *action:* intercalates with DNA and prevents its functioning; *uses:* Hodgkins disease, acute leukemia, neuroblastoma, multiple myeloma, bladder cancer, carcinomas of the lung, GI tract, ovary, breast.

doxycycline hyclate (dok′sisī′klēn hī′klāt), *n* brand names: Doryx, Doxy-Caps, Vibra-Tabs; *drug class:* tetracycline, broad-spectrum tetracycline antibiotic; *action:* inhibits protein synthesis in microorganisms; *uses:* rickettsial diseases, Lyme disease, *Chlamydia trachomatis and pneumonae,* gonorrhea, lymphogranuloma venereum, uncommon gram-negative and gram-positive organisms, localized aggressive periodontitis.

drachm (dram), *n* See dram.

draft, *n* See draw.

drag, *n* the lower, or cast, side of a denture mold or flask, to which the cope is fitted. The base of the cast is embedded in plaster or stone, with the remainder of the denture pattern exposed to be engaged by the plaster or stone in the cope (the upper part of the flask).

drain, *n* **1.** a substance that provides a channel for release or discharge from a wound. *v* **2.** to release or remove a fluid substance.

drain, cigarette, *n* See drain, Penrose.

drain, Penrose (cigarette), *n.pr* a thin-walled rubber tube through which a piece of gauze has been pulled.

drainage, *n* the placement or creation of a pathway from a deep lesion to the surface of the body to provide an avenue for the body to expel the byproducts of an infection or inflammation.

dram (drachm), *n* a unit of weight that equals the eighth part of the apothecaries' ounce. Symbol 3.

draught (draft), *n* See draw.

draw (draft, draught), *n* the taper or divergence of the walls of a preparation for insertion of a cemented restoration.

dressing, chemically cured, *n* a protective covering that contains the ingredients and accelerator necessary to initiate a chemical process upon application to a wound.

dressing, Coe-pak, *n.pr* the brand name of a commonly used chemical-cured dressing that is easy to place and remove. It is available as a pliable paste.

dressing, collagen (kol′əjin), *n* a protective covering made of natural materials that are particularly suited for application over moist or bleeding wounds.

dressing, Kirkland cement, *n.pr* a surgical dressing applied to the tissue after periodontal surgery; consists of zinc oxide, tannic acid, and powdered rosin, admixed with a liquid composed of lump rosin, sweet almond oil, and eugenol.

dressing, PerioCare, *n.pr* the brand name of a commonly used chemical-cured dressing that provides comfortable protection and is easy to apply and remove; available as a pliable paste-gel.

dressing, postoperative surgical, *n* a protective obtundent dressing applied to the teeth and tissues after surgical periodontal therapy. In general, dressings have no curative properties, but may assist healing by protecting the tissues after surgery. Also known as *periodontal dressing.*

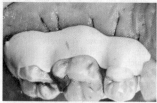

Postoperative surgical dressing. (Rose/Mealey/Genco, 2004)

dressing, pressure, *n* a protective covering applied with pressure on top of a wound in order to stop bleeding or to hold a tissue flap or graft in place.

dressing, Ward's, *n.pr* See Ward's Wonderpack.

DRG, *n* the abbreviation for diagnosis-related group, also dorsal root ganglion.

drift, *n* See tooth, drifting.

drill, *n* a cutting instrument for boring holes by rotary motion.

drill, bibevel **(bībev′əl),** *n* a drill with two flattened sides and the end cut in two beveled planes.

drill, spear-point, *n* a drill with a tri-beveled, or three-planed, point.

drill, trephine **(trifin′),** *n* a surgical drill with a hollow cutting head used to remove a circular section of bone or other tissue; also used to remove failed dental implants.

drill, twist, *n* a drill with one or more deep spiral grooves that extend from the point to the smooth part of the shaft. This term most often refers to bone cutting drills used in the preparation of parallel dental implant osteotomy sites.

drilling, *n* a colloquial term for boring a hole into a tooth with a rotary cutting instrument during cavity preparation. See also preparation, cavity.

drip, *n* the continuous slow intravenous introduction of fluid containing nutrients or drugs.

dronabinol (Delta -9-tetrahydrocannabinol), *n brand name:* Marinol; *drug class:* cannabinoid; *action:* stimulates cannabinoid receptor in the brain and reduces nausea and vomiting; *uses:* nausea and anorexia in AIDS patients, nausea and vomiting due to chemotherapy.

droperidol (drōper′adol), *n* a butyrophenone drug used in neuroleptanalgesia and preanesthetic medication.

droplet spread, *n* transmission of an infection through the projection of oral and nasal secretions by coughing, sneezing, or talking.

dropsy (drop′sē), *n* See anasarca.

drowning, *n* asphyxiation because of submersion in a liquid.

drug(s), *n/n.pl* a substance used in the prevention, cure, or alleviation of disease or pain or as an aid in some diagnostic procedures.

drug absorption, *n* See absorption, drug.

drug abuse, *n* an excessive or improper use of drugs, especially through self-administration for non-medical purposes. This term has increased significance because of the enactment of the Comprehensive Drug Abuse Prevention and Control Act of 1970, which replaces the Harrison Narcotic Act. See also substance abuse.

drug combinations, *n.pl* the use of drugs together to enhance the properties of both to the benefit of the patient.

drug dependence, *n* a physical or psychologic state in which a person displays withdrawal symptoms if drug use is halted suddenly; can lead to addiction.

Drug Enforcement Administration (DEA), *n.pr* the federal agency charged with monitoring use and abuse of narcotics. It provides the drug schedules used to determine the addiction potential of dental drugs.

drug hypersensitivity, *n* an allergic reaction that occurs after exposure to a suspect medication. It may manifest with a fever or rash and in severe cases, organ damage or death. It is classified as (1) immediate or occurring rapidly after exposure, or (2) delayed or occurring several days after exposure.

drug idiosyncrasy (**id′ēōsing′krəsē**), *n* an unusual reaction to a drug due to an altered enzyme activity in the patient. The trait is hereditary. In some cases the term is used to characterize an unexplained reaction to a drug.

drug interaction, *n* a modification of the effect of a drug when administered with another drug. The effect may be an increase or a decrease in the action of either substance, or it may be an adverse effect that is not normally associated with either drug.

drug resistance, *n* the capacity of a microorganism to build a tolerance to a drug.

drug stability, *n* the length of time a drug retains its properties without loss of potency; usually referred to as shelf life.

drug therapy, *n* the use of a drug in the treatment of a patient with a specific disease or illness.

drug tolerance, *n* the body's ability to increasingly withstand the effects of the substance being used, thereby requiring larger quantities of said substance in order to bring about the desired result.

drug toxicity, *n* the critical or lethal reaction to an erroneous dosage of a medication. Drug toxicity may occur due to human error or intentional overdose in the case of suicide or homicide.

drugs, antibiotic, *n.pl* the chemical compounds obtained from certain living cells of lower plant forms, such as bacteria, yeasts, and molds. They are antagonistic to certain pathogenic organisms and have a lethal or growth-inhibiting effect on them.

drugs, antimicrobial, *n.pl* the drugs, including penicillin and its derivatives, used to combat viral, fungal, and parasitic infections.

drugs, antiseptic, *n.pl* the chemical compounds used to reduce the number of microorganisms in the area of application such as the oral cavity.

drugs, autonomic, *n.pl* the drugs that mimic or block the effects of stimulation of the autonomic nervous system.

drugs, desensitizing, *n.pl* the agents used to diminish or eliminate sensitivity of teeth, especially the dentin, to physical, chemical, thermal, or other irritants (e.g., strontium chloride, silver [ammoniacal] or potassium nitrate, sodium fluoride, formalin, zinc chloride). See also hypersensitivity, dentin.

drugs, endodontic, *n.pl* the drugs used in treating the dental pulp and dental periapical tissue.

drugs, generic, *n.pl* nonproprietary agents.

drugs, nonofficial, *n.pl* the drugs that are not listed in the United States Pharmacopeia (U.S.P.) or the National Formulary (N.F.).

drugs, official, *n.pl* the drugs listed in the U.S.P. or N.F.

drugs, officinal (**ōfis′inəl**), *n.pl* drugs that may be purchased without a prescription. More commonly called *over-the-counter (OTC) drugs.*

drugs, over-the-counter (OTC), *n.pl* the drugs that may be purchased without a prescription. Sometimes called nonlegend drugs because the label does not bear the prescription legend required on all drugs that may be dispensed only on prescription.

drugs, parasympathetic (**par′əsim′p əthet′ik**), *n.pl* drugs that mimic the action of the parasympathetic nervous system.

drugs, parasympatholytic (**per′ə sim′pəthōlit′ik**), *n.pl* the drugs that block nerve impulses passing from parasympathetic nerve fibers to postganglionic neuroeffectors or drugs that block muscarinic cholinergic agonists.

drugs, parasympathomimetic (**per′ əsim′pəthōmimet′ik**), *n.pl* the drugs that have an effect similar to that produced when the parasympathetic nerves are stimulated.

drugs, proprietary (**prəprī′iter′ē**), *n.pl* the drugs that are patented or controlled by a private organization or manufacturer.

drugs, psychoactive (**sī′kōak′tiv**), *n. pl* the drugs or other agents that have the capacity to become habit forming because of their influence on mood, behavior, or conscious thought; may be therapeutic or recreational.

drugs, sympathetic, *n.pl* the agents that imitate the sympathetic autonomic nervous system actions. They usually cause raised levels of alertness and anxiety. Various types are used in dentistry as vasoconstrictors in conjunction with local anesthetics. See also adrenergic agents.

dry field, *n* the isolation of a surgical or operating field from body fluids such as saliva and blood. A dry field is essential in the placement of some enamel sealants and restorative fillings.

Dry-foil, *n.pr* the brand name for tinfoil that is supplied with an adhesive powder or coating on one side.

dry heat, *n* a method of sterilization of suitable instruments using a well-calibrated and time-controlled convection oven.

dry ice, *n* a solid form of carbon dioxide, with a temperature of about −140° F.

dry socket, *n* See socket, dry and osteitis.

drying, for sealant application, *n* the removal of moisture from the affected area prior to applying a sealant.

DSM-V (Diagnostic and Statistical Manual of Mental Disorders), *n* a publication of the American Psychiatric Association that classifies mental conditions.

dual choice (dual option), *n* the federal legislation that requires employers to give their employees the option to enroll in a local health maintenance organization rather than in the conventional employer-sponsored health program.

dual impression technique, *n* See technique, impression, dual.

duct, *n* a small passage such as in glandular tissue.

duct, Bartholin's, *n* See duct, sublingual.

duct, frontonasal, *n* the drainage canal of each frontal sinus to the nasal cavity.

duct, intercalated, *n* a duct that is connected to an acinus of the salivary glands. See also acinus.

duct, nasopalatine **(nā′zōpal′ət ĭn),** *n* See cyst, nasopalatine.

duct, parotid, *n* the duct of the parotid gland; it passes lateral to the masseter muscle and enters the oral cavity through the buccal tissue adjacent to the maxillary first and second molars. Older term is *Stenson's duct.*

duct, right lymphatic, *n* the duct formed from the convergence of the lymphatics of the right arm and thorax and the right jugular trunk that drains this side of the head and neck.

duct, Stensen's, *n.pr* See duct, parotid.

duct, striated, *n* a part of the ductal system to which the intercalated ducts are connected in the lobules of the salivary gland.

duct, sublingual **(subling′gwəl),** *n* the duct associated with sublingual salivary gland. Located on the floor of the oral cavity, inferior to the tongue. Older term is *Bartholin's duct.*

duct, submandibular, *n* the excretory duct of the submandibular glands; opens into the oral cavity at the sublingual caruncle on the floor of the mouth, posterior to the mandibular incisor teeth. Older term is *Wharton's duct.*

duct, thoracic, *n* the lymphatic duct draining the lower half of the body and left side of the thorax and draining the left side of the head and neck through the left jugular trunk.

duct, thyroglossal, *n* the tube that connects the thyroid gland with the base of the tongue during prenatal development and later becomes obliterated.

duct, Wharton's, *n.pr* See duct, submandibular.

ductility (duktil′itē), *n* the property of a material that allows permanent deformation under tension without rupture. It is measured as a percentage increase in length on rupture compared with original length and is termed percentage elongation, or elongation.

due process, *n* the rules governing the fair practice of law. Due process dictates that everyone is equal in the eyes of the law, and it also states that the law must be fair and clearly stated to prevent arbitrary actions by the state.

Duke's test, *n.pr* See test, Duke's.

Duloxetine, *n* brand name: Cymbalta; *drug class:* antidepressant; *action:* blocks re-uptake of serotonin (to a greater degree) and norepinephrine (to a lesser degree) in the central nervous system; *uses:* depression, anxiety, fibromyalgia, neuropathic pain in the diabetic, chronic musculoskeletal pain.

duodenal ulcer, *n* a peptic ulcer located in the duodenum. See also ulcer, peptic.

duodenum (doo'ədē'nəm), *n* the first, shortest, and most fixed portion of the small intestine. The duodenum courses from the pyloric valve of the stomach and terminates in a junction with the jejunum at the duodenojejunal flexure.

duplication, *n* the procedure of accurately reproducing a cast or other object.

   duplication impression, *n* See duplication.

dust-borne organisms, *n.pl* the organisms, including pathogens, which enter an inhabited space attached to dust particles and contaminate the contents of the inhabited space or the respiratory tracts of the inhabitants.

duty, *n* that which is due from a person; that which a person owes to another; an obligation.

DVD, *n* the acronym for digital versatile disk or digital video disk. A high-density compact disk for storing large amounts of data, especially high-resolution audio-video material.

dwarf, pituitary (pitoo'iterē), *n* an individual who is of small stature as a result of a deficiency of growth hormones. Such dwarfs usually are well proportioned.

dwarfism, *n* deficient growth and development leading to small stature and often skeletal deformity. It may be associated with ovarian agenesis, pituitary insufficiency, mongolism, progeria, rickets, renal disease, dietary deficiency, achondroplasia, cleidocranial dysostosis, osteogenesis imperfecta, microcephaly, hydrocephaly, sexual precocity, and delayed adolescence.

dyclonine hydrochloride (dī'klən ēn), *n* a ketone-type liquid topical anesthetic agent that may be applied with a cotton swab or used as a lozenge.

dye, occlusal registration, *n* a water-soluble dye used as an aid in locating occlusal contacts. A valuable aid in effecting fine adjustments in the final phases of the selective grinding procedure.

dyes, dental biofilm detection, *n.pl* See disclosing solution.

dyes, treatment, *n.pl* the dyes used in medicine and dentistry in the treatment of diseased states, the most useful of which are the rosaniline dyes (e.g., gentian violet, crystal violet) and the fluorescein dyes (e.g., Mercurochrome), which possess antiseptic and protective properties.

dynamic relation, *n* See relation, dynamic.

dyphylline (dī'fəlin), *n brand names:* Dilor, Dyflex, Lufyllin; *drug class:* Xanthine derivative; *action:* relaxes smooth muscle of respiratory system and has anti-inflammatory effects by blocking phosphodiesterase and by blocking adenosine receptors; *uses:* bronchial asthma, bronchospasm in chronic bronchitis, COPD, emphysema.

dysarthria (disärth'rēə), *n* a speech impediment brought on by emotional distress, paralysis, or muscle spasticity.

dysautonomia, familial (dis'ôtōnō' mēə), *n* See syndrome, Riley-Day.

dyscrasia (diskrā'zhə, -zēə), *n* **1.** a morbid condition, especially one that involves an imbalance of component elements. *n* **2.** an abnormal composition of the blood, such as that found in leukemia and anemia.

dysdiadochokinesia (dis'dīad'ōkō kinē'zhə, -zēə), *n* a disturbance of musculoskeletal function. There is a disorganization in the reciprocal innervation of agonists and antagonists and a loss of the ability to stop one act in terms of rate, magnitude, and the direction of movement and immediately to follow it with another act diametrically opposite (e.g., alternately elevating and depressing the mandible). Another example is observed in the inappropriate use of the tongue during mastication when it is necessary to change, reverse, and modify the energy and direction of movement.

dysentery (dis'ənter'ē), *n* an inflammation of the intestine, especially of the colon, that may be caused by chemical irritants, bacteria, protozoa, or parasites. It is characterized by frequent and bloody stools and severe abdominal pain.

dysesthesia (dis'esthē'zhə, -zēə), *n* an impairment of the senses, especially the sense of touch. No sensation is painful with dysesthesia.

dysfunction (disfunk′shən), *n* (mal-function), an abnormality or impairment of function or the inability of a body, organ, or organ system to perform normally.

dysfunction, dental, *n* an abnormal functioning or impairment of the functioning of the dental organ.

dysfunction, endocrine, *n* an abnormality in the function of an endocrine gland, either by hypofunction or hyperfunction of the secretory elements of the gland.

dysfunction, immune, *n* a reduction in the function of the immune system most often associated with chronic fatigue syndrome (CFIDS), which causes prolonged periods of debilitating fatigue.

dysgeusia (disgyoo′zēə), *n* an abnormal or impaired sense of taste.

dysgnathia (disnā′thēə), *n* the abnormalities that extend beyond the teeth and include the maxilla, the mandible, or both. See also anomaly, dysgnathic.

dyslexia (dislek′sēə), *n* an impairment of the ability to read. These persons often reverse letters and words, cannot adequately distinguish the letter sequences in written words, and have difficulty determining left from right.

dyslipidema (dislip′idēmə), *n* a state characterized by irregular or elevated quantities of lipids or lipoproteins in the blood. Dyslipidemia can be the result of genetic predisposition or lifestyle issues such as poor diet.

dysmenorrhea (dis′menərē′ə), *n* painful menstruation.

dysmetria (dismē′trēə), *n* the loss of ability to gauge distance, speed, or power of movement associated with muscle function; (e.g., the patient is unable to control the force of closure and strikes the opposite occluding teeth with greater vigor than necessary).

dysmorphism (dismôr′fizəm), *n* an aberration of form.

dysostosis (disostō′sis), *n* defective ossification.

dysostosis, cleidocranial (Sainton's disease) (klī′dōkrā′nēəl), *n* See dysplasia, cleidocranial.

dysostosis, craniofacial, *n* See syndrome, Crouzon.

dysostosis, mandibulofacial (Treacher-Collins syndrome), *n* a developmental disturbance of the cranial bones and hypoplasias of the upper part of the face. The mandibular body is underdeveloped, but the ramus is hyperplastic. The teeth are crowded and malposed.

dysostosis multiplex, *n* See syndrome, Hurler's.

dyspepsia, *n* a vague feeling of epigastric discomfort, felt after eating. It is not a distinct condition but may be a sign of underlying intestinal disorder, such as peptic ulcer, gallbladder disease, or chronic appendicitis. The symptoms usually increase during periods of stress.

dysphagia (disfā′jēə), *n* difficulty in swallowing. It may be caused by lesions in the oral cavity, pharynx, or larynx; neuromuscular disturbances; or mechanical obstruction of the esophagus (e.g., dysphagia of Plummer-Vinson syndrome [sideropenic dysphagia], peritonsillar abscess, Ludwig's angina, and carcinoma of the tongue, pharynx, larynx).

dysphoria (disfōr′ēə), *n* a feeling of discomfort or restlessness. See also euphoria.

dysplasia (displā′zhə), *n* in general, an abnormality of formation or shape. Epithelial dysplasia is characterized by an abnormality of cell shape and size, hyperchromatic state, increased size of nuclei, and an increased rate of cell division and abnormal mitotic configurations.

dysplasia, anteroposterior (anteroposterior facial dysplasia), *n* an abnormal anteroposterior relationship of the maxillae and mandible to each other or to the cranial base.

dysplasia, cementoosseous, *n* a fairly common benign fibroosseous lesion (BFOL) that appears in the jawbone. They appear on radiographic examinations as highly visible areas of mixed radiolucent/radiopaque bone. The three categories of cementoosseous dysplasia are focal, periapical, and florid. Such lesions are easily diagnosed with radiographic examination and do not require a biopsy, which can damage adjacent bone tissue.

dysplasia, cleidocranial (Sainton's disease) **(klī′dōkrā′nēəl),** *n* a familial disease or congenital disorder characterized by failure to form, or retarded formation of, the clavicles; delayed closure of the sutures and fontanels; and delayed eruption of teeth, with formation of supernumerary teeth. It is characterized by underdevelopment of the maxillae, agenesis or aplasia of the clavicle, abnormalities in other skeletal bones and muscles, and irregularities of the dentition. The syndrome may be mutational or transmitted on an autosomal dominant basis.

dysplasia, craniofacial, n a disharmony between the cranium and the face.

dysplasia, dentinal, n a genetic disturbance of the dentin characterized by early calcification of the pulp chambers and root canals and by root deformity. It is differentiated from dentinogenesis imperfecta by the latter's characteristics of attrition and relative freedom from root resorption.

dysplasia, dentofacial, n a disharmony between teeth and bones of the face (e.g., crowding and spacing).

dysplasia, ectodermal (**ek'tōdur'məl**), n a group of diseases characterized by failure to form two or more ectodermal derivatives. Sweat glands and teeth may be missing (anhidrosis and hypodontia, respectively), and there may be scant hair, faulty fingernails, and malformation of the iris.

dysplasia, enamel, n a development abnormality of enamel tissue.

dysplasia, epithelial, n a histologic diagnosis that indicates disordered growth. It is considered a premalignant condition.

dysplasia, fibroosseous, n See dysplasia, fibrous.

dysplasia, fibrous (fibroosseous dysplasia), n a metabolic disturbance characterized by replacement of the bone marrow with fibrous tissue and slow, progressive remolding and enlargement of the bone. It may be monostotic (limited to one bone) or polyostotic (present in many bones). McCune-Albright syndrome shows polyostotic fibrous dysplasia and other symptoms. See also syndrome, McCune-Albright.

dysplasia, focal osseous, n See fibroma, periapical.

dysplasia, maxillomandibular (**mak'sōmandib'yələr**), n a disharmony between one jaw and the other.

dysplasia, osseous (**os'ēəs**), n a chronic reaction of the bone to injury characterized by replacement of the bone marrow with fibrous connective tissue, unilateral enlargement of the maxillae or mandible, and characteristic radiographic findings. It is similar or identical to monostotic fibrous dysplasia and ossifying fibroma.

dysplasia, polyostotic fibrous (**pol' ēostot'ik fīb'rəs**), n the disease of fibrous dysplasia occurring in more than one bone. See also dysplasia, fibrous; osteofibroma; and syndrome, Albright's.

dyspnea (**dispnē'ə**), n difficult, labored, or gasping breathing; inspiration, expiration, or both may be involved.

dystonia (**distō'nēə**), n any impairment of muscle tone. The condition commonly involves the head, neck, and tongue and often occurs as an adverse effect of a medication.

dystrophy (**dis'trōfē**), n a state of faulty nutrition. Often used to refer to the results of faulty nutrition, that is, wasting away.

E

E space, n the net difference between the combined mesiodistal width of the primary canine, primary first molar, and primary second molar and that of the permanent canine, first premolar, and second premolar. In the mandible the mean leeway space is 3.4 mm, and in the maxilla it is 1.9 mm. Also called *leeway space.*

Eames' **technique** (**ēmz**), n See technique, Eames'.

e-antigen, n a peptide present in blood infected with the hepatitis B virus. The e-antigen is indicative of an actively reproducing hepatitis B virus and probable liver damage.

early childhood caries (ECC), *n.pl* the presence of one or more decayed, missing (due to caries), or filled tooth surfaces in any primary tooth in a child under the age of six years. In children under three years of age, any sign of smooth-surface caries is severe early childhood caries (S-ECC).

early and periodic screening, diagnosis, and treatment (EPSDT), *n. pr* service for persons under twenty-one years of age for medical, dental, and vision care paid by Medicaid.

Early Head Start program, *n* federal program that promotes the economic and social well-being of pregnant women and their children up to age three.

early-onset, *adj* describes a condition that has occurred before the normally prescribed time (e.g., early-onset Alzheimer's refers to the presence of Alzheimer's disease in persons younger than the age of 65, the average age of onset.)

earnings report, *n* a statement issued by a company showing its earnings or losses over a given period. The earnings report lists the income earned, expenses, and net result. Also called *income statement.*

ears, hemifacial microsomia in, *n* a craniofacial malformation consisting of unilateral mandibular hypoplasia, macrostomia, and ear deformities, often associated with ocular and vertebral anomalies (*oculoauriculovertebral spectrum,* for which this term is sometimes used synonymously). Most cases are sporadic, but instances of autosomal dominant or recessive inheritance have been reported.

eating disorders, *n.pl* the two major eating disorders are anorexia nervosa and bulimia nervosa. Binge eating disorder (BED) is a more recently described syndrome characterized by repeated episodes of binge eating, similar to those of bulimia nervosa, in the absence of inappropriate compensatory behavior.

EBIT, *n* the abbreviation for *earnings before interest and taxes.*

eburnation (ē'burnā'shən), *n* an increase in bony density into an ivory-like mass. See also osteitis, condensing and dentin eburnation.

eccentric (eksen'trik), *n* **I.** a deviation from the normal or conventional.

adj **2.** away from the central or reference position.

eccentric checkbite, *n* See record, interocclusal, eccentric.

eccentric jaw relation, *n* See relation, jaw, eccentric.

eccentric occlusion, *n* See occlusion, eccentric.

eccentric position, *n* See position, eccentric.

ecchymosis (ek'imō'sis), *n* a discoloration of mucous membranes caused by a diffuse extravasation of blood. See also bruise.

echocardiogram, *n* a visual representation, produced through ultrasound waves, of the heart's structure and movement.

echocardiography (ek'ōkar'dēog'rə fē), *n* a diagnostic procedure for studying the structure and motion of the heart using ultrasonic waves that pass through the heart and are reflected backward, or echoed, when they pass from one type of tissue to another.

echolalia (ek'ōlā'lyə), *n* an uncontrollable reiteration of a word or phrase recently stated by another individual.

echoviruses (ECHO virus), *n.pl* an enteric pathogen associated with fever and mild respiratory disease; sometimes may produce an aseptic meningitis.

ecology, *n* the study of the interaction between living organisms and their environment.

econazole nitrate (topical), *n brand names:* Ecostatin, Spectazole; *drug class:* local antifungal; *action:* interferes with fungal cell membrane by inhibiting ergosterol synthesis, leading to an increase in permeability and leaking of cell nutrients; *uses:* tinea pedis, tinea cruris, tinea corporis, tinea versicolor, cutaneous candidiasis.

economics, *n* in dentistry, a broad term that covers all the business aspects of dental practice.

ecosystem, *n* the sum total of all living and nonliving things that support the chain of life events within a particular area.

ecstasy (MDMA, 3-4-methylenedioxymethampheta-mine), *n* synthetic drug with amphetamine-like and hallucinogenic properties. It is classified as a stimulant and is often used recreationally. Frequent users tend to neglect themselves, including their oral health.

ectoderm (ek′tədurm), *n* the outermost of the three primary cell layers of an embryo. The ectoderm gives rise to the nervous system, the organs of special sense, the epidermis, and epidermal tissue such as fingernails, hair, and skin glands.

ectodermal dysplasia (ek′tədurməl displā′zhə), *n* See dysplasia, ectodermal.

ectomesenchyme (ek′tōmez′ənk īm), *n* a mass of tissue consisting of neurocrest cells present in the early formation of an embryo. It eventually forms the hard and soft tissue of the neck and cranium.

ectomorph (ek′tōmôrf), *n* a constitutional body type (Sheldon's classification) characterized by long, fragile bones and a highly developed nervous system.

ectopia lentis, *n* a displacement of the lens of the eye.

ectopic (ektop′ik), *adj* occurring outside the expected or usual location; displaced.

ectopic eruption, *n* See eruption, ectopic.

ectopic pregnancy, *n* the implantation occurring outside the uterus.

ectropion (ektrō′pēon), *n* an eversion, or rolling outward, of the eyelid margin.

eczema (ek′zəmə), *n* an inflammatory skin disease characterized by vesiculation, inflammation, watery discharge, and the development of scales and crusts. The large variety of types can be distinguished according to location and causal agent.

ED50, *n* See dose, median effective.

edema (edē′mə), *n* the accumulation of fluid in the tissue or in the peritoneal or pleural cavities. Primary factors favoring edema are increased capillary hydrostatic pressure (increased venous pressure), decreased osmotic pressure of plasma (hypoproteinemia), decreased tissue tension and lymphatic drainage, increased osmotic pressure of tissue fluids, and increased capillary permeability. Additional renal and hormonal factors are important. Clinical manifestations may consist of a steady weight gain or localized or generalized swelling.

edema, angioneurotic **(an′jēōnerot′ ik),** *n* See angioedema.

edema, cardiac, *n* an edema caused by venous congestion in association with congestive heart failure; tends to appear first in such dependent parts as the legs.

edema, dependent, *n* an edema that changes its position with the posture of dependent parts (e.g., edema of the legs in progressive heart failure).

edema, Ehlers-Danlos syndrome, *n* a group of inherited disorders of the connective tissue; they were formerly classified into ten types, but more recently only six types are distinguished, varying widely in severity. The major manifestations include hyperextensible skin and joints, easy bruisability, friability of tissues with bleeding and poor wound healing, calcified subcutaneous spheroids, and pseudotumors.

edema of glottis **(glot′is),** *n* an edema caused by fluid accumulation in the soft tissue of the larynx. The condition, usually inflammatory, may result from an infection, injury, allergy, or inhalation of toxic substances.

edema, periorbital **(per′ēor′bitəl),** *n* an edema of the eyelids in association with local injury, allergic reactions, hypoproteinemia, trichinosis, and myxedema.

edema, pitting, *n* a persistent indentation of the skin when pressure is applied to an edematous area.

edentulism (ēden′tūlizəm), *n* the condition of being edentulous, without teeth.

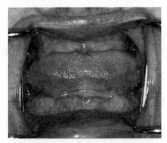

Edentulism. (Zarb et al, 2013)

edentulous (ēden′tūləs), *adj* without teeth; lacking teeth.

edge strength, *n* See strength, edge.

edge-to-edge bite, *n* See occlusion, edge-to-edge.

edge-to-edge occlusion, *n* See occlusion, edge-to-edge.

edgewise appliance, *n* See appliance, edgewise.

EDP, *n* the abbreviation for *electronic data processing.*

Edtac, *n* the brand name for a chelating agent used to soften calcified tissue.

education, *n* the act or process of imparting or acquiring knowledge, skill, or judgment.

education, continuing, *n* education that occurs after the completion of a course of study leading to a degree. Usually taken in short (1- to 2-day) courses covering a specific topic or procedure.

education, dental, *n* the formal education necessary to become qualified to practice dentistry; typically 4 years of full-time study in an accredited school of dentistry.

education of patient, *n* effective communication between the dental professional and the patient concerning dentistry and the principles of treatment and prevention. The procedure of increasing the patient's knowledge of the oral cavity and its care to the point where the reasons for proposed dental services are understood.

education, predental, *n* the formal education necessary to qualify for placement in a dental curriculum, typically 4 years of full-time study at the baccalaureate level.

educational status, *n* the level of education and skill obtained within a discipline or profession, usually referred to as a generalist or specialist in a discipline.

effect, *n* the result of an action.

effect, heel (anode heel effect), *n* the variation of intensity over the cross section of a useful radiographic beam, caused by the angle at which radiographs emerge from beneath the surface of the focal spot, which causes a differential attenuation of photons composing the useful beam.

effect of external radiation on bone, *n* See osteoradionecrosis.

effect of function on bone, *n* See law, Wolff's.

effect, photoelectric, *n* the process by which radiographic images are produced when the energy of an incident photon is absorbed as the result of bound electron ejection.

effect, wedging, *n* an effect produced by food impaction that forces the teeth apart.

effective half-life, *n* See life, radioactive.

effectiveness, *n* the degree to which action(s) achieves the intended health result under normal or usual circumstances.

effector (ēfek′tur), *n* **1.** a motor or secretory nerve ending in an organ, gland, or muscle; consequently called an *effector organ.* *n* **2.** an on-the-job organ of the body that responds to stimulations asking for corrections. Antonym: receptor.

efferent (ef′ərənt), *adj* conveying away from a center toward the periphery.

efferent nerves, *n.*pl See nerves, efferent.

efferent nervous system, *n* the motor nerve system which carries information from the brain or spinal cord to muscles or glands.

efferent vessel, *n* see vessel, efferent.

efficacy (clinical) (ef′ikəsē), *n* the ability to provide a clinically measurable effect, preferably beneficial.

efficiency, *n* the operation of a dental practice in such a way that both business and professional services are performed in a minimal amount of time without sacrificing quality of work, sympathetic attitude, and kindliness.

eH, *n* the symbol for oxidation reduction potential, which is regarded as a significant factor in the protection of the body against anaerobic bacteria. The eH of living tissue of pH level 7.4 is about 0.12 volt.

Ehlers-Danlos syndrome (ā′lurz-dan′lus), *n.pr* a hereditary disorder of connective tissue, marked by hyperplasticity of skin, tissue fragility, and hypermotility of joints. Minor trauma may cause a gaping wound with little bleeding. Sprains, dislocations, and synovial effusions are common. See also syndrome, Ehlers-Danlos.

EIA, *n* the abbreviation for *enzyme immunoassay*; better known as ELISA for enzyme-linked immunosorbent assay, used to detect a protein based on its antigenic properties (e.g., used to determine the presence of HIV antibody against HIV in the blood.)

Eikenella corrodens (īkənelə kə rod'ənz), *n.pr* a gram-negative, rod-shaped, facultatively anaerobic bacteria that is part of the normal flora of the oral cavity but may become an opportunistic pathogen in immunocompromised patients.

ejector (ijektər), *n* by common usage, a device used to remove debris and fluids by negative pressure. Another term is *aspirator.* See also aspirator.

ejector, saliva, *n* a device (containing a removable tip) that is attached to a vacuum supply to remove saliva from a dental field of operation.

ejector, saliva, tip, *n* a removable tip, made of metal, glass, rubber, plastic, or a combination of these, that is attached to a saliva ejector and bent to fit over lower teeth and reach the floor of the oral cavity.

elastic, *adj* referring to property of a solid substance that permits recovery of its shape after a deformation resulting from force application.

elastic deformation, *n* See deformation, elastic.

elastic impression, *n* See impression, elastic.

elastic, intermaxillary, *n* See elastic, maxillomandibular.

elastic, intramaxillary, *n* an elastic band used within either the maxillary or mandibular arch.

elastic limit, *n* See limit, elastic.

elastic, maxillomandibular, *n* an elastic band used between the maxillary and mandibular dentitions.

elastic memory, *n* **1.** the property of a material such as wax that enables it, after being warmed, bent, and cooled, to return to its original form upon rewarming. *n* **2.** a rubber plastic band used to apply force to the teeth.

elasticity (ilastis'itē), *n* the quality or condition of being elastic.

elasticity, modulus of (Young's modulus), *n* a measurement of elasticity obtained by dividing stress below the proportional limit by its corresponding strain value. A measure of stiffness.

elastomer (ēlas'tōmur), *n* a soft, rubberlike material; synthetic rubber. A rubber base impression material (e.g., silicone, mercaptan).

elastosis (ē'lastō'sis), *n* a degeneration of the elastic tissue; found on the vermilion border of the lip (lower lip) and sun-exposed skin. It is associated with actinic cheilitis.

elastosis, senile, *n* a dermatologic disease that results from degeneration of the elastic connective tissue.

elder abuse, *n* the infliction of physical, sexual, or emotional trauma on an elder.

elderly, *adj* used to describe a person who is beyond middle age and approaching old age. Also called *senior citizens.* See also geriatric dentistry.

electrical trauma to the mouth, *n* See burn, oral electrical.

electric pulp tester, *n* an electrical device (usually battery operated) that can cause a small electrical stimulus to be passed through a tooth. Some dentists feel that the device is useful in helping to determine pulp vitality in a tooth.

electroanesthesia (ilek'trōanesthē'zēə, -zhə), *n* local or general anesthesia induced by electric current.

electrocardiography (ilek'trōkar'dēog'rəfē), *n* a method of recording electrical activity generated by the heart muscle.

electrochemistry, *n* chemical reactions that elicit electrical potentials, and electrical potentials that initiate chemical reactions.

electrocoagulation (ēlek'trōkoag'yōōla'shən), *n* the use of electrically generated heat to destroy tissue by coagulation necrosis. Usually a platinum wire electrode or loop is used.

electroconvulsive therapy, *n* the induction of a brief convulsion by passing an electric current through the brain for the treatment of affective disorders, especially in patients resistant to psychoactive drug therapy.

electrode (ēlek'trōd), *n* an instrument with a point or a surface from which a current can be discharged into or received from the body of a patient or a solution.

embrasure, labial, n an embrasure that opens toward the lips.

embrasure, lingual, n an embrasure that opens toward the tongue.

embrasure, occlusal, n an embrasure that opens toward the occlusal surface or plane.

embryo (em′brēō), n an organism in the earliest stages of development; the stage between the time of implantation of the fertilized ovum until the end of the seventh or eighth week of prenatal development.

embryoblast layer (em′breoblast′), n a group of cells near the embryonic axis of the blastocyst that develop into the embryo.

embryology (em′brēol′əjē), n the study of the origin, growth, development, and function of an organism from fertilization to birth.

embryonic cell layers, n the germ layers derived from the increased number of embryonic cells.

embryonic folding, n the folding of the embryo that places the tissues in their proper positions for further embryonic development.

embryonic period (em′breon′ik pe′reod), n the stage between the second and eighth week of prenatal development, during which differentiation of organs and organ systems occurs.

Emdogain, n brand name of an enamel matrix derivative used for tissue regeneration. See also enamel matrix derivative.

emergence profile, n the axial contour of a tooth or crown as it relates to the adjacent soft tissue.

emergency, n an unforeseen occurrence or combination of circumstances that calls for immediate action or remedy; pressing necessity.

emergency cart/kit, n a portable container holding all the equipment and medicines that one would need to assist a patient in case of a medical crisis.

emergency medicine, n a branch of medicine concerned with the diagnosis and treatment of conditions resulting from trauma or sudden illness.

emergency prevention, n the procedures necessary to avoid creating a life-threatening crisis for a patient.

emergency training, n the system of imparting knowledge and skills to be used in case of an accident or an unforeseen occurrence.

emergency treatment, n treatment that must be rendered to the patient immediately for the alleviation of the sudden onset of an unforeseen illness or injury that, if not treated, would lead to further disability or death.

emergency treatment, burns, n the immediate, urgent care given to a burn victim to stabilize the individual until further medical assistance can be found.

emergency treatment, cortical deficiency, n the immediate, urgent care given to an individual experiencing adrenal crisis to stabilize that individual until further medical assistance can be found.

emergency treatment, facial fractures, n the immediate, urgent care given to a patient with facial fractures to stabilize the individual until further medical assistance can be found.

emergency treatment, heart failure, n the immediate, urgent care given to a patient experiencing heart failure to stabilize the individual until further medical assistance can be found.

emery (em′ərē), n an aluminum-based abrasive agent. Two types are aluminum oxide and levigated alumina. Emery is not suitable for polishing dental enamel. Also called *corundum.*

emesis (em′əsis), n the sudden expulsion of gastric contents through the esophagus into the pharynx. The act is partly voluntary and partly involuntary. See also vomiting.

emetic (əmet′ik), n a drug that induces vomiting.

EMF, n the abbreviation for *erythrocyte-maturing factor.*

emigration, n movement of erythrocytes or leukocytes through the walls of the vessels that carry them.

eminence, n a tubercle or rounded elevation on the bony surface.

eminence, frontal, n the prominence of the forehead.

eminence, retromylohyoid **(em′inəns, ret′rōmī′lōhī′oid),** n the distal end of the lingual flange of a mandibular denture. It occupies the retromylohyoid space.

eminenectomy (em′inenek′tōmē), n the operative removal of the anterior articular surface of the glenoid fossa.

emollient (ēmĭ′lēənt), *n* an agent that is soothing to the skin or mucous membrane; makes the skin softer or smoother.

emotion, *n* a complex feeling or state (affect) accompanied by characteristic motor and glandular activities; feelings; mood.

emotional, *adj* describing a person experiencing an emotion; manifesting emotional behavior, rather than logical, rational behavior; describing a person who is easily or excessively given to emotion.

empathy, *n* the quality of putting oneself into the psychologic frame of reference of another, so that the other person's feeling, thinking, and acting are understood and to some extent predictable. A desirable trust-building characteristic of a helping profession. It is embodied in the sincere statement, "I understand how you feel." Empathy is different from sympathy in that to be empathetic one understands how the person feels rather than actually experiencing those feelings, as in sympathy.

emphysema (em′fĭzē′mə), *n* **1.** a swelling caused by air in the tissue spaces. In the oral and facial regions it may be caused either by air introduced into a tooth socket or gingival crevice with the air syringe, or by blowing of the nose. *n* **2.** a permanent dilation of the respiratory alveoli.

employee, *n* a person who, under the direction and control of the employer, performs services for remuneration.

Employee Retirement Income Security Act *(ERISA),* *n.pr* a federal act, passed in 1974, that sets minimum standards for most voluntarily established pension and health plans in private industry to provide protection for individuals in these plans.

employer-sponsored plan, *n* a program supported totally or in part by an employer or group of employers to provide dental benefits for employees. The plan may be administered directly by the employer or another person or group under a contractual arrangement. Part of the cost may be borne by the employee.

employment, *n* **1.** to be engaged in work for hire. *n* **2.** use of a specific tool or technique in the accomplishment of a task.

empyema (em′pīē′mə, em′pēē′mə), *n* the presence of suppuration in a cavity, hollow organ, or space (e.g., the pleural cavity).

emulsifier (imul′səfĭər), *n* an agent such as gum arabic or egg yolk used to suspend droplets of oil in a water-based solution. An agent to maintain any element or particle in suspension within a fluid medium.

emulsion (ēmul′shən), *n* a colloidal dispersion of one liquid in another. See also suspension.

emulsion, digestive, *n* the suspension of fat globules, usually in the bile acid of the small intestine, and their resulting breakdown into smaller particles as part of the digestive process. See also emulsifiers.

emulsion, double, *n* a suspension of sensitive silver halide salts impregnated in gelatin and coated on both sides of a radiographic film base.

emulsion, silver, *n* a suspension of sensitive silver halide salts impregnated in gelatin and used for coating photographic plates and radiographic films.

emulsion, single, *n* a suspension of sensitive silver halide salts impregnated in gelatin and coated on only one side of a radiographic film base.

enalapril maleate (enal′əpril mālēāt), *n brand names:* Vasotec, Vasotec IV; *drug class:* angiotensin-converting enzyme (ACE) inhibitor; *actions:* selectively suppresses renin-angiotensin-aldosterone system; inhibits ACE; prevents conversion of angiotensin I to angiotensin II, leading to dilation of arterial and venous vessels and other beneficial effects due to the reduction of angiotensin II; *uses:* hypertension, heart failure, asymptomatic dysfunction of the left ventricle, to protect the kidney in diabetic patients.

enamel (inam′əl), *n* **1.** the hard, glistening tissue covering the anatomic crown of the tooth. It is composed mainly of hexagonal rods of hydroxyapatite, sheathed in an organic matrix (approximately 0.15%) and oriented with their long axes approximately at right angles to the surface. *n* **2.** the outermost layer or covering of the coronal portion of the tooth that overlies and protects the dentin.

enamel bonding, *v* See bonding, enamel.

enamel dysplasia, *n* the faulty development of enamel due to many factors.

enamel hypocalcification (**hī′pōka l′səfikā′shən**), *n* a hereditary condition in which the enamel of the tooth has formed without adequate amounts of mineralization, leaving the surface of the tooth brittle and often stained.

enamel lamellae (**ləmel′ē**), *n.pl* the incompletely calcified, microscopic structures present in the enamel. They may extend to the dentinoenamel junction and beyond.

enamel matrix, *n* the mineral structure of enamel, secreted by ameloblasts.

enamel, mottled, *n* See fluorosis, chronic endemic dental.

enamel, opacity, (white spot) (**ōpas′ itē**), *n* a visibly lighter area on a tooth's surface; may be caused by fluorosis, or demineralization.

enamel organ, *n* the portion of a developing tooth germ that produces enamel.

enamel pearl, *n* See pearl, enamel.

enamel rod, *n* crystaline structural unit of enamel.

enamel spindles, *n.pl* tubular projections from the dentinoenamel junction into the enamel, caused by penetration by odontoblasts before the junction is formed.

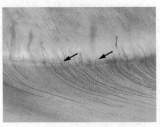

Enamel spindles. (Bath Balogh/Fehrenbach, 2011)

enamel tufts, *n.pl* the brush-shaped projections from the dentinoenamel junction into the enamel, caused by crystallization defects.

enamel epithelium, *n* See epithelium, enamel.

enamel matrix derivative (EMD), *n* an extract of porcine fetal tooth material used to biomimetically stimulate the soft and hard tissues surrounding teeth to regrow following tissue destruction in a process known as regeneration. EMD has been helpful to stimulate healing in reconstructive periodontal surgery and in replanting avulsed teeth.

enameloma, *n* See pearl, enamel.

enanthem (**enan′thəm**), *n* See enanthema.

enanthema (**enanthem**) (**en′anthē′ mə**), *n.pl* lesions involving the mucous membrane.

encephalitis (**ensef′əlītis**), *n* an inflammatory condition of the brain.

encounter form, *n* a document or record used to collect data about given elements of a patient visit to a dental office or similar site that can become part of a patient record or be used for management purposes or for quality review activities.

end organ, *n* the expanded termination of a nerve fiber in muscle, skin, mucous membrane, or other structure.

end organ, proprioceptor, *n.pl* the sensory end organs, located mainly in the muscles, tendons, and labyrinth, that provide information on the movements and position of the body. Four specific end organs are the muscle spindles; Golgi corpuscles, stimulated by tension; Pacini's corpuscles, stimulated by pressure; and bare nerve endings, stimulated by pain.

end organ, sensory, *n* the sensory nerve fibers that end peripherally as either unmyelinated fibers or special structures called receptors. Receptors are situated in the skin, mucous membranes, muscles, tendons, joints, and other structures and also in such special sense organs as those for vision, hearing, smell, and taste. The receptors are organized into a system that relates them to the environment: exteroceptors, interoceptors, and proprioceptors.

end points, *n.pl* **1.** the preestablished steps that, when completed, mark the achievement of a treatment goal. *n.pl* **2.** the clinical indications that a specific infectious condition has been lessened or eliminated altogether.

end section, *n* the distal portion of a twin-wire labial arch wire, consisting of a tube in which the anterior section of the labial arch is engaged.

end-bulb, *n* See end-feet.

end-feet (boutons terminaux, endbulb), *n.pl* the small, terminal enlargements of nerve fibers that are in contact with the dendrites or cell bodies of other nerve cells; the synaptic endings of nerve fibers.

end-plate, *n* the terminal fibers of the motor nerves to the voluntary muscles. The nerve endings lose their myelin sheaths as they enter the sheaths of striated muscle fibers, at which point they ramify across the muscle fiber like the roots of a tree.

end-plate, motor, *n* the end-plate by which impulses from nerves are transmitted to the muscle fibers. It is a modification of the sarcolemma and is continuous with it. The end-plate potential generated by the nerve impulse activates the muscle impulse.

end-stage disease, *n* See disease, end-stage.

end-to-end bite, *n* See occlusion, edge-to-edge.

end-to-end occlusion, *n* See occlusion, edge-to-edge.

endemic, *adj* peculiar to a specific location or region, or within a specific group of people.

ending, *n* a termination; the point at which something is concluded.

ending, annulospiral, *n* a nerve ending, associated with an intrafusal muscle fiber, that is stimulated by a stretch impulse resulting from the extension of a muscle. The ending is in the form of a gradual spiral around the length of the intrafusal muscle fiber in the muscle spindle and is connected to the coarse myelinated fibers.

ending, flower spray, *n* a sensory nerve ending that is attached to the distal end of an intrafusal muscle fiber and that is stimulated when the muscle fiber contracts, pulling on the nerve ending.

ending, free nerve, *n* the peripheral terminal of the sensory nerve.

endocarditis, bacterial (BE) (en'dō kahrdī'tis), *n* an inflammation of the heart (endocardium) valves and lining of the heart as a result of a bacterial infection. The term *subacute (SBE)* is no longer used. See also endocarditis, infective and premedication, antibiotic.

endocarditis, infective (IE), *n* includes viral, fungal, and bacterial infections of heart valves. Bacterial infection is by far the most common.

endocardium (en'dōkär'dēəm), *n* the innermost lining and connective tissue bed of the heart's chambers. It consists of smooth muscle cells, elastin, and collagen fibers.

endochondral bone, *n* See bone, endochondral.

endocrine (en'dōkrin'), *adj* refers to either the gland that secretes directly into the systemic circulation or the substance secreted.

endocrine disease, *n* an abnormal condition caused by some malfunction of an endocrine gland.

endocrine system, *n* the interrelated nature of the physiologic function of endocrine glands.

endocrinology (en'dōkrinol'əjē), *n* the study of the anatomy, physiology, biochemistry, and pathology of the endocrine system and the treatment of endocrine problems.

endocytosis (en'dōsītō'sis), *n* the uptake of materials from the extracellular environment into the cell.

endoderm, *n* the layer in the trilaminar embryonic disc derived from hypoblast layer.

endodontally involved (en'dōdon't əlē), *adj* pertaining to disease of the dental pulp and dental periapical tissue.

endodontic implant, *n* a metallic implant extending through the root canal into the periapical bone structure to increase support and retention of the tooth.

endodontic techniques, *n.pl* procedures used in pulpless teeth or teeth that are to be made pulpless.

endodontics (en'dōdon'tiks), *n* the speciality of dentistry which is concerned with the morphology, physiology, and pathology of the dental pulp and periradicular tissue. Its study and practice encompass the basic and clinical sciences, including biology of the normal pulp; the etiology, diagnosis, prevention, and treatment of diseases and injuries of the pulp; and associated periradicular conditions. One of the nine recognized specialities in dentistry.

endodontist (en'dōdon'tist), *n* a dental professional who practices endodontics as a specialty.

endodontology (endodontia, pulp canal therapy, root canal therapy) (en'dōdontol'ōjē), *n* the division of dental science that deals with the causes, diagnosis, prevention, and treatment of diseases of the dental pulp and their sequelae.

endogenous (endoj'ənəs), *adj* originating within.

endolith (en'dōlith), See denticle.

endometrium, *n* the uterine mucous membrane lining.

endoneurium, *n* connective tissue that surrounds each axon by a layer of connective tissue.

endonuclease (en'dōnoo'klēās'), *n* an enzyme (nuclease) that cleaves polynucleotides at interior bonds, producing polynucleotide or oligonucleotide fragments.

endophthalmitis (en'dofthəlmī'tis), *n* an inflammation of the tissue of the eyeball.

enophthalmos (en'əfthal'məs), *n* backward displacement of the eye in the bony socket caused by traumatic injury or developmental defect.

endophytic (en'dofit'ik), *adj* growing inward or on the inner surface of a structure.

endoplasmic reticulum *(ER)*, *n* an extensive network of membrane enclosed tubules in the cytoplasm of a cell.

endorphins (endor'fins), *n.pl* substances produced in the brain and pituitary gland. The three endorphins, called alpha-, beta-, and gamma-endorphin, are subsequences of the 91-amino-acid peptide hormone, beta-lipotropin. Beta-endorphin reduces pain sensations by binding to opioid receptors in the nervous system. The function of alpha- and gamma-endorphin is not well understood.

endoscopy (endos'kəpē), *n* the visualization of the interior of organs and cavities of the body with an illuminated, flexible optical tube.

endoscopy, gastrointestinal, *n* the visualization of the interior of the stomach and intestines with an illuminated, flexible optical tube.

endoscopy, periodontal, *n* the use of a small fiber-optic endoscope attached to a specially designed dental instrument, such as an explorer, showing subgingival deposits in a magnified view.

endosseous (endos'ēəs), *adj* refers to any object, such as a dental implant, placed or contained within a bone.

endosteal, *n* a thin membrane of cells that line the bone's mandullary cavity.

endosteal implants, *n.pl* See implants, endosteal.

endosteum (endos'tēəm), *n* a thin layer of connective tissue that lines the walls of the bone marrow cavities and haversian canals of compact bone and covers the trabeculae of cancellous bone. It has both osteogenic and hematopoietic potencies and, like the periosteum, takes an active part in the healing of fractures.

endothelioma (en'dōthē'lēō'mə), *n* See sarcoma, Ewing's.

endothelium (en'dōthē'lēəm), *n* the layer of simple squamous epithelial cells that line the heart, the blood and lymph vessels, and the serous cavities of the body.

endotoxin (en'dōtok'sin), *n* a nondiffusible lipid polysaccharide-polypeptide complex formed within bacteria (some gram-negative bacilli and others); when released from the destroyed bacterial cells, endotoxin is capable of producing a toxic manifestation within the host.

endotracheal (en'dōtrā'kēəl), *adj* describes placement of an object within the trachea, or windpipe. (E.g., an endotracheal tube is placed in the trachea and acts as an artificial airway.)

Endur, *n.pr* the brand name for a two-paste diacrylate resin adhesive used as a bonding agent in orthodontics.

enema, *n* a procedure in which a solution is introduced into the rectum for cleansing or therapeutic purposes.

energy, *n* the capacity for doing work.

energy, atomic, *n* the energy that can be liberated by changes in the nucleus of an atom.

energy binding, *n* the energy represented by the difference in mass between the sum of the component parts and the actual mass of the nucleus of an atom.

energy dependence, *n* the characteristic response of a radiation detector to a given range of radiation energies or wavelengths as compared with the response of a standard free-air chamber. Emulsions also show energy dependence.

energy excitation, *n* the energy required to change a system from its ground state to an excited state. With each excited state there is associated a different excitation energy. See also excitation.

energy ionizing, *n* the average energy lost by ionizing radiation in producing an ion pair in a gas. (For air, ionizing energy is approximately 33 V.)

energy kinetic, *n* the energy possessed by a mass because of its motion.

energy nuclear, *n* See energy, atomic.

energy photon (hv), *n* the electromagnetic energy in the form of photons, with a value in ergs equal to the product of their frequency in cycles per second and Planck's constant (E-hv).

energy potential, *n* the energy inherent in a mass because of its position with reference to other masses.

energy radiant, *n* the energy of electromagnetic waves, such as radio waves, visible light, x-rays, and gamma rays.

engine, dental, *n* an electric motor that, by means of a continuous-cord drive over pulleys, activates a handpiece that holds a rotary instrument.

engineering controls, *n.pl* devices or controls developed to provide safer administration of local anesthetics (safety syringes, sharps disposal containers, recapping devices, etc.)

engineering, dental, *n* the application of physical, mechanical, and mathematical principles to dentistry.

Engman's disease, *n* See dermatitis, infectiosa eczematoides.

enkephalin (enkef'əlin), *n* one of two pain-relieving pentapeptides produced in the body.

enlargement, *n* an increase in size.

enlargement, Dilantin, n.pr See hyperplasia, gingival, Dilantin.

enlargement, idiopathic, n gingival enlargement, of unknown causation, clinically characterized by a firm, rounded thickening of the attached gingival tissue and histologically characterized by connective tissue hyperplasia.

enlargement, parotid (pərot'id), *n* a swelling of the parotid glands observed most frequently in those with anorexia and bulimia.

enolase (e'nolās), *n* an enzyme characterized by its crystalline structure and role in carbohydrate utilization.

enostosis (en'ostō'sis), *n* a bony growth located within a bone cavity or centrally from the cortical plate. See also osteoma.

enoxacin (enok'səsin), *n brand name:* Penetrex; *drug class:* fluoroquinolone antibiotic; *action:* a broad-spectrum bactericidal agent that inhibits the enzyme deoxyribonucleic acid (DNA) gyrase, needed for replication of DNA; *uses:* uncomplicated urethral or cervical gonorrhea, uncomplicated and complicated urinary tract infections.

enrollee, *n* an individual covered by a benefit plan. See also beneficiary.

Entamoeba gingivalis (en'təmē'bə), *n* a genus of protozoan found in the oral cavity; repeatedly, but not conclusively, associated with the initiation and continuation of periodontitis.

enteral (en'tərəl), *adj* directly into the gastrointestinal tract; (e.g., pertaining to tube feedings that may be necessary when a patient cannot ingest food orally).

enteric coating (enter'ik), *n* See coating, enteric.

enteritis (en'təri'tis), *n* an inflammation of the mucosal lining of the small intestine.

Enterobacter cloacae (en'tərōbak' tər klōā'sē), *n.pr* a common species of bacteria found in human and animal feces, dairy products, sewage, soil, and water. It is rarely the cause of disease.

Enterobacteriaceae (en'tərōbak'ti r'ēā'sēē'), *n.pr* a family of aerobic and anaerobic bacteria that includes both normal and pathogenic enteric microorganisms such as *Escherichia, Klebsiella, Proteus,* and *Salmonella.*

Enterobius vermicularis (en'tərō' bēəs vərmik'yəlar'is), *n* a parasitic worm that resides in the large intestine, more commonly found in children, which may cause pruritis in the anal region. It can be contracted from contact with fomites or by ingesting or inhaling immature forms of the worm. Also called *pinworm.*

enterococcus (en′tərō′kok′əs), *n* any *Streptococcus* bacterium that inhabits the intestinal tract.

entropion (entrō′pēon), *n* the inversion, or infolding, of the eyelid margin.

entry, port of, *n* the point on the body through which infectious microorganisms may enter, such as the eyes, nose, respiratory tract, or open wound.

enucleate (enoo′klēāt), *v* to remove a lesion in its entirety.

enunciation (inun′sēā′shən), *n* an auxiliary function of teeth, particularly those in the anterior sector of the dental arch; the formation of sounds as in speech.

enuresis (enūrē′sis), *n* involuntary urination (e.g., during general anesthesia, at night).

environment (envī′rənment, envī′urnment), *n* the aggregate of all the external conditions and influences affecting the life and development of an organism.

environment, extracellular, n the external, or interstitial, environment provided and maintained for the tissue cells.

environment, oral, n all oral conditions present and their influences.

environmental health, *n* the various aspects of substances, forces, and conditions in and about a community that affect the health and well-being of the population.

environmental pollutants, *n.pl* the substances and conditions, including noise, that adversely affect the health and well-being of the people within a community.

environmental pollution, *n* the presence of substances and conditions that adversely affect the health and well-being of people within a community; usually substances in the air and water supply.

Environmental Protection Agency (EPA), *n.pr* a federal agency charged with the approval and overseeing of the use and disposal of hazardous materials. Workplace management of hazardous materials falls under the jurisdiction of the Occupational Safety and Health Administration (OSHA).

EPA registered, adj indicates that an object or substance has been approved

by the Environmental Protection Agency.

environmental tobacco smoke (ETS/passive smoke), *n* the gaseous by-product of burning tobacco products, including but not limited to commercially manufactured cigarettes and cigars; contains toxic elements harmful to the health of adults and children exposed to it. Also called *secondhand smoke.*

enzyme (en′zīm), *n* a protein substance that acts as a catalyst to speed up metabolic and other processes involving organic materials. Some enzymes function within cells; others function in the extracellular fluids and tissue spaces and organs. They are active in all major tissue functions, such as cellular respiration, muscle contraction, digestive processes, and energy consumption, and are produced intracellularly.

enzyme-linked immunosorbent assay (ELISA), n a species-specific serologic laboratory procedure used to identify microorganisms infecting or inhabiting a tissue or organ system. Its dental use is in the identification of pathogens involved in periodontal disease.

eosin (e′osin), *n* one of a pair of dyes used to color tissue samples to augment visibility under a microscope. The dyes are rose-colored, causing the cytoplasm to appear pink.

eosinophil (ē′əsin′əfil), *n* See leukocyte, eosinophilic.

eosinophilia (ē′əsin′əfil′ēə), *n* an absolute or relative increase in the normal number of eosinophils in the circulating blood. Various limits are given (e.g., absolute eosinophilia if the total number exceeds 500 mm^3) and relative if greater than 3% but total less than 500 mm^3. It may be associated with skin diseases, infestations, hay fever, asthma, angioneurotic edema, adrenocortical insufficiency, and Hodgkin disease.

eosinophilic granuloma, *n* See granuloma, eosinophilic.

EPA, *n.pr* See Environmental Protection Agency.

ephebodontics (əfe′bodon′tiks), *n* adolescent dentistry. See also pedodontics.

ephedrine sulfate (ifed′rin sul′fāt), *n brand name:* generic; *drug class:*

adrenergic, mixed direct and indirect effects; *actions:* causes increased contractility and heart rate by acting on β-receptors in heart; also acts on α-receptors, causing vasoconstriction in blood vessels; *uses:* shock, increase perfusion and bronchodilation, hypotension, narcolepsy, myasthenia gravis.

ephelis (əfē′lis), *n* a circumscribed macular collection of pigment in the epidermis or oral mucosa. An increased amount of melanin pigment is seen in the region of the basal layer of cells. Also called freckle.

epiblast layer, *n* the superior layer in the bilaminar disc.

epicanthic fold (ep′ikan′thik), *n* a characteristic crease in the eyelid; seen in persons with Down syndrome.

epicondyle, *n* the small prominence that is located above or upon a condyle.

epicondylitis (ep′ikon′dəli′tis), *n* a painful repetitive strain injury of the elbow characterized by inflammation or lesions in the muscles or tendons where they attach to the bone. Often known as "tennis elbow" when it affects the outside of the joint or "golfer's elbow" when it affects the inside of the joint.

epicranial aponeurosis, *n* the scalpel tendon from which the frontal belly of the epicranial muscle arises.

epidemic, *adj* spreading rapidly and widely among many individuals in a single location or region; illnesses labeled epidemic are those that occur beyond normal expectations and are usually traceable to a single source.

epidemiologic survey, *n* See research, epidemiologic survey.

epidemiology (ep′idē′mēol′əjē), *n* the science of epidemics and epidemic diseases, which involve the total population rather than the individual. The aim of epidemiology is to determine those factors in the group environment that make the group more or less susceptible to disease.

epidemiology, indices in, *n.pl* the data collection tools that aid in the measurement and evaluation of disease indicators and conditions; classification systems featuring numbered scales against which a specific population may be compared.

epidermis (ep′ider′mis), *n* the superficial, avascular layers of the skin.

epidermoid cyst, *n* a common, benign, variable, subcutaneous swelling lined by keratinizing epithelium and filled with a cheesy material composed of sebum and epithelial debris.

epidermolysis bullosa (ep′idurmol′isis), *n* a group of acquired autoimmune and hereditary mucocutaneous diseases characterized by formation of bullae and possible scarring and deformity at affected sites, depending on the variant present.

epiglottis (ep′iglot′is), *n* an elastic cartilage, covered by mucous membrane, that forms the superior part of the larynx and guards the glottis during swallowing.

epiglottic swelling, *n* the posterior swelling that develops from the fourth branchial arches and marks the development of the future epiglottis.

epilepsy (ep′ilep′sē), *n* a group of neurologic disorders characterized by recurrent episodes of convulsive seizures, sensory disturbances, abnormal behavior, and loss of consciousness. Most epilepsy is of an unknown etiology but may be associated with cerebral trauma, brain tumors, vascular disturbances, or chemical imbalance. Drugs used in the treatment of symptoms (e.g., hydantoin sodium, diphenylhydantoin sodium) may promote gingival hyperplasia.

epiloia (epiloi′ə), *n* See syndrome, Bourneville-Pringle.

epinephrine (ep′inef′rin), *n* a hormone secreted by the adrenal medulla that stimulates α_1, α_2, β_1, β_2, and β_3 adrenergic receptors. Its multiple effects include stimulation of hepatic glycogenolysis, causing an elevation in the blood sugar, vasodilation of blood vessels of the skeletal muscles, vasoconstriction of the arterioles of the skin and mucous membranes, relaxation of bronchiolar smooth muscles, and stimulation of heart action. Used in local anesthetics for its vasoconstrictive action to prolong the anesthesia action, provide hemostasis, and reduce systemic complications.

epinephrine/epinephrine bitartrate/ epinephrine HCl, *n brand names:* EpiPen Jr., Bronkaid Mist, Primatene

Mist; *drug class:* adrenergic agonist, catecholamine; *action:* stimulates α_1, α_2, β_1, β_2 and β_3 adrenergic receptors, producing bronchodilation and cardiac stimulation and vasoconstriction; *uses:* acute asthmatic attacks, hemostasis, bronchospasm, anaphylaxis, allergic reactions, cardiac arrest, as a vasopressor. Recommended for the dental office or clinic emergency kit. See EpiPen.

EpiPen, *n.pr* the brand name for an autoinjector containing epinephrine, used to treat severe allergic reactions. Dose is fast-acting and can be self administered.

epiphysis (epifʹisis), *n* the terminal portion of a long bone. The epiphysis is separated from the diaphysis during growth by a cartilaginous zone that serves as a growth center. Once ossification unites the epiphysis with the diaphysis, growth is completed.

epispinal (epispiʹnəl), *adj* located on the spinal column.

epistaxis (epʹistakʹsis), *n* bleeding from the nose cause by local irritation of mucous membranes, violent sneezing, fragility of the mucous membrane, or of the arterial walls, chronic infection, trauma, hypertension, leukemia, vitamin K deficiency, or, most often, picking the nose. Also called *nosebleed.*

epithelial (epʹithēʹlēəl), *adj* pertaining to the epithelium.

epithelial attachment (EA), *n* See attachment, epithelial.

epithelial cells, *n.pl* cells that form the epithelial tissue that lines both the inner and outer surfaces of the body; serve a protective function and also aid in absorption and secretion.

epithelial cuff, attached, *n* the portion of gingiva that overlies the band of attached epithelium around a tooth.

epithelial cuff, implant, *n* the portion of gingiva that overlies the band of attached epithelium around an implant or abutment.

epithelial desquamation, anesthetic **(desʹkwəmāʹshən),** *n* the ulceration and shedding of oral epithelial tissue that occurs as the result of prolonged exposure to topical anesthesia.

epithelial inclusion, *n* the bits of epithelial tissue introduced into bone crypts during perforation osteotomies. See also osteotomy, perforation.

epithelial layers, *n* the number and type of layers present in epithelium.

epithelial rests of Malassez **(maləsəʹ),** *n* the remnants of Hertwig's epithelial root sheath within the periodontal ligament.

epithelioma (epʹithēʹlēōʹmə), *n* an epithelial neoplasm.

epithelioma adenoides cysticum, *n* multiple trichoepitheliomas.

epithelioma, basal cell, *n* See carcinoma, basal cell.

epithelium (epithelia) (epʹithēʹlēəm), *n* the layer of cells lining a body cavity or the outer surface of the body; cells may be ciliated or unciliated, and may be squamous (flat, scale-like), cuboidal (cube-shaped), or columnar (column-shaped).

epithelium, basement membrane of, *n* See membrane, basement.

epithelium, desmosomes of **(dezʹmosōmzʹ),** *n* an electron microscopic finding of intercellular bridges that serve to attach adjacent epithelial cells to each other.

epithelium, enamel, inner (IEE), *n* the innermost layer of cells (ameloblasts) of the enamel organ that deposit the organic matrix of the enamel on the crown of the developing tooth. Also the innermost layer of Hertwig's epithelial root sheath.

epithelium, enamel, outer (OEE), *n* the outermost layer of cells of the enamel organ. It is separated from the inner enamel epithelium in the area of the developing crown by the stratum intermedium and stellate reticulum and lies immediately adjacent to the inner enamel epithelium in the area of the developing root.

epithelium, enamel, reduced (REE), *n* combined enamel epithelium; the remains of the enamel organ after enamel formation is complete. After eruption of the tip of the crown, that part of the combined epithelium remaining on the enamel surface is called the epithelial attachment.

epithelium, gingival, *n* a stratified squamous epithelium consisting of a basal layer; it is keratinized or parakeratinized.

epithelium, hyperplastic, *n* an increase in thickness, with alterations in structure, produced by proliferation of cellular elements of epithelium.

epithelium, oral, *n* the epithelial covering of the oral mucosa. Composed of stratified squamous epithelium of varying thickness and varying degrees of keratinization.

epithelium, pocket, *n* the epithelium that lines the periodontal pocket. Its most prominent characteristics are the presence of hyperplasia and ulceration.

epithelium, pseudostratified (soo′dō strat′ifĭd), *n* a type of epithelium in which there appears to be several layers (or strata) of cells, but all cells actually are resting on the base layer; often ciliated and occurs only in mucosa.

epithelium, simple, *n* the epithelium that consists of a single layer of cells.

epithelium, squamous (skwā′məs), *n* a type of epithelium consisting of flat, scalelike cells.

epithelium, simple squamous, *n* the lining of the blood and lymphatic vessels, heart, and serous cavities and important interfaces in the lungs and kidneys.

epithelium, stratified, *n* the epithelium that consists of two or more layers.

epithelium, stratified squamous, *n* the variety of epithelium covering the oral mucosa and dermal surfaces; composed of layers of cells oriented 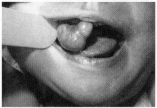 parallel to the surface. The various layers of cells in order from basement membrane to surface are stratum germinativum, stratum spinosum (prickle cell layer), and stratum lucidum (in dermal epithelium). The gingival epithelium generally exhibits some degree of keratinization, variable from parakeratinization to orthokeratinization within the layers of the stratum granulosum (granular layer) and stratum corneum (keratin layer).

epithelium, sulcal, *n* the stratified squamous epithelium forming the covering of the soft tissue wall of the gingival sulcus, or crevice. Extends from the gingival margin to the line of attachment of the epithelium to the tooth surface.

epithelialization **(epithelization)** (ep′əthē′lēəlizā′shən), *n* the natural act of healing by secondary intention; the proliferation of new epithelium

into an area devoid of it but that naturally is covered by it.

epizootic fever (ep′izōot′ik), *n* another name for foot and mouth disease in cloven-foot animals; also known as aphthous fever; caused by a type of coxsackievirus, uncommon in the United States. The disease in humans is characterized by malaise, fever, headache, itchy skin, and a sensation of xerostomia despite heavy salivation. Vesicles appear in the oral cavity, around the lips, and on the hands and feet. Oral vesicles and ulcers resolve within approximately 10 days.

eplerenone, *n brand name:* Inspra; *drug class:* aldosterone antagonist; *action:* blocks aldosterone receptors, leading to increase sodium and water excretion and blocking other effects of aldosterone; *uses:* heart failure, hypertension.

epoxy resin (ēpok′sē, əpok′sē), *n* See resin, epoxy.

Epstein's pearls, *n.pr* white, ricelike, keratin-filled lesions of the midline hard palate mucosa. See also cyst, palatal, of the newborn.

Epstein-Barr virus *(EBV)*, *n.pr* a herpesvirus associated with Burkitt's lymphoma and reported in cases of infectious mononucleosis.

epulis (epŭ′lis), *n* a benign tumor (tumescence) of the gingiva.

epulis, congenital of newborn, *n* a raised or pedunculated lesion located on the anterior gingivae of the newborn. It is histologically similar to granular cell myoblastoma. Also called *gingival granular cell lesion*.

Congenital epulis of the newborn. (Dean/Avery/McDonald, 2011)

epulis fissuratum (fisŏŏrat′əm), *n* a curtainlike fold of excess tissue associated with the flange of a denture.

Also called *inflammatory fibrous hyperplasia, redundant tissue.*

epulis, giant cell, *n* See granuloma, giant cell reparative, peripheral.

epulis granulomatosa (gran'yəlō 'mətō'sə), *n* a tumorlike mass of red, easily bleeding, infected granulation tissue that occurs as a result of exuberant reparative phenomena. Seen arising from tooth sockets or is associated with exfoliating necrotic bone. See granulation tissue.

equal protection, *n* clause set out in the Fourteenth Amendment of the U.S. Constitution that dictates that state governments cannot pass or enforce any laws based solely on a specific classification of person by race, gender, religion, ethnicity, or age.

EQUATOR (Enhancing the Quality and Transparency of Health Research), *n.pr* guidelines for the development and reporting of research.

equilibration (ēkwil'ibrā'shən), *n* the act of placing a body in a state of equilibrium.

equilibration diagnostic, *n* See diagnostic equilibration.

equilibration, mandibular, *n* the act or acts performed to place the mandible in a state of equilibrium.

equilibration, occlusal, *n* the modification of occlusal forms of teeth by grinding, with the intent of equalizing occlusal stress and of harmonizing cuspal relations in function.

equilibration of mounted casts, *n* an equilibration of the occlusion of mounted casts made of a patient for the purpose of observing and recording what must be done to adjust the natural occlusion.

equilibration, proper, *n* See proper equilibration.

equilibrator (ēkwil'ibrātur), *n* an instrument or device used in achieving or maintaining a state of equilibrium.

equilibrium (ē'kwilib'rēəm), *n* a state of balance between two opposing forces or processes.

equilibrium, functional, *n* the state of homeostasis within the oral cavity existing when biologic processes and local environmental factors, including the forces of mastication, are in a state of balance.

equilibrium, juvenile occlusal (joo' vənīl əkloo'səl), *n* one of the six eruptive phases of dentition, and the first of three postfunctional stages of eruption of the entire dentition. It occurs at or near adolescence when permanent teeth continue to erupt into the oral cavity in response to the vertical growth of the ramus.

equipment, *n* the nonexpendable items used by the dental staff in the office in the performance of professional duties.

equity, *n* a free and reasonable claim or right; fairness; impartiality. The money value of a property or of an interest in a property in excess of claims or liens against it; a risk interest or ownership right in property.

equivalent, *n* a state where there is an equal in force, value, measure, or effect; corresponding in function.

equivalent, aluminum, *n* the thickness of pure aluminum affording the same radiation attenuation, under specified conditions, as the material or materials being considered.

equivalent, concrete, *n* the thickness of concrete having a density of 2.35 g/cm^3 that would afford the same radiation attenuation, under specified conditions, as the material or materials being considered.

equivalent, lead, *n* the thickness of pure lead that would afford the same radiation attenuation, under specified conditions, as the material or materials being considered.

erbium (Er) (ur'bēəm), *n* a rare earth, metallic element with an atomic number of 68 and an atomic weight of 167.26.

erectile tissue, *n* the thin walled vessels in the nasal cavity that are capable of considerable engorgement.

erg (urg), *n* a unit of energy equal to the energy consumed by 1 dyne acting through 1 cm, which is equal to 10^{-7} joule.

ergocalciferol (vitamin D$_2$), *n brand names:* Calciferol, Drisdol; *drug class:* vitamin D; *action:* stimulates intracellular vitamin D receptor leading to typical vitamin D effects; *uses:* hypoparathyroidism, familial hypophosphatemia, vitamin D-resistant rickets.

ergonomics, *n* the study of workplace design and the physical and psychologic impact it has on workers. It is about the fit between people, their work activities, equipment, work systems, and environment to ensure that workplaces are safe, comfortable and efficient and that productivity is not compromised.

ergotamine tartrate (ur′got′əmēn tar′trāt), *n brand names:* Ergomar, Ergostat; *drug class:* α-adrenergic blocker; *action:* α-adrenergic blocker constricts blood vessels by direct action and vascular smooth muscle in peripheral and cranial blood vessels, contracts uterine muscle; *uses:* vascular headache (migraine or histamine), cluster headache.

ERISA, *n.pr* the acronym for the *Employee Retirement Income Security Act of 1974.* See also Employee Retirement Income Security Act.

erosion (ērō′zhən), *n* the chemical or mechanicochemical destruction of tooth substance, the mechanism of which is incompletely known, which leads to the creation of concavities of many shapes at the junction of teeth. The surface of the cavity, unlike dental caries, is hard and smooth.

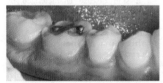

Erosion. (Neville, et al, 2009)

error, *n* a violation of duty; a fault; a mistake in the proceedings of a court in matters of law or of fact.

error, legal, n a mistaken judgment or incorrect belief as to the existence or effect of matters of fact, or a false or mistaken conception or application of the law.

error, numerical, n the amount of loss or precision in a quantity; the difference between an accurate quantity and its calculated approximation. Errors occur in numerical methods; mistakes occur in programming, coding, data transcription, and operating; malfunctions occur in computers and are caused by physical limitations of the properties of materials.

error of measurement, n the deviation of an individual score or observation from its true value, caused by the unreliability of the instrument and the individual who is measuring.

error, sampling, n any mistake in drawing a sample that keeps it from being unrepresentative; selection procedures that are biased; error introduced when a group is described on the basis of an unrepresentative sample.

error, variance, n that part of the total variance caused by anything irrelevant to a study that cannot be experimentally controlled.

eruption (erup′shən), *n* the migration of a tooth in the alveolar process of the maxilla or mandible into the oral cavity.

eruption, active, n the movement of a developing tooth from its area of development in the jaw into the oral cavity to become part of the dental arch.

eruption, continuous, n the normal occlusal progression of teeth noted throughout a lifetime.

eruption cyst, n a dentigerous cyst that causes a clinically evident bulging of the overlying alveolar ridge. See also cysts, eruption.

eruption, delayed, n the failure of the teeth to erupt from the gingival tissue at the usual developmental time. Often associated with hypothyroidism or impaction.

eruption, ectopic (ektop′ik), n the abnormal direction of tooth eruption, most common to mandibular first and third molars, which sometimes leads to abnormal resorption of the adjacent tooth.

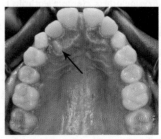

Ectopic eruption. (Courtesy Dr. Flavio Uribe)

eruption, forced, *n* **1.** the orthodontic eruption of a tooth that has fractured under the gingival margin to achieve adequate tooth structure for a proper full coverage restoration. *n* **2.** the process of erupting a periodontally compromised tooth in order to develop the bone. The tooth will later be extracted for the placement of an endosseous dental implant..

eruption hematoma, *n* an eruption cyst that is blood-filled, visualized as a bluish purple area of elevated tissue of the overlying alveolar ridge.

eruption, lingual, *n* the eruption of permanent teeth on the lingual side of primary teeth that have not yet been exfoliated.

eruption, passive, *n* the gradual increasing exposure of the clinical crown by apical migration of the gingiva that occurs after tooth eruption (i.e., gingival margin recedes apically rather than tooth moving coronally) often seen with aging and in the absence of clinical evidence of inflammation.

eruption sequestrum **(erup'shən səkwes'trēəm)**, *n* a needlelike piece of calcified tissue that is located over the gingival tissue of an erupting tooth.

eruption, surgical, *n* the surgical removal of tissue covering an abnormally unerupted tooth to allow its natural progress into position.

eruptive gingivitis, *n* See gingivitis, eruptive.

erysipelas **(er'isip'ələs)**, *n* an infectious skin disease characterized by redness, swelling, vesicles, bullae, fever, pain, and lymphadenopathy. It is caused by a species of group A β-hemolytic streptococci.

Erysipelothrix (er'əsip'əlothriks'), *n* a gram-positive bacterium that does not produce spores and has cell walls.

erythema **(er'ithē'mə)**, *n* a patchy, circumscribed, or marginated macular redness of the skin or mucous membranes caused by hyperemia or inflammation.

erythema, linear gingival (LGE) **(er'əthē'mə lin'ēer jin'jəvəl)**, *n* a gingival condition observed **immunocompromised** individuals (e.g., HIV infected, AIDS) that is characterized by an intensely red linear band that affects both labial and proximal tissue

and extends 2 to 3 mm apically from the gingival margin. The condition does not predictably respond to plaque removal.

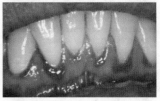

Linear gingival erythema. (Daniel/Harfst/Wilder, 2008)

erythema multiforme complex, *n* an acute, inflammatory mucocutaneous disease of uncertain etiology (although occasionally related to drug administration), characterized by erythematous macules, papules, vesicles, and bullae that appear on the skin and not infrequently on the oral mucosa. See also syndrome, Stevens-Johnson.

erythema infectiosum, *n* See disease, fifth.

erythematous/atrophic *Candida* **(er'əthem'ətəs ātrō'fik kandē'də)**, *n* a skin disease characterized by patches of smooth, red tissue on the tongue, palate, or oral mucosa. Most commonly seen in people with AIDS.

erythredema polyneuropathy **(əri th'redē'mə pol'ēnūrop'əthē)**, *n* See acrodynia.

erythremia **(Osler's disease, polycythemia rubra, polycythemia vera, primary polycythemia, Vaquez' disease) (er'ithrē'mēə)**, *n* a myeloproliferative disease characterized by a marked increase in the circulating red blood cell mass. Erythremia may represent a neoplastic growth of erythropoietic tissue. Neutrophilia, thrombocytopenia, and splenomegaly are common. Manifestations include plethora, vertigo, headache, and thrombosis.

erythrityl tetranitrate **(ərith'ritəl tetrəni'trāt)**, *n brand name:* Cardilate; *drug class:* organic nitrate; *actions:* causes relaxation of vascular smooth muscle; decreases preload/afterload, which is responsible for decreasing left ventricular end diastolic pressure; systemic vascular resistance; improved exercise tolerance; *uses:* chronic stable angina pectoris, prophylaxis of angina pain.

erythroblastosis fetalis (ərith′rō blastō′sis fētal′is), *n* an excessive destruction of red blood cells begun before or shortly after birth in the fetus or newborn. It may be caused by an Rh factor reaction. After birth the skin is yellow, and the teeth may be markedly discolored.

Erythrocin, *n.pr* the brand name for erythromycin.

erythrocyte (ərith′rōsīt), *n* a red blood cell; a nonnucleated, circular, biconcave, discoid, hemoglobin-containing, oxygen-carrying formed element circulating in the blood.

erythrocyte count, *n* the number of red blood cells per cubic millimeter of blood.

erythrocyte indices, *n.pl* the standard values of red blood cell numbers, morphologic characteristics, and behavior in comprehensive hematologic laboratory testing.

erythrocyte sedimentation rate (ESR), *n* the rate at which red blood cells settle in a pipette of unclotted blood, measured in millimeters per hour. It is used as an index of inflammation.

erythrocytosis (secondary polycythemia) (ərith′rōsītō′sis), *n* an increased circulating red blood cell mass resulting from compensatory effort to meet reduced oxygen content. May be seen in persons living at high altitudes, as well as in persons with emphysema, pulmonary insufficiency, and heart failure.

erythromycin (ərith′rōmī′sin), *n* an antibiotic produced by a strain of *S. erythroeus,* only active against several oral and respiratory tract organisms, useful for upper and lower respiratory tract, skin, and soft tissue infections of mild to moderate severity. It is no longer recommended by the American Heart Association and the American Dental Association for treatment of bacterial endocarditis in patients hypersensitive to penicillin.

erythromycin base (et al.), *n* brand *names:* E-mycin, Ery-Tab, et al.; *drug class:* macrolide antibiotic; *action:* binds to 50S ribosomal subunits of susceptible bacteria and suppresses protein synthesis; *uses:* infections caused by *N. gonorrhoeae,* mild to moderate respiratory tract, skin, soft tissue infections caused by *S. pneumoniae, C. diphtheriae, B. pertussis,* syphilis, Legionnaire's disease, *H. influenzae.*

erythroplakia (ərith′ropla′keə), *n* a flat red patch or lesion of unknown etiology on the oral or pharyngeal surfaces with a high risk of cancer or epithelial dysplasia present at the time of discovery.

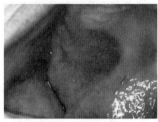

Erythroplakia.   (Regezi/Sciubba/Jordan, 2012)

erythroplasia of Queyrat (ərith′rō plā′zhə əv kərat′, kārī′), *n.pr* a form of intraepithelial carcinoma. The oral lesions are usually seen as dental biofilm (dental plaque) with a bright, velvety surface.

erythropoiesis (ərith′rōpoiē′sis), *n* the process in which red blood cells are formed.

erythrosin (ərith′rosēn), *n* a red dye used to reveal dental biofilm (dental plaque) deposits on teeth; administered in both tablet and liquid form. See also disclosing solution.

escharotic (es′kïrot′ik), *n* a caustic or corrosive agent that has the strength to burn tissue.

Escherichia coli (E. coli) **(eshə rik′ēə kō′lī),** *n.pr* a species of coliform bacteria normally present in the intestines and common in water, milk, and soil can become a pathogen at other body sites.

esculin (es′kəlin), *n* a glucoside from horse-chestnut bark; used as a sunburn protective.

esmolol, *n* brand *name:* Brevibloc; *drug class:* selective beta₁ adrenergic receptor blocker; *action:* inhibits the effects of agonists on the beta₁ receptor; *uses:* rapid treatment of supraventricular tachycardia, procedure-induced tachycardia or hypertension.

esophageal atresia (isof´əjē´əltrē´ zhə), *n* an abnormal esophagus that ends in a blind pouch or narrows to a thin cord and thus fails to provide a continuous passage to the stomach. It is usually a congenital anomaly.

esophageal stenosis (isof´əjē´əl stən ō´sis), *n* a narrowing or restriction of the lumen of the esophagus that slows or impedes the passage of fluid and foods from the oral cavity to the stomach.

esophagitis (isof´əjītis), *n* an inflammation of the mucosal lining of the esophagus caused by infection or irritation of the mucosa by reflux of gastric juice from the stomach.

esophagus (isof´əgəs), *n* the muscular canal extending from the pharynx to the stomach.

essence (es´ens), *n* an alcoholic solution of an essential oil.

essential oil, *n* See oil, essential.

essentials oils mouthrinses, *n.pl* mouthwashes made from thymol, menthol, eucalyptol, and methyl salicylate in combination with alcohol that are available over the counter for use in controlling dental biofilm (dental plaque) and gingivitis. See also mouthwash.

estate, *n* one's interest in land or other property.

estate planning, *n* a detailed, written-out plan (usually arrived at with the advice of estate counselors) in which all the financial affairs of the dental professional are clearly stated and provisions are made for alterations when changing conditions warrant it.

estazolam (estaz´olam), *n* brand name: ProSom; *drug class:* benzodiazepine, sedative-hypnotic; *action:* produces central nervous system (CNS) depression by interaction with benzodiazepine receptor, thereby enhancing the effect of γ-aminobutyric acid (GABA) in the CNS; *use:* insomnia.

ester (es´tur), *n* a compound formed from alcohol and an organic acid, in which the alcoholic OH forms a covalent bond with the carbonyl carbon of the acid.

ester linkage, *n* the bond between organic acids and alcohols.

ester, anesthetics, *n* a class of local anesthetics that are metabolized by plasma cholinesterase and commonly produce allergic reactions.

esterase (es´tərās), *n* an enzyme that catalyzes the hydrolysis of an ester into its alcohol and acid.

esterified estrogens, *n.pl* brand names: Estabs, Estratab, Menest; *drug class:* semisynthetic estrogens, principally estrone; *action:* stimulate estrogen receptors resulting in characteristic changes in the function of the female reproductive system; *uses:* menopause, breast cancer, prostatic cancer, hypogonadism, ovariectomy, primary ovarian failure.

esthetic zone, *n* the visible area seen upon full smile, including the teeth, gingiva, and lips.

esthetics (esthet´iks), *n* the branch of philosophy dealing with beauty, especially with the components thereof; (i.e., color and form). Can also be spelled *aesthetics.*

esthetics, dentistry, *n* the skills and techniques used to improve the art and symmetry of the teeth and face to enhance the appearance as well as the function of the teeth, oral cavity, and face.

esthetics, denture, *n* the cosmetic effect, produced by a denture, that affects the desirable beauty, charm, character, and dignity of the individual.

esthetics, denture base, *n* the esthetically proper tinting, contouring, and festooning of the gingival tissue portion of a denture base.

esthetics, gingival tissue (gingival tissue esthetics), *n* **1.** the balance and harmony in color, contour, shape, and texture of soft tissue. *n* **2.** see esthetics, denture base.

estimate, *n* the anticipated fee for dental services to be performed.

estimated average requirement (E.A.R.), *n* the accepted standard level of nutrients that an average person requires. The basis for the Recommended Daily Allowance is established by the U.S. government.

estoppel (estop´əl), *n* a preclusion, in law, that prevents a person from alleging or denying a fact because of his or her own previous act or allegation.

estradiol, *n* brand names: Estrace, Estraderm, Evamist, Alora; *drug* *class:* estrogen; *action:* stimulates estrogen receptors resulting in characteristic changes in the function of the female reproductive system; *uses:* menopause, hypogonadism in females, breast cancer, prostate cancer, prevention of postmenopausal osteoporosis.

estrin (es'trin), *n* the generic term for the ovarian estrogens estriol, estrone, and estradiol.

estrogens (es'trōjenz), *n.pl* the collective term for substances capable of producing estrus. The term also applies to the estrogenic hormones in women. Estradiol is the principal human estrogen. Synthetic or semisynthetic estrogens include, hexestrol, and ethinyl estradiol.

eszopiclone, *n brand name:* Lunesta; *drug class:* sedative hypnotic; *action:* selectively stimulates GABA$_A$ receptors at the alpha$_1$ subunit of the chloride channel, also called the BZ$_1$ receptor; *use:* insomnia.

etanercept, *n brand name:* Enbrel; *drug class:* anti TNF-α; *action:* binds TNF-α and inhibits its action at its receptor; *uses:* arthritis (rheumatoid and some other forms), ankylosing spondylitis, plaque psoriasis.

etch, acid, *v* See acid etching.

etching, *n* a process used to decalcify the superficial layers of enamel as a step in the application of sealants or bonding agents in preventive dentistry, restorative dentistry, and orthodontics. The agent of choice is phosphoric acid in concentrations of 30% to 40%.

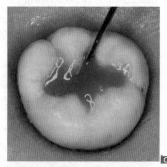

Tooth being etched. (Freedman, 2012)

ethacrynate sodium/ethacrynic acid (eth'akrin'āt), *n brand name:* Edecrin Sodium; *drug class:* loop diuretic; *action:* acts on loop of Henle by blocking the sodium/potassium/chloride co-transporter, thereby increasing excretion of sodium, potassium, and chloride; *uses:* pulmonary edema, edema in congestive heart failure, liver disease, nephrotic syndrome, ascites, hypertension.

ethambutal HCl (ētham'byootol), *n brand name:* Myambutol; *drug class:* antitubercular; *action:* inhibits arabinosyl transferase III, resulting in inhibition of cell wall in mycobacteria; *use:* pulmonary tuberculosis, as adjunct.

ethane (eth'ān), *n* a constituent of natural and "bottled" gases.

ethics (eth'iks), *n* **1.** the science of moral obligation; a system of moral principles, quality, or practice. *n* **2.** the moral obligation to render to the patient the best possible quality of dental service and to maintain an honest relationship with other members of the profession and mankind in general.

ethics, dental, *n* See ethics, professional.

ethics, professional, *n* the principles and norms of proper professional conduct concerning the rights and duties of health care professionals themselves and their conduct toward patients and fellow practitioners, including the actions taken in the care of patients and family members.

ethinyl estradiol (eth'inil es'trə dī'ol), *n brand names:* Estinyl; *drug class:* semi-synthetic estrogen; *action:* stimulates estrogen receptors resulting in characteristic changes in the function of the female reproductive system and other tissues.; *uses:* birth control (with a progestin), menopause, prostate cancer, breast cancer.

ethionamide (eth'ēon'əmīd'), *n brand name:* Trecator-SC; *drug class:* antitubercular; *action:* bacteriostatic against Mycobacterium tuberculosis; inhibits mycolic acid synthesis and thereby, cell wall synthesis; *uses:* pulmonary, extrapulmonary tuberculosis when other antitubercular drugs have failed.

ethmoid bone, *n* a single midline cranial bone of the skull.

ethmoid bone, orbital plate of the, *n* the plate that forms most of the medial orbital wall.

ethnic group, *n* a population of individuals organized around an assumption of common cultural origin.

ethnocentrism, *n* belief that one's own culture or traditions are better than that of other cultures.

ethosuximide **(eth′ōsuk′səmīd′),** *n brand name:* Zarontin; *drug class:* anticonvulsant; *actions:* suppresses spike wave formation in absence seizures (petit mal); decreases amplitude, frequency, duration, spread of discharge in minor motor seizures; *use:* absence seizures (petit mal).

ethyl acetate, abuse of (eth′əl as′ətāt), *n* the recreational, often compulsive inhaling of the fumes of a liquid solvent, especially those found in paint thinners. See also huffing.

ethyl aminobenzoate (eth′əl əme ′noben′zoāt), *n* an ester-type anesthetic agent formulated for surface application as a liquid, gel, ointment, or spray; the most widely used topical numbing agent.

ethyl chloride (eth′il klôr′īd), *n* (C_2H_5Cl) a colorless liquid that boils between 12° and 13° C. It acts as a local, topical anesthetic of short duration through the superficial freezing produced by its rapid vaporization from the skin. Ethyl chloride is used occasionally in inhalation therapy as a rapid, fleeting general anesthetic, comparable to nitrous oxide but somewhat more dangerous.

ethylene (olefiant gas, CH_2CH_2) (eth′ilēn), *n* a colorless gas of slightly sweet odor and taste.

ethylene oxide sterilization, *n* a process that uses gas to sterilize instruments, equipment, and materials that would otherwise be damaged by heat or liquid chemicals. Effective at room temperature. Requires between 10 and 16 hours to be effective. The gas must penetrate the material. The gas is highly toxic and must be vented before opening the sealed sterilizing unit. Sterilized materials must also be well aerated before using.

etidocaine HCl (local), *n brand names:* Duranest, Duranest MPF; *drug class:* amide, local anesthetic; *actions:* inhibits sodium channels and sodium ion fluxes across membranes;

decreases rise of depolarization phase of action potential; blocks nerve action potential; *uses:* local dental anesthetic, peripheral nerve block, caudal anesthetic, central neural block, vaginal block.

etidronate disodium (ē′tədrō′nāt dīsō′dēəm), *n brand name:* Didronel; *drug class:* bisphosphonate antihypercalcemic; *actions:* decreases bone resorption and new bone development; *uses:* Paget's disease, heterotopic ossification.

etiology (ē′tēol′əjē), *n* **1.** causative factors. *n* **2.** the factors implicated in the causation of disease. *n* **3.** the study of the factors causing disease.

etiology, local factors, *n* the environmental influences that may be implicated in the causation or perpetuation of a disease process.

etiology, systemic factors, *n* generalized biologic factors that are implicated in the causation, modification, or perpetuation of a disease entity. Within the oral cavity, the actions of the systemic factors are modified by interaction with local factors.

etodolac (ētō′dəlak), *n brand name:* Lodine; *drug class:* nonsteroidal antiinflammatory; *action:* inhibits prostaglandin synthesis by interfering with cyclooxygenase, which is needed for biosynthesis; *uses:* mild to moderate pain, osteoarthritis.

etoposide, *n brand names:* VePesid, Etopophos; *drug class:* antineoplastic; *action:* inhibits topoisomerase II and forms free radicals, thereby inhibiting or damaging DNA; *uses:* testicular cancer, lung cancer, lymphomas, Kaposi's sarcoma.

Eubacterium (ū′baktē′rēəm), *n.pr* a genus of anaerobic, non-spore forming, nonmotile bacteria containing straight or curved gram-positive rods that usually occur singly, in pairs, or in short chains. They usually metabolize carbohydrates and may be pathogenic.

eugenol (yōō′jənol), *n* **1.** an allyl guaiacol obtainable from oil of cloves. Used with zinc oxide in a paste for temporary restorations, bases under restorations, and impression materials. Believed to have a palliative effect on dental pulp and possibly a limited germicidal effect. *n* **2.** a colorless or pale yellow liquid obtained from clove oil; has a clove odor and pungent, spicy taste. Used as the liquid portion of zinc oxide and eugenol cements and in toothache medications.

eugnathia (ūnā′thēə), *n* the normal or proper relationship of the jaws to each other.

euphemism, *n* the substitution of a mild, inoffensive, relatively uncontroversial word or phrase for the accurate word or phase in an effort to make an explanation more understandable for a particular audience. Dentists use euphemisms frequently to explain treatments to younger patients. For example, the dentist may say "tooth vitamins" for "fluoride treatment" or the "whistle" instead of "high speed handpiece."

euphoria (ūfôr′ēə), *n* a sense of well-being or normalcy. Pleasantly mild excitement.

euphoric (ūfôr′ik), *n* a substance that produces an exaggerated sense of well-being.

eupnea (ūpnē′ə), *n* a situation with easy or normal respiration.

europium (yŏŏrō′pēəm), *n* a rare earth metallic element with an atomic number of 63 and an atomic weight of 151.96.

eustachian tube (ūstā′shən), *n* a tube, lined with mucous membrane, that joins the nasopharynx and the middle ear cavity, allowing equalization of the air pressure in the middle ear with atmospheric pressure. Also called the *auditory tube.*

Eutectic Mixture of Local Anesthetics *(EMLA)* (ūtek′tik), *n brand names:* EMLA, Oraqix; *drug class:* topical anesthetic; *action:* a topical anesthetic (blocks sodium channels in nerves) made from equal parts of lidocaine and prilocaine; *uses:* applied as a cream on unbroken skin, then covered with an occlusive dressing, to kill pain prior to venipuncture, intramuscular injections, intravenous cannulation, or minor skin procedures. See lidocaine HCl (topical), prilocaine hydrochloride.

euthanasia (ū′thənā′zhə), *n* an act of deliberately bringing about the death of a person who is suffering from an incurable disease or condition; also called *mercy killing.* Active euthanasia is illegal in most jurisdictions;

passive euthanasia, or the withholding of some life support systems, has legal standing in some jurisdictions.

euthyroidism (ūthī′roidizəm), *n* a state of normal thyroid function.

evacuation system, *n* a centralized vacuum system connected to each dental operating unit, used to keep the oral cavity clear of water, saliva, blood, and debris, generally operating at a high volume, high velocity, and low pressure.

evacuator tip, *n* a stainless steel or plastic tip which attaches to high-velocity tubing on a dental unit; used to evacuate large volumes of fluid and debris from the oral cavity.

evaluation, *n* to make a judgment or appraisal of a condition or situation. In dentistry, used to describe the clinical judgment of a patient's dental health or an appraisal of staff performance.

evaluation studies, *n.pl* the control study of the comparative value of different treatment modalities or medications.

Evans blue, *n.pr* a diazo dye used for the determination of the blood volume on the basis of the dilution of a standard solution of the dye in the plasma after its intravenous injection.

evidence, *n* the proof presented at a trial by the parties through witnesses, records, documents, and concrete objects for the purpose of inducing the court or jury to believe their contentions.

evidence, radiographic, *n* the shadow images depicted in radiographs.

evidence-based care, *n* a philosophy of treatment that relies on up-to-date, germane research as its foundation.

evoked potential, *n* an electrical response in the brainstem or cerebral cortex that is elicited by a specific stimulus. This property of the brain may be used to monitor brain function during surgery.

evulsed tooth (ivul′st), *n* See tooth, avulsed.

evulsion, nerve, *n* See avulsion, nerve.

evulsion, tooth, *n* See avulsion, tooth.

Ewing's sarcoma, *n.pr* See sarcoma, Ewing's.

Ewing's tumor, *n.pr* See sarcoma, Ewing's.

examination, *n* **1.** inspection; search; investigation; inquiry; scrutiny; testing. *n* **2.** the inspection or investigation of part or all of the body to measure and evaluate the state of health or disease. The examination may include visual inspection, percussion, palpation, auscultation, and measurement of mobility as well as various laboratory and radiographic procedures.

examination, anteroposterior extraoral radiographic, *n* an examination in which the film is placed at the posterior direction with the rays passing from the anterior to the posterior direction to record images.

examination, bite-wing intraoral radiographic, *n* radiography in which an intraoral radiograph records on a single film the shadow images of the outline, position, and mesiodistal extent of the crowns, necks, and coronal third of the roots of both the maxillary and mandibular teeth and alveolar crests.

examination, body section extraoral radiographic, *n* a radiographic procedure of various internal layers of the head and body accomplished by the synchronized movement of the roentgen-ray tube and film in parallel planes but in opposite directions from each other. Also known as *tomography, laminagraphy, planigraphy,* and *stratigraphy.*

examination, bregmamentum extraoral radiographic **(breg′məmen′təm),** *n* radiography in which the film is placed beneath the chin, with the rays directed downward through the junction of the coronal and sagittal sutures (bregma) to the chin (mentum).

examination, cephalometric extraoral radiographic **(sef′əlōmet′rik),** *n* See cephalometric radiography.

examination, clinical, *n* **1.** the visual and tactile scrutiny of the tissue of and surrounding the oral cavity. *n* **2.** the formal testing of the dental professional student to determine whether his or her skills meet or exceed established standards.

examination, complete, *n* a methodical, complete assessment of an individual involving basic and supplementary procedures as well as evaluation of the plan for preventive care.

examination, extradental intraoral radiographic, *n* an examination in which the receptor is placed between the teeth and the tissue of the cheek or lip for the exploration or localization of the internal structures of these tissues.

examination, extraoral radiographic, *n* an examination of the oral and paraoral structures by exposing receptors placed extraorally, in contrast to intraorally.

examination, gingival, *n* the observation of the primary visual symptoms of periodontal disease, including color changes, changes in surface texture, deviations from normal contour and structure, tissue tone, and vitality, presence or absence of clefts, and the position of attachment.

examination, intraoral, *n* an examination of all the structures contained within the oral cavity.

examination, intraoral radiographic, *n* the examination of the oral and paraoral structures by exposing receptors placed within the oral cavity.

examination, lateral facial extraoral radiographic, *n* an examination by means of a lateral head receptor.

examination, lateral head extraoral radiographic, *n* an examination in which the receptor is placed parallel to the sagittal plane of the head.

examination, lateral jaw extraoral radiographic, *n* an examination in which the receptor is placed adjacent to the mandible.

examination, limited, *n* an assessment typically conducted during an emergency situation for the management of a critical medical condition.

examination, mental extraoral radiographic, *n* an examination in which the receptor is placed beneath the chin, and the radiation is directed through the long axis of the mandibular central incisors while the oral cavity is open.

Examination, National Board Dental Hygiene (NBDHE), *n.pr* See National Board Dental Hygiene Examination.

examination, oblique occlusal intraoral radiographic, *n* an exploratory examination of the maxillae or mandible using an occlusal type of receptor placed between the teeth. The rays are directed obliquely downward or upward (usually 60° to 75° in the vertical plane) and parallel to the sagittal plane.

examination, panoramic extraoral radiographic, n a type of extraoral radiographic procedure in which the beam source and film rotate in a synchronized manner about the head, exposing oral structures sequentially with simultaneous exposure of corresponding areas of the receptor, producing a wide view of oral structures.

examination, periapical intraoral radiographic, n the basic intraoral examination, showing all of a tooth and the surrounding periodontium.

examination, posteroanterior extraoral radiographic, n an examination in which the receptor is placed anteriorly, with the rays passing from the posterior to the anterior direction.

examination, profile extraoral radiographic, n a lateral head examination to show the profile of bone and soft tissue outline. It uses a decrease in milliampere seconds or an increase in target-receptor distance for recording the soft tissue image.

examination, radiographic, n 1. the production of the number of radiographic images necessary for the radiologic interpretation of the part or parts in question. *n* 2. the study and interpretation of radiographic images of the oral cavity and associated structures.

examination, stereoscopic extraoral radiographic, n a radiographic examination in conjunction with a stereoscope for localization. Exposures of two receptors are made, with identical placement of each film adjacent to the part in question and with a different angulation for each exposure.

examination, temporomandibular extraoral radiographic, n an examination in which the receptor is placed adjacent to the area to be examined, with the rays directed through a point that is 2.5 inches (6.25 cm) above the tragus of the opposite external ear, with a vertical angulation of 15° and a horizontal angulation of 5° downward. Various other techniques and angulations are used, including laminagraphy, in examining this area.

examination, true occlusal topographic intraoral radiographic, n the radiography of the maxillae or mandible using an occlusal type of receptor placed between the teeth, with the rays directed at right angles to the plane of the receptor or through the long axis of the teeth adjacent to the part in question.

examination, Waters extraoral radiographic, n.pr the posteroanterior examination of the paranasal sinuses. The receptor is placed in contact with the nose and chin, with the rays directed at right angles to the plane of the receptor.

excavator (eks′kəvātur), *n* an instrument used to remove diseased tissue from teeth and to prepare the resulting cavity for treatment. Such instruments include hoes, spoons, and angle formers.

excavator, spoon, n a paired hand instrument intended primarily to remove carious material from a cavity.

excess, *n* more than is necessary, useful, or specified.

excess, marginal, n a condition in which the restorative material extends beyond the prepared cavity margin.

excess overhang, n a gingival margin excess.

excipient (eksip′ēənt), *n* an ingredient included in a pharmaceutical preparation for the purpose of improving its physical qualities. See also binder; filler; vehicle.

excision (eksizh′ən), *n* the act of cutting away or taking out.

excision, local, n an excision limited to the immediate area of the lesion in question.

excision, radical, n an excision involving not only the lesion in question but also anatomic parts remote from the site.

excision, wide, n an excision involving the lesion in question and immediately adjacent anatomic structures.

excitant (eksīt′ənt), *n* an agent that stimulates the activity of an organ.

excitation (eksītā′shən), *n* the addition of energy to a system, thereby transferring it from its ground state to an excited state.

exclusions, *n.pl* the dental services not covered under a dental benefits program.

exclusive provider organization (EPO), *n* a dental benefits plan that provides benefits only if care is rendered by institutional and professional providers with whom the plan contracts (with some exceptions for emergency and out-of-area services).

excursion, lateral, *n* the movement of the mandible from the centric position to a lateral or protrusive position.

execute, *v* to finish; accomplish; fulfill. To carry out according to certain terms.

exercise, *n* the performance of physical activity for the purpose of conditioning the body, improving health, or maintaining fitness or as a means of therapy for correcting a deformity or restoring the organs and bodily function to a state of health.

exercise, orofacial myotherapeutic, *n* See therapy, myofunctional.

exercise prosthesis, *n* See prosthesis, exercise.

exertion, *n* vigorous action, a great effort, a strong influence.

exfoliation (eksfō'lēā 'shən), *n* the physiologic loss of the primary dentition. Also called *shedding.*

exhalation (ekshəlā'shən), *n* giving off or sending forth in the form of vapor; expiration.

exhaustion (egzôs'chən), *n* the loss of vital and nervous power from fatigue or protracted disease.

exhibit (egzib'it), *n* a paper, document, or object presented to a court during a trial or hearing as proof of facts, or as otherwise connected with the subject matter, and which, on being accepted, is marked for identification and considered a part of the case.

exit, port of, *n* the means by which infectious microorganisms may leave the body, such as secretions of mucus, blood, saliva, or other fluids.

exocrine (ek'sokrin), *adj* exuding outside the body, from a duct.

exocytosis (ek'sōsītō'sis), *n* the active transport of material from a vesicle out into the extracellular environment.

exodontics (ek'sōdon'tiks), *n* the science and practice of removing teeth from the oral cavity as performed by dental professionals.

exogenous (eksoj'ənəs), *adj* originating or caused by aspects external to a body.

exophthalmos (ek'softhal'mōs), *n* an abnormal protrusion of the eyeball. It is characteristic of toxic (exophthalmic) goiter.

exophytic (ek'sofit'ik), *adj* developing externally.

exostosis (pl. exostoses) (ek'sostō'sis), *n* (hyperostosis) a bony growth projecting from a bony surface.

exotoxin (ek'sōtoksin), *n* the toxic material formed by microorganisms and subsequently released into their surrounding environments.

expanded duty auxiliary, *n* a person trained (and possibly licensed or certified) to carry out dental procedures more complex than the responsibilities usually delegated to dental auxiliaries.

expanded polytetrafluoroethylene (ePTFE) (ekspan'did pol'ētet' rəflöör'ōeth'əlēn), *n* a stretched polymer of tetrafluoroethylene that allows passage of fluids but not cells; it is used as a nonabsorbable suture material and in guided tissue and bone regeneration as a nonresorbable membrane.

expansile infrastructure endosteal implant (ikspan'sil in'frəstruk'chər endos'tēəl), *n* an intraosseous implant device designed to enlarge or open after its insertion into the bone to provide retention.

expansion (ekspan'shən), *n* an increase in extent, size, volume, or scope.

expansion, delayed (secondary expansion), *n* **1.** an expansion occurring in amalgam restorations as a result of moisture contamination. *n* **2.** an expansion exhibited by amalgam that has been contaminated by moisture during trituration or insertion.

expansion, dental arch, *n* the therapeutic increase in circumference of the dental arch by buccal or labial movement of the teeth.

expansion, hygroscopic, *n* an expansion, caused by absorption of water during setting of an investment, used to compensate for the shrinkage of metal from the molten to the solid state.

expansion, secondary, *n* See expansion, delayed.

expansion, setting, *n* an expansion that occurs during the setting or hardening of materials such as amalgam and gypsum products.

expansion, skeletal, *n* approach undertaken in patients with transverse maxillary width deficiency, prior to closure of mid-palatal suture in the adolescent or with surgery in the adult.

expansion, thermal, *n* an expansion caused by heat. Thermal expansion of the mold is one of the important factors in achieving adequate compensation for the contraction of cast metal when it solidifies.

expansion, thermal coefficient, *n* a number indicating the amount of expansion caused by each degree of temperature change. The rate of change in restorative materials and tooth substance should be relatively the same.

experience rating, *n* a determination of the premium rate for a particular group partially or wholly on the basis of that group's own experience. Age, sex, use, and costs of services provided determine the premium.

experiment, *n* a trial or special observation made to confirm or disprove something doubtful; an act or operation undertaken to discover some unknown principle or effect or to test, establish, or illustrate some suggested or known truth.

experimental approach, research study also known as a clinical trial that studies an experimental treatment or intervention.

experimental group, *n* the group of participants in a clinical study who receive the actual drug or treatment being studied. See also controlled clinical trial.

expert, *n* a person who has special skill or knowledge in a particular subject, such as a science or art, whether acquired by experience or study; a specialist.

expert system, *n* a computer program that follows a logical pathway or algorithm to a conclusion in a manner that mimics what an expert in the field would follow.

expert testimony, *n* the sworn statements of a person with special knowledge about a subject under consideration by a court of law.

expert witness, *n* a person who has special knowledge of a subject about which a court requests testimony to educate the court and the jury in the subject under consideration.

expiration (ek′spərā′shən), *n* **1.** the act of breathing forth or expelling air from the lungs. *n* **2.** a cessation.

expiration date, *n* **1.** the date on which a dental benefits contract expires. *n* **2.** the date an individual ceases to be eligible for benefits.*n* **3.** the date that the Food and Drug Administration (FDA) requires pharmaceutical manufacturers to provide on all their products. For the majority of drugs sold in the United States, these dates range from 12 to 60 months from the date they are manufactured.

explanation of benefits, *n* a written statement to a beneficiary, from a third-party payer, after a claim has been reported, indicating the benefits and charges covered or not covered by the dental benefits plan.

exploration, *n* **1.** an examination by touch, either with or without instruments. (E.g., a carious lesion is explored with a special explorer, but the mucobuccal fold may be explored with the finger.) *n* **2.** the process of examination of a surface, with or without the use of instruments, to determine the condition or the surface depth of a defect or other similar diagnostic parameters.

explore, *v* to investigate.

explorer, *n* a dental instrument with a slender head that is honed to a fine point, used to conduct a tactile examination and appraisal of pits and fissures, carious lesions, root surfaces, and margins of restoration.

explorer, 11/12-type, *n* a type with a paired working end and long lower shank whose specially angled tip design makes it suited for use in either shallow depressions or deep pockets.

explorer, cowhorn, *n* a type so named because of the shape of its shank that is used to examine teeth for calculus, caries, and restoration margins. Also called *pigtail explorer.*

explorer, curved shank, *n* a type used to examine proximal tooth surfaces for calculus and caries, which, because of its arc, allows easier access to back teeth.

explorer, Orban No. 20, *n.pr* a type that is used to detect calculus, caries, lesions, and cemental changes on the subgingival surfaces of a tooth.

explorer, pigtail, *n* See explorer, cowhorn.

explorer, periodontal, *n* a fine, thin instrument that is easily adapted around the root surfaces and is used to locate deposits of calculus.

explorer, pocket, *n* See explorer, Orban No. 20.

explorer, sickle, *n* a hand-activated assessment tool, so named because of the distinctive shape of its shank, that is used to examine fissures and the surfaces of natural teeth, restorations, and sealants; not suited for exploration inferior to the gingival margin.

explorer, straight, *n* a type with an unpaired working end and short lower shank that is used to examine caries inferior to the gingival margin and in restorations with irregular margins; not suited to detecting calculus inferior to the gingival margin.

explorer, TU-17, *n.pr* a type that is used to detect calculus, caries, lesions, and cemental changes on the subgingival surfaces of a tooth; may be adapted for use on selected supragingival surfaces.

explorers, paired, *n.pl* two identical explorers with contralateral curves that are used to examine opposite tooth surfaces superior to the gingival margin; mirrored-image explorers.

explosion, *n* a violent, noisy outbreak caused by a sudden release of energy.

exposure **(iksp** o **'zhər)**, *n* uncovering; subjection to viewing or radiation.

exposure, accidental pulp, *n* a pulp exposure unintentionally created during instrumentation.

exposure, air, *n* the radiation exposure measured in a small mass of air under conditions of electronic equilibrium with the surrounding air, (i.e., excluding backscatter from irradiated parts or objects).

exposure, cariogenic **(karēōjen'ik),** *n* an incident in which teeth come into contact with foods that tend to create

a favorable environment for development of dental caries.

exposure, carious pulp, *n* a pulp exposure occasioned by extension of the carious process to the pulp chamber wall.

exposure, chronic, *n* a radiation exposure of long duration, either continuous (protraction exposure) or intermittent (fractionation exposure); usually referring to exposure of relatively low intensity.

exposure, cumulative, *n* the total accumulated exposure resulting from repeated radiation exposures of the whole body or of a particular region.

exposure, double, *n* the two superimposed exposures on the same radiographic or photographic film.

exposure, entrance, *n* an exposure measured at the surface of an irradiated body, part, or object. It includes both primary radiation and backscatter from the irradiated underlying tissue or material.

exposure, erythema **(erəthē'mə),** *n* the radiation exposure necessary to produce a temporary redness of the skin. The exposure required varies with the quality of the radiation to which the skin is exposed.

exposure incident, *n* an event in which a health care professional's potential for infection is heightened after coming into contact with a patient's blood, body fluids, mucous membranes, or broken skin.

exposure, mechanical pulp, *n* See exposure, pulp, surgical.

exposure, parenteral, *n* exposure of the internal systems of the body due to the puncturing of the skin by a needle or other sharp instrument.

exposure, protraction, *n* the continuous exposure to radiation over a relatively long period at a low exposure rate.

exposure, pulp, *n* an opening through the wall of the pulp chamber uncovering the dental pulp.

exposure, radiographic, *n* a measure of the x or γ radiation to which a person or object, or part of either, is exposed at a certain place, this measure being based on its ability to produce ionization. The unit of x- or γ-radiation exposure is the roentgen (R).

exposure, radiographic, entrance (surface), n the radiation exposure measured at the external surface of a person or object that has been irradiated. Measurement includes both backscatter radiation from the exposed tissue and primary radiation.

exposure rate, output, n the exposure to radiation at a specified point per unit of time, usually expressed in roentgens per minute.

exposure, surface, n See exposure, entrance.

exposure, surgical pulp, n (mechanical pulp exposure) the pulp exposure created intentionally or unintentionally during instrumentation.

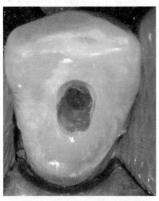

Surgical exposure of pulp. (Hargreaves/Cohen, 2011)

exposure, threshold, n the minimum exposure that will produce a detectable degree of any given effect.

exposure time, n the time during which a person or object is exposed to radiation, expressed in one of the conventional units of time.

express, v to state distinctly and explicitly and not leave to inference; to set forth in words.

exsufflation (ek'suflā'shən), n the forced discharge of the breath.

extension (iksten'shən), n **1.** an enlargement in boundary, breadth, or depth. n **2.** the process of increasing the angle between two skeletal levers having end-to-end articulation with each other; the opposite of flexion.

extension base, n See base, extension.

extension base, gingiva, attached, n a gingival extension operation; a surgical technique designed to broaden the zone of attached gingiva by repositioning the mucogingival junction apically.

extension base, groove, n the enlargement of a cavity preparation outline to include a developmental groove.

extension base of benefits, n an extension of eligibility for benefits for covered services, usually designed to ensure completion of treatment commenced before the expiration date. Duration is generally expressed in terms of days.

extension base, ridge, n an intraoral surgical operation for deepening the labial, buccal, or lingual sulci.

extension for prevention, n a principle of cavity preparation promoted by G.V. Black. To prevent the recurrence of decay, he advocated extension of the preparation into an area that is readily polished and cleaned. The philosophy is no longer used in dentistry.

extenuate (iksten'ūāt'), v to lessen; to mitigate.

external, adj the outer side of the wall of a hollow structure.

external oblique line (ōblēk'), n See line, external oblique.

external pin fixation, n See appliance, fracture.

external traction, n See traction, external.

exteroceptors (ek'stərōsep'turz), n.pl the sensory nerve end receptors that respond to external stimuli; located in the skin, oral cavity, eyes, ears, and nose.

extirpation, pulp (ek'sturpā'shən), n See pulpectomy.

extracellular (eks'trəsel'ulər), adj taking place outside of a cell.

extracellular matrix, n an amorphous or structured substance produced by cellular activity that lies within the tissue but outside the cell.

extracoronal (ek'strəkôr'ōnəl), adj pertaining to that which is outside, or external to, the body of the coronal portion of a natural tooth.

extracoronal retainer, n See retainer, extracoronal.

E

extract (ek´strakt), *n* a concentrate obtained by treating a crude material, such as plant or animal tissue, with a solvent, evaporating part or all of the solvent from the resulting solution, and standardizing the resulting product.

extraction, *n* the removal of a tooth from the oral cavity by means of elevators and/or forceps.

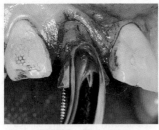

Extraction. (Block, 2011)

extraction, serial, *n* the extraction of selected primary teeth over a period of years (often ending with removal of the first premolar teeth) to relieve crowding of the dental arches during eruption of the lateral incisors, canines, and premolars.

extraoral, *adj* literally, outside the oral cavity.

extraoral anchorage, *n* orthodontic force applied from a base outside the oral cavity. See also anchorage, extraoral.

extrapolate (ekstrap´ōlāt), *v* to infer values beyond the observable range from an observed trend of variables; to project by inference into the unexplored.

extrasystole (ek´strəsis´tōlē), *n* a heartbeat occurring before its normal time in the rhythm of the heart and followed by a compensatory pause.

extravasation (ekstrav´əzā´shən), *n* the escape of a body fluid out of its proper place (e.g., blood into surrounding tissue after rupture of a vessel, urine into surrounding tissue after rupture of the bladder).

extremity (ikstrem´itē), *n* an arm or a leg; the arm may be identified as an upper extremity, and the leg as a lower extremity.

extrinsic (ikstrin´sik), *adj* originating outside; not inherent or essential.

extroversion (ek´strəvur´zhən), *n* a tendency of the teeth or other maxillary structures to become situated too far from the median plane.

extrude (ekstrōod´), *v* to elevate; to move a tooth coronally.

extrusion (ikstroo´zhən), *n* the movement of teeth beyond the natural occlusal plane that may be accompanied by a similar movement of investing tissue. See also eruption, continuous.

extubate (eks´toobāt), *v* to remove a tube, usually an endotracheal anesthesia tube or a Levin gastric suction tube.

extubation (eks´toobā´shən), *n* the removal of a tube used for intubation.

exudate (eks´ōōdāt), *n* the outpouring of a fluid substance, such as exudated suppuration or tissue fluid.

exudate, purulent **(eks´ōōdāt pyür´ələnt),** *n* pus or suppuration that exudes from the gingival tissue and contains a mixture of enzymes, dead tissue, bacteria, and leukocytes, primarily neutrophils.

exudates, gingival, *n* the outpouring of an inflammatory exudate from the gingival tissue.

exudation (eks´oodā´shən), *n* See exudate.

eye, *n* one of a pair of organs of sight, contained in a bony orbit at the front of the skull.

eye, assessment of, *n* an examination of the eyes—which includes an observation of pupil size, sclera color, the relative location of the eyeball, and use of corrective eyeware—to determine the presence of disease.

eye-ear plane, *n* See plane, Frankfort horizontal.

eye loupes, *n* the low-magnification lenses that allow the wearer to visualize small details, such as the teeth and oral cavity.

eye wash station, *n* a cleansing receptacle set apart for the purpose of emergencies in which the eyes must be quickly flushed with water.

eyeglass, postmydriatic (pōst´mid´r eat´ik), *n* a disposable protective eyewear made of pliable plastic material, handed out by ophthalmologists to patients whose pupils have been dilated during a mydriatic examination.

eyelids, *n.pl* a moveable fold of thin skin over the eye. The orbicularis oculi muscle and the oculomotor nerve control the opening and closing of the eyelid.

eyewear, protective, *n* **1.** the goggles or safety glasses that are worn to protect the eyes from dust and debris while using dental powders or trimmers in the preparation of a study cast. *n* **2.** the goggles or safety glasses worn to protect the dental care worker or the patient from accidental eye exposure to blood or other body fluids, or to prevent accidental injury from dental instruments. Pediatric patients or patients with sensitive eyes may be given shaded glasses or goggles to protect the eyes from the brightness of the dental examination lamp.

ezetimibe, *n brand name:* Zetia; *drug class:* cholesterol absorption inhibitor; *action:* binds the cholesterol transporter in the intestine and reduces plasma cholesterol ; *use:* hypercholesterolemia.

fabrication (fab′rikā′sh ən), *n* the construction or making of a restoration.

face, *n* the front of the head from the chin to the brow, including the skin and muscles and structures of the forehead, eyes, nose, oral cavity, cheeks, and jaws.

face, changeable area of, the part of the face from the nose to the chin.

face form, n See form, face.

face, instrument blade, n See instrument blade face.

face shield, n.pl a type of protective eyewear sometimes used by oral health care workers in place of safety glasses. Although intended to cover the face completely for high-spatter treatments such as polishing and scaling, they may have limited impact resistance and should not be considered a replacement for protective breathing masks.

face-bow, *n* a caliper-like device that is used to record the relationship of the maxillae to the temporomandibular joints (or opening axis of the mandible) and to orient the casts in this same relationship to the opening axis of an articulator.

face-bow adjustable axis, n See facebow, kinematic.

face-bow, kinematic (hinge-bow) (kinəmat′ik), n a face-bow attached to the mandible with caliper ends (condyle rods) that can be adjusted to permit the accurate location of the axis of rotation of the mandible.

facet (fas′et), *n* a flattened, highly polished wear pattern, as noted on a tooth.

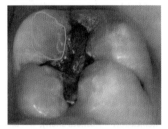

Facet of wear (*circled***).** (Dawson, 2007)

facial angle, *n* an anthropomorphic expression of the degree of protrusion of the lower face, assessed by the measured inclination of the facial plane in relation to the Frankfort horizontal reference plane.

facial artery, *n* one of a pair of tortuous arteries that arise from the external carotid arteries, divide into four cervical and five facial branches, and supply various organs and tissue in the head. The cervical branches of the facial artery are the ascending palatine, tonsillar, glandular, and submental. The facial branches are the inferior labial, superior labial, lateral nasal, angular, and muscular.

facial asymmetry (āsim′ətrē), *n* the variation in the configuration of one side of the face from the other when viewed in relation to a projected mid-sagittal line.

facial bones, *n.pl* the bones of the face, which include the frontal, nasal, maxillary, zygomatic, and mandibular bones.

who teach within an institution of learning.

FAD, *n* abbreviation for *flavin adenine dinucleotide.*

failure, *n* a deficiency; an inefficiency as measured by some legal standard; an unsuccessful attempt.

failure to thrive, n the abnormal retardation of the growth and development of an infant resulting from conditions that interfere with normal metabolism, appetite, and activity.

faint, *n* a state of syncope, or swooning.

false light, *n* a misleading fashion in which a person is depicted before the public that a reasonable person finds offensive and damaging.

false negative aspiration, *n* a perceived negative aspiration during the administration of a local anesthetic where the needle tip lies within a blood vessel and is butting up against the wall of the vessel, preventing the entrance of blood into the cartridge.

falsify, *v* to forge; to give a false appearance to anything, as to falsify a record.

famciclovir (famsī′klōvēr), *n* brand name: Famvir; *drug class:* antiviral; *action:* converted to active metabolite, penciclovir triphosphate, which inhibits viral DNA synthesis and replication; *uses:* acute herpes zoster (shingles) infection, herpes labialis, genital herpes.

family, *n* **1.** a group of people related by heredity, such as parents, children, and siblings. The term is sometimes broadened to include related by marriage or those living in the same household, who are emotionally attached, interact regularly, and share concerns for the growth and development of the group and its individual members. *n* **2.** a category of animals or plants situated on a taxonomic scale between order and genus. *n* **3.** the legal definition varies, depending on the jurisdiction and purpose for which the term is defined.

family counseling, n a program that consists of providing information and professional guidance to members of a family concerning specific health matters.

family deductible, n a deductible that is satisfied by combined expenses of all covered family members. A plan with a $25 deductible may limit its application to a maximum of three deductibles, or $75, for the family, regardless of the number of family members.

family dentistry, n the branch of dentistry that is concerned with the diagnosis and treatment of dental problems in people of either sex and at any age. Family dental professionals were formerly known as *general practitioners,* and therefore family dentistry does not constitute one of the specialty areas of dentistry.

family history, n a part of the medical history process; practitioner should ask patient about history of diseases or serious illness in family to determine if the patient might be predisposed to certain illnesses.

family membership, n a membership that includes spouses and/or dependents.

family unit, n an insured group member and dependents who are eligible for benefits under a dental care contract; an accounting unit.

famotidine (fəmō′tədēn′), *n* brand names: Pepcid, Pepcid IV; *drug class:* H_2-histamine receptor antagonist; *action:* inhibits histamine at H_2 receptor site in parietal cells, which inhibits gastric acid secretion; *uses:* short-term treatment of active duodenal ulcer, gastric ulcer, heartburn.

fascia (fash′ēə) (pl. fasciae), *n* the fibrous connective tissue of the body that may be separated from other specifically organized fibrous structures such as the tendons, the aponeuroses, and the ligaments. Fascia generally covers and separates muscles and muscle groups.

fascia, buccopharyngeal, n the deep cervical fascia that encloses the entire upper portion of the alimentary canal.

fascia, investing, n the most external layer of the deep cervical fascia.

fascia masseteric-parotid (fash′ēə mas′iter′ik-pərot′id), n the fascia that covers the masseter, a cheek muscle that closes the jaw. Also known as the *masseteric fascia.*

fascia, pterygoid, n the deep fascia located on the medial surface of the medial pterygoid muscle.

fascia, temporal, n the deep fascia covering the temporalis muscle down to the zygomatic arch.

fascia, vertebral, n the deep cervical fascia that covers the vertebrae, spinal column, and associated muscles.

fascia, visceral, n the deep cervical fascia that is a single midline tube running down the neck.

fascial, *adj* relating to the fascia.

fasciitis **(fəsi'tis),** n a tumorlike growth occurring in submucosal tissue in the oral cavity, usually in the cheek. A benign lesion sometimes mistaken for fibrosarcoma. Fasciitis consists of young fibroblasts and numerous capillaries. It grows rapidly and may regress spontaneously.

fasciculi, *n.pl* nerve fibers bundled together into groups.

fast, v to abstain from ingesting food for a specific period, usually for diagnostic, therapeutic, or religious purposes.

fast-set powder, n an irreversible, hydrocolloid material used to make impressions of a patient's dentition; this alginate material has a working time of 1.25 minutes and a setting time of 1 to 2 minutes (as opposed to a working time of 2 minutes and a setting time of 4.5 minutes with a normal-set powder).

fast green, n a green dye used to reveal dental biofilm (dental plaque) deposits on teeth; consists of F. D. & C. Green No. 3 in concentrations of either 5% or 2.5%.

fat, n **1.** a substance composed of lipids or fatty acids and occurring in various forms or consistencies ranging from oil to tallow. n **2.** a type of connective tissue containing stored lipids.

fat embolism **(em'bɔliz'əm),** n a circulatory condition characterized by the blocking of an artery by an embolus of fat that enters the circulatory system after the fracture of a long bone, or less commonly, after traumatic injury to fatty tissue or to a fatty liver.

fatal outcome, n a consequence that results in death. The course of a disease that results in the death of the patient.

fate, n a synonym for the more modern term *biotransformation.* See also biotransformation.

fatigue, n a condition of cells or organs under stress, resulting in a diminution or loss of an individual's capacity to respond to stimulation.

fatigue, dental materials, n dysfunction due to damage caused by recurring use or stress.

fatigue, muscle, n a peripheral phenomenon caused by the failure of the muscle to contract when stimuli from the nervous system reach it. Occurs when muscle activity exceeds tissue substrate and oxygenation capacity.

fatigue strength, n the ability of a material to withstand repeated stress. In dental work, the fatigue strength of materials used in fillings and dentures is an important consideration because patients will repeatedly stress their fillings and dentures when eating.

fatty acid, n an organic acid produced by the hydrolysis of neutral fats.

fauces **(fô'sēz),** n the archway between the pharyngeal and oral cavities; formed by the tongue, anterior and posterior tonsillar pillars, and soft palate.

faucial pillars (fô'shəl), *n.pl* the vertical folds of tissue created by muscles that create the fauces, which surround the palatine tonsils. See anterior faucial pillar; posterior faucial pillar; tonsil, palatine.

FDA, *n.pr* the abbreviation for the Food and Drug Administration. See also Food and Drug Administration.

F. D. & C., n See Food, Drug, and Cosmetic Act.

fear, n an emotion, generally considered negative and unpleasant, that is a reaction to a real or threatened danger; fright. Fear is distinguished from anxiety, which is a reaction to an unreal or imagined danger.

febrile (feb'rəl), *adj* pertaining to or characterized by an elevated body temperature. A body temperature of over 100° F is commonly regarded as febrile.

feces (fē'sēz), n the waste or excrement from the digestive tract that is formed in the intestine and expelled through the rectum. It consists of water, food residue, bacteria, and secretions of the intestines and liver.

Fede's disease, See disease, Riga-Fede.

Federal Tort Claims Act, *n.pr* a statute passed in 1946 that allows the federal government to be sued for the wrongful action or negligence of its employees. The act, for most purposes, eliminates the doctrine of governmental immunity, which formerly prohibited or limited the bringing of suit against the federal government.

Fédération Dentaire Internationale (F. D. I.) Two-Digit System (fā′dārāsyŏn dônter′ en′ternäs′yō näl′), *n.pr* a recognized method used to identify and designate permanent and primary and deciduous teeth within the oral cavity. The first digit represents the quadrant number (1-4) starting with the maxillary right quadrant, moving around the maxillary arch to the left, then down and back to the right, and ending with the mandibular right quadrant. The second digit represents each tooth in the quadrant, numbered distally from the midline. Also called the *International System.*

fee, *n* the compensation for services rendered or to be rendered; payment for professional services.

fee, customary, n a fee is customary if it is in the range of the usual fees charged by dental professionals of similar training and experience for the same service within the specific and limited geographic area (i.e., the socioeconomic area of a metropolitan area or of a county).

fee-for-service plan, n a plan providing for payment to the dental professional for each service performed rather than on the basis of salary or capitation fee.

fee, reasonable, n a fee is considered reasonable if, in the opinion of a responsible dental association's review committee, it is the usual and customary fee charged for services rendered, considering the special circumstances of the case in question.

fee schedule, n **1.** a list of maximum dollar allowances for dental procedures that apply under a specific contract. *n* **2.** a list of the charges established or agreed to by a dental professional for specific dental services.

fee, usual, n the fee customarily charged for a given service by an individual dental professional to a private patient.

feedback, *n* the constant flow of sensory information back to the brain. When feedback mechanisms are deficient because of sensory deprivation, motor function becomes distorted, aberrant, and uncoordinated.

Feer's disease (fārz), *n.pr* See erythredema polyneuropathy.

felbamate, *n brand name:* Felbatol; *drug class:* anticonvulsant; *action:* anticonvulsant action is unclear; *uses:* alone or as an adjunct therapy in partial seizures.

feldspar (feld′spär), *n* a crystalline mineral of aluminum silicate with potassium, sodium, barium, or calcium—$NaAlSi_3O_8$ or $KAlSi_3O_8$. Feldspar melts over a range of 1,100° F to 2,000° F (593.5° C to 1093.5° C). An important constituent of dental porcelain.

feldspar, orthoclase ceramic, n a clay found in large quantity in the solid crust of the earth. It acts as a filler and imparts body to the fused dental porcelain.

felodipine (fəlŏ′dəpēn′), *n brand names:* Plendil, Renedil; *drug class:* calcium channel blocker; *actions:* inhibits calcium ion influx across cell membranes of cardiac muscle and smooth muscle of blood vessels, produces relaxation of coronary vascular smooth muscle, dilates coronary arteries, decreases SA node automaticity and AV node conduction, *use:* essential hypertension, alone or with other antihypertensives.

felony, *n* a crime declared by statute to be more serious than a misdemeanor and deserving of a more severe penalty. Conviction usually requires imprisonment in a penitentiary for longer than 1 year.

felypressin (fel′ipres′in), *n brand name:* Octapressin; *drug class:* vasopressin analogue; *actions:* helps to contain anesthetic in a specific area by reducing systemic absorption, decreasing blood flow, and prolonging effectiveness; *use:* an ingredient (that in some countries) is added to a local anesthetic for the purpose of constricting blood vessels. It is not available in the United States.

fenestration, in alveolar plate, (fenestrā′shən, alvē′ələr), *n* a round or oval defect in the facial alveolar bony plate that results in parital exposure of the root (or implant) by bone.

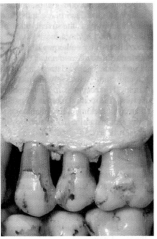

Fenestration. (Perry/Beemsterboer, 2007)

fenoprofen calcium, *n brand name:* Nalfon; *drug class:* nonsteroidal antiinflammatory; *action:* inhibits prostaglandin synthesis by interfering with cyclooxygenase needed for biosynthesis; *uses:* mild to moderate pain, osteoarthritis, rheumatoid arthritis, acute gout, dysmenorrhea.

fentanyl (fen'tənil), *n brand names:* Abstral Actiq, Duragesic, Fentora, Ionsys; *drug class:* narcotic analgesic; *action:* interacts with opioid receptors in the central nervous system to alter pain perception; *uses:* management of chronic pain when opioids are necessary, by a variety of routes and methods of administration.

fermentable, *adj* the ability to undergo a chemical reaction in the presence of an enzyme that results in the creation of either acid or alcohol; in the oral cavity, the ability to create acid in dental biofilm (dental plaque).

fermentation (fur'məntā'shən), *n* a chemical change that is brought about in a substance by the action of an enzyme or microorganism, especially the anaerobic conversion of foodstuffs to certain products such as acetic fermentation, alcoholic fermentation.

ferric sulfate, *n* an iron salt that coagulates blood. It is advocated by some dentists as a pulp capping agent for pulpotomies in primary teeth.

Ferrier's separator (fer'ēurz), *n.pr* See separator, Ferrier's.

ferritin (fer'itin), *n* the compound iron-appoferritin, which is produced in the intestine and stored primarily in the liver, spleen, and bone marrow. It eventually becomes a component of hemoglobin and can be measured to estimate the body's iron levels.

ferromagnetic   (fer'ōmagnet'ik), *adj* pertaining to substances that exhibit unusually strong magnetic properties; ironlike substances.

ferrous fumarate/ferrous gluconate/ferrous sulfate, *n brand names:* Femiron, Feostat; *drug class:* hematinic, iron preparation; *action:* replaces iron stores needed for red blood cell development; *uses:* iron deficiency anemia, prophylaxis for iron deficiency in pregnancy.

fertility, *n* the ability to reproduce.

fertilization, *n* the process by which the sperm penetrates the ovum during the preimplantation period.

ferule (fer'əl), *n* a protective ring (usually of metal) around a natural tooth root used to join an artificial crown. Also spelled *ferrule.*

ferrule effect, *n* dental crown preparations should have a circumference of very slightly tapered healthy dentin with minimum of 2 mm height above the prepared margin to minimize the risk of inadequate retention and/or fracture under function.

festoon(s)   (festoon'), *n/n.pl*   a carving in the base material of a denture that simulates the contours of the natural tissue being replaced by the denture.

festoon, gingival, *n* the distinct rounding and enlargement of the margins of the gingival tissue found in early gingival involvement.

festoons, McCall's, *n.pr* enlargements of the gingival margins that may be associated with occlusal trauma.

festooning   (festoon'ing), *n* the process of carving the base material of a denture or denture pattern to

in groups that function as the mode of attachment of the tooth to the alveolus and form the periodontal ligament.

fibers, Sharpey's, *n.pr* the collagen fibers of the periodontal ligament that become incorporated into the cementum or alveolar bone.

fibers, transseptal, *n.pl* a part of the collagen fibers of the periodontal ligament that extends from the supraalveolar cementum of one tooth horizontally through the interdental attached gingiva above the septum of the alveolar bone to the cementum of the adjacent tooth. Also called *interdental fibers.*

fiberoptic light, *n* a miniaturized light source that uses the property of flexible fiberglass strands to conduct light over long distances with little or no distortion; used in intraoral application, such as a light attached directly to the dental handpiece.

fiberoptics (fībərop′tiks), *n* the technical process by which an internal organ or cavity can be viewed, using glass or plastic fibers to transmit light through a special tube designed to magnify and reflect an image of the surface of the internal region under observation.

fibrillation (fib′rilā′shən), *n* a local quivering of muscle fibers.

fibrillation, atrial, *n* a cardiac arrhythmia caused by disturbed spread of excitation through atrial musculature.

fibrillation, auricular (ôrik′ūlur), *n* an uncoordinated, independent contraction of the heart that results in marked irregularity of heart action.

fibrillation, ventricular, *n* an uncoordinated, independent contraction of the ventricular musculature resulting in cessation of cardiac output.

fibrinogen (fībrin′əjən) (factor I, profibrin), *n* a soluble plasma protein (globulin) that is acted on by thrombin to form fibrin. The normal level is 200 to 400 mg/100 ml in plasma. Coagulation is impaired if the concentration is less than 100 mg/100 ml. Another form called *tissue fibrinogen,* which has the power of clotting the blood without the presence of thrombin, occurs in body tissue.

fibrinokinase (fī′brinōki′nās) (fibrinolysokinase, lysokinase), *n* an activator of plasminogen better known now as *plasminogen activator.*

fibrinolysin (fī′brinol′isin), *n* See plasmin.

fibrinolysis (fī′brinol′isis), *n* the continual process of fibrin decomposition during the removal of small fibrin clots by the action of enzyme fibrinolysin.

fibrinolysokinase, *n* See fibrinokinase.

fibrinolytic agents, *n.pl* agents that increase the breakdown of fibrin.

fibroblast (fī′brōblast), *n* a cell found within fibrous connective tissue, varying in shape from stellate (young) to fusiform and spindle shaped. Associated with the formation of collagen fibers and intercellular ground substance of connective tissue.

fibroblast, of periodontal ligament, *n* a cell that plays an important role in formation and remodeling of fibrous matrix and intercellular substance.

fibroblastoma (fī′brōblastō′mə), *n* a tumor arising from an ordinary connective tissue cell or fibroblast. The tumor may be a fibroma or a fibrosarcoma.

fibroblastoma, neurogenic, *n* See neurofibroma.

fibroblastoma, perineural, *n* See neurilemoma and neurofibroma.

fibrocystic disease, *n* See disease fibrocystic.

fibroma (fībrō′mə), *n* a benign mesenchymal tumor composed primarily of fibrous connective tissue.

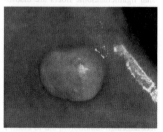

Irritation fibroma. (Courtesy Dr. James Sciubba)

fibroma, ameloblastic, *n* a mixed tumor of odontogenic origin characterized by the simultaneous proliferation of both the epithelial and mesenchymal components of the tooth germ without the production of hard structure.

fibroma, calcifying, n See fibroma, ossifying.

fibroma, cementifying, n an intrabony lesion not associated with teeth, composed of a fibrous connective tissue stroma containing foci of calcified material resembling cementum; a rare odontogenic tumor composed of varying amounts of fibrous connective tissue with calcified material resembling cementum. Central lesion of the jaws.

fibroma, desmoplastic (dez'məplas' tik), n a fibrous bone tumor, usually benign, found most commonly in children and young adults.

fibroma, irritation, n a localized peripheral, tumorlike enlargement of connective tissue caused by prolonged local irritation and usually seen on the gingiva or buccal mucosa.

fibroma, neurogenic, n See neurilemoma; neurofibroma.

fibroma, odontogenic, n a central odontogenic tumor of the jaws, consisting of connective tissue in which small islands and strands of odontogenic epithelium are dispersed. A mesodermal odontogenic tumor composed of active dense or loose fibrous connective tissue; contains inactive islands of epithelium.

fibroma, ossifying, n a benign neoplasm of bone characterized by unilateral swelling and fibroblastic and osteoblastic activity in marrow spaces. An aggressive variant of this lesion has been described and is termed juvenile ossifying fibroma or juvenile active ossifying fibroma.

fibroma, periapical (benign periapical fibroma, fibrous dysplasia, first-state cementoma, focal osseous dysplasia, traumatic osteoclasia), n a benign connective tissue mass formed at the apex of a tooth with a normal pulp.

fibroma, peripheral odontogenic, n a fibrous connective tissue tumor associated with the gingival margin and believed to originate from the periodontium. Often contains areas of calcification. Localized fibromatosis gingivae.

fibroma, peripheral ossifying, n a type of reactive gingival growth that

appears most commonly in teenagers and young adults. They can be surgically removed, but rate of recurrence is high.

fibroma, with myxomatous degeneration, n See fibromyxoma.

fibromatosis (fī′brōmətō′sis), n a gingival enlargement believed to be a hereditary condition that is manifested in the permanent dentition and characterized by a firm hyperplastic tissue that covers the teeth. Differentiation between this and diphenylhydantoin (Dilantin) hyperplasia is based on a history of drug ingestion.

fibromatosis gingival, n a generalized enlargement of the gingivae caused by an overproduction of collagen. May be idiopathic, inherited, or associated with a syndrome.

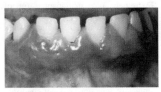

Gingival fibromatosis. (Rose/Mealey/Genco, 2004)

fibromatosis, idiopathic, n See fibromatosis gingival.

fibromyalgia (fī′brōmīal′jēə), n a debilitating chronic syndrome characterized by diffuse or specific muscle, joint, or bone pain; fatigue; and a wide range of other symptoms, as well as tenderness on palpation at various sites.

fibromyxoma (fibroma with myxomatous degeneration), (fī′brōmi ksō′mə) n a fibroma that has certain characteristics of a myxoma; a fibroma that has undergone myxomatous degeneration. Combination of both fibrous and myxomatous elements.

fibro-osseous (fīb′rō-os′ēəs), adj composed of bony and fibrous tissue; often associated with lesions of the jaw.

fibrosarcoma (fī′brōsärkō′mə), n a malignant mesenchymal tumor, the basic cell type being a fibroblast. Most fibrosarcomas are locally infiltrative and persistent but do not metastasize.

F

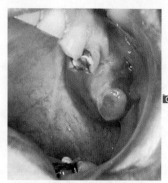

Fibrosarcoma. (Sapp/Eversole/Wysocki, 2004)

fibrosarcoma, odontogenic, n an extremely rare malignant form of odontogenic fibroma.

fibrosis (fĭbrō'sĭs), *n* **1.** the process of forming fibrous tissue, usually by degeneration (e.g., fibrosis of the pulp). The process occurs normally in the formation of scar tissue to replace normal tissue lost through injury or infection. *n* **2.** an abnormal condition in which fibrous connective tissue spreads over or replaces normal smooth muscle or other normal organ tissue. Fibrosis is most common in the heart, lung, peritoneum, and kidney.

fibrosis, diffuse hereditary gingival, n an uncommon form of severe gingival hyperplasia considered to be of genetic origin. The tissue is pink, firm, dense, and insensitive and has little tendency to bleed.

fibrosis, hereditary gingival, n an uncommon form of severe gingival hyperplasia that may begin with the eruption of the deciduous or permanent teeth and is characterized by a firm, dense, pink gingival tissue with little tendency toward bleeding.

fibrotomy (fĭbrō'təmē), *n* an orthodontic surgical procedure in which the gingival fibers around a tooth are severed in order to prevent the orthodontically corrected tooth from relapsing.

fibrous dysplasia, *n.pl* See dysplasia, fibrous.

fibrous encapsulation, *n* the process in which an implant (or other implanted material) becomes surrounded by fibrous connective tissue during tissue healing process as opposed to osseointegration where the implant is surrounded and in intimate contact with the bone.

fibula (fĭb'yələ), *n* one of the two bones of the lower leg, lateral to and smaller in diameter than the tibia. The proportion to its length, it is the most slender of the long bones and presents three borders and three surfaces for attaching various muscles, including the peronei longus and brevis and the soleus longus.

fiduciary (fĭdoo'shēerē), *n* a person who has a duty to act primarily for another's benefit, as a trustee. Also, pertaining to the good faith and confidence involved in such a relationship.

field, *n* an area, region, or space.

field block, n See block, field.

field, operating, n the area immediately surrounding and directly involved in a treatment procedure (e.g., all the teeth included in a rubber dam application for the restoration of a single tooth or portions thereof).

field, radiation, n the region in which radiant energy is being propagated.

field of view, n the area that is captured during radiographic imaging procedures.

fifth disease, *n* an infectious disease primarily found in children that is caused by transmission of the human parvovirus B19 through the upper respiratory tract. Symptoms include fever and a skin rash that begins on the cheeks and spreads to other body surfaces. Also called *erythema infectiosum.*

fight or flight response, *n* the body's primitive, automatic, inborn response that prepares the body to "fight"or "flee" from perceived attack, harm, or threat to survival.

filament (fĭl'əmənt), *n* **1.** a fine, threadlike fiber. *n* **2.** an individual manufactured toothbrush bristle.

filament, curved, n a single toothbrush bristle, manufactured to bend with the curve of the dental surface, designed to assist contact with the gingival line when used at a 45° angle.

filament, end rounded, *n* refers to the manufactured shaping of an individual toothbrush bristle with an exceptionally rounded tip designed to protect teeth and gums during brushing.

filamentous bacilli, morphologic form of (filəmen'təs bəsil'ē), *n* the clustered strands of narrow filaments, rounded at one end and tapered at the other, which are characteristic of the filamentous bacilli.

file, *n* **l.** a metal tool of varying size and form with numerous ridges or teeth on its cutting surfaces; may be push-cut or pull-cut; used for smoothing or dressing down metals and other substances. *n* **2.** a collection of records; an organized collection of information directed toward some purpose such as patient demographic data. The records in a file may or may not be sequenced according to a key contained in each record. *v* **3.** to reduce by means of a file.

file, gold, *n* a file designed for removing surplus gold from gold restorations; may be pull-cut or push-cut.

file, Hirschfeld-Dunlop, *n.pr* a periodontal file used with a pull stroke for the removal of calculus; available in various angulations for approach to different surfaces of teeth.

file, periodontal, *n* an instrument with multiple, angled cutting edges used to roughen the surface of a smooth calculus deposit before removal with a curet.

file, root canal, *n* a small metal hand instrument with tightly spiraled blades used to clean and shape the canal.

file, sharpening, *n* a difficult honing procedure requiring special tools designed to address the file's numerous parallel ridges.

file-access safeguards, *n.pl* the methods of limiting certain users' access to particular data.

filing, *n* the act of using a file to shape or smooth an object, usually metal.

filled resin, *n* See resin, composite.

filled sealant, *n* See resin, composite and resin-filled.

filled teeth, indices and scoring methods for, *n.pl* See index, DEF and index, DMF.

filling, *n* a material used to fill a space. See also restoration.

filling, dental, *n* a colloquial term for restoration.

filling, "ditched," *n* the marginal failure of amalgam restorations caused by fracture of either the material or the tooth structure itself in that area.

filling, material, *n* See material, filling.

filling, postresection, *n* See filling, retrograde.

filling, retrograde (postresection filling, retrograde obturation), *n* a restoration placed in the apical portion of a tooth root to seal the apical portion of the root canal.

filling, root canal, *n* material placed in the root canal system to seal the space previously occupied by the dental pulp.

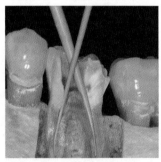

Root canal filling. (Hargreaves/Cohen/Berman, 2011)

filling, technique, *n* See technique, filling.

filling, treatment, *n* a temporary filling, usually of a sedative nature, used to allay sensitive dentin before the final restoration of the cavity.

film, *n* a thin, flexible, transparent sheet of cellulose acetate or similar material coated with a light-sensitive emulsion.

film base, *n* See base, film.

film, bite-wing (interproximal film) (BWX), *n* See examination, bitewing, intraoral radiographic and radiograph, bite-wing.

film emulsion, *n* See emulsion, silver.

film fault, *n* a defective result in a radiograph; usually caused by a chemical, physical, or electrical error in its production.

film fault, black spots, *n.pl* the spots caused by dust particles or developer on the films before development; also caused by outdated (expired) film.

film fault, blurred, *n* a fault caused by film or patient movement during exposure, bent film during exposure, double exposures, or flowing of emulsion during processing in excessively warm solution.

film fault, clear radiographic, *n* the result of treating the film with fixer before developing or by excessive washing. The problem can be prevented by following appropriate processing procedures.

film fault, dark, *n* a fault caused by overexposure of the film to radiation, film fog from extended development, accidental exposure to light (light leaks in film packet or dark room), or an unsafe darkroom light.

film fault, distorted, *n* See distortion, film-fault.

film fault, dyschroic fog, *n* a fogging of the radiograph, characterized by the appearance of a pink surface when the film is viewed by transmitted light and a green surface when the film is seen by reflected light. It usually is caused by an exhaustion of the acid content of the fixing solution (incomplete fixation).

film fault, fogged, *n* a fault caused by stray radiation, use of expired film, or an unsafe darkroom light.

film fault, light, *n* a fault caused by underexposure, underdevelopment (expired or diluted developing solution), development in temperatures that are too cold, or accidental use of a wrong film speed.

film fault, reticulation, *n* a network of corrugations produced because of an excessive difference in temperature between any two of the three darkroom solutions.

film fault, roller marks on, *n.pl* the dark lines on films caused by contaminated chemicals in automatic film processing units. Prevented by cleaning and replenishing the developer and fixer solutions regularly.

film fault, stained, *n* a fault caused by contaminated solutions, improper rinsing, exhausted solutions, improper washing, contamination by improper handling of the emulsions during or after processing, or film hangers containing dried fixer on the clips.

film fault, static electricity, *n* an image in the emulsion that has the appearance of black lightning streaks. Caused by rapid opening of the film packet or transfer of static electricity from the technician to the film.

film fault, white spots, *n* a fault caused by air bubbles clinging to the emulsion during development or by fixing solution spotted on the emulsion before development.

film hanger, *n* an instrument or device for holding radiographic film during processing procedures.

film holder, cardboard, *n* See cassette, cardboard.

film image, *n* the shadow of a structure as depicted on a radiographic or photographic emulsion.

film immersion method, *n* a procedure for processing radiographic films involving submerging the films in a sodium hypochlorite solution for anywhere between 30 seconds and 5 minutes. The solution should be 5.25% sodium hypochlorite.

film, interproximal, *n* See film, bitewing.

film mounting, *n* the placement of radiographs in an anatomic sequence on a suitable carrier for illumination and study.

film packet, *n* a small, lightproof, moisture-resistant, sealed paper or plastic envelope containing one or two intraoral films, a piece of black paper for light protection, and a lead foil backing to help prevent backscattered radiation. A variety of sizes of film packets are available.

film placement, *n* the positioning of the radiographic film to receive the image cast by the roentgen rays.

film processing, *n* a chemical transformation of the latent image, produced in a film emulsion by exposure to radiation, into a stable image visible by transmitted light. The usual procedure is basically a selective reduction of affected silver halide salts to metallic silver grains (development), followed by the selective removal of unaffected silver halide (fixation), washing to remove the processing chemicals, and drying.

film, processing, acids in, *n* chemicals that arrest the process of film development and also neutralize leftover developer.

film processing, automatic, *n* a fast and efficient method of processing in which the film is mechanically transferred from the developer to the fixer, is washed, and finally is dried.

film processing, rapid, *n* the use of high-speed chemicals or elevated temperatures to reduce processing time.

film speed (film sensitivity), *n* the amount of exposure to light or roentgen rays required to produce a given image density. It is expressed as the reciprocal of the exposure in roentgens necessary to produce a density of 1 above base and fog; films are classified on this basis in six speed groups, between each of which is a twofold increase in film speed.

film thickness, *n* the thickness of a layer of material, particularly in reference to dental cements. In standardization tests, film thickness is the minimal thickness or layer obtained under a specific load.

film, radiographic, *n* older term was *x-ray.* See survey, radiographic.

Filoviridae (fĭ'lōvĭr'idā), *n* a major virus family, to which both the Marburg and Ebola viruses belong. Viruses in this family have a single-stranded RNA molecular structure with complex symmetry.

filter, *n* a material placed in the useful beam to absorb preferentially the less energetic (less penetrating) radiations. See also filtration.

filter, added, *n* a filter added to the inherent filter.

filter, compensating, *n* a filter designed to shield less dense areas so that a more uniform image quality will be produced.

filter, inherent, *n* the filtration introduced by the glass wall of the radiographic tube, any oil used for tube immersion, or any permanent tube enclosure in the path of useful beam.

filter, orange, *n* the recommended safelight filter for darkroom illumination when processing intraoral film only. Also called *filter type ML-2.*

filter, red, *n* the recommended safelight filter for darkroom illumination when processing either intraoral or extraoral film. Also called *filter type GBX-2.*

filter, total, *n* the sum of inherent and added filters.

filtration (filtrā'shən), *n* the use of absorbers for the selective attenuation of radiation of certain wavelengths from a useful primary beam of x-radiation.

filtration, built-in, *n* the filtration put into effect by nonremovable absorbers deliberately built into the tubehead assembly to increase the inherent beam filtration.

filtration, external, *n* the action of absorbers external to the tube-head assembly, consisting of added filtration plus the attenuating effect of materials of which any closed-end cone such as a pointer cone may be made. See also filter, added.

financial management, *n* the management or control of the money or cash flow of a business or enterprise.

financial support, *n* the funding of a project to assist in its accomplishment.

finasteride, *n brand names:* Proscar, Propecia; *drug class:* synthetic steroid; *action:* competitive inhibitor of 5 α-reductase, which converts testosterone into dihydrotestosterone (DHT) in the prostate gland; *uses:* symptomatic benign prostatic hyperplasia, male pattern hair loss.

findings, radiographic (roentgenographic findings), *n* the recorded radiographic evidence of normal and deviated anatomic structures.

fineness, *n* a means of grading alloys with regard to gold content. The fineness of an alloy is designated in parts per thousand of pure gold, pure gold being 1000 fine.

finger, *n* any one of the five digits of the hand.

pigments. They are found in soil and fresh and salt water; some species are pathogenic.

flavonoids (flā'vənoidz'), *n.pl* a group of substances containing the plant pigment flavone. There is no known requirement for them. They have antioxidant and other potentially beneficial effects. Also known as *bioflavonoid.*

flavoxate HCl, *n brand name:* Urispas; *drug class:* antispasmodic, antimuscarinic anticholinergic; *action:* relaxes smooth muscles in urinary tract; *uses:* relief of nocturia, incontinence, suprapubic pain, dysuria.

flecainide acetate, *n brand name:* Tambocor; *drug class:* antidysrhythmic (Class IC); *actions:* blocks sodium channels and decreases conduction in all parts of the heart with greatest effect on His-Purkinje system; *uses:* life-threatening ventricular dysrhythmias, sustained supraventricular tachycardia, paroxysmal supraventricular tachycardia, atrial fibrillation.

flexibility, *n* the property of elastic deformation under loading.

flexible benefits, *n.pl* a benefits program in which an employee has a choice of credits or dollars for distribution among various benefit options (e.g., health and disability insurance, dental benefits, child care, pension benefits). See also cafeteria plans and flexible spending account.

flexible spending account *(FSA),* *n* an employee reimbursement account primarily funded with employee designated salary reductions. Funds are reimbursed to the employee for health care (medical and/or dental), dependent care, and/or legal expenses and are considered a nontaxable benefit.

flexion (flek'shən), *n* the bending of a joint between two skeletal members to decrease the angle between the members; opposite of extension.

flexion-extension reflex, n See reflex, flexion-extension.

flexure (flek'shur), *n* the quality or state of being flexed.

flexure, clasp, n the flexure of a retentive clasp arm to permit passage over the surveyed height of contour, thus permitting the seating or removal of the clasp.

flexure, mandibular, n the change in shape of the mandible caused by the pterygoid muscles contracting during opening and protrusion movements.

floater, *n* one or more spots that appear to drift in front of the eye, caused by a shadow cast on the retina by vitreous debris.

floor of cavity, *n* See cavity floor.

flora (flôr'ə), *n.pl* the bacteria living in various parts of the alimentary canal.

flora, fusospirochetal, n.pl the microorganisms *F. fusiforme* and *B. vincentii.* Present in most individuals as normal inhabitants of the oral cavity. Believed by some to be the primary and by others the secondary cause of necrotizing ulcerative gingivitis (NUG).

flora, normal oral, n.pl the varying types of bacteria that are usually present in the oral cavity.

flora, oral, n.pl the microorganisms inhabiting the oral cavity. They are usually saprophytic in nature and live together in a symbiotic relationship. Some are potentially pathogenic, assuming a pathologic role when adverse local or systemic factors such as increased body temperature influence the symbiotic balance of the microorganic flora.

floss, *n* a waxed or unwaxed string or tape used to remove dental biofilm (dental plaque) from the interproximal and contact areas of the teeth. Its regular and proper use is essential to good oral hygiene and prevention of both dental caries and periodontal disease.

floss cleft, n a narrow gap created in the gingival tissue between the teeth by floss that is repeatedly positioned incorrectly so that it presses against the gingiva.

floss cuts, prevention of, n the patient care information centered around the protection of injury to the gingival tissue, particularly the interdental papilla. Instruction includes careful attention to the angle and thickness of floss used, as well as proper flossing technique.

floss, expanded PTFE dental, n one of three varieties of filament-based dental hygiene tools; consists of a waxy artificial chemical called polytetrafluoroethylene; tends to resist shredding and breaking.

floss, tape, n thicker floss.

floss, threader, n oral hygiene auxiliary used to access the interproximal area under bridges and orthodontic appliances with dental floss.

floss, tufted dental, n a floss made from alternating sections of traditional thin fiber and thicker tufted fiber that is especially suited to removing dental biofilm (dental plaque) from teeth separated by wide spaces.

▶ **flossing,** n the mechanical cleansing of interproximal tooth surfaces with stringlike, waxed or unwaxed dental floss or tape.

🖸 *flossing aids,* n.pl the commercially available devices designed to make flossing easier and more effective, particularly in places that are tight or difficult to reach. These include plastic holders and threaders.

flow, n to move in a manner similar to a liquid stream.

flow, dental material, n the continued deformation or change in shape under a static load, as with waxes and amalgam.

flow, traffic, n the pattern of office personnel and patient movement from one area within the office to another.

flowchart, n a graphic representation of a sequence of operations using symbols to represent the operations. Flowcharts often symbolize the most important steps of the process without detailing the algorithm of the way the work is to be performed.

flowmeter, n a physical device for measuring the rate of flow of a gas or liquid, such as with nitrous oxide.

fluconazole (flookon′əzōl), n brand name: Diflucan; *drug class:* azole antifungal; *action:* inhibits ergosterol biosynthesis; *uses:* oropharyngeal candidiasis, urinary candidiasis, cryptococcal meningitis, coccidioidomycosis, vaginal candidiasis.

fluctuation (fluk′choowā′shən), n a wavelike motion produced in soft tissues in response to palpation or percussion. Fluctuation is caused by a collection of fluids or exudates in the tissues.

flucytosine (floosī′təsēn′), n brand name: Ancobon; *drug class:* pyrimidine antifungal; *action:* converted to fluorouracil after entering fungi, which inhibits DNA and RNA synthesis; *uses: Candida* infections, cryptococcal meningitis.

fludrocortisone acetate (floo′drōk or′tisōn′ as′ətāt), n brand name: Florinef Acetate; *drug class:* glucocorticoid, with greater mineralocorticoid activity; *action:* promotes increased reabsorption of sodium and loss of potassium from renal tubules; *uses:* adrenal insufficiency, salt-losing adrenogenital syndrome.

fluid (floo′id), n a liquid or gaseous substance.

fluid, crevicular, n a clear, usually unnoticeable fluid that can serve as a defense mechanism against infection by carrying antibodies and other therapeutic substances between the connective tissue and sulcus or pocket. Also called *gingival sulcus fluid* or *sulcular fluid.*

fluid delivery, n the continual fluid stream of an ultrasonic instrument, either over or through the vibrating tip, which is necessary to maintain a stable instrument temperature throughout a procedure.

fluid, dentinal, n the fluid content within the dentinal tubules of the dentin of the tooth.

fluid, lacrimal, n a watery secretion of the lacrimal gland, commonly called tears. The fluid is secreted into the lacrimal lake, an area located between the eyeball and the upper eyelid. It helps bathe the sensitive cornea. Tearing can result from eye irritation, or during periods of emotional distress.

fluid, synovial, n See synovial fluid.

fluid, total body, n all the fluids contained in the body. There are two main types: the intracellular fluid, which is contained totally within the cells, and the extracellular fluid, which is contained entirely outside the cells.

fluid wax, n See wax, fluid.

flumazenil (floo′mazənil′), n brand name: Romazicon; *drug class:* benzodiazepine receptor antagonist; *action:* antagonizes actions of benzodiazepines on the central nervous system; *use:* reversal of sedative effects of benzodiazepines.

flunisolide (floonis′əlīd′), *n brand names:* Oral INH aerosol, AeroBid; *drug class:* synthetic glucocorticoid; *action:* binds to steroid receptors, long-acting synthetic adrenocorticoid with antiinflammatory activity; *use:* rhinitis (seasonal or perennial).

fluocinonide (floo′əsin′ənīd′), *n brand names:* Licon, Lidex, Lidex-E, Vanos; *drug class:* topical corticosteroid; *action:* interacts with steroid cytoplasmic receptors to induce antiinflammatory effects; possesses antipruritic, antiinflammatory actions; *uses:* psoriasis, eczema, contact dermatitis, pruritus, oral lichen planus lesions.

fluorapatite (flôrap′ətīt), *n* a member of the family of minerals that make up the basic structure of bones and teeth; basically a hydroxyapatite form in which fluoride ions replace hydroxyl ions.

fluorapatite crystal **(kris′təl),** *n* the crystalline structure that occurs after hydroxyapatite changes into fluorapatite as a result of the tooth being exposed to fluoride.

fluorescein (flôres′ēin), *n* in dentistry, a dye applied to teeth to reveal dental biofilm (dental plaque). In ophthalmology, it is used to discover corneal lesions.

fluorescence (fləres′əns), *n* the emission of radiation of a particular wavelength by certain substances as the result of absorption of radiation of a shorter wavelength.

fluorescent screen, *n* See screen, intensifying.

fluorhydroxyapatite (flôr′hīdrok′sē ap′ətīt), *n* a member of the family of minerals that make up the basic structure of bones and teeth. It is formed when small amounts of fluoride and teeth mineral react. When higher concentrations of fluoride are involved, the result is the formation of calcium fluoride.

fluoridate (flôr′idāt), *v* to add fluoride to a water supply.

fluoridated salt, *n* a compound of sodium chloride with fluoride added; not considered as effective as fluoridated water.

fluoridation (floor′idā′shən), *n* **1.** the process of adding fluoride to a public water supply to reduce dental caries. *n* **2.** the use of a fluoride to prevent caries and promote remineralization; may be by means of communal water supplies; oral hygiene preparations for home use; or topical applications.

fluoride(s) (floor′īd), *n/n.pl* a salt of hydrofluoric acid, commonly sodium or stannous (tin).

fluoride dietary supplements, **n.pl** the orally administered nutritional additives of the chemical fluoride; often taken by individuals without regular access to a fluoridated water supply; available as chewable tablets, drops, pills, and in combination with vitamin supplements. See also fluoride drops.

fluoride drops, **n** a supplemental liquid form of the chemical fluoride. They can be administered to children from 6 months to 3 years of age but are not usually recommended because most children are exposed to normal levels of fluoride in their water systems at home and school and in their beverages.

fluoride, stannous, **n** a compound of tin and fluorine used in dentifrices to prevent caries.

fluoride tablets/lozenges, **n.pl** the supplemental forms of the chemical fluoride. Tablets must be chewed, and lozenges must be held in the oral cavity until dissolved in order to benefit from the fluoride's contact with the teeth.

fluoride toxicity, **n** poisoning as a result of ingesting too much fluoride. Symptoms range from upset stomach to death.

fluoride varnish, **n** a topical resin containing fluoride that is thinly applied to the tooth surface and used as a preventive treatment for caries. Can also be used as a desensitizing agent to treat dentinal hypersensitivity by temporarily blocking dentinal tubules.

fluorides, topical, **n.pl** the salts of hydrofluoric acid (usually sodium or tin salts) that may be applied in solution to the exposed dental surfaces to prevent dental caries and promote remineralization. They can be applied by trays or mouthrinses or by techniques such as paint-on.

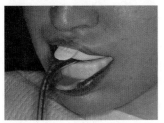

Topical fluoride (being applied with a tray). (Dean/Avery/McDonald, 2011)

brown mottled appearance to the enamel of developing teeth.

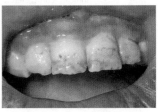

Fluorosis. (Courtesy Dr. Charles Babbush)

fluorides, topical, paint-on technique, n a professionally administered procedure in which the exposed dental surfaces are coated with a fluoride solution or gel or varnish to prevent caries and promote remineralization.

fluorine (flŏŏr'ēn), n an element of the halogen family and the most reactive of the nonmetals. Its atomic number is 9, and its atomic weight is 19. Small amounts of sodium fluoride added to the public water supply will reduce the incidence of dental caries, particularly among children. Excessive amounts of fluoride can mottle tooth enamel and cause osteosclerosis. Acute fluoride poisoning can cause death.

fluoroscope (flôr'əscōp), n a device consisting of a fluorescent screen mounted in a metal frame covered with lead glass. In the presence of a roentgen ray, the screen glows in direct proportion to the intensity of the remnant x-radiation, producing visual impressions of the densities traversed.

fluorosis (flərō'sis), n an enamel hypoplasia caused by the ingestion of excess fluoride during the time of enamel formation. General term for chronic fluoride poisoning.

fluorosis, chronic endemic dental (mottled enamel), n an enamel defect caused by excessive ingestion of fluoride, possibly in the water supply (usually 2 to 8 ppm) during the period of tooth calcification. Affected teeth appear chalky white on eruption and later turn brown.

fluorosis, dental, n an abnormal condition resulting from the ingestion of too much fluoride, causing a white or

fluorosis, index of dental, n a classification system for determining the presence and severity of chronic fluoride poisoning in which the enamel on individual teeth is rated against a 0 to 4 scale with 0 representing normal enamel and 4 severely damaged enamel. This index may be used by communities to adjust the levels of fluoride in their water systems.

fluorouracil topical (flŏŏr'əyŏŏr 'əsil), n brand names: Carac, Efudex, Fluoroplex; drug class: topical pyrimidine antineoplastic; action: inhibits synthesis of DNA and RNA in susceptible cells; uses: keratosis, basal cell carcinoma.

Fluothane, n.pr the brand name for halothane.

fluoxetine (flŏŏok'sətēn'), n brand name: Prozac; drug class: antidepressant; action: inhibits CNS neuron uptake of serotonin but not norepinephrine; use: depressive disorders.

fluoxymesterone (flŏŏok'sēmes'tə rōn'), n brand names: Android-F, Halotestin; drug class: androgenic anabolic steroid; actions: increases weight by building body tissue; increases potassium, phosphorus, chloride, nitrogen levels; increases bone development; uses: impotence from testicular deficiency, hypogonadism, palliative treatment of female breast cancer.

fluphenazine decanoate/fluphenazine enanthate/fluphenazine HCl (floofen'əzēn' dec'anō'āt), n brand name: Prolixin; drug class: phenothiazine antipsychotic; action: blocks dopamine receptors in the cerebral cortex, hypothalamus, and limbic system; uses: psychotic disorders, schizophrenia.

flurandrenolide (flŏŏr'andren'əlīd), *n brand names:* Cordran, Cordran SP; *drug class:* topical corticosteroid; *action:* binds to glucocorticoid receptor leading to an anti-inflammatory and antipruritic effect; *uses:* corticosteroid-responsive dermatoses, pruritus.

flurazepam HCl (flŏŏraz'əpam), *n brand name:* Dalmane; *drug class:* benzodiazepine, sedative-hypnotic; *action:* produces central nervous system depression by interaction with benzodiazepine receptor to facilitate action of inhibitory neurotransmitter γ-aminobutyric acid (GABA); *use:* insomnia.

flurbiprofen (flŏŏrbip'rəfen), *n brand name:* Ansaid; *drug class:* nonsteroidal antiinflammatory; *actions:* inhibits prostaglandin synthesis by interfering with cyclooxygenase needed for biosynthesis; possesses analgesic, antiinflammatory, antipyretic properties; *uses:* acute, long-term treatment of rheumatoid arthritis, osteoarthritis.

flurbiprofen sodium, n brand name: Ocufen; *drug class:* nonsteroidal antiinflammatory ophthalmic; *action:* inhibits cyclooxygenase necessary for biosynthesis of prostaglandins; *uses:* inhibition of intraoperative miosis, corneal edema.

flush, *n* **1.** a blush or sudden reddening of the face and neck caused by vasodilation of small arteries and arterioles. *n* **2.** a sudden, subjective feeling of heat. *n* **3.** a sudden, rapid flow of water or other liquid. *adj* **4.** a structure that is even or level, as with a surface; forming the same plane. *adj* **5.** to place in direct contact; squarely.

flush terminal plane, n a type of terminal plane relationship in which the primary maxillary and mandibular second molars are in an end to end relationship in centric occlusion.

flutamide (floo'təmīd'), *n brand name:* Eulexin; *drug class:* antiandrogen; *actions:* interferes with testosterone at cellular level, inhibits androgen uptake and androgen binding to its receptor; *use:* metastatic prostatic carcinoma.

fluticasone propionate (flŏŏtik'əsōn prō'pēənāt'), *n brand names:* Cutivate (topical), Flonase (nasal spray); *drug class:* synthetic corticosteroid; *actions:* stimulates steroid cytoplasmic receptors to induce antiinflammatory effects, possesses antipruritic, antiinflammatory actions; *uses:* topical for inflammation of corticosteroid-responsive skin disorders, spray for seasonal and perennial allergic rhinitis.

fluting (floo'ting), *n* **1.** the elongated developmental depressions along the root branches of tooth root surfaces of certain teeth. *n* **2.** in periodontology, the reshaping or grooving of bone into furcation or interdental defect areas, as part of treatment during osseous periodontal surgery.

flutter, *n* a quick, irregular motion.

fluvastatin sodium (floo'vəstat'ən sōdēəm), *n brand name:* Lescol; *drug class:* cholesterol-lowering agent; *action:* inhibits HMG-CoA reductase enzyme, which reduces cholesterol synthesis; *use:* hypercholesterolemia.

fluvoxamine maleate (flŏŏvak'səm ēn' mā'lēāt), *n brand name:* Luvox; *drug class:* selective serotonin reuptake inhibitor antidepressant; *action:* selectively inhibits reuptake of serotonin in central nervous system neurons; *use:* obsessive-compulsive disorder.

flux (fluks), *n* a substance or mixture used to promote fusion, especially the fusion of metals or minerals. Used principally in dentistry as an inclusion in ceramic materials and in soldering and casting metals.

flux, casting, n a flux that increases fluidity of the metal and helps to prevent oxidation.

flux, ceramic, n a flux used in the manufacture of porcelain and silicate powders.

flux, reducing, n a flux that contains powdered charcoal to remove oxides.

flux, soldering, n a ceramic material such as borax, boric acid, or a combination, in paste, liquid, or granular form; used to keep metallic parts clean while they are being heated during a soldering procedure. It is a solvent for metallic oxides and will flow over the parts to be soldered at temperatures well below the fusion temperature of solder, but it becomes separated from the solid metal by the molten solder.

FMIA, *n.pr* See angle, Frankfort mandibular incisor.

focal infection, *n* the site or origin of an infectious process. Endodontically treated teeth have frequently been accused of being the source of septicemias, often without justification. See also infection, focal.

focal spot, *n* See spot, focal.

focal trough, *n* in panoramic radiography, the curved zone in which structures are reasonably well defined. Patients must be aligned in panoramic radiography so that the maxillary and mandibular arches fall within the focal trough of the machine.

focal-receptor distance, *n* See distance, target-receptor.

focus group, *n* a demographic target group of people used to gather opinions or data descriptive of the population represented by the sample selected.

fog (fogging), *n* See film fault, fogged.

fog, chemical, *n* See film fault.

fog, dyschroic, *n* See film fault, dyschroic fog.

fog, light, *n* See film fault.

fog, radiation, *n* the film darkening caused by radiation from sources other than intentional exposure to the primary beam; (e.g., receptor may be exposed to scatter radiation, or accidental exposure may occur if stored receptor is not protected from radiation).

foil, *n* a very thin, flexible sheet of metal, usually gold, platinum, or tin.

foil, adhesive, *n* a tin foil that is covered on one side with powdered gum arabic or karaya gum.

foil assistant, *n* See foil holder.

foil, cohesive gold, *n* a gold foil that has been annealed or had a surface so completely pure so that it will cohere or weld at room temperature.

foil, corrugated gold, *n* a gold foil made by burning gold foil sheets between paper in the absence of air.

foil cylinder, *n* a cylinder of gold foil formed by repeatedly folding a sheet of foil into a narrow ribbon, which is then rolled into cylindrical form.

foil, gold (fibrous gold), *n* pure gold that has been rolled and beaten from ingots into a very thin sheet. Thickness usually varies from 1/40,000 inch (No. 2 foil) to 1/20,000 inch (No. 4 foil). Classified as cohesive, semicohesive, or noncohesive. One of the oldest restorative materials, the most permanent if used properly, and the yardstick by which all others are measured. It is compacted or condensed into a retentive cavity form piece by piece, using this metal's property of cold welding.

foil holder (foil assistant), *n* an instrument used to retain a foil pellet in place while it is being condensed or to retain a bulk of gold while additions to it are made.

foil, lead, *n* a component of the intraoral film packet included to shield the film from backscattered radiation.

foil, noncohesive gold, *n* a gold foil that will not cohere at room temperature because of the presence on its surface of a protecting or contaminating coating. If the coating is a volatile substance, such as ammonia, the foil may be rendered cohesive by heating or annealing it to remove the protection.

foil passer (foil carrier), *n* a pointed or forked instrument used to carry pellets of gold foil through an annealing flame or from the annealing tray to the prepared cavity for compaction.

foil pellet, *n* See pellet, foil.

foil, platinized gold (plat'ənīzd), *n* a form rolled or hammered from a "sandwich" made of platinum placed between two sheets of gold; used in portions of foil restorations where greater hardness is desired.

foil, platinum, *n* pure platinum rolled into extremely thin sheets. A precious-metal foil whose high fusing point makes it suitable as a matrix for various soldering procedures; also suitable for providing the internal form of porcelain restorations during fabrication.

foil, tin, *n* a base-metal foil used as a separating material, or protective covering (e.g., between the cast and denture base material during flasking and curing procedures).

folate (fō'lāt), *n* a form of folic acid that helps transport single carbon units between molecules.

fold, *n* a doubling back of a tissue surface.

fold, mucobuccal (mucobuccal reflection), *n* the depth of the oral mucosa from the mandible or maxillae to the cheek.

structure; that which initiates, changes, or arrests motion.

force and stress, *n* the pressure forcibly exerted on the teeth and on their investing and supporting tissues that is detrimental to tissue integrity. In occlusal trauma, the production of lesions of the attachment apparatus depends on an interrelationship of the strength, duration, and frequency of the application of the force.

force, centrifugal, *n* a force that tends to recede from the center.

force, chewing, *n* the degree of force applied by the muscles of mastication during the mastication of food.

force, component of, *n* **1.** one of the factors from which a resultant force may be compounded or into which it may be resolved. *n* **2.** one of the parts of a force into which it may be resolved.

force, condensing, *n* **1.** the force required to compress gold-foil pellets, facilitating their cohesion, to fabricate or build up a gold-foil restoration. *n* **2.** the force required to compact or condense a plastic material (e.g., amalgam, wax).

force, constant, *n* a continuous force or pressure applied to the teeth.

force, counter-dislodgement, *n* pressure that comes into play when food is evenly distributed in the oral cavity so that contact between the maxillary and mandibular teeth is equalized on both sides during mastication.

force, denture-dislodging, *n* an influence that tends to displace a denture from its intended position on supporting structures.

force, denture-retaining, *n* an influence that tends to maintain a denture in its intended position on its supporting structures.

force, electromotive, *n* the difference in potential in a roentgen-ray tube between the cathode and anode; usually expressed in kilovolts.

force, intermittent, *n* a force or pressure (applied to the teeth) that is alternated with a period of passiveness or rest.

force, line of, *n* the direction of the power exerted on a body.

force, masticatory, *n* the force applied by the muscles attached to the mandible during mastication.

force, occlusal (occlusal load), *n* **1.** the result of muscular forces applied on opposing teeth. *n* **2.** the force transmitted to the teeth and their supporting structures by tooth-to-tooth contact or through a bolus of food or other interposed substance.

force, shear, *n* commonly employed as a calculation of the physical stress a material can bear, it refers to the type of force that is expressed parallel to the face of an object.

force, tensile, *n* the type of force manifested in an extension of an object itself. A stretched rubber band is an example of tensile force.

forced expiratory volume (FEV), *n* the volume of air that can be forcibly expelled in a fixed time after full inspiration.

forceps (for′seps), *n* **1.** a colloquial term for an instrument used for grasping or applying force to teeth, tissues, or other objects, such as when they are extracted. *n* **2.** an instrument used for grasping and holding tissues or specific structures.

forceps, bone, *n* the force used for grasping or cutting bone.

forceps, chalazion, *n* a thumb forceps with a flattened plate at the end of one arm and a matching ring on the other. Originally used for isolation of eyelid tumors. It is useful for isolation of lip and cheek lesions, such as a mucocele, to facilitate removal.

forceps, dental extracting, *n* forceps used for grasping teeth.

forceps, hemostatic, *n* an instrument for grasping blood vessels to control hemorrhage.

forceps, insertion, *n* See forceps, point.

forceps, lock, *n* See forceps, point.

forceps, Magill, *n.pr* a tongs-shaped tool used to remove objects from the oral cavity.

forceps, mosquito, *n* a small hemostatic forceps.

forceps, point (lock forceps, insertion forceps), *n* a device used in filling root canals that securely holds the filling cones during their placement.

forceps, rubber dam clamp, *n* forceps whose beaks are designed to engage holes in the rubber dam retainer to facilitate its placement, adjustment, or removal.

forceps, suture, n See needle holder.

forceps, thumb, n the forceps used for grasping soft tissue; used especially during suturing.

forceps, tissue, n a thumb forceps; an instrument with one or more fine teeth at the tip of each blade for controlling tissues during surgery, especially during suturing.

Fordyce granules (for'dīs gran'ūlz), *n.pr* small, elevated, yellowish areas on the oral mucosa and lips that occur in more than 80% of the population. They are the result of ectopic sebaceous glands and are not considered abnormal. Also called *Fordyce spots.*

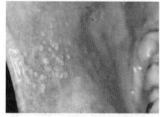

Fordyce's granules. (Neville, et al, 2009)

Fordyce's spots, *n.pr* See Fordyce granules.

forecasting, n the attempt to predict the future on the basis of expert opinion, market research, trend projection, leading indicators, and other modalities.

foregut, n the anterior portion of the future digestive tract or primitive pharynx that forms the oropharynx.

forehead, n the portion of the face directly above the orbits and extending posteriorly/superiorly to the hairline or crown of the head.

foreign body, n an object or substance found in the body in an organ or tissue in which it does not belong under normal circumstances, such as a bolus of food in the trachea or a particle of dust in the eye. See also body, foreign.

forensic (fəren'sik), *adj* pertaining to the law or to legal proceedings.

forensic anthropology, n the use of anatomic structures and physical characteristics to identify a subject for legal purposes.

forensic dentistry, n see dentistry, forensic.

foreshortening, n See distortion, vertical.

forging, n working or shaping heated metal.

fork, face-bow, n the part of the face-bow assembly used to attach an occlusion rim or transfer record of maxillary teeth to the face-bow proper.

form, n the configuration, shape, or particular appearance of anything.

form, acquaintance, n a registration sheet for new patients on which data (e.g., the patient's name and address) are recorded and that contains a statement of the policies of the specific dental professional's office or clinic and the responsibilities of the office or clinic to the patient.

form, anatomic, n the natural shape of a part.

form, anatomic charting, n one of three types of manually recorded dental documentation, features a graphic template displaying a representation of each tooth, as well as the roots and gingival tissues. Design provides for note taking associated with each tooth. The form becomes part of the patient's legal health records and is useful for planning patient care and ascertaining legal questions regarding treatment, and is relied upon for patient identification in the event of an emergency. See also form, examination.

form, arch, n the shape of the dental arch. See also arch, dental.

form, convenience, n the modifications necessary, beyond basic outline form, to facilitate proper instrumentation for the preparation of the cavity or insertion of the restorative material; also the placing of starting points or slight undercuts to retain the first portions of restorative material while succeeding portions are placed.

form, examination, n the written documentation recording the thorough assessment of the oral cavity and surrounding structures. The form should include patient history and descriptions of observed abnormalities of visible characteristics. Also called *record form.*

form, face, n the outline form of the face from an anterior frontal view.

form, functional, n the shape that permits optimal performance.

form, geographic charting, n one of three types of manually recorded dental documentation, describes each tooth by either a number or a letter within a quadrant. The gingival tissues and roots of the teeth are not included, making this chart unsuitable for periodontal assessment.

form, message, n a checklist form, by means of which dental office staff can quickly make a record of telephone communications for the dental staff to look at later.

form, occlusal, n the form of the occlusal surface of a tooth, a row of teeth, or dentition.

form, outline, n the shape of the area of the tooth surface included within the cavosurface margins of a prepared cavity.

form, posterior tooth, n the distinguishing contours of the occlusal surface of the various posterior teeth.

form, registration, n a form used to gather personal (nonprofessional) data about a patient.

form, resistance, n the shape given to a prepared cavity to enable the restoration and remaining tooth structure to withstand masticatory stress.

form, retention, n the provision made in a cavity preparation to prevent displacement of the restoration.

form, root, n the shape of the root of the tooth. It is capable of being modified by such factors as resorption and cemental apposition.

form, tooth, n the characteristics of the curves, lines, angles, and contours of various teeth that permit their identification and differentiation.

formaldehyde (formal′dəhīd′), n a toxic, pungent water-soluble gas used in the aqueous form as a disinfectant, fixative, or tissue preservative.

formalin (for′məlin), n a clear aqueous solution of formaldehyde. A 37% solution is used to fix and preserve tissues for histologic and pathologic study.

format, n a predetermined computer arrangement of characters, fields, lines, page numbers, punctuation marks, and the like.

formative evaluation, n internal examination of a program's process, usually conducted while planning the program.

former, angle, n See angle former.

former, crucible, n See sprue former.

former, sprue, n See sprue former.

formocresol (for′mōkres′ol), n *brand name:* Buckley's Formo Cresol; a compound consisting of formaldehyde, cresol, glycerin, and water used in vital pulpotomy of primary teeth and as a temporary intracanal medicament during root canal therapy.

formoterol, n *brand names:* Foradil, Perforomist; (Arformoterol, Brovana, is the R,R- enantiomer of formoterol, and has similar action and uses.) *drug class:* selective beta$_2$ adrenergic receptor agonist; *action:* stimulates beta$_2$ adrenergic receptors in the lung, causing bronchodilation and reduced inflammation; *uses:* asthma (formoterol), chronic obstructive pulmonary disease (arformoterol).

fortified (fôrtə′fīd), *adj* containing additives more potent than the principal ingredient.

forward protrusion, n See protrusion, forward.

foscarnet sodium/phosphonoformic acid (foskär′nət sōdēəm fos′fōnōfor′mik), n *brand name:* Foscavir; *drug class:* antiviral; *actions:* antiviral activity is produced by selective inhibition at the pyrophosphate binding site on virus-specific DNA polymerases, inhibits replication of all known herpesviruses; *uses:* CMV retinitis in AIDS, herpes simplex, acyclovir-resistant varicella-zoster.

Foshay's test, *n.pr* See test, Foshay's.

fosinopril (fosin′ōpril), n *brand name:* Monopril; *drug class:* angiotensin-converting enzyme (ACE) inhibitor; *action:* selectively suppresses renin-angiotensin-aldosterone system; *uses:* hypertension, heart failure, to protect the kidney in diabetic patients.

fossa(e) (fos′ə), n a pit, hollow, or depression on a tooth or bone.

fossa, articular, n a concave structure situated adjacent to the articular eminence on the temporal bone of the skull. Bone that is part of the articulating area of the temporomandibular joint.

fossa, canine, n the fossa in the canine maxilla superior to the apex of the canine tooth.

fossa, central, n a fossa located at the convergence of the cusp ridges in a central point on the occlusal surface of posterior teeth.

fossa, depth of, n on the occlusal table, the distance from the top of the shorter cusp downward into the bottom of the fossa.

fossa, infratemporal, n the fossa inferior to the temporal fossa and infratemporal crest on the greater wing of the sphenoid bone.

fossa, lacrimal, n fossa the fossa of the frontal bone that contains the lacrimal gland.

fossa, lateral, n a shallow, concave area of peritoneum on the rear wall of the abdominal cavity, bordered by the lateral umbilical fold and the inguinal ligament.

fossa, lingual, n a fossa on the lingual surface of certain anterior teeth.

fossa, mental, n a depression located between the alveolar and mental ridges of the roots of the incisors.

fossa, nasal, n See cavity, nasal.

fossa, pterygopalatine (ter'igōpal'ət īn), n a depression located between the maxilla and the sphenoid bone in the anatomy of the skull.

fossa, pterygoid, n a fossa between the medial and lateral pterygoid plates of the sphenoid bone.

fossa, sublingual, n a depression found underneath the tongue, adjacent to the sublingual glands.

fossa, submandibular, n a depression found underneath the internal oblique ridge, which houses the submandibular salivary gland.

foundation, n **1.** a charitable organization usually established to allocate private funds to worthy projects or to provide other services. n **2.** in dentistry, any device or material added to a remaining tooth structure to enhance the stability and retention of an overlying cast restoration. May be a pin retainer of amalgam, plastic cement, or a casting.

four-handed dentistry, n See dentistry, four-handed.

fovea, palatine (fō'vēə), n a small depression at the junction between the hard and soft palates; plays a role in the gag reflex.

fovea, pterygoid, n a depression on the anterior surface of the condyle of the mandible.

Fox scissors, n.pr See scissors, Fox.

Fox's knife, n.pr See knife, Goldman-Fox.

fractionation (frak'shənā'shən), n **1.** the separation of a substance into its basic constituents. n **2.** the process of isolating a pure culture by successive culturing of a small portion of a colony of bacteria. n **3.** the process of isolating different components of living cells by centrifugation. n **4.** the process of administering a dose of radiation in smaller units over time to minimize tissue damage.

fracture, n a break or rupture of a part. In the oral region, fracture is most often seen in teeth and bones.

fracture, avulsion, n the loss of a section of bone.

fracture, blow-out, n a fracture involving the orbital floor, its contents, and the superior wall of the maxillary antrum, in which orbital contents are incarcerated in the fracture area, producing diplopia.

fracture, bulk, n a fracture or failure in the amalgam of a restoration. An improperly finished restoration by the dental professional, poor cavity design, or improper loading of the restoration can lead to a bulk fracture.

fracture, cementum, n the tearing of fragments of the cementum from the tooth root.

fracture, clasp, n failure of a clasp arm because of stresses that have exceeded the elastic limit of the metal from which the arm was made.

fracture, closed reduction of, n a reduction and fixation of fractured bones without making a surgical opening to the fracture site.

fracture, comminuted, n a fracture in which the bone has several lines of fracture in the same region; a fracture in which the bone is crushed and splintered.

fracture, compound, n a fracture in which the bony structures are exposed to an external environment.

fracture, craniofacial dysjunction (transverse facial fracture), n a complex fracture in which the facial bones are separated from the cranial bones; a LeFort III fracture.

fracture, dislocation, n a fracture of a bone near an articulation, with dislocation of the condyloid process.

fracture, fissured, n a fracture that extends partially through a bone, with no displacement of the bony fragments.

fracture fixation, n the fractured fragments of bone are stabilized in close proximation to promote healing.

fracture, greenstick, n a fracture in which the bone appears to be bent; usually only one cortex of the bone is broken.

fracture, Guérin's **(gāraz′),** *n.pr* a LeFort I fracture of the facial bones in which there is a bilateral horizontal fracture of the maxillae.

fracture, impacted, n a fracture in which one fragment is driven into another portion of the same or an adjacent bone.

fracture, indirect, n a fracture at a point distant from the primary area of injury caused by secondary forces.

fracture, intraarticular, n a fracture of the articular surface of the condyloid process of a bone.

fracture, intracapsular, n a fracture of the condyle of the mandible occurring within the confines of the capsule of the temporomandibular joint.

fracture, LeFort, *n.pr* a transverse fracture involving the orbital, malar, and nasal bones.

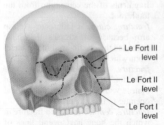

Lefort fractures. (Bagheri, 2008)

- Le Fort III level
- Le Fort II level
- Le Fort I level

fracture, mandibular, n breaks through the mandibular bone. Also known as *fractures of the jaw.*

fracture, midfacial, n fractures of the zygomatic, maxillary, nasal, and associated bones.

fracture, nasal-orbital-ethmoid (NOE), n fracture that occurs when the nose is subjected to severe trauma from the front, rather than from the side. The blunt force trauma buckles the medial orbital walls and fragments the thin nasal, lacrimal, ethmoid, and frontal bones.

fracture, orbital, n, breakage of any of the seven facial bones in the eye socket (orbit), a cup-shaped arrangement of bones surrounding the eye, which normally protect the eye from injury. They are caused by blunt trauma.

fracture, pyramidal, n a fracture of the midfacial bones, with the principal fracture lines meeting at an apex in the area of the nasion; a LeFort II fracture.

fracture, root, n a microscopic or macroscopic cleavage of the root in any direction.

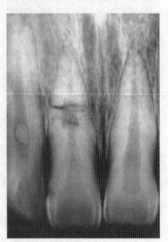

Root fracture. (Sapp/Eversole/Wysocki, 2004)

fracture, simple, n a linear fracture that is not in communication with the exterior.

fracture, stress, n **1.** a type of stress usually occurring from sudden, strong, violent, endogenous force, such as a simple fracture of the fibula in a runner. n **2.** the fracture of metallic parts as a result of fatigue of prolonged or frequent stress.

fracture, tooth, n a traumatic injury to a tooth that manifests itself as a chip, crack, or break. Manifestations may also include dislocation or complete displacement of a tooth.

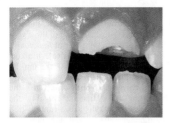

Tooth fracture. (Robinson/Bird, 2007)

fracture toughness, *n* the quality of the material used for brackets that indicates its ability to withstand applied force without cracking.

fracture, transverse facial, *n* See fracture, craniofacial dysjunction.

fracture,   zygomaticomaxillary *n* fracture composed of a set of three bone fractures. The first portion of the tripod fracture involves the maxillary sinus, including the anterior and postero-lateral walls and the floor of the orbit. The second portion involves the zygomatic arch. The third portion involves the lateral orbital rim, usually including the lateral orbital wall or the zygomaticofrontal suture. Also known as *tripod or malar fracture.*

Fragile X syndrome *(FXS)* *n.pr* a genetic syndrome that is the most commonly known single-gene cause of autism and the most commonly inherited cause of intellectual disability. Also called *Martin-Bell syndrome* or *Escalante syndrome.*

fragilitas ossium (frajil'ētəs os'ēəm), *n* See osteogenesis imperfecta.

fragment, *n* a broken or disconnected part of a larger whole, such as a tooth or root.

frail elderly, *n.pl* older persons (usually over the age of 75 years) who are afflicted with physical or mental disabilities that may interfere with the ability to independently perform activities of daily living.

frame, *n* a structure, usually rigid, designed to give support or attachment to a part, or to immobilize a part.

frame, implant, *n* See substructure, implant.

frame, occluding (ōkloo'ding), *n* a device for relating casts to each other for the purpose of arranging teeth or for use in making an index of the occlusion of dentures; an articulator. See also articulator.

frame, rubber dam, *n* See holder, rubber dam.

framework, *n* the skeletal metal portion of a removable partial denture around which and to which the remaining units are attached.

franchise dentistry, *n* **1.** the practice of dentistry under a brand name, the rights of which have been purchased from another dental professional or dental practice. Under a franchise license agreement, the franchiser may use the brand name, marketing products, and treatment techniques for a sum of money, as long as certain rules and regulations of the franchise are adhered to. *n* **2.** a system for marketing a dental practice, usually under a brand name, where permitted by state laws. In return for a financial investment or other consideration, participating dental professionals may also receive the benefits of media advertising, a national referral system, and financial and management consultation.

Francisella (fransīsel'ə), *n* a type of gram-negative eubacteria with cell walls. It requires oxygen to survive.

F. tularensis (too'ləren'sis), *n.pl* the bacteria that causes the circulatory disease tularemia, which can be contracted via contaminated food or drink, physical contact, spray, or bug bite. Symptoms include fever, headache, swelling of the lymph nodes, and other pain or discomfort.

Frankel appliance, *n.pr* See appliance, Frankel removable orthodontic.

Frankfort horizontal plane, *n.pr* See plane, Frankfort horizontal.

Frankfort-mandibular incisor angle, *n.pr* See angle, Frankfort-mandibular incisor.

F-ratio (F-test), *n* a value used in determining whether the difference between two variables is statistically significant or stable. A larger variance is divided by a smaller variance, both of which are the results of analysis of variance procedures. The value for F is looked up in a table that shows the probability of occurrence of a ratio of this size.

fraud, *n* an intentional perversion of truth for the purpose of inducing another, in reliance on it, to part with something valuable or to surrender a legal right; deliberate deception; deceit; trickery.

fraudulent concealment, *n* the deliberate attempt to withhold information or to conceal an act to avoid contractual responsibility. Fraudulent concealment as applied to health care providers arises when a treating doctor conceals from an aggrieved patient that a previous treating doctor may have committed malpractice.

freckle, *n* See ephelis.

free gingiva, *n* See gingiva, free.

free gingival crest, *n* the most superficial portion of the marginal gingiva.

free gingival groove, *n* See groove, gingiva, free.

free gingival margin, *n* See margin, gingival.

free mandibular movement, *n* See movement, mandibular, free.

free radical, *n* a compound with an unpaired electron or proton. It is unstable and reacts readily with other molecules.

free-end, *n* See base, extension.

freedom of choice, *n* a provision in a dental benefits program that permits the insured to choose any licensed dental professional to provide his/her dental care and receive full benefits under the program.

freeway space, *n* See distance, interocclusal.

freeze drying, *n* the freezing of heat-sensitive liquid materials in a vacuum to preserve the characteristics of the substrate and remove the volume of water or liquid by sublimation.

fremitus (frem′itus), *n* the palpable vibrations of nonvascular origin that can be noted by placing the hand on the chest. See also thrill.

Fremitus, dental, n an abnormal mobility of a tooth in occlusal contact, best detected by placing a fingernail on the tooth and feeling the tooth movement compared to others. A symptom of excessive tooth contact, and/or reduced periodontal attachment.

frenal pull, charting (frē′nul), *n* notations made to a patient's chart concerning evidence of the forces 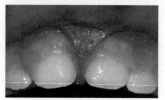 exerted by frenums, both on the maxillary and mandibular arches.

frenectomy (frənek′tōmē), *n* **1.** the excision of a frenum. *n* **2.** the surgical detachment and/or excision of a frenum from its attachment into the mucoperiosteal covering of the alveolar processes. Other term: *frenotomy.*

frenoplasty (frē′nōplas′tē), *n* a correction of an abnormal frenum by repositioning it.

frenotomy (frənot′əmē), *n* the cutting of a frenum; possibly the release of ankyloglossia (tongue-tie), although this is not the preferred method of treatment. More common term: *frenectomy.*

frenotomy, traumatic (frənot′əmē trəmat′ik), n a laceration of an oral frenum, usually the maxillary labial frenum, due to trauma. Most commonly seen in children.

Traumatic frenectomy. (Courtesy Dr. Beth Schulz-Butulis)

frenulum (fren′ūlum), *n* See frenum.

frenum (frē′num), *n* a vertical band of oral mucosa that attaches the cheeks and lips to the alveolar mucosa of the mandibular and maxillary arches, limiting the motions of the lips and cheeks. Older term: *frenulum.*

frenum, abnormal (enlarged labial frenum), n a labial frenum appearing to be unusually heavy, broad, or attached too near the crest of the ridge that may be an etiologic factor in periodontal disease involving the marginal gingivae.

frenum, buccal, n the vertical band(s) of oral mucosa connecting the residual alveolar ridge to the cheek in the premolar region. They exist in both the maxillary and mandibular arches and separate the labial vestibule from the buccal vestibule.

frenum, enlarged labial, n See frenum, abnormal.

frenum, labial, n the vertical band of oral mucosa connecting the lip of the residual alveolar ridge near the midline of both the maxillary and mandibular arches.

frenum, lingual, n the vertical band of oral mucosa connecting the tongue with the floor of the oral cavity and the alveolar or residual alveolar ridge. See ankyloglossia.

frequency, n the number of cycles per second of a wave or other periodic phenomenon. Frequency indicates the energy of a particular radiation.

frequency polygon, n a graphic representation of a frequency distribution constructed by plotting each frequency above the score or midpoint of a class interval laid out on a base line and connecting the points so plotted by a straight line.

Frey syndrome (frī), *n.pr* See syndrome, Frey.

friable (frī'əbəl), *adj* brittle or fragile; easily damaged.

fricative (frik'ətiv), n a speech sound made by forcing the airstream through such a narrow opening that audible high-frequency air currents or vibrations are set up (e.g., sounds of s, z, f, and v.)

friction (frik'shən), n the resistance to movement as one object is moved across the other, usually creating heat.

Friedman's test (frēd'mənz), *n.pr* See test, pregnancy.

fringe benefits, *n.pl* the benefits, other than wages or salary, provided by an employer for employees (e.g., health insurance, vacation time, disability income).

frit (frit), n a partly or wholly fused porcelain that has been plunged into water while hot. The mass cracks and fractures, and from this "frit," dental porcelain powders are made.

frontal, *adj* in anatomy, referring to the body's frontal plane or to the forehead or frontal bone.

frontal [(PA) cephalometric radiograph,] n a cephalometric radiograph made with the subject facing the receptor (posteroanterior [PA] view); the axis between the ears is parallel to the receptor and perpendicular to the radiographic beam.

frontal bone, n a single cranial bone that forms the front of the skull from above the orbits posteriorly to a junction with the parietal bones at the coronal suture.

frontal lobe, n the largest of five lobes constituting each of the two cerebral hemispheres. The frontal lobe lies beneath the frontal bone. The frontal lobe significantly influences personality and is associated with the higher mental activities, such as planning, judgment, and conceptualizing.

frontal region, n the region of the head that includes the forehead and supraorbital area.

frontal sinus, n See sinus(es), frontal.

frovatriptan, n *brand name:* Frova; *drug class:* antimigraine; *action:* agonist at the serotonin 5-HT $_{1A/1B}$ receptor, whose stimulation leads to reduced pain nerve activity in the brain as well as reduced inflammation around nerves and less vasodilation of cerebral blood vessels; *use:* migraine headache.

frozen sections, n a histologic section of tissue that has been frozen by exposure to dry ice.

fructose (fruk'tōs), n a yellowish-to-white, crystalline, water-soluble, levorotatory ketose monosaccharide that is sweeter than sucrose and is found in honey, several fruits, and combined in many disaccharides and polysaccharides. Also called *fruit sugar* and *levulose.*

fructose intolerance, n an inherited disorder marked by an absence of enzymes needed to metabolize fructose. Symptoms include sweating, tremors, confusion, and digestive distress with vomiting, and failure of infants to grow.

fulcrum, extraoral (fōōl'krəm), n a stabilizing support point outside the oral cavity against which the hand or finger is placed for leverage during a dental procedure in order to ensure precise control of the instrument; usually the chin or cheek.

fulcrum, intraoral, n a stabilizing support point within the oral cavity against which a finger is placed for leverage during treatment in order to ensure precise control of the instrument; usually a tooth that is in close proximity to the one being treated.

fulcrum line, n See line, fulcrum.

fulguration (ful'gyərā'shən), n the destruction of soft tissue by an electric spark that jumps the gap from an electrode to the tissue without the electrode touching the tissue. See also electrocoagulation.

g, *n* See gram.

gabapentin (gab'ə-pen'tin), *n brand name:* Neurontin; *drug class:* antiepileptic; *actions:* blocks the α2δ calcium channel and prevents depolarization in certain parts of the central nervous system; *uses:* neuropathic pain, partial seizures.

gadolinium (Gd) (gadlin'ēəm), *n* a rare-earth metallic element with an atomic number of 64 and an atomic weight of 157.25. It is used as a phosphor to intensify radiography screens.

gag, *n* a surgical device for holding the oral cavity open.

gag reflex, *n* a normal neural reflex elicited by touching the soft palate or posterior pharynx. The response is a symmetric elevation of the palate, a retraction of the tongue, and a contraction of the pharyngeal muscles. It is used as a test of the integrity of the vagus and glossopharyngeal nerves.

gagging, *n* an involuntary retching reflex that may be stimulated by something touching the posterior palate or throat region.

gait (gāt), *n* a manner of walking; a cyclic loss and regaining of balance by a shift of the line of gravity in relationship to the center of gravity. A person's gait is as characteristic and as individual as a fingerprint.

gait, cerebellar, *n* an unsteady, irregular gait characterized by short steps and lurching from one side to the other; most commonly seen in multiple sclerosis or other cerebellar diseases.

gait, festinating, *n* a gait characterized by rigidity, shuffling, and involuntary hastening. The upper part of the body advances ahead of the lower part. It is associated with paralysis agitans and postencephalitic Parkinson's syndrome.

gait, sensor ataxic, *n* an irregular, uncertain, stamping gait. The legs are kept far apart, and either the ground or the feet are watched, because there has been a loss of knowledge of the position of the lower limbs. This gait

is caused by an interruption of the afferent nerve fibers and may be associated with tabes dorsalis and sometimes with multiple sclerosis and other lesions of the nervous system.

gait, spastic, *n* a slow, shuffling gait in which the patient appears to be wading in water. Knee and hip movements are restricted. This gait may be associated with multiple sclerosis, syphilis, combined systemic disease, or other diseases affecting the spinal pyramidal tracts.

gait, staggering, *n* a reeling, tottering, and tipping gait in which the individual appears as if he may fall backward or lose his balance. It is associated with alcohol and barbiturate intoxication.

gait, waddling, *n* an exaggerated alteration of lateral trunk movements, with an exaggerated elevation of the hip, suggesting the gait of a duck; characteristic of progressive muscular dystrophy.

galactin (gəlak'tin), *n* See hormone, lactogenic.

galactosamine, *n* a chondrosamine; a derivative of galactose, occurs in various mucopolysaccharides, notably of chondroitin sulfuric acid and B blood group substance.

galactose (gəlak'tōs), *n* a simple sugar found in the dextrorotatory form in lactose (milk sugar), nerve cell membranes, sugar beets, gums, seaweed, and, in the levorotatory form, in flaxseed mucilage. Galactose, a white crystalline substance, is less sweet and less soluble in water than glucose but is similar in other properties.

galactosemia (gəlak'tose'meə), *n* an inherited condition that prevents normal metabolism of galactose because of a lack of the galactose-*l*-phosphate uridyl transferase enzyme.

gallic acid (gal'ik), *n* an astringent used topically, made from tannic acid or nutgalls, and chemically known as 3,4,5-trihydroxybenzoic acid.

gallium (gal'ēəm), *n* a metallic element with an atomic number of 31 and an atomic weight of 69.72. It is used in high temperature thermometers, and its radioisotopes are used in total body scanning procedures.

galvanic current, *n* See current, galvanic.

galvanic skin response (GSR), *n* a reaction to certain stimuli as indicated by a change in the electric resistance of the skin. The GSR is used in some polygraph examinations.

galvanism, *n* See current, galvanic.

galvanotherapy, *n* See ionization.

gamma globulins, *n.pl* plasma proteins that are essential antibodies that circulate in the immune system. The most significant gamma globulins are antibodies or immunoglobulins. See also immunoglobulins.

gamma rays, *n.pl* an electromagnetic radiation of short wavelength emitted by the nucleus of an atom during a nuclear reaction. Composed of high-energy photons, gamma rays lack mass and an electric charge and travel at the speed of light.

ganciclovir (gansī′klōvir), *n brand names:* Cytovene, Vitrasert, Zirgan; *drug class:* antiviral; *action:* inhibits replication of most herpes viruses by selective inhibition of human cytomegalovirus (CMV) DNA polymerase and by direct incorporation into viral DNA; *uses:* CMV-retinitis in patients with AIDS, systemic CMV infections.

▣ **ganglion(ia) (gang′glēon),** *n/n.pl* an accumulation of neuron cell bodies outside the central nervous system.

ganglion, basal, *n* a group of forebrain nuclei that, with the related structures of the brain, play an important role in the regulation of muscle tone and motor control. The cell groups of these ganglia and their respective nerve tracts are classified as the *extrapyramidal motor system* to differentiate them from the *pyramidal motor system,* which goes directly from the cerebral cortex to the lower motor neuron. Disease associated with the basal ganglia is manifested by three principal motor abnormalities: disturbance of muscle tone, derangement of movement, and loss of associated or automatic movement.

ganglion, ciliary, *n* a parasympathetic nerve ganglion in the posterior part of the orbit. The ciliary ganglion receives preganglionic fibers from the region of the oculomotor nucleus and sends postganglionic fibers via short ciliary nerves to (1) the constrictor muscle of the iris (constriction of pupil) and (2) circular fibers of the ciliary muscle (accommodation for vision).

ganglion, otic, *n* a ganglion located medial to the mandibular nerve just below the foramen ovale in the infratemporal fossa. It supplies the sensory and secretory fibers for the parotid gland. Its sensory fibers arise from the facial and glossopharyngeal nerves.

ganglion, pterygopalatine, *n* the ganglion associated with the greater petrosal nerve and branches of the maxillary nerve.

ganglion, sphenopalatine (sfē′nōpal ′ətīn), *n* a ganglia located deep in the pterygopalatine fossa that is intimately associated with the maxillary nerve. It lies distal and medial to the maxillary tuberosity. Its fibers supply the oral mucosa of the oropharynx, tonsils, soft and hard palates, and nasal cavity. The mucous and serous secretions of all the oral mucosa of the oropharynx are also mediated by this ganglion.

ganglion, submandibular, *n* a ganglion located on the medial side of the mandible between the lingual nerve and the submandibular duct. The submandibular ganglion is distributed to the sublingual and submandibular glands. The sensory fibers arise from the lingual branch of the trigeminal nerve (i.e., the chorda tympani of the facial nerve).

ganglion, trigeminal (trī′jem′ən əl), *n* a cluster of nervous tissue located on the root of the fifth cranial (trigeminal) nerve.

ganglionectomy (gang′lēōnek′tə mē), *n* the excision of a ganglion.

ganglionitis, acute posterior (gang ′glēənītis), *n* See herpes zoster.

▣ **gangrene (gang′grēn),** *n* the death of tissue en masse, usually the result of loss of blood supply, bacterial invasion, and subsequent putrefaction (e.g., gangrene of the pulp is total death and necrosis of the pulp). All types require the removal of the necrotic tissue before healing can progress.

gangrene, dry, *n* a late complication of diabetes mellitus that is already complicated by arteriosclerosis in which the affected extremity becomes cold, dry, and shriveled and eventually turns black.

gangrene, gas, *n* the necrosis accompanied by gas bubbles in soft tissue after trauma or surgery. It is caused by anaerobic microorganisms such as various species of *Clostridium,* particularly *C. perfringens.* If untreated, it is rapidly fatal.

gangrene, moist, *n* a condition that may follow a crushing injury or an obstruction of blood flow by an embolism, tight bandages, or a tourniquet. This form of gangrene has an offensive odor, spreads rapidly, and may result in death in a few days.

Gantrisin, *n.pr* the brand name for sulfisoxazole, an antibacterial sulfonamide, which is effective in the treatment of acute, recurrent, or chronic urinary tract infections, meningococcal meningitis, and acute otitis media.

gap arthroplasty, *n* the surgical correction of ankylosis by creation of a space between the ankylosed part and the portion in which movement is desired.

gap, interocclusal, *n* See distance, interocclusal.

Gardasil HPV vaccine, *n* a vaccine that protects against human papillomavirus.

Gardner-Diamond's syndrome, *n. pr* a condition resulting from autoerythrocyte sensitization, marked by large, painful, transient ecchymoses that appear without apparent cause but often accompany emotional upsets, various collagen disorders, and abnormalities of protein metabolism. Treatment includes topical and systemic corticosteroids. Also called *autoerythrocyte sensitization syndrome.*

gargoylism, *n* See syndrome, Hurler's.

GAS, *n* See syndrome, general adaptation.

gas, *n* a fluid with no definite volume or shape whose molecules are practically unrestricted by cohesive forces.

gas, laughing, *n* colloquial term for *nitrous oxide.* See also nitrous oxide.

gas, noble, *n* a gas that will not oxidize; the inert gases (e.g., helium and neon).

gas, olefiant, *n* a machine that uses ethylene oxide gas to sterilize objects that cannot withstand high temperatures, such as soft plastic and cloth.

gasometer (gasäm′ətur), *n* a calibrated instrument or vessel for measuring the volume of gases; used in clinical and physiologic investigation for measuring respiratory volume.

gastric acid, *n* the hydrochloric acid secreted by the gastric glands in the stomach; aids in the preparation of food for digestion.

gastric intrinsic factor (GIF), *n* a substance secreted by the gastric mucosa that is essential for the intestinal absorption of vitamin B_{12}; also known as *intrinsic factor.*

gastric juice, *n* the digestive secretions of the gastric glands in the stomach, consisting mainly of pepsin, hydrochloric acid, rennin, and mucin.

gastric mucosa, *n* the lining of the stomach.

gastrinoma, *n* a gastrin-secreting tumor associated with the Zollinger-Ellison's syndrome.

gastritis (gastrī′tis), *n* an inflammation of the lining of the stomach that occurs in both acute and chronic forms. Acute gastritis may be caused by aspirin or other antiinflammatory agents, corticosteroids, drugs, foods, condiments, and alcohol and chemical toxins. The symptoms are anorexia, nausea, vomiting, and discomfort after eating. Chronic gastritis is usually a sign of underlying disease, such as peptic ulcer or pernicious anemia.

gastritis, atrophic, *n* a chronic form of gastritis with atrophy of the mucous membrane and destruction of the peptic glands, sometimes associated with pernicious anemia or gastric carcinoma.

gastroenteritis (gas′trōen′təri′tis), *n* an inflammation of the stomach and intestines accompanying numerous gastrointestinal (GI) disorders. Symptoms are anorexia, nausea, vomiting, abdominal discomfort, and diarrhea.

gastroenterology (gas′trōen′tərol ′əjē), *n* the study of diseases affecting the GI tract, including the esophagus, stomach, intestines, rectum, gallbladder, and bile duct.

gastroesophageal reflux disease (GERD) (gas′trōisof′əjē′əl), *n* a backflow of the contents of the stomach into the esophagus that is often the result of incompetence of the lower esophageal sphincter. Gastric juices are acid and therefore produce burning pain in the esophagus and possibly demineralize the teeth.

gastrointestinal disease, *n* an abnormal state or function of the GI system.

🔲 **gastrointestinal system,** *n* the chain of organs of the GI tract, from the oral cavity to the anus.

gastroscopy (gastros′kəpē), *n* the visual inspection of the interior of the stomach by means of a flexible fiberoptic tube inserted through the oral cavity and passing the length of the esophagus into the stomach.

gastrostomy (gastros′təmē), *n* the surgical creation of an artificial opening into the stomach through the abdominal wall, used to feed a patient who has cancer of the esophagus or other kind of barrier to oral feeding.

gate-keeper system, *n* a managed care concept used by some alternative benefit plans, in which enrollees elect a primary care dental professional, usually a general practitioner or pediatric dental professional, who is responsible for providing nonspecialty care and managing referrals, as appropriate, for specialty and ancillary services.

gauge, *n* an instrument used to determine the dimensions or caliber of an object.

gauge, Boley, *n.pr* a vernier type of instrument used for measuring in the metric system. It is accurate to tenths of millimeters.

gauge, leaf, *n* a device for measuring the distance between two objects. A leaf gauge consists of a series of thin strips of plastic or metal, each calibrated and arranged in a sequential fashion in ascending or descending thicknesses, usually expressed in millimeters or fractions of millimeters. In dentistry, the leaf gauge is used to measure interocclusal space or the magnitude of an interocclusal interference.

gauge, undercut, *n* an attachment used in conjunction with a dental cast surveyor to measure the amount of infrabulge of a tooth in a horizontal plane.

gauze strip, for flossing, *n* a folded 6- to 8-inch pieces of sterile gauze used to clean abutment teeth, teeth located at the end of a row, the space underneath dental appliances that cannot be completely removed, and between teeth that are exceptionally far apart.

gel (jel), *n* a colloid in solid form, jellylike in character. Hydrocolloid impression materials are examples of gels.

gel, brush-on, fluoride, *n* a gelatinous preparation used to promote remineralization of teeth and discourage further demineralization, intended to augment daily brushing and flossing. Formulas contain either 1.1% sodium fluoride or 0.4% stannous fluoride in a glycerin base.

gel strength, *n* See strength, gel.

gel time, *n* See time, gel.

gelatin, *n* a protein formed from collagen by boiling in water. Medically, gelatin is used as a hemostat, a plasma substitute, and a protein food adjunct in severe cases of malnutrition. Gelatin is used in the manufacture of capsules and suppositories. It is also used in the production of radiographic films as the medium for suspending the crystal salts on the surface of the acetate film.

gelation time (jelā′shən), *n* See time, gel.

gemfibrozil (jemfi′brəzil′), *n brand name:* Lopid; *drug class:* antihyperlipidemic; *action:* reduces plasma triglycerides and very-low-density lipoproteins; *uses:* type IIb, IV, and V hyperlipidemia.

gemination (jem′ənā′shən), *n* the formation of two teeth from a single tooth germ.

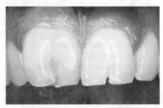

Gemination. (Neville et al., 2009)

gene, *n* the biologic unit of inheritance, consisting of a particular nucleotide sequence within a DNA molecule that occupies a precise locus on a chromosome and codes for a specific polypeptide chain.

gene, homeobox (ho′meoboks′), *n* a gene containing a DNA sequence called the homeobox, which is very similar between species and encodes a DNA-binding domain in the resulting protein molecule. Homeobox genes usually play a role in controlling development of the organism.

gene locus, *n* See locus, gene.

gene, sex-linked, *n* a gene located in a sex chromosome.

gene therapy, *n* a procedure that involves injection of "health genes" into the bloodstream of a patient to cure or treat a hereditary disease or similar illness.

general oral health assessment index *(GOHAI),* *n* a 12-question oral health assessment with five possible Likert-style answers to each question.

general supervision, *n* a circumstance of treatment in which the dental professional must diagnose and authorize the work to be performed on the patient by the dental staff but is not required to be on the premises while the treatment is carried out.

generated path (chew-in), *n* See path, generated occlusal.

generator, *n* one who or which begets, causes, or produces.

generator, electric, *n* a device that converts mechanical energy into electrical energy.

generator, radiographic, *n* a device that converts electrical energy into electromagnetic energy (photons).

genetic counseling, *n* the process of advising a patient with a genetic disease, or child-bearing parents of a patient with a genetic disease, about the probabilities and risks of future genetic accidents in conception, and counseling such persons about future family planning.

genetic disease, *n* a disease that is caused by a defect or anomaly in the genetic inheritance of the patient.

genetic effects of radiation (jənet′ik), *n.pl* the changes produced in the individual's genes and chromosomes of all nucleated body cells, both somatic and gonadal, because of exposure to radiation. The more common meaning relates to the effect produced in the reproductive cells. Radiation received by the gonads before the end of the reproductive period has the potential to add to the number of undesirable genes present in the population.

genetic marker, *n* a specific gene that produces a readily recognizable genetic trait that can be used in family and population studies or in linkage analysis.

genetic testing, *n* the analysis of a person's DNA, usually to determine predispositions for or diagnoses of certain inherited conditions. See also DNA.

genetics, *n* the science that deals with the origin of the characteristics of an individual.

genial tubercle, *n* See tubercle, genial.

genioplasty (jē′nēōplastē), *n* a surgical procedure, performed either intraorally or extraorally, to correct deformities of the mandibular symphysis.

genital wart (condyloma acuminatum), *n* a soft, wartlike growth found on the warm, moist skin and mucous membranes of the genitalia, caused by a papillomavirus, usually types 6 and 11, and transmitted by sexual contact. Also called *acuminate wart.*

genome (jē′nōm), *n* the total gene complement of a set of chromosomes found in higher life forms.

genome, human, *n* the complete set of genes in the chromosomes of each cell.

genotype (jē′nōtīp), *n* the aggregate of ordered genes received by offspring from both parents; e.g., a person with blood group AB is of genotype AB.

gentamicin sulfate, *n* (ophthalmic), *brand names:* Genoptic, Gentamicin Pediatric, Gentak; *drug class:* aminoglycoside antiinfective ophthalmic; *action:* inhibits bacterial ribosomal protein synthesis; *use:* systemic or eye infections caused by several aerobic bacteria, chiefly gram-negatives.

gentian violet (jen′shən), *n* See violet, gentian.

geographic tongue, *n* See tongue, geographic.

geometric unsharpness, *n* an impairment of image definition resulting from the geometric penumbra. See also penumbra, geometric and radiograph beam.

geometry of radiographic beam, *n* the effect of various factors on the spatial distribution of radiation emerging from a radiographic generator or source. See also law, inverse square;

penumbra, geometric; and radiographic beam.

geriatric assessment, *n* the evaluation of the physical, mental, and emotional health of elderly patients.

geriatric dentistry, *n* a branch of dentistry that deals with the special and unique dental problems of the elderly. See also elderly.

geriatrics (jer′ēat′riks), *n* the department of medicine or dentistry that treats health problems peculiar to advanced age and the aging, including the clinical problems of senescence and senility.

germ cell, *n* a sexual reproductive cell in any stage of development; that is, an ovum or spermatozoon or any of their preceding forms.

germanium *(Ge)* **(jərmā′nēəm),** *n* a metallic element with some nonmetallic properties. Its atomic number is 32 and its atomic weight is 72.59.

germicide (jur′misīd), *n* a substance capable of killing a wide variety of microorganisms; more specifically, one capable of killing all microorganisms, except for spores, with which it is in contact for a standard period.

germinal center, *n* the center region of the lymphatic nodule of a lymph node where the lymphocytes mature.

gerodontics (jer′ōdon′tiks), *n* the branch of dentistry that deals with the diagnosis and treatment of the dental conditions of aging and aged persons.

gerodontology (jer′ōdontol′ōjē), *n* See gerodontics.

gerontology (jer′ontol′əje), *n* the comprehensive (physical, psychologic, and social) study of aging.

gestation, *n* the period of development between conception and birth.

gestational age, *n* the age of a fetus or newborn, usually expressed in weeks dating from the first day of the mother's last menstrual period.

giant cell, *n* an abnormally large tissue cell. It often contains more than one nucleus and may appear as a merger of several normal cells.

giantism, *n* excessive growth resulting in a stature larger than the range that is normal for age and race.

giantism, infantile, n excessive growth occurring before adolescence.

giantism, primary, n excessive growth not attributable to a definite cause.

giantism, secondary, n excessive growth secondary to a disorder of the adrenal, pineal, gonadal, or pituitary gland.

Giardia **(jēär′dēə),** *n* a common genus of the flagellate protozoans. Many species normally inhabit the digestive tract and cause inflammation in association with other factors that produce rapid proliferation of the organism.

giardiasis (jēärdī′əsis), *n* an inflammatory intestinal condition caused by overgrowth of the protozoan *G. lamblia.* The source of infection is usually contaminated water. Also called *traveler's diarrhea.*

GIF, *n* See gastric intrinsic factor.

Gillies′ operation, *n.pr* See operation, Gillies′.

Gillmore needle, *n.pr* See needle, Gillmore.

Gilson fixable-removable bar, *n.pr* See connector, cross arch bar splint.

gingiva(e) (jin′jivə), *n/n.pl* the fibrous tissue that immediately surrounds the teeth. Colloquial term is *gums.*

gingiva, adequate attached (AAG), n the amount of attached gingival tissue needed to prevent recession of the gingival tissue.

gingivae, attached, n the portion of the gingivae extending from the free gingival groove, which demarcates it from the marginal (free) gingivae, to the mucogingival junction, which separates it from the alveolar mucosa. This tissue is firm, dense, stippled, and tightly bound down to the underlying periosteum, tooth, and bone.

gingivae, attached, extension, n See extension, gingiva, attached.

gingiva, detached by calculus, n the recession and ultimate disconnection of gingival tissue from tooth surfaces that occurs as the result of the presence of large amounts of calculus.

gingivae, erythemic **(erəthē′mik),** *n.pl* the unusually red gingival tissue that may be caused by either inflammation or excessive blood in the tissue. The condition may occur as a result of excess vitamin A.

gingivae, free, n.pl an older term for the unattached coronal portion of the gingiva that encircles the tooth to

epinephrine; others are impregnated with an astringent.

gingival shrinkage, n the reduction in size of gingival tissue, principally by diminution of edema, usually as a result of therapeutic elimination of subgingival deposits and curettement of the soft tissue wall of the pocket.

gingival stippling, n a series of small depressions characterizing the surface of healthy gingivae, varying from a smooth velvet to that of an orange peel.

gingival sulcus, n the space between the free gingiva and the tooth.

gingival surface texture, n the texture of the attached gingivae, which normally is stippled. In inflammatory conditions, the edema, cellular infiltration, and concomitant swelling cause loss of the surface stippling, and the gingivae take on a smooth, shiny, edematous appearance.

gingival third, n the most apical one third of a given clinical crown or of an axial surface cavity or preparation.

gingival topography, n the form of the healthy gingival tissue. The marginal gingivae and interdental papillae have a characteristic shape.

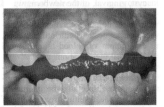 gingivectomy (jin′jivek′təmē), n the surgical or laser excision of unsupported gingival tissue to the level at which it is attached, creating a new gingival margin apical in position to the old.

gingivectomy in edentulous area, n the elimination of periodontal pockets surrounding abutment teeth; requires the removal of gingival tissue on the adjacent edentulous area.

gingivitis (jin′jivī′tis), n an inflammation of the gingival tissue; a major classification of periodontal disease.

gingivitis and malposed teeth, n the malposition may predispose the gingivae to inflammation by permitting food impaction or impingement, providing irregular spaces in which calculus may be deposited, and making oral hygiene difficult.

gingivitis, bacteria in, n the causative organisms in gingival inflammation. The common chronic forms of gingivitis, from a bacterial standpoint, are nonspecific, with the exception of acute necrotizing ulcerative gingivitis, in which there is an apparent specificity of the bacterial flora; the fusospirochetal organisms.

gingivitis, bismuth, n a metallic poisoning caused by bismuth given for treatment of systemic disease; characterized by a dark, bluish line along the gingival margin.

gingivitis, chronic atrophic senile, n gingival inflammation characterized by atrophy and areas of hyperkeratosis; found primarily in elderly women.

gingivitis, desquamative (des′kwəm ā′tiv), n an inflammation of the gingivae characterized by a tendency of the surface epithelium to desquamate. The condition is a clinical entity, not a pathologic entity. Older term: *gingivosis.*

gingivitis, eruptive (ērup′tiv), n the gingival inflammation occurring at the time of eruption of the primary or permanent teeth.

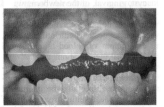

Eruptive gingivitis. (Newman/Takei/ Klokkevold, 2012)

gingivitis, fusospirochetal, n See gingivitis, necrotizing ulcerative.

gingivitis gravidarum, n See gingivitis, pregnancy.

gingivitis, hemorrhagic, n the gingivitis characterized by profuse bleeding, especially that associated with ascorbic acid deficiency or leukemia.

gingivitis, herpetic, n an inflammation of the gingivae caused by herpesvirus. See also gingivostomatitis, herpetic.

gingivitis, hormonal, n the gingivitis associated with endocrine imbalance. The endocrinopathy is modified, in most instances, by the influence of local environmental factors.

gingivitis, hyperplastic, n the gingivitis characterized by proliferation of the various tissue elements; May be accompanied by dense infiltration of inflammatory cells.

gingivitis, idiopathic, n a gingival inflammation of unknown causation.

gingivitis, infectious, n a gingivitis not caused by plaque, but instead originating from bacteria, fungi, or viruses.

gingivitis, inflammatory cells in, n the inflammatory cells are, for the most part, lymphocytes, plasma cells, and some histiocytes, because the gingival inflammatory process is usually chronic and progressive in nature. With acute exacerbations, polymorphonuclear leukocytes are also present.

gingivitis, marginal, n an inflammation of the gingivae localized to the marginal gingivae and interdental papillae.

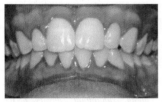

Marginal gingivitis. (Neville et al., 2009)

gingivitis, menstrual cycle–associated, n gingival inflammation that occurs during ovulation as a result of hormone level changes.

gingivitis, necrotizing ulcerative, n a form of necrotizing periodontal disease with an inflammation of the gingivae characterized by necrosis of the interdental papillae, ulceration of the gingival margins, the appearance of a pseudomembrane, pain, and a fetid odor. Synonyms: fusospirochetal gingivitis, NUG, trench oral cavity, ulcerative gingivitis, ulceromembranous gingivitis, Vincent's gingivitis, Vincent's infection.

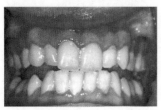

Necrotizing ulcerative gingivitis. (Ibsen/Phelan, 2009)

gingivitis, nephritic, n membrane form of stomatitis and gingivitis associated with a failure of kidney function. It is accompanied by pain, ammonia-like odor, and increased salivation. Also called *uremic gingivitis* and *uremic stomatitis*.

gingivitis, non–plaque-induced, n a gingivitis caused by factors other than plaque, such as allergic reaction, dermatologic disease, a genetic condition, infectious agents, response to a foreign body, or physical trauma.

gingivitis, plaque-induced, n a gingivitis caused by the accumulation of plaque.

gingivitis, pregnancy, n an enlargement of hyperplasia of the gingivae resulting from a hormonal imbalance during pregnancy. Synonyms: gingivitis gravidarum, hormonal gingivitis.

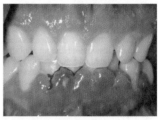

Pregnancy gingivitis. (Ibsen/Phelan, 2009)

gingivitis, puberty, n an enlargement of the gingival tissue as a result of an exaggerated response to irritation resulting from hormonal changes.

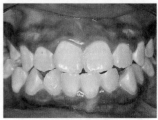

Puberty gingivitis. (Zitelli/McIntire/Nowalk, 2012)

gingivitis, scorbutic, n a gingivitis associated with vitamin C (ascorbic acid) deficiency.

gingivitis, systemic disease–induced, n a gingivitis occurring as a complication of a systemic disease, such as type 1 diabetes mellitus or acute leukemia.

gingivitis, uremic, n See gingivitis, nephritic.

gingivoplasty (jin'jivōplastē), *n* the surgical contouring of the gingival tissue to secure the physiologic architectural form necessary for the maintenance of tissue health and integrity.

gingivosis (jin'jivō'sis), *n* a noninflammatory degenerative condition of the gingivae. This older term is applied to desquamative gingivitis.

gingivostomatitis (jin'jivōstō'mətī'tis), *n* an inflammation that involves the gingivae and the oral mucosa.

gingivostomatitis, acute herpetic, n See stomatitis, herpetic, acute.

gingivostomatitis, herpetic, n an inflammation of the gingivae and oral mucosa caused by primary invasion of herpesvirus. Herpetic gingivostomatitis occurs mainly in childhood. One attack gives immunity to generalized stomatitis but not isolated lesions (herpetic lesions), unless an adult has had an isolated upbringing. The symptoms are red and swollen gingivae; red mucosa, which soon shows vesicles and ulcers; painful oral cavity; and elevated temperature. The course is about 14 days.

gingivostomatitis, membranous, n a disease, or group of diseases, in which false membranes form on the gingivae and oral mucosa. The membranes are a grayish white color and are surrounded by a narrow red margin. Detachment of the membrane leaves a raw, bleeding surface. One cause is mixed pyogenic infection, in which S. viridans and Staphylococcus organisms predominate.

gingivostomatitis, white folded, n See nevus spongiosus albus mucosa.

ginglymus (hinge joint) (jing'gliməs), *n* a joint that allows motion around an axis.

glabella (gləbel'ə), *n* the smooth, elevated area on the frontal bone between the supraorbital ridges; the most anterior point on the frontal bone.

gland(s), *n/n.pl* an organ producing a specific product or secretion.

gland, parotid salivary, n the largest of the major salivary glands. Its anterior position is situated between the ramus of the mandible, its posterior portion between the mastoid process and sternocleidomastoid muscle, and inferior to the zygomatic arch. It is irregularly wedge shaped, with the lateral surface flattened and the medial aspect more or less pointed toward the pharyngeal wall. Its secretion, which is serous, travels the parotid duct (Stenson's duct) to empty into the oral cavity at the ductal opening at the parotid papillae on the buccal mucosa opposite the maxillary molar teeth.

gland, pituitary (hypophysis), n an endocrine gland located at the base of the brain in the sella turcica. The pituitary gland is composed of two parts: the pars nervosa, which is an extension of the anterior part of the hypothalamus, and the pars intermedia, which is an epithelial evagination of secretory tissue from the stomodeum of the embryo. By its structural and functional relationships with the nervous system and endocrine glands, it acts as a mediator of both the nervous system and endocrine system.

gland, sublingual salivary, n the smallest of the major salivary glands. It lies inferior to the floor of the oral cavity bilateral to the lingual frenum and is in contact with the sublingual depression on the inner side of the mandible. Its numerous ducts open directly into the oral cavity bilateral to the lingual frenum and join to form the sublingual duct (duct of Bartholin's), which enters into the submandibular duct (Wharton's duct). Its secretion is mucous in nature.

gland, submandibular salivary, n a major salivary gland that has an irregular form and is situated in the submandibular space, bordered anteriorly by the anterior belly of the digastric muscle and posteriorly by the stylomandibular ligament. Its mucoserous section is carried by the submandibular duct (Wharton's duct), whose openings lie at a small papilla (submandibular caruncle) bilateral to the lingual frenum.

gland, thymus, n See thymus.

gland, thyroid, n See thyroid gland.

glands, Blandin and Nuhn's, n.pr See spots, Fordyce's.

glands, endocrine, n.pl a gland of internal secretion; a hormonesecreting gland (e.g., the pituitary gland, thyroid gland, parathyroid glands, adrenal glands, ovaries, and testes).

glands, lacrimal, n.pl the ducted (exocrine) glands that produce lacrimal fluid, commonly called *tears.* See also lacrimal apparatus.

glands, minor salivary, n.pl the glands located at the posterior aspect of the dorsum of the tongue posterior to the circumvallate papillae (von Edner's) and along the lateral surface of the tongue; also located in the palate, floor of mouth, labial mucosa, and buccal mucosa. The secretion is mucous, and they do not have named ducts. Older term: *accessory salivary glands.* See also salivary glands, von Edner's.

glands, parathyroid, n See parathyroid glands.

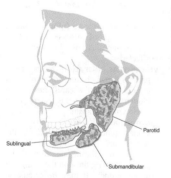

glands, salivary, n.pl the glands in the oral cavity that secrete saliva. Three major salivary glands contribute their secretions to form the whole saliva. The minor mucous glands found within oral mucosa contribute a lesser amount. The major salivary glands are the parotid, submandibular, and sublingual.

Parotid
Sublingual
Submandibular

Salivary glands. (Daniel/Harfst/Wilder, 2008)

glands, salivary, von Ebner, n.pr the minor secretory glands located at the base of the circumvallate papillae on the posterior dorsal surface of the tongue. Also known as *Ebner glands.*

Glasgow Coma Scale (GCS), *n* a standardized system for assessing the degree of consciousness in the critically ill and for predicting the duration and ultimate outcome of coma, primarily in patients with head injuries. It involves eye opening, verbal response, and motor response.

glass, bioactive, *n* a form of glass that encourages bone growth. The compound consists of silica (glass) and other materials (often including calcium) in powder or molded form. In dental offices, bioactive glass is often used to repair bone structures during extractions or other procedures.

glass ionomer cement (īon′əmər), *n* a dental cement of low strength and toughness produced by mixing a powder prepared from a calcium aluminosilicate glass and a liquid prepared from an aqueous solution of prepared polyacrylic acid; used mainly for small restorations on the proximal surfaces of anterior teeth and for restoration of eroded areas at the gingival margin.

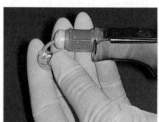

Glass ionomer cement. (Hatrick/Eakle/Bird, 2011)

glass, lead, *n* the lead-impregnated glass used in windows of control booths and protective shields to protect clinicians when taking radiographs.

glatiramer acetate (glahtear ′ameer as′ətāt), *n* a medication used to decrease or stop a relapse of multiple sclerosis. It is typically used to treat individuals resistant to the effects of interferon-β.

glaucoma (gloukō′mə), *n* an abnormal condition of elevated pressure within the eye because of obstruction of the outflow of aqueous humor.

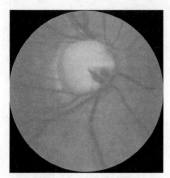

Glaucoma. (Patton/Thibodeau, 2013)

glaucoma, acute, *n* a condition that occurs if the pupil in an eye with a narrow angle between the iris and cornea dilates markedly, causing the folded iris to block the exit of aqueous humor from the anterior chamber. Also called *closed angle glaucoma.*

glaucoma, chronic, *n* a condition that is much more common than closed-angle glaucoma and is often bilateral. Open-angle glaucoma develops slowly and is genetically determined and progressive with age. The obstruction is believed to occur within the canal of Schlemm. Also called *chronic* or *primary glaucoma.*

glaze, *n* a critical stage in the final firing of dental porcelain when complete fusion takes place, with the formation of a thin, vitreous, glossy surface, or glaze.

glenoid (glē′noid), *n* the fossae in the temporal bone in which condyles of the mandible articulate with the skull.

gliadin (glī′ədin), *n* a protein substance that is obtained from wheat and rye. Its solubility in diluted alcohol distinguishes gliadin from glutenin.

glide(s), *n* **1.** the passage of one object over another as guided by their contacting surfaces. *n.pl* **2.** the sounds *w, wh,* and *y,* which are voiced as bilabial and palatal glides, respectively. The rapid movement of the lips or tongue from a set position toward a neutral vowel (*u,* as in up).

glide, mandibular, *n* the side-to-side, protrusive, intermediate movement of the mandible that occurs when the teeth or other occluding surfaces are in contact.

gliding occlusion, *n* See occlusion, gliding.

glimepiride (glimep′ərīd), *n brand name:* Amaryl; *drug class:* oral antidiabetic; *action:* a second-generation sulfonylurea, blocks ATP-dependent potassium channels in the beta cells of the pancreas and increases insulin release; *use:* non–insulin-dependent (type 2) diabetes.

glioma (glē′ōmə), *n* the largest group of primary tumors of the brain, composed of malignant glial cells.

glipizide (glip′izīd), *n brand name:* Glucotrol; *drug class:* oral antidiabetic (second generation); *action:* causes functioning β cells in pancreas to release insulin, leading to a drop in blood glucose levels; *use:* stable adult-onset diabetes mellitus (type 2).

globin (glō′bin), *n* a group of four globulin protein molecules that become bound by the iron in heme molecules to form hemoglobin or myoglobin.

globulin (glob′yəlin), *n* a class of proteins.

globulin, antihemophilic, *n* See factor VIII.

globulin, antihemophilic A, *n* See factor VIII.

globulin, antihemophilic B, *n* See factor IX.

glomerular disease (glōmer′yələr), *n* a group of diseases in which the glomerulus of the kidney is affected.

glomerular filtration, *n* the renal process in which fluid in the blood is filtered across the capillaries of the glomerulus and into the urinary space of Bowman's capsule.

glomerular filtration rate, *n* a kidney function test in which the results are determined from the amount of ultrafiltrate formed by plasma flowing through the glomeruli of the kidney. It may be calculated from the use of an inulin injection or by estimating it from the creatinine clearance value.

glomerulus (glōmer′yələs), *n* a cluster of blood vessels or nerve fibers, such as the cluster of blood vessels in the kidney that function as filters of the plasma portion of the blood.

glossalgia (glôsal′jēə), *n* painful sensations in the tongue.

glossectomy (glôsek′təmē), *n* the surgical removal of the tongue, a portion of the tongue, or a lesion of the tongue.

glossitis (glôsī′tis), *n* an inflammation of the tongue.

glossitis areata exfoliativa, *n* See tongue, geographic.

glossitis, atrophic, *n* the atrophy of the glossal papillae, resulting in a smooth tongue. The tongue may be pallid or erythematous and may appear small or enlarged. It may be associated with anemias, pellagra, vitamin B–complex deficiencies, sprue, or other systemic diseases or may be local in origin. Because atrophy may be one phase, and circumscribed, painful, glossal excoriations may be another phase of one or more of the same systemic disease(s), much confusion in terminology has arisen (e.g., Moeller's glossitis; Hunter's glossitis; slick, glazed, varnished, glossy, smooth, or bald tongue; chronic superficial erythematous glossitis; glossodynia exfoliativa; beefy tongue; and pellagrous glossitis).

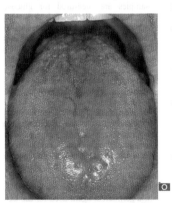

Atrophic glossitis. (Regezi/Sciubba/Pogrel, 2000)

glossitis, benign migratory, *n* See tongue, geographic.

glossitis exfoliativa, *n* See glossitis, Moeller's.

glossitis, interstitial sclerous, *n* nodular, lobulated, indurated tongue associated with terminal syphilis. Synonym: Clarke-Fournier's glossitis.

glossitis, median rhomboid, *n* See atrophy, central papillary.

glossitis migrans, *n* See tongue, geographic.

glossodynia (glôs′ōdī′nēə), *n* painful sensations in the tongue; a sensation of burning in the tongue; a sore tongue.

glossopharyngeal air space (glos′ôf ərin′jēəl er spās), *n* the empty area between the tongue and the pharynx at the back of the throat.

glossopharyngeal nerve (glos′ôfəri n′jēəl), *n* See nerve, glossopharyngeal (IX).

glossoplasty (glôs′ōplastē), *n* a surgical procedure performed on the tongue.

glossoplegia (glôs′ōplē′jēə), *n* a paralysis of the tongue; may be unilateral or bilateral.

glossoptosis, *n* a downward displacement of the tongue; a severe displacement may occlude the airway.

glossopyrosis (glôs′ōpīrō′sis), *n* a burning sensation of the tongue.

glossorrhaphy (glôsôr′əfē), *n* the suture of a wound of the tongue.

glossotomy (glôsot′əmē), *n* an excision or incision of the tongue.

glottal (glot′əl), *adj* pertaining to, or produced in or by, the glottis. The sound of *h* is a voiceless glottal fricative. The airstream on the exhalation phase moves unimpeded through the larynx, pharynx, and oral cavities.

glottis (glot′is), *n* the vocal apparatus of the larynx, consisting of the true vocal cords (vocal folds and the opening between them [rima glottidis]).

gloves, *n.pl* the gloves used as an essential part of barrier protection in health care delivery.

gloves, examination, *n.pl* nonsterile gloves most frequently worn by dental personnel during patient care. They are usually made of latex or vinyl. Gloves containing no latex can be used when the practitioner has a sensitivity to latex. They are discarded after single use.

gloves, over, *n.pl* gloves made of light, clear plastic which can be worn over contaminated examination gloves to prevent contamination of

renal disease, and in patients taking adrenocorticosteroids.

glycosylated hemoglobin assay, *n* a laboratory test to determine the amount of glucose in the blood that is permanently bound to a molecule of hemoglobin; helps prevent development of long-term complications by monitoring glycemic control over a longer period.

Gm, *n* See gram.

gnathion (nā'thēon), *n* the lowest point in the inferior border of the mandible at the median plane. It is a point on the bony border palpated from below and naturally lies posterior to the tegumental border of the chin.

gnathodynamometer (nath'ōdī 'nəmom'ətur), *n* an instrument used for measuring biting pressure.

gnathodynamometer, bimeter, *n* a gnathodynamometer equipped with a central bearing point of adjustable height.

Gnathograph (nath'ōgraf), *n.pr* an articulator that resembles the Hanau instrument but differs mainly by having a provision for increasing the intercondylar distance, an important determinant of groove directions in the occlusal surfaces of teeth.

Gnatholator (nāth'əla'tər), *n.pr* an articulator design that has since been succeeded by an improved instrument called the *Simulator* (or *Gnathosimulator*).

gnathologic instrument, *n* a term often used as a synonym for an articulator. Any dental instrument used for diagnosis and treatment, such as a probe for determining the depth of a periodontal pocket, is a gnathologic tool.

gnathology (nāthol'əjē), *n* the study of the functional and occlusal relationships of the teeth; sometimes also used to identify a specific philosophy of occlusal function.

gnathoschisis (nathos'kisis), *n* See jaw, cleft.

gnathostatics (nath'ōstat'iks), *n* a technique of orthodontic diagnosis based on relationships between the teeth and certain landmarks on the skull. See also cast, gnathostatic.

goal, *n* the purpose toward which an endeavor is directed, such as the outcome of diagnostic, therapeutic,

and educational management of a patient's health problem.

goblet cells, *n* the cells in respiratory mucosa that produce the mucus that keeps the respiratory mucosa moist.

goggles, *n* the protective eyewear worn by dental personnel and patients during dental procedures.

goiter (goi'tur), *n* an enlargement of the thyroid gland.

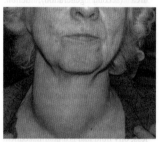
Goiter. (Little/Falace/Miller/Rhodus, 2013)

goiter, colloid (endemic goiter, iodine deficiency goiter, simple goiter), *n* a visible enlargement of the thyroid gland without obvious signs of hypofunction or hyperfunction of the gland resulting from inadequate intake or an increased demand for iodine.

goiter, endemic, *n* See goiter, colloid.

goiter, exophthalmic, *n* a disease of the thyroid gland consisting of hyperthyroidism, exophthalmos, and goitrous enlargement of the thyroid gland. A diffuse primary hyperplasia of the thyroid gland of obscure origin; may occur at any age. It produces nervousness, muscular weakness, heat intolerance, tremor, loss of weight, lid lag, and absence of winking and may lead to thyrotoxic heart disease and thyroid crisis. Also called *Graves' disease.*

goiter, iodine deficiency, *n* See goiter, colloid.

goiter, nodular, nontoxic, *n* the recurrent episodes of hyperplasia and involution of colloid goiter, which result in a multinodular goiter. Symptoms are related to pressure.

goiter, simple, *n* See goiter, colloid.

goitrogens (goi'trōjenz), *n.pl* the agents such as thiouracil and related antithyroid compounds that are capable of producing goiter.

gold, *n* a precious or noble metal; yellow, malleable, ductile, nonrusting; much used in dentistry in pure and alloyed forms.

gold alloys, *n.pl* an alloy that contains gold; usually alloyed with copper, silver, platinum, palladium, and zinc. The alloying of gold enhances certain properties such as hardness, or creates a lower melting point for gold solder.

gold, cohesive, *n* gold usually manufactured in thin sheets of foil, that has been treated to cause it to cohere, or stick together. This allows it to be easily formed into a variety of shapes.

gold compound, *n* a drug containing gold salts, usually administered with other drugs in the treatment of rheumatoid arthritis. Various radioisotopes of gold have been used in diagnostic radiology and in the radiologic treatment of certain malignant neoplastic diseases.

gold, crystal, *n* See gold, mat.

gold, fibrous, *n* See foil, gold.

gold file, *n* See file, gold.

gold foil, *n* See foil, gold.

    gold foil cylinder, *n* See foil cylinder.

    gold foil pellet, *n* See pellet, foil.

gold, inlay, *n* **1.** an alloy, principally gold, used for cast restorations. Desired physical properties may be obtained by selecting those with varying ingredients and/or proportions. Acceptable alloys are classified by the American Dental Association (ADA) specifications according to Brinell hardness: Type A—soft, Brinell 40 to 75; Type B—medium, Brinell 70 to 100; Type C—hard, Brinell 90 to 140. *n* **2.** an intracoronal cast restoration of gold alloy fabricated outside the oral cavity and cemented into the prepared cavity.

gold knife, *n* See knife, gold.

gold, mat, *n* a noncohesive form of pure gold prepared by electrodeposition. It is sometimes used in the base of restorations and then veneered or overlaid with cohesive foil. Also called *crystal gold* and *sponge gold.*

gold, powdered, *n* the fine granules of pure gold, formed by atomizing the molten metal or by chemical precipitation. For clinical use, powdered gold is available either as clusters of the granules or as pellets of the powder contained in an envelope of gold foil.

gold saw, *n* See saw, gold.

gold sodium thiosulfate, *n* an antirheumatic used in the treatment of rheumatoid arthritis.

gold, sponge, *n* See gold, mat.

gold, white, *n* a gold alloy with a high palladium content. It has a higher fusion range, lower ductility, and greater hardness than a yellow gold alloy.

Golden Proportions, *n* a mathematical proportion as a representation of esthetic perfection.

Goldent, *n.pr* the brand name for a direct gold restorative material. It consists basically of varying amounts of powdered gold contained in a wrapping or envelope of gold foil.

Goldman-Fox knife, *n.pr* See knife, Goldman-Fox.

Golgi apparatus (gōl'jē), *n.pr* the small membranous structures found in most cells, composed of various elements associated with the formation of carbohydrate side chains of glycoproteins, mucopolysaccharides, and other substances. Also called *Golgi body* or *Golgi complex.*

Golgi's corpuscles (gol'jēz), *n.pr* See corpuscle, Golgi's.

gomphosis (gämfō'sis), *n* a form of joint in which a conical body is fastened into a socket, as a tooth is fastened into the jaw.

gonad (gō'nad), *n* an ovary or testis, the site of origin of eggs or spermatozoa.

gonadotrophin (gōnad'ōtrōf'in), *n* See gonadotropin.

gonadotropin (gonadotropic hormone) (gōnad'ōtrōp'in), *n* a gonad-stimulating hormone derived either from the pituitary gland (e.g., follicle-stimulating hormone [FSH] and luteinizing hormone [LH], which is also an interstitial cell-stimulating hormone [ICSH]) or from the chorion (e.g., chorionic gonadotropin, which is found in the urine of pregnant women).

gonadotropin, chorionic, *n* See hormone, pregnancy.

gonion (Go), *n* the most posteroinferior point of the angle of the mandible near the inferior border of the ramus.

gonorrhea (gon′ərē′ə), *n* a sexually transmitted disease of the genitourinary tract caused by *Neisseria gonorrhoeae* that is spread by direct contact with an infected person or fluids containing the infectious microorganism. It may also affect the conjunctiva, oral tissue, and other tissue and organ systems.

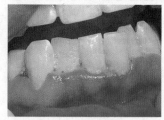

Gonorrhea. (Neville/Damm/Allen, 2009)

good faith, *n* honesty of intention. Generally, not a sufficient defense in a dental malpractice lawsuit.

good samaritan legislation, *n* the statutes enacted in some states protecting health care professionals from liability for aid rendered in emergency situations, unless there is a showing of willful wrong or gross negligence.

goodwill, *n* the intangible assets of a firm established by the excess of the price paid for the ongoing concern over its book value.

gothic arch tracer, *n* See tracer, needle point.

gothic arch tracing, *n* See tracing, needle point.

gout, *n* a disease associated with an inborn error of uric acid metabolism that increases production or interferes with the excretion of uric acid. Excess uric acid is converted to sodium urate crystals that precipitate from the blood and become deposited in joints and other tissue. The great toe is a common site for the accumulation of urate crystals. It can be exceedingly painful, with swelling of a joint, and may be accompanied by chills and fever.

gown, *n* the protective garment worn by a health care provider designed to prevent the spread of infection between the health care provider and the patient.

gr, *n* See grain.

grace period, *n* a specified time, after a plan's premium payment is due, in which the protection of the plan continues subject to actual receipt of the premium within that time.

graft, *n* a slip or portion of tissue used for implantation. See also donor site; recipient site.

graft, allo-, n a graft between genetically dissimilar members of the same species.

graft, allogenic, n a graft using tissue from the same species (i.e., person to person). See also allograft.

graft, alloplast (al′əplast′), n a graft of an inert metal or plastic material.

graft, auto-, n See graft, autogenous.

graft, autogenous (ôtoj′ənəs), n a graft taken from one portion of an individual's body and implanted into another portion of the individual's body.

graft, autogenous bone, n the bone that is removed from one area of a patient's body and transplanted into another area that requires additional bony material. Such bone grafts are advantageous because they contain live active cells that promote bone growth.

graft, bone, n the transplantation of healthy bone tissue to a defective bone cavity so that the new bone tissue meets the surrounding, unaffected surface and promotes healing and new growth.

graft, bone, allograft, n a bone graft using tissue obtained from an individual other than, but of the same species as, the host of the bone graft; sources include human cadavers, living relatives, and nonrelatives. Also called *allogeneic graft* and *homograft.*

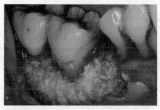

Allograft bone graft. (Courtesy Dr. Flavio Uribe)

G

graft, bone, autogenous, n See graft, autogenous.

graft, composite, n a transplant involving living tissue made of different materials, such as skin and cartilage.

graft donor site, n the site from which graft material is taken.

graft, filler, n the filling of defects, such as bone chips used to fill a cyst.

graft, free, n a graft of tissue completely detached from its original site and blood supply.

graft, full-thickness, n a skin graft consisting of the full thickness of the skin with none of the subcutaneous tissue.

graft, gingival, n a graft in which a thin piece of tissue is taken from the palate of the oral cavity, or moved over from adjacent areas, to provide a stable band of soft tissue around a tooth or implant.

graft, hetero-, n See graft, heterogenous.

graft, heterogenous (het′əraj′ən əs), n a graft implanted from one species to another.

graft, homo-, n See graft, homogenous.

graft, homogenous (həmoj′ənəs), n a graft taken from a member of a species and implanted into the body of a member of the same species.

graft, iliac, n a bone graft whose donor site is the crest of the ilium. Various locations of the iliac crest duplicate areas of the mandible and curvatures of the midfacial skeleton.

graft, iso-, n a graft between individuals with identical or histocompatible antigens.

graft, kiel, n a denatured calf bone used to fill defects or restore facial contour.

graft, mucosal, n a split-thickness graft involving the mucosa.

graft, onlay bone, n a graft in which the grafted bone is applied laterally to the cortical bone of the recipient site, frequently to improve the contours of the chin or the malar eminence of the zygomatic bone.

graft, particulate, n a surgical tissue implant or graft consisting of various particles; e.g., used in the stimulation of bone growth.

graft, pedicle (ped′ikəl), n a stem or tube of tissue that remains attached near the donor site to nourish the graft during advancement of a skin graft.

graft, ramus, n the surgically removed bone taken from the ascending ramus of the mandible for the purpose of transplantation.

graft, split-thickness, n a graft with varying thickness containing only mucosal elements and no subcutaneous tissue.

graft, swaging, n a procedure analogous to bone grafting; also referred to as a *contiguous transplant,* which involves a greenstick fracture of bone bordering on an infrabony defect and the displacement of bone to eliminate the osseous defect.

graft, Thiersch's skin (tērsh′əz), n. pr a split-thickness skin graft containing cutaneous and some subcutaneous tissue, the line of cleavage through the rete peg layer.

graft-versus-host disease *(GVHD),* n See disease, graft-versus-host (GVHD).

grain (gr), n **1.** a unit of weight equal to 0.0648 g. **2.** a crystal of an alloy.

grain boundary, n the junction of two grains growing from different nuclei, impinging and causing discontinuity of the lattice structure. Important in corrosion and brittleness of metals.

grain growth, n See growth, grain.

gram *(Gm, g),* n the basic unit of mass of the metric system. Equivalent to 15.432 gr.

gram-negative, n having the pink color of the counterstain used in Gram's method of staining microorganisms. Staining property is a common method of classifying bacteria. See also Gram's stain.

gram-positive, n retaining the violet color of the stain used in Gram's method of staining microorganisms. Staining property is a common method of classifying bacteria. See also Gram's stain.

Gram's stain, n.pr a sequential process for staining microorganisms in which a violet stain is followed by a wash and then a counterstain of safranin. Gram-positive organisms appear violet or blue; gram-negative organisms appear rose pink.

granisetron, n brand names: Kytril, Sancuso; drug class: antiemetic; action: blocks serotonin 5-HT3 receptors; *uses:* chemical- or radiation-induced nausea.

granular layer, *n* the layer superficial to the prickle cell layer in some forms of keratinized epithelium that appears because of drying of tissue. See also stratum granulosum.

granulation tissue, *n* a soft, pink, fleshy projections that form during the healing process in a wound not healing by first intent. It consists of many capillaries surrounded by fibrous collagen. Overgrowth is termed *proud flesh.* In dentistry, such tissue is evident at the opening to a fistulous tract or at the site of a recent tooth extraction.

granules, sulfur, *n.pl* See actinomycosis.

granulocyte (gran′yəlōsīt′), *n* a type of leukocyte (white blood cell) characterized by the presence of cytoplasmic granules.

granulocyte colony stimulating factor (G-CSF), *n brand name:* Neupogen; *drug class:* myeloid growth factor; *action:* stimulates cell membrane receptors in neutrophils; *uses:* cancer patients receiving myelosuppression therapy or receiving bone marrow transplant, chronic neutropenia. Also known as *filgrastim.*

granulocyte/macrophage colony stimulating factor (GM-CSF), *n brand name:* Leukine; *drug class:* myeloid growth factor; *action:* stimulates cell membrane receptors in granulocytes, monocytes, and to a certain extent, erythrocytes, and megakaryocytes; *uses:* to stimulate myeloid tissue in certain cases of bone marrow transplant, acute myelogenous leukemia patients. Also known as *sargramostim.*

granulocytopenia (gran′ūlōsī′tōpē ′nēə), *n* a deficiency in the number of granulocytic cells in the bloodstream. See also agranulocytosis.

granuloma (gran′ūlō′mə), *n* a painless, benign and expansile lesion usually anterior to the mandibular first molar tooth that rarely crosses the midline and contains variable numbers of multinucleated, osteoclast-like giant cells.

granuloma, central giant cell, n a painless, benign, expansile lesion on bone, usually on the anterior mandible, less frequently crossing the midline of the mandible. It usually contains a number of multinucleated giant cells.

granuloma, *chronic, n* (chronic apical periodontitis) a chronic inflammatory tissue surrounding the apical foramina as a result of irritation from within the root canal system.

granuloma, dental, n a mass of granulation tissue surrounded by a fibrous capsule attached at the apex of a pulp-involved tooth. It produces a radiolucency that is fairly well demarcated.

granuloma, eosinophilic (ē′əsin′əfil ′ik), *n* a granulomatous inflammatory disease of unknown etiology, usually monofocal in bone but sometimes affecting soft tissue. Sheets of histiocytes and masses of eosinophils characterize the lesion histologically. See also disease, Langerhans cell.

granuloma, giant cell peripheral, n an inflammatory lesion located near the gingival margin. It takes the shape of a mushroom, has a smooth, glossy surface, bleeds easily, and tends to reoccur after removal. It generally occurs in the third trimester of pregnancy. See also granuloma, pyogenic and granuloma, central giant cell.

granuloma inguinale (ing′gwināl′), *n* a sexually transmitted disease characterized by ulcers of the skin and subcutaneous tissue of the groin and genitalia. It is caused by infection with *C. granulomatis,* a small, gramnegative, rod-shaped bacillus.

granuloma, pyogenic, n a tumorlike mass of granulation tissue produced in response to minor trauma in some individuals. It is not suppuration producing, as the name suggests, but is highly vascular and bleeds readily. They are histologically identical to pregnancy granulomas, but they may be found in either gender in any location, and may occur at any age. Some prefer the term *lobular capillary hemangioma* to describe a pyogenic granuloma, as it more accurately describes the histologic findings.

graph   305   grinding, selective

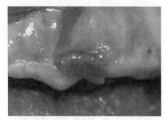

Pyogenic granuloma. (Courtesy Dr. James Sciubba)

granuloma, reticuloendothelial (ritik′yəlōen′dōthē′lēəl), *n* See disease, lipoid storage.

graph, *n* a diagram used to compare numerical relationships.

graphite, *n* a soft carbon substance with a metallic black or gray sheen and a greasy feel. It is used in pencils, as a constituent of lubricants, and for making refractories such as crucibles in which to melt gold and other metals.

grasp, *n* the manner in which an instrument is held.

grasp, finger, n a modification of the palm and thumb grasp. It is more useful with modern, smaller-handled instruments. The handle is held by the four flexed fingers rather than allowed to rest in the palm, and the thumb is used to secure a rest. Used when working indirectly on the maxillary arch.

grasp, instrument, n a method of holding the instrument with the fingers in such a manner that freedom of action, control, tactile sensitivity, and maneuverability are secured. The most common grasp is the pen grasp.

grasp, modified pen, n a method for holding instruments that is designed to enhance control and sensitivity. The grasp consists of the tips of the thumb, index finger, and middle finger holding the instrument while the ring finger provides support. See also grasp, pen.

grasp, palm-and-thumb, n a grasp that is similar to the hold on a knife when one is whittling wood. The handle rests in the palm and is grasped by the four fingers, while the thumb rests on an adjoining object.

grasp, pen, n a grasp in which the instrument is held somewhat as a pen is held, with the handle in contact with the bulbous portion of the thumb and index finger and the shank in contact with the radial side of the bulbous portion of the middle finger (not crossing the nail), while the handle rests against the phalanx of the index finger.

grasp, pincer, n the grasping an object between the thumb and forefinger. The ability to perform this task is a milestone of fine motor development in infants, usually occurring from 9 to 12 months of age.

gratis, *adj* free, without reward or consideration.

Graves′ disease, *n.pr* See goiter, exophthalmic.

gravity, specific, *n* a number indicating the ratio of the weight of a substance to that of an equal volume of water.

Gray (Gy), *n* a unit of measurement for an absorbed dose of radiation, from the French *Systéme International d′Unités;* converts to the traditional rad by the formula 100 rad = 1 Gy.

greater palatine foramen, *n* See foramen, greater palatine.

grid, *n* a device used to prevent as much scattered radiation as possible from reaching a receptor during the production of a radiograph. It consists essentially of a series of narrow lead strips closely spaced on their edges and separated by spacers of low-density material.

grid, crossed, n an arrangement of two parallel grids rotated in position at right angles to each other. See also grid, parallel.

grid, focused, n a grid in which the lead foils are placed at an angle so that they all point toward a focus at a specified distance.

grid, moving, n a grid that is moved continuously or oscillated throughout the making of a radiograph.

grid, parallel, n a grid in which the lead strips are oriented parallel to each other.

grid, Potter-Bucky, n.pr a grid using the principle of the moving grid, with an oscillating movement.

grid, stationary, n a nonoscillating or nonmoving grid; the image of its strips will be visible on the radiograph for which it is used.

grinding, selective, *n* a modification of the occlusal forms of teeth by grinding at selected places to improve function.

grinding-in, *n* the process of correcting errors in the centric and eccentric occlusions of natural or artificial teeth.

griseofulvin microsize/griseofulvin ultramicrosize (gris′ēōful′vin mī′krōsīz′ ul′trəmī′krōsīz′), *n brand names:* Fulvicin U/F, Grifulvin V, Gris-PEG; *drug class:* antifungal; *action:* arrests fungal cell division at metaphase; binds to human keratin, making it resistant to disease; *uses:* dermatophyte fungal infections: tinea corporis, tinea pedis, tinea cruris, tinea barbae, tinea capitis, tinea unguium if caused by the dermatophytes *(Epidermophyton, Microsporum,* or *Trichophyton).*

grit, *n* the measurement of the abrasive particle size.

groin, *n* each of two areas where the abdomen joins the thighs.

groove, *n* a linear channel or sulcus.

groove, abutment, n a transverse groove that may be cut in the bone across the alveolar ridge to furnish positive seating for the implant framework and to prevent tension of the tissue.

groove, branchial, n See branchial grooves.

groove, central, n the most prominent developmental groove on posterior teeth, which generally travels mesiodistally and separates the occlusal table buccolingually.

groove, developmental, n a fine depressed line in the enamel of a tooth that marks the union of the lobes of the crown in its development.

groove, gingiva, free, n the shallow line or depression on the surface of the gingiva at the junction of the free and attached gingivae.

groove, interdental, n a linear, vertical depression on the surface of the interdental papillae; functions as a spillway for food from the interproximal areas.

groove, labiomental, n a natural indentation in the chin, just below the lips, that takes its form from the muscles and bones lying beneath the skin.

groove, lingual, n a furrow or channel that forms on the tongue side of selected anterior teeth.

groove, linguogingival, n vertical groove on the lingual surface of certain anterior teeth that originates in the lingual pit and extends cervically and slightly distal onto the cingulum.

groove, marginal, n a developmental groove that forms across the marginal ridges of posterior teeth.

groove, mylohyoid, n a groove on the mandible in which the mylohyoid nerve and blood vessels travel.

groove, nasolacrimal **(groov nā′zōlak′rəmal),** *n* a linear depression that extends from the eye to the olfactory sac in an embryo and separates the lateral nasal process from the maxillary process.

groove, retention, n a groove formed by opposing vertical constrictions in the preparation of a tooth that provides improved retention of the restoration.

groove, supplemental, n a secondary groove that is a shallower, more irregular linear depression and that branches from the developmental grooves on the lingual surface of anterior teeth and the occlusal table on posterior teeth.

groove, triangular, n the grooves that separate a marginal ridge from the triangular ridge of a cusp and which at the termination of the ridges form the triangular fossae.

ground, electrical, *n* an electrical connection with the earth (or other ground).

ground state, *n* the state of a nucleus, an atom, or a molecule when it has its lowest energy. All other states are termed *excited.*

ground substance, *n* See matrix.

ground substance, of bone, n a major component of bone consisting of proteoglycans that contain chondroitin sulfate and hydroxyapatite. More recently called *intercellular substance.*

grounded, *adj* pertaining to an arrangement whereby an electrical circuit or equipment such as a radiographic generator is connected by an electrical conductor with the earth or some similarly conducting body.

group, blood, *n* See blood groups.

group function, *n* See function, group.

group practice, *n* the association of several health care providers to complement, facilitate, and extend their scope of health care delivery, not possible in a sole or single practice. See also practice, group.

group purchase, *n* the purchase of dental services, either by postpayment or prepayment, by a large group of people.

growth, *n* an increase in size.

growth and development, *n* the process of *growth* is defined as an increase in size; *development* is defined as a progression toward maturity. Thus the terms are used together to describe the complex physical, mental, and emotional processes associated with the "growing up" of children.

growth factor, *n* the chemical messengers that induce cell growth by tissue type (e.g., osteoinductive factor, epidermal growth factors).

growth failure, *n* a lack of normal physical and psychologic development as a result of genetic, nutritional, pathologic, or psychosocial factors. See also failure to thrive.

growth, grain, *n* a phenomenon resulting from heat treatment of alloys. In excessive amounts, this growth produces undesirable physical properties.

growth hormone (GH), *n* a single-chain peptide secreted by the anterior pituitary gland in response to growth hormone releasing factor (GHRF) from the hypothalamus. Growth hormone promotes protein synthesis in all cells, increased fat mobilization and use of fatty acids for energy, and decreased use of carbohydrates. Growth hormone (generic names: somatrem and somatropin) is also used as a drug. *Brand names:* Protropin, Saizen, Genotropin, Accretropin, Valtropin. *Use:* replacement therapy in those lacking growth hormone.

GTT, *n* See test, glucose tolerance.

guaiacol, *n* catecholomonomethyl ether, which is used as an expectorant and intestinal disinfectant.

guaifenesin (gwī′əfen′əsin), *n brand names:* Anti-Tuss, Robitussin; *drug class:* expectorant; *action:* acts as an expectorant by stimulating mucosal reflex to increase production of less viscous lung mucus; *use:* dry, nonproductive cough.

guanabenz acetate (gwän′ə benz), *n brand name:* Wytensin; *drug class:* centrally acting antihypertensive; *action:* stimulates central α_2-adrenergic receptors, resulting in decreased sympathetic outflow from the brain; *use:* hypertension.

guanadrel sulfate (gwän′ədrel), *n brand name:* Hylorel; *drug class:* antihypertensive; *action:* inhibits sympathetic vasoconstriction by inhibiting release of norepinephrine, depleting norepinephrine stores in adrenergic nerve endings; *use:* hypertension.

guanethidine sulfate (gwäneth′idēn), *n brand name:* Ismelin; *drug class:* antihypertensive; *action:* inhibits norepinephrine release, depleting norepinephrine stores in adrenergic nerve endings; *use:* moderate to severe hypertension.

guanfacine HCl (gwän′fəsēn), *n brand names:* Tenex, Intuniv; *drug class:* antihypertensive; *action:* stimulates central α_2-adrenergic receptors, resulting in decreased sympathetic outflow from the brain; *use:* hypertension.

guanosine (gwän′əsēn), *n* a compound derived from a nucleic acid, composed of guanine and a sugar, D-ribose. Guanosine is a major molecular component of the nucleotides guanosine monophosphate and guanosine triphosphate and of DNA and RNA.

guanosine triphosphate (GTP), *n* a high-energy nucleotide, similar to adenosine triphosphate, that functions in various metabolic reactions such as the activation of fatty acids and the formation of the peptide bond in protein synthesis.

guaranty (gar′əntē), *n* a contract that some certain and designated thing shall be done exactly as it is agreed to be done.

guard, bite, *n* an acrylic resin appliance designed to cover the occlusal and incisal surfaces of the teeth of a dental arch to stabilize the teeth and/or provide a flat platform for the unobstructed excursive glides of the mandible. See also plane, bite.

guard, night, *n* See guard, bite.

guard, mouth, *n* a resilient intraoral device worn during participation in contact sports to reduce the potential for injury to the teeth and associated tissue.

guardian, *n* a person appointed to take care of the person or property of another; one who legally has the care and management of the person or the property or both of a child until the child attains adulthood.

guardian ad litem, *n* a person appointed by the court to represent a child's or incapacitated person's best interests during legal proceedings.

Guérin's fracture (gāranz′), *n.pr* See fracture, Guérin's

guidance, *n* a mechanical or other means for controlling the direction of movement of an object.

guidance, angle, *n* See angle, incisal guidance.

guidance, condylar, *n* See guide, condylar.

guidance, condylar, inclination, *n* See guide, condylar, inclination.

guidance, developmental, *n* the comprehensive orofacial orthopedic control over the growth of the jaws and eruption of the teeth, with the objective of optimizing the achievement of the genetic potential of the individual. It requires a combination of carefully timed active appliance therapy and supervisory examinations, including radiography and other diagnostic records, at various stages of development. It may be required throughout the entire period of growth and maturation of the face, beginning at the earliest detection of a developing malformation.

guidance, incisal, *n* the influence on mandibular movements of the contacting surfaces of the mandibular and maxillary anterior teeth.

guide, *n* a device for directing the motion of something.

guide, adjustable anterior, *n* an anterior guide, the superior surface of which may be varied to provide desired separation of the casts in various eccentric relationships.

guide, anterior, *n* the part of an articulator contacted by the incisal guide pin to maintain the selected separation of the upper and lower members of the articulator. The guide influences the changing relationships of mounted casts in eccentric movements. See also guide, incisal.

guide, condylar (condylar guidance), *n* the mechanical device on an articulator; intended to produce guidance in articulator movement similar to that produced by the paths of the condyles in the temporomandibular joints.

guide, condylar, inclination (condylar guidance inclination), *n* the angle of inclination of the condylar guide mechanism of an articulator in relation to the horizontal plane of the instrument.

guide, incisal, *n* the part of an articulator that maintains the incisal guide angle. Also called an *anterior guide.*

guide, incisal, adjustment, *n* an occlusal adjustment that produces a minimum of overbite (vertical overlap) and a maximum of overjet (horizontal overlap), eliminates fremitus and racking effects on the anterior segment of teeth in the protrusive glide, and attains maximal incisive group function.

guide, incisal, angle, *n* See angle, incisal guide.

guide plane, *n* a fixed or removable orthodontic appliance designed to deflect the functional path of the mandible and alter the positions of specific teeth.

guidelines, *n.pl* a set of standards, criteria, or specifications to be used or followed in the performance of certain tasks.

gum(s), *n* the colloquial term for the fibrous and mucosal covering of the alveolar process or ridges or gingiva(e). See also gingiva.

gum pads, *n* edentulous segments of the maxillae and mandible that correspond to the underlying primary teeth.

gumboil, *n* an older term for an abscess of the gingiva and periosteum resulting from injury, infection, impacted food particles, or periapical infection. The gingival tissue is characteristically red, swollen, and tender. The abscess may rupture spontaneously, or it may require incision, as well as treatment of the underlying cause. See also abscess.

gumma (gum′ə), *n* a granulomatous, soft and slightly compressible lesion of tertiary syphilis. The palate and tongue are sites of predilection in the oral region. A similar lesion occurring with tuberculosis is designated a tuberculous gumma.

gummy smile, *n* condition in which gingival tissue is located more on the cervical third of the crowns than is normal, resulting in teeth that appear shorter and "gummy."

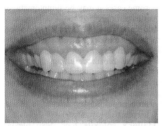

Gummy smile. (Courtesy Dr. Flavio Uribe)

Gunn's syndrome, *n.pr* See splint, Gunning's.

gutta-percha (gut′ə-pur′chə), *n* the coagulated juice of various tropical trees that has certain rubberlike properties. Used for temporary sealing of dressings in cavities; also used in the form of cones for filling root canals and in the form of sticks for sealing cavities over treatment.

gutta-percha, baseplate, *n* the gutta-percha combined with fillers and coloring materials and rolled into sheets that are used as temporary bases for denture construction.

gutta-percha points, *n.pl* the fine, tapered cylinders of gutta-percha used, because of their radiopacity, for radiographic ascertainment of pocket depth and topography; used also as a root canal filling material.

gutta-percha, temporary stopping, *n* the gutta-percha mixed with zinc oxide and white wax. Used for temporary sealing of dressings in cavities.

gynecologist (gī′nikol′əjist), *n* a physician whose practice of medicine focuses on the care of women, including the treatment of conditions related to the female genitourinary tract, endocrine system, and reproductive organs.

gypsum (jip′sum), *n* the dihydrate of calcium sulfate ($CaSO_4$-$2H_2O$). α-hemihydrate and β-hemihydrate are derived from gypsum. See also plaster of paris.

h II., *n* See hemophilia B.

h.s., *n* Latin phrase for "at bedtime"; used in writing prescriptions.

habilitation, *n* See rehabilitation.

habit, *n* the tendency toward an act that has become a repeated performance, relatively fixed, consistent, easy to perform, and almost automatic. Once learned, habits may occur without the intent of the person or may appear to be out of control and be difficult to change. In dentistry, habits such as bruxism, clenching, digit sucking, tongue thrusting, and lip and cheek biting may produce injury to the teeth, their attachment apparatus, oral mucosa, mandibular and temporomandibular musculature, and articulation.

habituation, *n* a state in which an individual involuntarily tends to continue the use of a drug. Generally refers to the state in which an individual continues self-administration of a drug because of psychologic dependence without physical dependence.

Haemophilus **(hēmof′iləs),** *n* a genus of gram-negative pathogenic bacteria, frequently found in the respiratory tract of humans and other animals. *Haemophilus* are generally sensitive to cephalosporins, tetracyclines, and sulfonamides.

H. influenzae, *n* a small, gram-negative, nonmotile, parasitic bacterium that occurs in two forms, encapsulated and nonencapsulated, and in six types: A, B, C, D, E, and F. Almost all infections are caused by the encapsulated type B organisms. It is found in the throats of 30% of healthy, normal people. It may cause destructive inflammation of the larynx, trachea, and bronchi in children and debilitated older people.

Hageman factor (hä′gəmən), *n* See factor XII. (not current)

hair covering, *n* a part of an overall contamination-limiting strategy. Hair should be pulled back from the shoulders and face. Longer hair may be completely concealed beneath a cap made from an approved material.

who have enough hearing left for practical use.

hard palate, See palate, hard.

hardener, *n* an ingredient (potassium alum) of the photographic and radiographic fixing solution that serves to harden the gelatin of the film to prevent softening and swelling of the gelatin.

hardening, *n* the process of setting or becoming firm.

hardening, age, *n* the precipitation of intermetallic compounds that alters certain physical properties in alloys; usually brought about through heat treatment.

hardening, precipitation, n See tempering.

hardening solution, n See solution, hardening.

hardening, strain, n an increase in proportional limit resulting from distortion of the space lattice and fracture of grain boundaries through cold working. Ductility is markedly reduced.

hardening, work, n the hardening of a metal by cold work, such as repeated flexing.

hardness (of a substance), *n* the ability of a material to resist an indenting type of load.

hardness (of radiographs), n a term used to indicate in a general way the quality of x-radiation, with hardness being a function of the wavelength; the shorter the wavelength, the harder the x-radiation.

hardness, Mohs, n a relative scratch resistance of minerals based on an arbitrary scale: 10, diamond; 9, corundum; 8, topaz; 7, quartz; 6, orthoclase; 5, apatite; 4, fluorite; 3, calcite; 2, gypsum; and 1, talc.

hardness tests, See tests, hardness.

hardware, *n* the mechanical, magnetic, electronic, and electric devices or components of a computer.

harelip (cheiloschisis, cleft lip, congenital cleft lip) (her'lip), *n* an older term for a congenital nonunion or inadequacy of soft and hard tissue related to the lip. The deformity may be extensive enough to involve the nose, alveolar process, hard palate, and velum. The extent of the deformity varies among individuals. Various classifications have been established to identify the extent of a

cleft. A rare midline cleft may occur in the lower lip at the embryonal junction of the two mandibular processes. See also lip, cleft and lip, congenital cleft.

harmony, functional occlusal, *n* an occlusal relationship of opposing teeth in all functional ranges and movements that provides the greatest masticatory efficiency without causing undue strain or trauma on the supporting tissue.

harmony, occlusal, *n* the nondisruptive relationship of an occlusion to all its factors (e.g., the neuromuscular mechanism, temporomandibular joints, teeth and their supporting structures).

hashish, abuse of (hash'ish, həshēsh), *n* a regular use of the cannabis derivative hashish for reasons other than recognized medical applications. Street names are *hash* and *soles.*

Hatch clamp, *n* See clamp, gingival, Hatch. (not current)

hatchet, *n* an angled cutting hand instrument in which the broad side of the blade is parallel with the angle(s) of the shank. Used to develop internal cavity form. May be bibeveled or single beveled like a chisel, in which case the instrument is paired with another.

haversian system, *n* See osteon.

Hawley retainer, *n.pr* See retainer, Hawley.

hay fever, *n* an acute seasonal allergic rhinitis, stimulated by tree, grass, or weed pollens. Also called *allergic rhinitis.*

hay rake, *n* See appliance, hay rake.

hazard communication plan, *n* a set of written standards designed to reduce workplace illness and injury by ensuring that all employees are familiar with the names and potential hazards of the chemicals they handle and understand the precautions necessary for protecting themselves and others against any possible risks.

hazard, radiation, *n* the hazard that exists in any area in which a person is subject to radiation.

hazardous waste, *n* any material, gas, liquid, or solid substance that has the potential to cause injury or illness; that in an unprotected state poses a risk to the environment, including plant or animal life.

HDL, *n* the abbreviation or acronym for *high-density lipoproteins*. HDL molecules are considered a protective factor in coronary heart disease.

head, *n* the rounded surface projecting from a bone by a neck.

head covering, *n* a part of an overall contamination limiting strategy, a protective accessory that conceals most of the hair and head

Head Start Program, *n.pr* a federally funded comprehensive child development program that serves low income preschool-aged children and families. Oral health care is included.

head, steeple, See oxycephalia.

head tilt–chin lift maneuver, *n* a maneuver used to open the airway of an unconscious patient. The maneuver is performed by placing the palm of one hand on the patient's forehead and applying gentle backward pressure. The fingers of the other hand are placed on the bony part of the chin and the chin is lifted forward. This maneuver lifts the tongue from the back of the throat and reestablishes the airway.

headache, *n* a pain in the cranial vault resulting from intracranial, extracranial, or psychogenic causes: intracranial vascular dilation; space-occupying lesions; diseases of the eyes, ears, and sinuses; extracranial vascular dilation; sustained muscular contraction; hysteria; certain habit patterns (clenching); and reaction to stress.

headache, cluster, *n* See neuralgia, facial, atypical.

headache, lower-half, *n* See neuralgia, facial, atypical.

headache, migraine, *n* a vascular type of headache, typically unilateral in the temporal, frontal, and retroorbital area, but may occur midface. It is described as throbbing, burning, pulsating, exploding, or pressure and may become generalized and persist for hours or days. Onset of pain is usually preceded by prodromal symptoms that may include visual disturbances, scotomas, vomiting, and nausea. A migraine headache is usually considered to be a psychophysiologic (psychosomatic) disorder.

headcap, *n* the part of an extraoral orthodontic appliance that engages the

back of the head, incorporating the skull as a source of resistance for tooth movement, and gives attachment to the intraoral element of the appliance.

headcap, plaster, *n* a cap that is constructed of plaster-of-Paris gauze and embodies points for applying fixation and traction appliances in the treatment of mandibular and maxillofacial injuries.

headgear, *n* the apparatus encircling the head or neck and providing attachment for an intraoral appliance in use of extraoral anchorage.

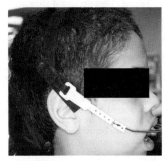

Headgear. (Courtesy Dr. Flavio Uribe)

headgear, radiologic, *n* a device that is used to protect the head from injury by radiation.

healing cap, *n* a device used during the second stage of dental implantation. It consists of a cylindrical head on the superior part and two downwardly projecting legs that are inserted into an anchor. It protects the area before the insertion of permanent prosthesis.

health, *n* a bodily state in which all parts are functioning properly. Also refers to the normal functioning of a part of the body. A state of normal functional equilibrium; homeostasis.

health, ASA classification, *n.pr* a classification system for ranking the level of a patient's physical health, established by the American Society of Anesthesiologists (ASA). Patients are classified as ASA I, indicating a patient in a normal state of health, with no apparent disease. ASA II indicates a patient with a mild

H

disease. ASA III indicates a patient with a serious disease, which may limit normal activity but does not cause incapacitation. ASA IV indicates a patient with a life-threatening and incapacitating disease. ASA V indicates a declining patient who is not expected to live beyond a day, regardless of medical attention. ASA E indicates emergency status when added to any of the normal status designations.

health assessment, *n* an evaluation of the health status of an individual by performing a physical examination after obtaining a health history. Various laboratory and functional tests may also be ordered to confirm a clinical impression or to screen for possible disease involvement.

health behavior, *n* an action taken by a person to maintain, attain, or regain good health and prevent illness. Health behavior reflects a person's health beliefs.

health care clearing house, *n* an entity used to process or aid in the processing of information; may also be called a repricing company, billing service, community health information system, community health management information system, or "value-added" switch or network.

health care operations, *n.pl* the functions performed by a health care provider, health care plan, or health care clearing house to conduct administrative and business management activities.

health care professional, *n* a person who by education, training, certification, or licensure is qualified to and is engaged in providing health care.

health care provider, *n* an individual who provides health services to health care consumers (patients).

health education, *n* an educational program directed to the general public that attempts to improve, maintain, and safeguard the health care of the community.

health hazard, *n* a danger to health resulting from exposure to environmental pollutants such as asbestos or ionizing radiation, or to a lifestyle influence such as cigarette smoking or chemical abuse.

health history, *n* previously diagnosed physical or mental condition of

an individual. Also called *medical history.* See also health assessment and chart, history.

health information, *n* recorded information in any format (e.g., oral, written, or electronic) regarding the physical or mental condition of an individual, health care provision, or health care payment. See also health assessment and health, patient.

health information, individually identifiable, *n* recorded information in any format (e.g., oral, written, or electronic) regarding the physical or mental condition of an individual, health care provision, or health care payment. It contains demographic information able to specifically distinguish an individual. In some cases, this information may not be considered "protected." See also health information, protected.

health information, protected (PHI), *n* recorded information in any format (e.g., oral, written, or electronic) regarding the physical or mental condition of an individual, health care provision, or health care payment. It contains demographic information able to specifically distinguish an individual. See also health information, individually identifiable.

Health Insurance Portability and Accountability Act (HIPAA), *n.pr* a public law enacted by Congress in 1996, consisting of two parts. Title I of the act protects workers and their families from the loss of health insurance coverage should they change or lose their jobs. Title II of the act calls for the establishment of national standards for electronic health care records, as well as national identities for health care providers, health insurance plans, and employers. In addition, Title II protects the privacy and security of an individual's health information.

health maintenance organization (HMO), *n* a legal entity that accepts responsibility and financial risk for providing specified services to a defined population during a defined period at a fixed price. An organized system of health care delivery that provides comprehensive care to enrollees through designated providers. Enrollees are generally assessed a monthly payment for health care services and may be required to remain in the program for a specified amount of time.

health, patient, n the state of bodily soundness of the patient; the patient's absolute or relative freedom from physical and mental disease.

health physics, n the study of the effects of ionizing radiation on the body and the methods for protecting people from the undesirable effects of radiation.

health policy, n **1.** a statement of a decision regarding a goal in health care and a plan for achieving that goal (e.g., to prevent an epidemic, a program for inoculating a population is developed and implemented). *n* **2.** a field of study and practice in which the priorities and values underlying health resource allocation are determined.

health promotion, n an educational program or effort directed at a targeted population to improve, maintain, and safeguard the health of that segment of society. See also health education.

health resources, n all materials, personnel, facilities, funds, and anything else that can be used for providing health care and services.

health risk, n a disease precursor associated with higher than average morbidity or mortality. The disease precursors may include demographic variables, certain individual behaviors, familial and individual histories, and certain physiologic changes.

health risk appraisal, n a process of gathering, analyzing, and comparing an individual's prognostic characteristics of health with a standard age group, thereby predicting the likelihood that a person may develop prematurely a health problem associated with a high morbidity and mortality rate.

Healthy People National Health Objectives, *n.pr* science-based health objectives developed by the Department of Health and Human Services that are revised every 10 years and are used to guide the activities of the public health programs in the United States. The Healthy People objectives are to (1) increase quality and years of healthy life, and (2) eliminate health disparities. Enhancing oral health is an important goal.

hearing, *n* the sense by which sound perception occurs; happens after sound waves are converted into impulses of the nerves and translated by the brain.

hearing aid, *n* an electronic device used to amplify and shape waves of sound entering the external auditory canal.

hearing aid, behind-the-ear, n an electronic device, situated over the ear, for amplifying and shaping sound waves entering the external auditory canal.

hearing aid, eyeglass model, n an electronic device, attached to the eyeglasses' thickened temple bar, for amplifying and shaping sound waves entering the external auditory canal.

hearing disorders, *n.pl* a structural or functional impairment of the ability to detect and recognize sound.

hearing disorders, indications of, n. pl symptoms such as an inability to pay attention or respond appropriately to spoken dialogue, heightened focus, increased use of a specific ear, frequent requests for repetition of spoken statements, and abnormal quality of speech.

hearing disorders, types of, n.pl classifications include a loss of central, mixed, sensorineural, or conductive hearing.

hearing loss, *n* a reduction in the acuity to detect and recognize sound.

hearing loss, conductive, n a hearing impairment of the outer or middle ear caused by abnormalities or damage within the conductive pathways leading to the inner ear.

hearing loss, mixed, n a hearing impairment that is the result of damage to both conductive pathways of the middle ear and the nerves or sensory hair cells of the inner ear.

hearing loss, sensorineural **(sen′so-rēner′əl),** *n* a hearing impairment of the inner ear resulting from damage to the sensory hair cells or the nerves that supply the inner ear.

hearsay, *n* **1.** the testimony given by a witness who relates not what is known personally but what others have stated. *n* **2.** the evidence that does not derive its value solely from the credit of the witness, but rests mainly on the veracity and competency of other persons and is admitted in court only in specified cases, from necessity.

heart, *n* the muscular pump that maintains and regulates the flow of blood through the body.

heart, artificial, *n* a mechanical device that acts to pump blood to and from the body tissue during repair of the heart.

heart attack, *n* See myocardial infarction; thrombosis, coronary; or occlusion, coronary.

heart block, *n* the condition in which the muscular interconnection between the auricle and ventricle is interrupted so that the auricle and ventricle beat independently of each other.

heart, compression of, *n* See massage, cardiac.

heart defect, *n* a fault in the structural integrity of the heart.

heart defect, congenital, *n* the structural errors in the heart formed during embryonic and fetal life.

heart disease, *n* a disorder in the normal functioning of the heart.

heart disease, dental concerns, *n.pl* the special considerations taken to eliminate oral disease by maintaining an elevated level of oral health and prevent infective endocarditis, an infection of the heart valves that may be caused by bacteremia created during dental treatments. Heart disease has also been linked with increased levels of periodontal disease.

heart disease, ischemic, *n* See disease, heart, ischemic.

heart disease risk factors, *n.pl* the hereditary, lifestyle, and environmental influences that increase one's chances of developing heart disease.

heart massage, *n* See massage, cardiac.

heart murmur, *n* the sound of blood flowing back through a defective heart valve. Two types are possible: organic or functional.

heart, normal, *n* a heart without anatomic defects that could cause an impairment in the function of the organ.

heart rate, *n* the rate or tempo of heart contractions recorded in beats per minute.

heart sounds, *n.pl* the normal noises produced within the heart during the cardiac cycle that can be heard over the precordium and may reveal abnormalities in cardiac structure or function. The use of the stethoscope over the left side of the chest is a common clinical technique to assess heart function. The typical sounds are a rhythmic lub dup; abnormal sounds include clicks, murmurs, rubs, snaps, and gallops.

heart surgery, *n* a surgical procedure involving the heart, performed to correct acquired or congenital defects, replace diseased valves, open or bypass blocked vessels, or graft a prosthesis or a transplant in place.

heart valves, *n.pl* one of the four structures within the heart that prevent backflow of blood by opening and closing with each heartbeat. They include two semilunar valves, the aortic and pulmonary; the mitral, or bicuspid, valve; and the tricuspid valve. They permit the flow of blood in only one direction, and any one of the valves may become defective, permitting the backflow associated with heart murmurs.

heart failure (härt′ fālyur), *n* a sudden, sometimes fatal, cessation of the heart's action.

heart failure, acute, *n* a rapid and marked impairment of cardiac output.

heart failure, congestive, *n* a clinical syndrome resulting from chronic cardiac decompensation associated with left- or right-sided heart failure. Left-sided failure may result from rheumatic mitral valvular disease, aortic valvular disease, systemic hypertension, or arteriosclerotic disease. Manifestations include orthopnea, paroxysmal dyspnea, pulmonary edema, cough, and cardiac asthma. Right-sided failure results most commonly from pulmonary congestion and hypertension associated with left-sided failure but may result from anemia, myocarditis, beriberi, or dysrhythmia. Manifestations include peripheral pitting edema, ascites, cyanosis, oliguria, and hydrothorax.

heartburn, *n* a painful burning sensation in the esophagus just below the sternum. It is usually caused by the reflux of gastric contents into the esophagus, but may be caused by gastric hyperacidity or peptic ulcer.

heat, *n* the state of a body or matter that is perceived as being opposite of cold and is characterized by elevation of temperature.

heat, applied, *n* the therapeutic application of wet or dry heat to increase circulation and produce hyperemia, accelerate the dissolution of infection and inflammation, increase absorption from tissue spaces, relieve pain, relieve muscle spasm and associated pain, and increase metabolism.

   heat, applied, and cold, *n* the most commonly employed physical agents in dental practice. They modify the physiologic processes and have both a systemic and a local effect. The principal effect on the tissue is mediated by the alteration in the circulatory mechanisms. Properly used, they have a salutary therapeutic result. Improperly used, they may produce serious pathologic consequences.

   heat, applied, contraindications, *n. pl* the conditions that preclude the use of heat application: peripheral neuropathy, conditions in which maximum vasodilation and inflammation are already present, acute inflammatory conditions in which more swelling will cause acute pain and pulpitis, septicemia, and malignancies.

   heat, applied, general physiologic effects, *n.pl* the physiologic effects of generally applied wet or dry heat; increase in body temperature, generalized vasodilation, rise in metabolism, decrease in blood pressure, increase in pulse rate and circulation, and increase in depth and rate of respiration.

   heat, applied, local physiologic effects, *n.pl* the physiologic effects of locally applied wet or dry heat to the intraoral or extraoral tissue: increase in caliber and number of capillaries, increased absorption resulting from capillary dilation, increased lymph formation and flow, relief of pain, relief of spasm, increase of phagocytes, and a rise in local metabolism.

heat loss, metabolic causes, *n.pl* the biologic factors that influence heat loss: redistribution of blood vasodilation and vasoconstriction, variations in blood volume, tendency

of fat to insulate the body, and evaporation.

heat loss, physical causes, *n.pl* the physical factors that influence heat loss: radiation, convection, and conduction; evaporation from the lungs, skin, and mucous membranes; the raising of inspired air to body temperatures; and the production of urine and feces.

heat production, metabolic causes, *n.pl* the chemical factors of the body that cause heat production: specific dynamic action of food, especially protein, that results in a rise of metabolism; a high environmental temperature that, by raising temperatures of the tissue, increases the velocity of reactions and thus increases heat production; and stimulation of the adrenal cortex and thyroid glands by the hormones of the pituitary glands.

heat treatment, See treatment, heat.

heat stable, *adj* heat resistant. Also called *thermostabile.*

heavy function, *n* See function, heavy.

hebephrenia (hē′bəfrē′nēə), *n* a form of schizophrenia in which the individual behaves like a child (e.g., inappropriate laughter and silliness).

heel effect, *n* See effect, heel.

Heerfordt's syndrome, *n.pr* See fever, uveoparotid.

height of contour, *n* See contour, height of.

height, ramus, *n* the measurement of the expanse of a ramus. It is used to calculate the correct age of infants and toddlers with undetermined age statistics.

Heimlich maneuver (hīm′lik), *n.pr* an emergency procedure for dislodging food or other obstruction from the trachea to prevent asphyxiation. The choking person is grasped from behind by the rescuer, whose fist, thumb side in, is placed just below the victim's sternum and whose other hand is placed firmly over the fist. The rescuer then pulls the fist firmly and abruptly into the epigastrium, forcing the obstruction up the trachea.

Heimlich sign, *n.pr* a universal distress signal that a person is choking and unable to speak, made by grasping the throat with a thumb and index finger, thereby attracting the attention of others nearby.

HeLa cells, *n* the first successful immortal cell culture, created in 1951 at Johns Hopkins University in Baltimore. HeLa cells were cultured from a sample of cervical cancer cells of a woman named Henrietta Lacks and are still used today in research laboratories all over the world. Cell culture research has been valuable to create vaccines and develop gene therapies.

Helicobacter pylori **(hel′ikōəbak′t ər),** *n* a gram-negative, spiral-shaped bacteria that is active as a human gastric pathogen. It is associated with lesions or gastritis or peptic ulcers. See also ulcer, peptic.

helium *(He)* **(hē′lēum),** *n* a colorless, odorless, tasteless gas; one of the inert gaseous elements. Atomic number, 2; atomic weight, 4.003. Used in medicine as a diluent for other gases.

helix, *n* the superior and posterior free margin of the auricle.

hellac base, See base, shellac. (not current)

helminths **(hel′minths),** *n.pl* the parasitic worms that cause disease and illness in humans such as tapeworm, pinworm, and trichinosis. They are usually transmitted via contaminated food, water, soil, or other objects. Adult worms live in the intestines and other organs. Minor infections may be asymptomatic, whereas stronger cases may cause dietary deficiencies or digestive, muscular, and nervous disorders.

Helsinki declaration (accords), *n. pr* a declaration signed by the representatives of member nations of the Conference on Security and Cooperation in Europe in Helsinki, Finland. The principle and practice of informed consent in health care grew from the Helsinki accords.

hemangioameloblastoma **(hēman′jēōəmel′ōblastō′mə),** *n* a neoplasm in the jaw that has characteristics of ameloblastoma and hemangioma.

hemangioendothelioma **(hēman′jēōen′dōthē′lēō′mə),** *n* a vascular-derived tumor formed by proliferation of endothelium of the capillary vessels.

hemangiofibroma **(hēman′jēōfîbrō′mə),** *n* a benign neoplasm characterized by proliferation of blood channels in a dense mass of fibroblasts.

hemangioma **(hēman′jēō′mə),** *n* **1.** a benign neoplasm characterized by blood vascular channels. A cavernous form consists of large vascular spaces. A capillary form consists of many small blood vessels. *n* **2.** a benign tumor composed of newly formed blood vessels.

hemangiopericytoma **(hēman′jēōper′isītō′mə),** *n* a vascular tumor composed of pericytes.

hemarthrosis **(he′mahrthro′sis),** *n* the blood found in the cavity of a joint.

hemataerometer, *n* a device for determining the pressure of the gases in the blood. (not current)

hematemesis **(hē′mətem′esis),** *n* vomiting of blood.

hematocrit **(hēmat′ōcrit),** *n* (packed-cell volume), the percentage of the total blood volume composed of red blood cells (erythrocytes). Specific groups averaging: children, 32% to 65%; adult men, 42% to 50%; adult women, 36% to 45%.

hematogenous (hemətoj′ēnus), *adj* part of or originating in the blood, or distributed through the bloodstream.

hematogenous total joint replacement **(hemətoj′ēnus),** *n* the replacement of a diseased or damaged joint with an artificial joint. The joint replacement is considered hematogenous if it comes into contact with the bloodstream.

hematologic disorders, *n.pl* the diseases of the blood and blood-forming tissue.

hematology **(hē′mətol′əjē),** *n* the scientific study of blood and blood-forming tissue.

hematology tests, *n.pl* the diagnostic tests of the blood and its constituent parts.

hematoma **(hē′mətō′mə),** *n* a mass of blood in the tissue as a result of trauma or other factors that cause the rupture of blood vessels.

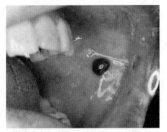

Hematoma. (Ibsen/Phelan, 2009)

hematoma, subdural, *n* a collection of extravasated blood trapped below the dural membranes of the brain causing pressure on the brain, resulting in pain and neural dysfunction. It may be life threatening.

hematopoiesis (hē'mətō'poiē'sis), *n* the normal formation and development of blood cells in the bone marrow.

hematosis (hē'mətō'sis), *n* the oxygenation or aeration of the venous blood in the lungs.

hematoxylin, *n* a dye or stain commonly used to treat tissue sections for microscopic examination, usually used in combination with eosin.

hematopoietic stem cell transplant, *n* see bone marrow transplant.

hematuria (hē'mətoo'rēə), *n* the presence of blood in the urine.

hematuria, gross, *n* the visible evidence of blood in the urine. It may occur from neoplasms of the kidney and bladder, hemorrhagic diathesis, hypertension with renal epistaxis, or acute glomerular nephritis.

hematuria, microscopic, *n* the demonstration of hematuria during the microscopic examination of centrifuged urine. It may result from the same causes as gross hematuria or from toxicity of drugs, embolic glomerulitis, vascular diseases, or chronic glomerular nephritis.

heme (hēm), *n* the pigmented, iron-containing, nonprotein portion of the hemoglobin molecule.

hemiachromatopsia (hem'ēak'rōmətō'zhə), *n* a state of being color blind in only one half of the visual field.

hemianesthesia (hem'ēan'esthē'zhə), *n* the anesthesia or loss of tactile sensibility on one side of the body.

hemiatrophy (hem'ēat'rōfē), *n* an atrophy of one half of the body, an organ, or a part (e.g., facial hemiatrophy).

hemidesmosome (hem'ēdez'mōsōm), *n* **1.** one half of a cell junction localized along the inferior aspect of the basal cell plasma membrane. *n* **2.** the connection site between the surface of the tooth and the epithelium as a part of the epithelial attachment as well as the interface between the epithelium and connective tissue.

hemifacial microsomia (HFM) (hem'ifā'shəl mī'krəsō'mēə), *n* a condition in which one side of the lower face fails to develop properly. It is characterized by the malformation of the ear on the affected side and defects in the structure of the mandible. It is the second most common birth defect after clefts. Also called *brachial arch syndrome, oral-mandibular-auricular syndrome, lateral facial dysplasia,* or *otomandibular dysostosis.*

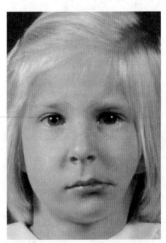

Hemifacial microsomia. (Proffit/Fields/Sarver, 2013)

hemiglossectomy (hem'ēglôsek'təmē), *n* the surgical removal of half of the tongue.

hemihydrate, *n* a chemical compound in which the number of water molecules is half that of the other portion of the compound. In dentistry, hemi-hydrates are used in the manufacture of crowns, inlays, bridges, and dental molds.

hemihypertrophy (hem′ēhīpur′trə fē), *n* an excessive growth of half of the body, an organ, or a part (e.g., hemihyperplasia of the tongue).

hemiplegia (hem′ēplē′jēə), *n* the paralysis of one side of the body.

hemisection (hem′ēsek′shən), *n* the complete sectioning through the crown of a tooth into the furcation region.

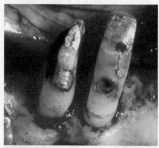

Hemisection. (Newman/Takei/Klokkev-old, 2012)

hemochromatosis (hē′mōkrō′mətō′sis), *n* an uncommon disorder, usually a complication of hemolytic anemia, that results in a surplus of iron deposits throughout the body. See also hemosiderosis, iron metabolism, siderosis, and thalassemia.

hemocyte, *n* a generic term referring to any cellular or formed element of the blood. Synonym: *hematocyte.*

hemodialysis (hē′mōdīal′isis), *n* a procedure in which impurities or wastes are removed from the blood. The patient's blood is shunted from the body through a machine for diffusion and ultrafiltration and returned to the patient's circulation. This procedure is used in treating renal failure and various toxic conditions. Without this, toxic wastes build up in the blood and tissue and cannot be filtered out by the ailing kidneys. This condition is known as uremia, which means "urine in the blood." Eventually, this waste buildup leads to death. Dental treatment should occur within 24 hours of hemodialysis. See also kidney failure.

hemodynamics, *n* the study of the physical aspects of blood circulation, including cardiac function and peripheral vascular physiology.

hemoglobin (hē′mōglōbin), *n* the oxygen-carrying red pigment of the red blood corpuscles. It is a reddish, crystallizable conjugated protein consisting of the protein globulin combined with the prosthetic group, heme.
hemoglobin A (HBA), *n* a normal hemoglobin. Also called adult hemoglobin.
hemoglobin estimation, *n* a determination of the hemoglobin content of the blood. By the Sahli method, 14 to 17 g/100 mL of blood is normal, and 15.1 Sahli units are taken as 100% for estimation of hemoglobin percentages.

hemoglobinopathy (hē′mōglō′binop′əthē), *n* a group of genetically determined diseases involving abnormal hemoglobin (e.g., sickle cell disease, in which hemoglobin S occurs, and hemoglobin C disease).
hemoglobinopathy, paroxysmal nocturnal, *n* an acquired hemolytic anemia of unknown cause characterized by increased hemolysis during sleep, resulting in the presence of hemoglobin in the urine on awakening.

hemogram, dental (hē′məgram′), *n* a simple blood test that measures the numbers, proportions and morphologic characteristics of the blood cells. In dentistry, hemograms are used to determine the amount of bleeding in the dental pulp after the treatment of caries.

hemohydremia, anhydremia, *n* a decrease in blood volume resulting from a decrease in the serum component of blood. It occurs in shock or any condition in which blood fluid is passed into the tissue and results in hemoconcentration. (not current)

hemolysin (hēmol′isin), *n* an antibody that causes hemolysis of red blood cells in vitro.

hemolysis (himol′isis), *n* the breakdown of red blood cells and the release of hemoglobin that occurs normally at the end of the life span of a red blood cell.

hemophilia (bleeder's disease) (hē′mōfil′ēə), *n* a sex-linked genetic disease manifested in males and characterized by severe hemorrhage.

hemophilia A (classic hemophilia), n a hemorrhagic diathesis resulting from a deficiency of antihemophilic globulin (AHG); inherited as a recessive sex-linked characteristic and characterized by recurrent bouts of bleeding from even trivial injury. The coagulation time is prolonged, but the bleeding time is normal.

hemophilia B (Christmas disease), n a hemorrhagic diathesis resulting from a deficiency of factor IX.

hemophilia, classic, n See hemophilia A.

hemopoiesis (hē′mōpōē′sis), n See hematopoiesis.

hemoptysis (hēmop′tisis), n the expectoration of blood, by coughing, from the larynx or lower respiratory tract.

hemorrhage (hem′ərəj), n the escape of a large amount of blood from the blood vessels in a short period; excessive bleeding.

hemorrhage, pulpal (hem′ərij pul′pəl), n bleeding in the pulp of a tooth. Such bleeding may occur during dental extractions and restorations and is often controlled by the application of a hemostatic agent.

hemorrhagic bone cyst, n See cyst, hemorrhagic.

hemorrhagic diathesis, n an inherited predisposition to any one of a number of abnormalities characterized by excessive bleeding.

hemosiderin (hē′mōsid′ərin), n an intracellular storage form of iron; the granules consist of an ill-defined complex of ferric hydroxides, polysaccharides, and proteins having an iron content of approximately 33% by weight. It appears as a dark yellow-brown pigment.

hemosiderosis (hē′mōsid′ərō′sis), n a focal or general increase in tissue iron stores without associated tissue damage.

hemostasis (hē′mōstā′sis), n the arrest of an escape of blood.

hemostat (hē′mōstat), n a procedure or device that stops the flow of blood.

hemostatic (hē′mōstat′ik), n an agent used to reduce bleeding from small blood vessels by speeding up the clotting of blood or by the formation of an artificial clot.

Hepadnaviridae **(hepad′nəvir′ĭdē),** n one of the major virus families, to which the hepatitis B virus belongs. Viruses in this family have a double-stranded incomplete circular molecular structure with icosahedral symmetry.

heparin/heparin calcium/heparin sodium, n *brand names:* Hep Lock, Heparin; *drug class:* anticoagulant; *actions:* acts in combination with antithrombin III (heparin cofactor) to inhibit thrombosis; inactivates factor Xa and inhibits conversion of prothrombin to thrombin; affects both intrinsic and extrinsic clotting pathways; *uses:* anticoagulant in thrombosis, embolism, coagulopathies, deep vein thrombosis, dialysis, maintenance of patency of indwelling intravenous lines.

heparinized lock system, n an indwelling intravenous system by which multiple daily intravenous accesses can be accomplished and multiple penetrations of the veins can be avoided. The heparin chamber prevents the formation of a clot or thrombus at the needle site.

hepatitis (hep′ətī′tis), n an inflammation of the liver.

hepatitis C, n a type transmitted largely by blood transfusion or percutaneous inoculation, such as with intravenous drug users with HCV sharing needles. The disease progresses to chronic hepatitis in up to 80% of the patients acutely infected.

hepatitis, chronic active, n a hepatitis with chronic portal inflammation with regional necrosis and fibrosis, which may progress to nodular postnecrotic cirrhosis.

hepatitis delta virus (HDV), n the infectious agent that causes delta hepatitis, but only in the presence of the hepatitis B virus.

hepatitis E, n a self-limited type of hepatitis caused by the hepatitis E virus (HEV) that may occur after natural disasters because of fecal-contaminated water or food. It is rare in the United States and can be fatal in pregnant women.

hepatitis, hepatitis A (infectious), n a viral hepatitis caused by HAV that is frequently epidemic in nature and has an incubation period of 1 to 4 or even 7 weeks. It is usually transmitted by the virus in fecal matter but may be transmitted by humans (transfusions, lacerations, needle punctures).

hepatitis, homologous serum (homologous serum jaundice, serum hepatitis, hepatitis B serum), n a viral hepatitis caused by HBV; clinically difficult to distinguish from epidemic infectious hepatitis. It is transmitted by human serum (through parenteral injection, transfusions, lacerations). The incubation period is 40 to 90 days or longer. Principal manifestations are jaundice, gastrointestinal symptoms, anorexia, and malaise.

hepatitis, non–A-E, n a viral infection of the stomach and intestines that is diagnosed by ruling out other forms of hepatitis. It may be transmitted orally, via injection, sexual contact, or fecal matter.

hepatitis, serum, n See hepatitis, homologous serum.

hepatitis, viral, n **1.** hepatitis caused by one immunologically unrelated viruses: hepatitis A virus; hepatitis B virus; n **2.** hepatitis caused by one of the following: HAV, HBV, HCV, HDV, HEV or non–A-E virus.

hepatomegaly, abnormal (hep′ətō meg′əlē), n an enlargement of the liver that is usually a sign of liver disease. It is usually discovered by percussion and palpation as part of a physical examination. It may be caused by hepatitis, fatty infiltration, alcoholism, biliary obstruction, or malignancy.

Herbst appliance, n.pr the only fixed, tooth-borne, functional orthodontic appliance in which jaw position is influenced by a pin-and-tube spring-loaded appliance that is cemented or bonded to the teeth.

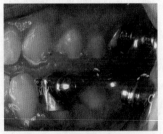

Herbst appliance. (Courtesy Dr. Flavio Uribe)

hereditary benign intraepithelial dyskeratosis (həred′iter′ē bənīn′ in′trəep′əthē′lēəl dis′kerətō′sis), n a hereditary disease seen in triracial isolates (whites, Native Americans, blacks). It involves the oral and ocular mucosa and may cause periodic seasonal keratoconjunctivitis.

hereditary gingival fibromatosis, n See fibromatosis, gingival.

hereditary opalescent dentin (həred′iter′ē ō′pəles′ənt den′tin), n a developmental disturbance in the formation of dentin, better known as dentinogenesis imperfecta. The teeth range from gray to brownish violet and are translucent or opalescent. The crowns fracture easily because of an abnormal dentinoenamel junction.

heredity (hered′itē), n the inheritance of resemblance, physical qualities, or disease from a familial predecessor; the passage of characteristics from one generation to its progeny by genetic linkage.

Hering-Breuer reflex (her′ing-broi′ur), n.pr See reflex, Hering-Breuer.

hermetic seal, n See seal, hermetic.

hernia (hur′nēə), n the protrusion of an organ through an abnormal opening in the muscle wall of the cavity that surrounds it. It may be congenital, may result from the failure of certain structures to close after birth, or may be acquired later in life because of obesity, muscular weakness, surgery, or illness.

hernia, hiatal (hī′ātəl), n a protrusion of a portion of the stomach upward through the diaphragm. The condition occurs in approximately 40% of individuals and most people display few, if any, symptoms. The major difficulty is gastroesophageal reflux, which is the backflow of the acid contents of the stomach into the esophagus.

hernia, inguinal (direct), n a protrusion of the intestines into an opening between the deep epigastric artery and the edge of the rectus muscle; (indirect) involves the internal inguinal ring and passes into the inguinal canal.

heroin (her′ōin), n a highly addictive alkaloid prepared from morphine. Use is prohibited by federal law because of its highly addictive properties and potential for abuse.

⊙ **herpangina (hur'panjī'nə),** *n* a viral disease of children, usually occurring in summer, and characterized by sudden onset, fever (100° to 105° F; 38° to 40.5° C), sore throat, and oropharyngeal vesicles. Herpangina results from Coxsackie A viruses and is self-limiting.

herpangina aphthous ulcer, n See aphthous pharyngitis.

herpes labialis (hur'pēz lā'bēal'is), *n* a disease of the lips caused by herpes simplex virus and characterized by vesicles that rupture, leaving ulcers. The local lesions are often called *fever blisters* or *cold sores.* Also called *herpes simplex of the lips.* See also herpes simplex.

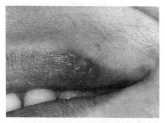

Hebes labialis. (Neville et al., 2009)

herpes simplex (hur'pēz sim'plex), *n* an infection caused by the herpes simplex virus. Primary infection, occurring most often in children between 2 and 5 years of age, may result in apparent clinical disease or such manifestations as acute herpetic gingivostomatitis, keratoconjunctivitis, vulvovaginitis, or encephalitis. Recurrent manifestations may include herpes labialis (fever blisters or cold

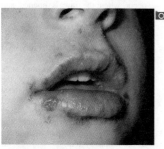

Herpes simplex. (Kliegman et al., 2011)

sores), dendritic corneal ulcers, or genital herpes simplex. See also herpes labialis and gingivostomatitis, herpetic.

herpes zoster (hur'pēz zos'tur), *n* an acute viral disease involving the dorsal spinal root or cranial nerve and producing unilateral vesicular eruption in areas of the skin corresponding to the involved sensory nerve. Pain is a prominent feature and may persist, although skin lesions subside in 1 to 2 weeks. It is caused by the varicella zoster virus, which is also responsible for childhood chickenpox. A vaccine against herpes zoster is now available. Colloquial term: *shingles.*

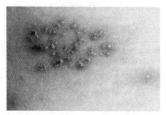

Herpes zoster. (Neville et al., 2009)

Herpesviridae **(hər'pēzvi'rīde),** *n* one of the major virus families, to which the herpes simplex, varicella zoster, and Epstein-Barr viruses belong. Viruses in this family have a double-stranded linear molecular structure with icosahedral symmetry.

herpetic lesion, *n* See lesion, herpetic.

herpetic whitlow (hurpet'ik hwit'lō), *n* See whitlow, herpetic.

⊙ **herringbone pattern,** *n* an image seen on a processed dental film that has been placed backwards in the mouth and exposed to radiation.

⊙ **Hertwig's (epithelial) root sheath,** *n* an elongation of the cervical loop, which helps determine the shape, size, and number of roots and which influences the formation of dentin in the root area during the developmental stages of a tooth. See also cervical loop.

heteresthesia (het'əresthē'zēə, -zhə), *n* a variation in the degree of cutaneous sensibility on adjoining areas of the body surface.

heterograft, *n* See graft, heterogenous.

heteropolysaccharides (het′ərōpol ′ēsak′ərīdz), *n.pl* the complex carbohydrates formed by combining carbohydrates with noncarbohydrates or carbohydrate derivatives; examples include pectin, lignin, glycoproteins, glycolipids, and mucopolysaccharides.

heterosexual, *n* **1.** a person with a sexual attraction to or preference for persons of the opposite gender. *adj* **2.** having erotic attraction to, predisposition to, or sexual activity with a person of the opposite gender.

heterotrophic (het′ərōtrof′ik), *adj* pertaining to an organism that must depend on others to provide sustenance; parasitic.

heterozygous (het′ərōzī′gus), *adj* a term indicating that genes lying at equivalent loci on chromosome pairs are different.

hexamethonium (heksəmethō nēəm), *n* a prototypic, but little used, drug that selectively blocks nicotinic cholinergic receptors in ganglions. It used to be used to treat hypertension. The classic description of "hexamethonium man" described the effects of ganglionic blockade.

hexosamine (heksō′səmēn), *n* the amine derivative (NH2 replacing OH) of a hexose such as glucosamine.

HGF, *n* See glucagon.

HIAA, *n.pr* the abbreviation for *Health Insurance Association of America.*

hiccup, *n* an involuntary spasmodic contraction of the diaphragm that causes a beginning inspiration that is suddenly checked by closure of the glottis, thus producing a characteristic sound.

hidradenoma, *n* a benign neoplasm derived from epithelial cells of sweat glands.

hidrocystoma (hī′drōsistō′mə), *n* a cystic form of sweat gland adenoma. A hidrocystoma is produced by the cystic proliferation of apocrine secretory glands. It is not uncommon, occurring in adult life in no particular age group, with males and females equally affected. The most common site is around the eye. Hidrocystomas are cured by surgical removal.

hierarchy (hī′ərär′kē), *n* **1.** system of persons or things ranked one above the other. *n* **2.** in psychology and psychiatry, an organization of habits or concepts in which simpler components are combined to form increasingly complex integrations.

hierarchy, Maslow's, See Maslow's hierarchy.

high blood pressure, *n* See hypertension.

high labial arch, *n* See arch, high labial.

high lip line, *n* See lip line, high.

high speed, *n* See speed, high.

high-pull headgear, *n* an apparatus designed to give an upward pull on the face-bow.

high-speed handpiece, *n* See handpiece, high-speed.

hilus (hī′lus), *n* an indentation appearing on an organ or other internal structure, such as a lymph node, at the point at which nerves and vessels enter. Also called *hilum.*

hinchazon (hinch′əzon), *n* See beriberi.

hindgut, *n* the posterior portion of the future digestive tract.

hinge axis, *n* See axis, hinge.

hinge axis, determination, *n* See axis, condylar, determination.

hinge axis, orbital plane, *n* See axis, hinge, orbital plane.

hinge axis point, *n* See point, hinge axis.

hinge movement, *n* See movement, hinge.

hinge position, *n* See position, hinge.

hinge-bow, *n* the kinematic facebow used to determine the location of the hinge axis. The hinge-bow is a three-piece instrument with independently adjustable arms controlled by micrometer screws that lengthen or shorten them. Other micrometer screws raise or lower the caliper points to find the spots in or on the skin near the tragi in which only rotary movements occur when the jaw is opened and closed at the rearmost point. See also facebow, kinematic.

HIPAA, *n.pr* See Health Insurance Portability and Accountability Act (HIPAA).

hippocampus (hip′ōkam′pəs), *n* a curved convoluted elevation of the floor of the inferior horn of the lateral ventricle of the brain. It is composed of gray substance covered by a layer of white fibers, or the alveus, and functions as an important component of the limbic system.

hippus, respiratory (hip′əs), *n* a dilation of the pupils occurring during inspiration and a contraction of the pupils occurring during expiration; often associated with pulsus paradoxus.

Hirschfeld-Dunlop file, *n.pr* See file, Hirschfeld-Dunlop.

Hirschfeld's method, *n.pr* See point, Hirschfeld's silver.

hirsutism (hir′sootizəm), *n* increased body or facial hair, which is especially noted in females.

histamine (his′təmēn′), *n* a compound found in all cells that is produced by the decarboxylation of histidine. It is released in allergic, inflammatory reactions and causes dilation of capillaries, decreased blood pressure, increased secretion of gastric juice, and constriction of smooth muscles of the bronchi and uterus.

histamine blocker, *n* a drug that blocks either the histamine H_1 or the H_2 receptor. H_1 receptor blockers have historically been termed *antihistamines* and include such drugs as diphenhydramine and chlorpheniramine. They are used to reduce inflammation and vasodilation caused by histamine. H_2 receptor blockers include such drugs as nizatidine and ranitidine. These drugs inhibit the release of stomach acid and are used in the treatment of gastroesophageal reflux disease and hyperacidity.

histidine (his′tidēn), *n* an essential amino acids for infants and children. See also amino acid.

histiocyte (his′tēəsīt′), *n* a large phagocytic cell found in the interstices of the tissue; of reticuloendothelial origin.

histiocytosis, acute disseminated, X, *n* See disease, Letterer-Siwe.

histiocytosis, chronic disseminated X, *n* See disease, Hand-Schüller-Christian.

histiocytosis, Langerhans cell (histiocytosis X, Langerhans cell disease), *n* a group of diseases characterized by a proliferation of abnormal histiocytoid cells. Includes: **(1)** Chronic disseminated histiocytosis (Hand-Schüller-Christian disease); **(2)** Acute disseminated histiocytosis (Letterer-Siwe disease); and **(3)** eosinophilic granulomas.

histiocytosis, nonlipid (his′tēōsītō′ sis), *n* See disease, Letterer-Siwe.

histoclasia, implant (his′tōklā′zēə), *n* a condition of the tissue existing in the presence of an implant, in which the implant is not directly involved. It is a condition of the oral mucosal tissue, in which the pathologic condition results from some external cause (e.g., calculus, attached prosthetic appliances).

histocompatibility (his′tokəmpat′i bil′itē), *n* the compatibility of the antigens of donor and recipient of transplanted tissue.

histocompatibility testing, n the determination of the compatibility of the antigens of donor and recipient before tissue transplantation. Usually follows a blood typing protocol.

histocytoma (his′tōsītō′mə), *n* a tumor composed of histiocytes.

histodifferentiation (his′tōdif′əren ′shēā′shən), *n* the process in which cells develop the distinctive characteristics of the tissue to which they are to belong.

histogenesis (his′tōjen′isis), *n* a series of integrated processes that occur during embryonic development wherein undifferentiated cells assume the characteristics of the various tissue contained in the human body. These undifferentiated cells comprise part of the three primary germ layers, the endoderm, mesoderm, and ectoderm.

histogram, *n* a bar graph; a graphic representation of a frequency distribution.

histology (histol′əjē), *n* microanatomy, which is the microscopic study of normal tissue and organs at the cellular level.

histology, oral, of soft tissue, n See epithelium, oral; lamina, propria; submucosa; and membrane, basement.

histomorphometry (his′tōmorfäm ′ətrē), *n* a method used to accurately quantify the level of cellular activity and the amount of existing bone mass. Such methods include bone biopsies performed to determine the underlying cause for osteoporosis.

histopathology (his′tōpəthol′əjē), *n* the microscopic study of abnormal tissue and organs at the cellular level.

histoplasmosis (his′tōplazmō′sis), *n* a disease caused by the fungus *H.*

capsulatum and affecting the reticulo-endothelial system. Ulceration of the oral mucosa may occur.

history, case, *n* a detailed and concise compilation of all physical, dental, social, and mental factors relative and necessary to diagnosis, prognosis, and treatment.

history, case, forms, n.pl questionnaires to aid the practitioner in taking medical history; should cover all aspects of patient's prior medical history; the American Dental Association distributes a basic health form that may provide a baseline.

history, case, hepatic disease, n as part of the process of taking a medical history, practitioner should ask patient for details and occurrences of liver disease or drug metabolism problems.

history case, self-medication, n as part of the medical history process, practitioner should ask patient for descriptions of the type and frequency of self-administered medication as well as any history of substance abuse. This information can help eliminate complications in patient treatment schedules.

histotoxic (his′tōtäk′sik), *adj* relating to poisoning of the respiratory enzyme system of the tissue.

HIV, *n* See human immunodeficiency virus (HIV).

HIV gingivitis (HIV-G), *n* an aggressive form of periodontal disease presenting with a distinct type of gingivitis found in HIV-infected patients, characterized by an intensely red linear erythremic band (LGE) around the free gingiva that extends 2 to 3 mm apically into the attached gingiva. The involved gingiva tends to bleed spontaneously and may be present even in AIDS patients with good oral hygiene.

HIV periodontitis (HIV-P), *n* an aggressive form of periodontal disease with all the characteristics of HIV-G combined with those of periodontitis: soft tissue ulceration and necrosis and rapid destruction of the periodontium and bone. The condition is very painful. HIV-P may resemble necrotizing ulcerative gingivitis (NUG). However, NUG is limited to the soft tissue, whereas HIV-P disease extends into the crestal bone.

HIV-1, *n* the abbreviation for *human immunodeficiency virus type 1,* which is widely recognized as the causal agent of acquired immunodeficiency syndrome (AIDS). HIV-1 is characterized by its cytopathic effect and affinity for the T4-lymphocyte.

HIV-2, *n* the abbreviation *for human immunodeficiency virus type 2,* which is related to HIV-1 but carries different antigenic components with differing nucleic acid composition. It shares serologic reactivity and sequence homology with the simian lentivirus simian immunodeficiency virus (SIV) and infects only T4-lymphocytes expressing the CD4 phenotypic marker.

HIV-G, *n* See HIV gingivitis.

HIV-P, *n* See HIV periodontitis.

HIV-wasting syndrome, *n* a constitutional disease associated with AIDS, also known as the *slim disease.* Patients in this subgroup have a history of fever of more than 1 month, involuntary weight loss of more than 10%, or diarrhea persisting for more than 1 month.

hives, *n* See urticaria.

Hodgkin's disease, *n.pr* See lymphoma, Hodgkin's.

hoe, *n* an angled instrument with the broad dimension of its blade perpendicular to the axis of the shank of the shaft.

hold, *v* to possess by reason of a lawful title.

hold harmless clause, n a contract provision in which one party to the contract promises to be responsible for liability incurred by the other party. Hold harmless clauses frequently appear in the following contexts: (1) Contracts between dental benefits organizations and an individual dental professional often contain a promise by the dental professional to reimburse the dental benefits organization for any liability organization incurs because of dental treatment provided to beneficiaries of the organization's dental benefits plan. This may include a promise to pay the dental benefits organization's attorney fees and related costs. (2) Contracts between dental benefits organizations and a group plan sponsor may include a promise by the dental benefits organization to assume responsibility for

hormones, antidiuretic (ADH, vasopressin), *n.pl* a hormone of the posterior pituitary gland that encourages reabsorption of water by stimulating the insertion of water channels (aquaporins) into the apical membrane of epithelial cells of the renal collecting duct. The hormone thus has an antidiuretic effect. It also raises blood pressure by its effect on the peripheral blood vessels. An absence of antidiuretic hormone causes diabetes insipidus.

hormones, antiinflammatory, *n.pl* See glucocorticoids.

hormones, catabolic, *n.pl* the hormones that stimulate the breakdown of macromolecules in the body releasing smaller molecules and energy as well as increasing blood glucose; examples include glucagon, epinephrine, steroid and growth hormones, and thyroxine.

hormones, chorionic gonadotropic, *n.pl* a glycoprotein secreted by placental tissue early in normal pregnancy. This protein is also found in the urine or blood in association with chorioepitheliomas and some neoplastic diseases of the testes.

hormones, corticosteroid, *n.pl* See steroid, adrenocortical.

hormones, corticotropic, *n.pl* hormones that stimulate the adrenal cortex. See also ACTH.

hormones, female sex, *n.pl* the hormones secreted by the ovary. They include two main types: the follicular, or estrogenic, hormones produced by the graafian follicle, and the progestational hormones from the corpus luteum.

hormones, follicle-stimulating, *n.pl* a pituitary tropic hormone that promotes the growth and maturation of the ovarian follicle and, with other gonadotropins, induces secretion of estrogens and possibly spermatogenesis.

hormones, gastrointestinal, *n.pl* the hormones that regulate motor and secretory activity of the digestive organs, including secretin and cholecystokinin.

hormones, gonadotropic, *n.pl* See gonadotropin.

hormones, growth (somatotropic hormone, somatotropin), *n.pl* a hormone that is secreted by the anterior lobe of the pituitary gland and that exerts an influence on skeletal growth. As long as the growth apparatus is functional, it is responsive to the effects of the hormone.

hormones, ketogenic, *n.pl* the term used to describe a factor of the anterior pituitary hormone responsible for ketogenic effect. It is probably not an entity differing from known pituitary hormones.

hormones, lactogenic (galactin, mammotropin, prolactin), *n.pl* a pituitary hormone that stimulates lactation.

hormones, luteal, *n.pl* See hormones, progestational.

hormones, luteinizing, *n.pl* a pituitary hormone that causes ovulation and development of the corpus luteum from the mature graafian follicle. It is called an *interstitial cell and stimulating hormone* because of its action on the testis in maintaining spermatogenesis and because of its role in the development of accessory sex organs.

hormones, male sex (androgenic hormone, C-19 steroids), *n.pl* the hormones found in the testes, urine, and blood. Included are testosterone found in the testes, androsterone excreted into the urine, and dehydro-3epiandrosterone found in the blood.

hormones, α-melanocyte-stimulating (α-MSH), *n.pl* a hormone of the anterior pituitary gland that increases melanin deposition by the melanocytes of the skin.

hormones, neurohypophyseal, *n.pl* the nonapeptides of the neural lobe of the pituitary gland: oxytocin and vasopressin.

hormones, parathyroid, *n.pl* the secretory product of the parathyroid glands that promotes bone resorption and increases renal reabsorption of calcium and magnesium and diminishes that of phosphate. Excessive secretion produces generalized bone resorption, formation of fibrous marrow in the spongiosa, and, in young individuals, hypocalcification of the teeth.

hormones, pituitary, *n.pl* See *hormones, adenohypophyseal* for anterior pituitary hormones. Vasopressin and oxytocin are secreted by the posterior lobe of the pituitary gland.

tissue, including the periodontal ligament, in which compression of the ligament between bone and tooth occurs as a result of orthodontic forces.

hyalinization of periodontal ligament, n a degenerative process resulting from long-continued occlusal trauma, in which the fibers become hyalinized into a homogeneous mass.

hyalinized (hī'ələnī'zd), *adj* refers to the transformation of a substance to a glasslike or transparent state. Hyalinized tissue is often found in the bronchial tubes of a person who has died of a viral respiratory infection.

hyaluronic acid (hī'əlōōron'ik), n a mucopolysaccharide that forms the gelatinous substance in the tissue spaces. Hyaluronic acid is the intercellular cementing substance found throughout the tissue of the body.

hyaluronidase (hī'əlyooron'ədās), n an enzyme that produces hydrolysis of hyaluronic acid, the cementing substance of the tissue. It is produced by certain pathogenic bacteria and also formed by sperm.

hybrid glass ionomers, n See resin modified glass ionomer cements.

hydralazine HCl, n brand name: Apresoline; *drug class:* antihypertensive, direct-acting peripheral vasodilator; *action:* preferentially dilates arterioles by activation of the nitric oxide/guanylate cyclase pathway in vascular smooth muscle; *use:* hypertension.

hydraulic pressure, n See pressure, hydraulic.

hydremia (hī'drē'mēə), n an increase in blood volume caused by an increase in serum volume. This may result from cardiac failure, renal insufficiency, pregnancy, or the intravenous administration of fluids.

hydroalcoholic (hī'drōal'kōhol'ik), *adj* containing both water and alcohol. See also *solution.*

Hydrocal (hī'drōkal), n the brand name for a gypsum product, a-hemihydrate, known as artificial stone. It is used for making casts.

hydrocele (hī'drōsel'), n an accumulation of fluid in any saclike cavity or duct, specifically in the tunica vaginalis testis or along the spermatic cord.

hydrocephalus (hī'drōsef'əlus), n an abnormal accumulation of cerebrospinal fluid in the cranial vault, resulting in a disproportionately large cranium.

hydrochloric acid, n a compound consisting of hydrogen and chlorine. Hydrochloric acid is secreted in the stomach and is a major component of gastric juice.

hydrochlorothiazide, n brand names: Esidrix, HydroDIURIL, Hydro-Par; *drug class:* thiazide diuretic; *action:* inhibits the sodium/chloride cotransporter in the distal tubule of the kidney and increases the excretion of water, sodium, and chloride; *uses:* edema, hypertension, congestive heart failure, nephrogenic diabetes insipidus.

hydrocodone (hī'drōkō'dōn), n a semisynthetic narcotic analgesic and antitussive with multiple actions similar to those of codeine. Hydrocodone is an ingredient in prescription analgesics and cough medicines.

hydrocodone bitartrate, n brand name: Hycodan; *drug class:* opioid derivative, narcotic analgesic; *actions:* stimulates opioid receptors in the central nervous system and in the periphery to reduce pain perception; acts directly on cough center in medulla to suppress cough; *uses:* hyperactive and nonproductive cough, mild to moderate pain.

hydrocolloid(s) (hī'drōkol'oid), n/n.pl **1.** the materials listed as colloid solids with water; used in dentistry as elastic impression materials. They can be reversible or irreversible. n **2.** an agar-base impression material.

hydrocolloid, irreversible (alginate), n a type whose physical condition is changed by a chemical action that is not reversible. It is an impression material that is elastic when set. See also alginate.

hydrocolloid, reversible (agar-agar type), n a type whose physical condition is changed by temperature. The material is made fluid by heat and becomes an elastic solid on cooling.

hydrocortisone (hī'drōkôr'tison), n a glucocorticosteroid secreted by the adrenal cortex in response to stimulation by ACTH. Hydrocortisone stimulates glucocorticoid receptors in the cell leading to multiple effects on protein, carbohydrate and lipid metabolism. Hydrocortisone stimulates gluconeogenesis and is antianabolic. It inhibits phospholipase A_2 and reduces inflammation, especially at pharmacologic doses and through multiple mechanisms. Its effects protect the body against stress. Also called *cortisol.*

hydrocortisone acetate/hydrocortisone sodium phosphate/hydrocortisone sodium succinate, *n brand names:* Solu-Cortef, Carmol, Cortenema; *drug class:* corticosteroid; *actions:* hydrocortisone stimulates gluconeogenesis, inhibits phospholipase A_2 and reduces inflammation. Antiinflammatory effects include inhibition of the production of leukotrienes and prostaglandins, suppression of macrophage and leukocyte migration; reduction of capillary permeability and inhibition of lysosomal enzymes; *uses:* severe inflammation, shock, adrenal insufficiency, ulcerative colitis, collagen disorders, certain anemias, adjunct in leukemias and lymphomas, rheumatic disorders, skin inflammation, pruritus.

hydrocortisone acetate/ hydrocortisone valerate, *n brand names:* Acticort, Cortaid, Cort-Dome, Dermacort, Westcort; *drug class:* topical corticosteroid; *actions:* interacts with steroid cytoplasmic receptors to induce antiinflammatory effects; possesses antipruritic, antiinflammatory actions; *uses:* psoriasis, eczema, contact dermatitis, pruritus.

hydrodynamic theory, *n* the principles of physics relating to the study of fluidity and the movement of particles within fluids.

hydrofluoric acid, *n* a compound consisting of hydrogen and fluorine. It is a very active, corrosive compound, used to etch glass and precious metals.

hydrogen (H), *n* a gaseous, univalent element. Its atomic number is 1 and its atomic weight is 1.008. It is the simplest and lightest of the elements and is normally a colorless, odorless, highly flammable diatonic gas.

hydrogen peroxide, *n* an unstable compound of hydrogen and oxygen that is easily broken down into water and oxygen. A 3% solution is used as a mild antiseptic for the skin and mucous membranes. More concentrated solutions may be used as a

whitening (bleaching) agent. It may be used to reduce gingival inflammation, but may not eliminate the responsible bacteria.

hydrogenation (hīdroj′ənā′shən), *n* the infusion of hydrogen into a compound. Also called *reduction.*

hydrokinetic activity (hī′drōkinet ′ik), *n* refers to the movement or source of movement that causes fluid to be in motion.

hydrolysis (hīdrol′isis), *n* **1.** a reaction between the ions of salt and those of water to form an acid and a base, one or both of which is only slightly dissociated; a process whereby a large molecule is split by the addition of water. The end products divide the water, the hydroxyl group being attached to one and the hydrogen ion to the other. *n* **2.** the splitting of a compound into two parts with the addition of the elements of water.

hydromorphone HCl (hī′drōmor′f ōn), *n brand names:* Dilaudid, Dilaudid-HP, Ex Algo; *drug class:* opioid derivative, narcotic analgesic; *action:* stimulates opioid receptors in the central nervous system and periphery, increasing the pain threshold, and inhibiting pain perception; *use:* moderate to severe pain.

hydrophilic (hī′drōfil′ik), *adj* having an affinity for water. Opposite of lipophilic. See also ointment, hydrophilic.

hydrophobic, *adj* refers to the resistance of a substance to combine with water. Hydrophobic substances, such as oil, are composed of nonpolar molecules, which tend to associate and repel water.

hydroquinone (hīdrōkwin′ōn), *n* **1.** a reducing agent used as an inhibitor in resin monomers to prevent polymerization during storage. *n* **2.** one of the two chemicals used as reducing agents in film-developing solutions. It is made from benzene (paradihydroxybenzene) and is sensitive to thermal changes. Above 70° F (21° C), the action of hydroquinone is rapid; below 60° F (15.5° C), hydroquinone becomes inactive. Its action is to control the contrast of the film.

hydrostatic pressure (hī′drōstat′ik), *n* See pressure, hydrostatic.

hydrotherapy (hī′drōther′əpē), *n* an empirical adjunct to oral

H

Manifestations are related to abnormalities of the bones, kidneys, and blood vessels. Skeletal changes are referred to as *generalized osteitis fibrosa cystica or von Recklinghausen's disease.* Brown tumors, which are essentially giant cell tumors, may develop generally, as well as in the jaws. Kidney changes include renal stones and nephrocalcinosis. Calcification of muscles in arteries occurs. Renal rickets is associated with secondary hyperparathyroidism in children with chronic renal disease. Laboratory findings include a high serum calcium level, low phosphorus level, and a normal or high alkaline phosphatase level. Renal impairment, such as occurs in secondary hyperparathyroidism, tends to nullify hypercalcemia because of an increased loss of calcium in the urine. *n* **2.** an abnormal increase in activity of the parathyroid glands, causing loss of calcium from the bones and resulting in tenderness in bones, spontaneous fractures, muscular weakness, and osteitis fibrosa. *n* **3.** excessive production of parathormone by the parathyroid gland (as in parathyroid hyperplasia and/or adenoma), resulting in increased renal excretion of phosphorus by lowering of the renal threshold for this substance. The pathologic changes produced are osteoporotic or osteodystrophic in nature as a consequence of withdrawal of calcium and phosphorus from osseous tissue.

hyperparathyroidism, brown node of, n See node, brown, of hyperparathyroidism.

hyperphagia (hī′pərfā′jēə), *n* a disorder marked by an abnormal appetite and excessive ingestion of food, even to the point of gastric pain and vomiting. It is associated with the malfunction of the hypothalamus and is often linked to conditions such as Kleine-Levin syndrome and central nervous disorders.

hyperphosphatemia (hī′purfos′fətē′mēə), *n* an increased concentration of inorganic phosphates in the blood serum. Hyperphosphatemia may occur in childhood and also in acromegaly, renal failure, and vitamin D intoxication. Normal adult range of serum inorganic phosphorus is 2.5 to 4.2 mg/100 mL.

hyperphosphaturia (hī′purfos′fətoo′rēə), *n* an excessive excretion of phosphate in the urine.

hyperpigmentation, *n* an unusual darkening of the skin. Causes include heredity, drugs, exposure to the sun, and adrenal insufficiency.

hyperpituitarism (hī′purpitoo′iteri zəm), *n* a condition caused by excessive production of the hormones secreted by the pituitary gland. An excess of the growth hormone results in giantism or acromegaly; an excess of ACTH produces Cushing's syndrome.

hyperplasia (hī′purplā′zēə, -zhə), *n* the abnormal multiplication or increase in the number of normal cells in normal arrangement in a tissue or organ, resulting in a thickening or enlargement of the tissue or organ.

hyperplasia, denture (denture hypertrophy), n an enlargement of tissue beneath a denture that is traumatizing the soft tissue.

hyperplasia, drug-induced gingival, n the swelling of fibrous gingival tissue most often seen with sustained use of the drugs phenytoin (an antiseizure medication), cyclosporine (an immunosuppressant), and nifedipine (a calcium blocking agent).

hyperplasia, focal fibrous, n a small, firm nodule originating in the fibrous connective tissue, which forms on the tongue, lower lip, or oral mucosa lining of the oral cavity as the result of injury or chronic irritation.

hyperplasia, gingival, n **1.** an enlargement of the gingival tissue resulting from proliferation of its cellular elements. Hereditary or inflammatory causes may be involved. *n* **2.** the proliferation of gingival epithelium to form elongated rete pegs and proliferation of fibroblasts with increased collagen formation in the underlying connective tissue; leads to nodular enlargement of the gingiva in diphenylhydantoin sodium therapy. *n* **3.** gingival enlargement, primarily produced by proliferation of connective tissue elements; often accompanied by gingival inflammation as a result of trauma to the hyperplastic tissue and coincidental with or following the ingestion of diphenylhydantoin sodium and other medications.

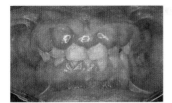

Gingival hyperplasia. (Regezi/Sciubba/Jordan, 2012)

hyperplasia, idiopathic gingival, n See fibromatosis gingivae.

hyperplasia, inflammatory fibrous, n See epulis fissurata.

hyperplasia, inflammatory papillary (inflammatory papillomatosis, multiple papillomatosis, papillary hyperplasia), n a condition of unknown cause but associated with the presence of maxillary dentures. Characterized by numerous red papillary projections on the hard palate.

hyperplasia, papillary, n a growth in the midline of the hard palate, usually in the relief area of a denture; characterized by a papillary, or raspberry, appearance.

hyperplasia, phenytoin-related gingival, n an enlargement of the gingivae caused by the use of phenytoin (Dilantin) in the management of epilepsy. Numerous other medications have also been associated with gingival hyperplasia.

hyperplastic tissue, *n* See tissue, hyperplastic.

hyperpnea (hī′purpnē′ə), *n* an abnormal increase in respiratory volume; an abnormal increase in the rate and depth of breathing.

hyperpotassemia (hī′purpot′əsē′mēə), *n* See hyperkalemia.

hyperproteinemia (hī′purprō′tēnē′mēə), *n* an abnormal increase in serum and plasma proteins.

hyperproteinuria (hī′purprō′tēn yoo′rēə), *n* See albuminuria.

hypersalivation, *n* See sialorrhea.

hypersensitive, *n* abnormally sensitive.

hypersensitiveness (hī′pursen′sitiv nes), *n* a state of altered reactivity in which the body reacts more strongly than normal to a foreign agent.

hypersensitivity, *n* **1.** an adverse reaction to contact with specific substances in quantities that usually produce no reaction in normal individuals. *n* **2.** an allergic tendency. In general, a tendency to react with unusual violence to stimuli. *n* **3.** a common complaint after periodontal therapy in which dentin may be exposed, resulting in pain in the teeth or sensitivity to heat, cold, and sweet substances.

hypersensitivity, atopic, n See atopy.

hypersensitivity, bacterial, n delayed inflammatory reaction resulting from previous sensitization of the host by an antigen.

hypersensitivity, delayed, n a type involving a latent period between the antigen introduction and the reaction; cellular reactions mediated by the T lymphocytes (e.g., tuberculosis and transplant reaction).

hypersensitivity, dentin, n refers to the pain caused by fractures, or gingival recession, which exposes the dentin of a tooth. This condition requires immediate treatment and can be corrected with topical agents or with periodontal or restorative procedures, such as gingival grafts or enamel bonding.

hypersensitivity, immediate, n a humoral reaction, mediated by the circulating B lymphocytes, which causes any of three immediate responses: anaphylactic hypersensitivity, cytotoxic hypersensitivity, and immune system hypersensitivity.

hypersensitivity reaction, cytotoxic, n a reaction in which the surface antigens of a cell join with an antibody, causing complement-mediated cell destruction, or other types of cell-membrane damage.

hypersensitivity reactions, immune complex, n.pl one of four types of hypersensitivity reactions to antigens in the body that acts as a barrier to disease. The reactions can cause tissue damage.

hypersensitization (hī′pərsen′sitizā ′shən), *n* the process of rendering abnormally sensitive or the condition of being abnormally sensitive.

hypersplenism (hī′pərsplen′izəm), *n* a syndrome consisting of splenomegaly and a deficiency of one or more types of blood cells.

hypersthenuria (hī′pursthenyoo′r ēə), *n* urine with an abnormally high

hypocalciuria (hī′pōkal′sēoo′rēə), *n* a decrease in urinary calcium. Normal values vary considerably but are roughly related to calcium intake. Various values are given (e.g., 100 to 200 mg/day on a normal diet, or 350 to 400 mg/day for calcium intake of 10 mg/kg of body weight in children). Hypocalciuria may occur in hypoparathyroidism, rickets, osteomalacia, metastatic carcinoma of the prostate, and renal failure. See also test, Sulkowitch's.

hypocapnia (hī′pōkap′nēə), *n* a deficiency of carbon dioxide in the blood.

hypocarbia, *n* See hypocapnia.

hypochloremia (hī′pōklôrē′mēə), *n* a decrease below normal of chloride concentration in the plasma. The normal range is 98 to 100 mEq/L. It may occur in adrenal insufficiency, persistent vomiting, renal failure, acute infections, and dehydration with sodium depletion.

hypochlorous acid, *n* a greenish-yellow liquid derived from an aqueous solution of lime. An unstable compound that decomposes to hydrochloric acid and water. Hypochlorous acid is used as a bleaching agent and disinfectant.

hypochondria (hī′pōkon′drēə), *n* anxiety about disease; a type of neurosis characterized by fear of disease or by simulated disease.

hypochondriasis (hī′pōkondrī′əsis), *n* See hypochondria.

hypochromia (hīpōkrō′mēə), *n* a reduced staining quality of cells, particularly pale staining red blood cells associated with hemoglobin deficiency.

hypodermoclysis (hī′pōdurmok′li sis), *n* a subcutaneous injection of fluid in large volume.

hypodontia (hī′pōdon′shēə), *n* a condition characterized by having fewer teeth than normal.

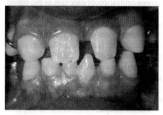
Hypodontia. (Neville et al., 2009)

hypoesthesia (hī′pōesthē′zēə, -zhə), *n* a decreased sensitivity to touch or pressure.

hypoestrogenism (hī′pōes′trōjeniz əm), *n* a diminished production of estrogenic substances by the ovaries, such as that which occurs during menopause. May produce desquamative lesions on the oral mucosa. See also gingivitis, desquamative.

hypofibrinogenemia (hī′pōfibrin ′ōjənē′mēə), *n* a reduction of fibrinogen in the blood. Excessive bleeding may occur following trauma. The deficiency of fibrinogen may be congenital or may result from faulty synthesis associated with liver disease and defibrinogenation resulting from disorders of pregnancy involving the placenta and amniotic fluid. The normal range is 200 to 600 mg/100 mL of plasma. Clotting deficiencies do not occur until the concentration falls below 75 mg/100 mL.

hypogammaglobulinemia (hī′pō gam′əglob′ūlinē′mēə), *n* a deficiency of gammaglobulin, usually manifested by recurrent bacterial infections.

hypogeusia (hī′pōgoo′zēə), *n* a decreased sense of taste.

hypoglossal nerve, *n* see nerve, hypoglossal.

hypoglycemia (hī′pōglīsē′mēə), *n* a condition existing when the concentration of blood sugar (true blood sugar) is 40 mg/100 mL or less. Symptoms may not occur even when the concentration is considerably less. Symptoms include nervousness, hunger, weakness, vertigo, and faintness. Hypoglycemia may occur in the fasting state or following the injection of insulin.

hypoglycemia, fasting, n a type occurring in the postabsorptive state; occurs in renal glycosuria, lactation, hepatic disease, and central nervous system lesions.

hypoglycemia, insulin, n a type resulting from improper administration of insulin. If hypoglycemia is severe, convulsions, coma, and death may occur. See also shock, insulin.

hypoglycemia, mixed, n a type occurring during the fasting state and after the ingestion of carbohydrates; occurs in idiopathic spontaneous hypoglycemia of infancy, in anterior pituitary and adrenocortical insufficiency, and with tumors of the islet cells of the pancreas.

hypoglycemia, reactive, *n* a type occurring after the ingestion of carbohydrates with an excessive release of insulin, as in functional hyperinsulinism.

hypoglycemia, spontaneous, *n* a type that is functional (e.g., renal glycosuria, lactation, and severe muscular exertion) or is caused by organic disease such as in hepatic disease and adrenocortical insufficiency.

hypoglycemic agents (hī′pōglīsē′mik), *n.pl* a large heterogeneous group of drugs prescribed to decrease or control the amount of glucose circulating in the blood; used in the prevention and treatment of diabetes.

hypogonadism (hī′pōgō′nadizəm), *n* a gonadal deficiency resulting from abnormalities of the testes and ovaries or to pituitary insufficiency. Manifestations include eunuchism, eunuchoidism, Fröhlich's syndrome, amenorrhea, and incomplete development or maintenance of secondary sex characteristics.

hypohidrotic ectodermal dysplasia (hī′pōhīdrot′ik ektōdur′məl displā′zhə), *n* a group of heritable conditions demonstrating abnormalities of at least two ectodermal derivatives, including hypotrichosis, hypodontia, abnormalities of the nails, hypohidrosis, craniofacial alterations, and abnormalities of the digits.

hypokalemia (hī′pōkəlē′mēə), *n* an abnormally low serum potassium level. Hypokalemia may occur in metabolic alkalosis, chronic diarrhea, Cushing's syndrome, primary aldosteronism, and excessive use of deoxycorticosterone, cortisone, or ACTH.

hypolarynx (hī′pōler′inks), *n* the infraglottic compartment of the larynx that extends from the true vocal cords to the first tracheal ring.

hypolethal (hī′pōlē′thəl), *adj* not quite lethal; said of dosage.

hypomagnesemia (hī′pōmag′nəsē′mēə), *n* a deficiency of magnesium in the blood serum (normal values range from 1.5 to 2.5 mEq/L). It may be associated with chronic alcoholism, starvation, and prolonged diuresis in congestive heart failure. Manifestations include muscular twitching, convulsions, and coma.

hyponasality (hī′pōnāzal′itē), *n* a lack of nasal resonance necessary to produce acceptable voice quality. The type of voice quality heard when the speaker's nose is occluded or the speaker is suffering from a severe cold.

hyponatremia (hī′pōnətrē′mēə), *n* an abnormally low concentration of sodium in the blood serum. It may develop in adrenocortical insufficiency and chronic renal disease or with extreme sweating.

hypoparathyroidism (hī′pōper′əthī′roidizəm), *n* a decrease in parathyroid function, usually the result of surgical removal. Symptoms include tetany, irritability, and muscle weakness. The serum calcium is low, the blood phosphorus elevated, the blood magnesium reduced, and the alkaline phosphatase normal.

hypopharyngoscope (hī′pōfəring′gōskōp), *n* an apparatus devised for bringing the inferior portion of the pharynx or hypopharynx into view.

hypopharynx (hī′pōfer′inks), *n* the division of the pharynx that lies below the superior edge of the epiglottis and opens into the larynx and esophagus.

hypophosphatasia (hī′pōfos′fətā′zhə), *n* a familial disease in which the children may have very low serum alkaline phosphatase levels, total or partial aplasia of the cementum, and an abnormal periodontal ligament in the primary teeth; a decreased phosphatase level that has been linked to a premature loss of primary teeth in children. Examination reveals absence, hypoplasia, or dysplasia of cementum.

hypophosphatemia (hī′pōfos′fətē′mēə), *n* an abnormally low concentration of serum phosphates. Blood phosphorus levels are low in sprue, celiac disease, and hyperparathyroidism and in association with an elevated alkaline phosphatase in vitamin D–resistant rickets and other diseases involving a renal tubular defect in resorption of phosphate.

hypophyseal portal system (hīpof′ə sē′əl), *n* the structure of blood vessels responsible for transportation of hormones between the hypothalamus and anterior pituitary gland.

hypophysis, *n* See gland, pituitary.

implant, shoulder of blade endosteal, *n* the unbroken surface of the wedge-shaped infrastructure that is widest and most superficial. This part is tapped during the seating of the implant.

implant, single-stage, *n* See implant, one-stage.

implant, single-tooth subperiosteal, *n* an implant designed to replace a single missing tooth; usually unsupported by adjacent natural teeth.

implant, spiral endosteal, *n* a screw type of implant, either hollow or solid, usually consisting of abutment, cervix, and infrastructure.

implant, staple, *n* a type of transosteal implant that allows the attachment of a lower denture to the abutments of two or four threaded posts that go transcortically from a curved plate, which has been inserted through a submental incision and fixed into place at the inferior border of the mandible, through to the canine areas of the alveolar crest of the mandible; retentive screws partially inserted into the inferior border affix the rest of the plate. Also known as a *mandibular staple implant* and *transmandibular implant.*

implant, stock, *n* an implant, usually endosteal, that is available in manufactured form in uniform sizes and shapes.

implant, strut of subperiosteal, *n* a thin, striplike component of an infrastructure.

implant, subperiosteal, *n* an appliance consisting of an open-mesh frame designed to fit over the surface of the bone beneath the periosteum.

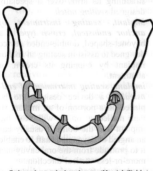

Subperiosteal implant. (Hatrick/Eakle/Bird, 2011)

implant, superstructure of, *n* a completed prosthesis that is supported entirely or in part by an implant. It may be a removable or fixed prosthesis, or may be a single crown or a complete arch splint.

implant, threaded, *n* an endosseous implant with threads resembling a screw; also known as a *screw-type implant.*

implant, transosteal (transos ′tēəl), *n* an implant that passes completely through the buccal and lingual aspects of a toothless ridge; also, an implant whose threaded posts pass completely through the mandible in the parasymphyseal region from the inferior border to the alveolar crest, allowing the attachment of a dental prosthesis. Also known as a *transosseous implant.* See also staple implant.

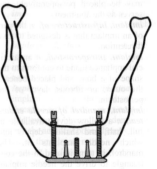

Transosteal implant. (Hatrick/Eakle/Bird, 2011)

implant, two-piece, *n* an implant, either end-osteal or subperiosteal, having its infrastructure and abutment in separate parts. Generally, the abutment, which is threaded, is screwed to the infrastructure some weeks after its incision, so that healing has taken place.

implant, two-stage, *n* an endosseous implant placed in the bone, with the soft tissue over the implant being sutured closed in a stage-one surgery to allow osseointegration of the implant. A second surgery is performed later in which the soft tissue over the submerged implant is removed in order to thread an abutment into the implant so that a prosthesis can be attached. Also known as a *submergible implant.*

implant, zygomatic **(zī'gəmat'ik),** *n* a long, screw-shaped endosseous implant first placed in the area of the former first maxillary molar up into the zygomatic bone following an intrasinusal trajectory and used as an alternative to bone augmentation of a severely atrophic maxilla.

implantation **(ĭm'plāntā'shən)** *n* the process during prenatal development; the embedding of a blastocyst in the endometrium.

implantology, oral **(im'plantol 'əjē),** *n* the art and science of dentistry concerned with the surgical insertion of materials and devices into, onto, and about the jaws and oral cavity for purposes of oral maxillofacial or oral occlusal rehabilitation or cosmetic correction.

implied, *adj* inferred; conceded.

implied consent, *n* assent to a clinical procedure that is recognized as an informed agreement by the patient, even if verbal or written consent is not explicitly given.

impression, *n* an imprint or negative likeness of an object from which a positive reproduction may be made.

impression, anatomic, *n* a type that records tissue shape without distortion.

impression, area, *n* See area, impression.

impression, boxing of an, *n* See boxing.

impression, bridge, *n* a type made for the purpose of constructing or assembling a fixed restoration, fixed partial denture, or bridge.

impression, cleft palate, *n* a type that records the upper jaw of a patient with a cleft (incomplete closure, or union) in the palate.

impression, closed oral cavity, *n* a type made while the oral cavity is closed and with the patient's muscular activity molding the borders.

impression, complete denture, *n* a type that records the edentulous arch made for the purpose of constructing a complete denture.

impression, composite, *n* a type consisting of two or more parts.

impression compound, *n* a hemoplastic material containing a mix of resin, filler, and lubricant components,

which is useful in obtaining an imprint or impression of the teeth.

impression coping, *n* a medical device used to mark the placement of a dental implant in an impression of the teeth.

impression, correctable, *n* an impression with a surface that is capable of alteration by the removal from or addition to some area of its surface or border.

impression, digital, *n* a computer-assisted method of using a mechanical or optical sensor to record the shape of teeth and tissues and storing these data in a digital format. This can eliminate the procedure of making a dental impression.

impression, dual, *n* See technique, impression, dual.

impression, duplicating, n See duplication.

impression, elastic, *n* a type made in a material that will permit registration of undercut areas by springing over projecting areas and then returning to its original position.

impression, final (secondary impression), *n* a type used for making the master cast.

impression, fluid wax, *n* an impression of the functional form of subjacent structures made with selected waxes that are applied (brushed on) to the impression surface in fluid form.

impression, functional, *n* a type that records the supporting structures in their functional form. See also structure, supporting, functional form of.

impression, hydrocolloid, *n* a type made of a hydrocolloid material.

impression, lower, *n* See impression, mandibular.

impression, mandibular (lower impression), *n* a type that records the mandibular arch and related tissue and dental structures.

impression, material, *n* See material, impression.

impression, maxillary (upper impression), *n* an impression of the maxillary jaw and related tissue and dental structures.

impression, mercaptan **(mərkap 'tan),** *n* a type made of mercaptan (polysulfide), a rubber-base elastic material.

impression, partial denture, *n* a type that includes part or all of a partially epithelium cells with concentric layers of keratin.

income, *n* the return in money from one's business, practice, or capital invested; gains, profit.

income tax, n a tax upon an adjusted gross income (individual or corporate) imposed as a major source of governmental revenue at the state and federal levels.

incompatibility (in′kəmpat′ibil′itē), *n* a disharmonious relationship among the ingredients of prescriptions or other drug mixtures.

incompatibility, chemical, n a situation in which two or more of the ingredients of a drug interact chemically, with resulting deterioration of the mixture.

incontinentia pigmenti, *n* See syndrome, Bloch-Sulzberger.

incubation (in′kūbā′shən), *n* the maintenance of an ideal environment with regard to temperature, light, air, and humidity so as to foster development of an organism or culture.

incubation period, *n* the lapsed time between exposure to an infectious agent and the onset of symptoms of a disease.

incubator (in′kūbātur), *n* a laboratory container with controlled temperature for the cultivation of bacteria.

incurred claims, *n.pl* the outstanding obligations of the insurer for dental services rendered to the insured.

indapamide (indap′əmīd′), *n* brand name: Lozol; drug class: diuretic, thiazide-like; action: acts on distal tubule by increasing excretion of water, sodium, chloride, potassium; uses: edema, hypertension.

indemnification schedule, *n* See table of allowances.

indemnity benefit, *n* a contract benefit that is paid to the insured to meet the cost of dental services received.

indemnity plan, *n* **1.** a plan that provides payment to the insured for the cost of dental care but makes no arrangement for providing care itself. *n* **2.** a dental plan in which a third-party payer provides payment of an amount for specific services regardless of the actual charges made by the provider. Payment may be made to enrollees or by assignment directly to

dental professionals. Schedule of allowances, table of allowances, and reasonable and customary plans are examples of indemnity plans.

index, *n* **1.** the ratio of a measurable value to another. *n* **2.** a core or mold used to record or maintain the relative position of a tooth or teeth to one another or to a cast. See also splint.

index, Broders's (Broders's classification), n.pr **1.** a system of grading of epidermoid carcinoma suggested by Broders. Tumors are graded from I to IV on the basis of cell differentiation. Grade I tumors are highly differentiated, with much keratin production. Grade IV tumors are poorly differentiated; the cells are highly anaplastic, with almost no keratin formation. *n.pr* **2.** the classification and grading of malignant neoplasms according to the proportion of malignant cells to normal cells in the lesion.

index, cardiac, n the minute volume of blood per square meter of body surface.

index, carpal, n the degree of ossification of the carpal bones noted in radiographs of the wrist; a method of determining the state of skeletal maturation.

index, cephalic, n head shape and size.

index, Dean's Fluorosis (flōörō′sis), n.pr the most commonly used system for classifying dental fluorosis. Ratings are assigned based on the most severe fluorosis seen on two or more teeth.

index, DEF (decayed, extracted, filled), n a dental caries index applied to the primary dentition in somewhat the same manner as the DMF index is used for classifying permanent teeth. Missing primary teeth are ignored in this index because of the uncertainty in determining whether they were extracted because of advanced caries or exfoliated normally.

index, DMF (decayed, missing, filled), n a technique for managing statistically the number of decayed, missing, or filled teeth in the oral cavity. Analysis may be based on the average number of DMF teeth (sometimes called DMFT) per person or the average number of DMF tooth surfaces (DMFS).

index, facial height, *n* the ratio of posterior facial height to anterior facial height.

index, gingiva and bone count (Dunning-Leach index), *n* an index that permits differential recording of both gingival and bone conditions to determine gingivitis and bone loss.

index, gingival (GI), *n* an assessment tool used to evaluate a case of gingivitis based on visual inspection of the gingivae that takes into consideration the color and firmness of gingival tissue along with the presence of blood during probing.

index, gingival bleeding (GBI), *n* an assessment tool used to verify the presence of gingival inflammation based on any bleeding that occurs at the gingival margin during or immediately after flossing.

index, gnathic, *n* the relationship of jaw size to head size.

index, icterus, *n* See test, Meulengracht's.

index, malocclusion, *n* a measure of the severity of a malocclusion, obtained by assigning values to a series of defined observations.

index, measuring, *n* an expression of relationship of one measurable value to another, or a formula based on measurable values.

index, missing teeth, *n* See index, DMF.

index, oral hygiene, simplified (Greene-Vermillion index), *n* an index made up of two components, the debris index and the calculus index, which are based on numerical determination representing the amount of debris or calculus found on six preselected tooth surfaces.

index, periodontal (Ramfjord index), *n* a thorough clinical examination of the periodontal status of six teeth, with an evaluation of the gingival condition, pocket depth, calculus and plaque deposits, attrition, mobility, and lack of contact.

index, periodontal disease (Russell index), *n* an index that measures the condition of both the gingiva and the bone individually for each tooth and arrives at the average status for periodontal disease in a given oral cavity.

index, plaque, *n* an assessment tool used to evaluate the thickness of plaque at the gingival margin that may be applied to selected teeth or to the entire oral cavity.

index, PMA (Schour-Massler index), *n* an index used for recording the prevalence and severity of gingivitis in schoolchildren by noting and scoring three areas: the gingival papillae (P), the buccal or labial gingival margin (M), and the attached gingiva (A).

index, Pont's, *n.pr* the relation of the width of the four incisors to the width between the first premolars and the width between the first molars.

index, Russell, *n.pr* See index, periodontal disease.

index, salivary Lactobacillus (lak'tō bəsil'əs), *n* a count of the lactobacilli per milliliter of saliva; used as an indicator of present dental caries activity. The test is of questionable value in individual patients, although its use in large groups has led to valuable information on caries activity.

index, saturation, *n* a number indicating the hemoglobin content of a person's red blood cells as compared with the normal content.

index, sulcus bleeding, *n* an assessment tool used to evaluate the existence of gingival bleeding in individual teeth and/or regions of the oral cavity upon gentle probing by assigning a score of 0–5, with 0 indicating a healthy appearance and no bleeding.

index, therapeutic, *n* the ratio of toxic dose to effective dose.

index, ventilation, *n* the index obtained by dividing the ventilation test by the vital capacity.

indication, *n* that which serves as a guide or warning.

indicator, *n* a mark or symptom specific to a condition or disease.

indicator, biologic, *n* a small quantity of harmless bacteria (*B. stearothermophilus*) placed into an object before sterilization, the subsequent death of which indicates that sterilization has taken place. See *B. stearothermophilus.*

indicator chemical, *n* a temperature-sensitive mark that changes color when a specific temperature has been reached. Used in the heat sterilization process but is by itself not proof that an object has been sterilized.

indicator diseases, *n* opportunistic infectious diseases or neoplastic diseases that are associated with primary immunodeficiency disease, such as caused by the retrovirus HIV-1.

indirect, contact, *n,* See contact, indirect.

indirect method, *n* See method, indirect restorative.

indirect pulp treatment, *n* a procedure for a tooth with a deep carious lesion and a diagnosis of reversible pulpitis, in which most but not quite all carious dentin is removed before placing the restoration. The goal is to restore the tooth to a healthy, functional state while avoiding any form of direct pulp therapy.

indirect retention, *n* See retention, indirect.

indirect vision, *n* See vision, indirect.

indium (In) (in′dēm), *n* a silvery metallic element with some nonmetallic chemical properties. Its atomic number is 49, and its atomic weight is 114.82. It is used in electronic semiconductors.

individual practice association (IPA), *n* **I.** an organization for the maintenance of the solo private practitioner as a lobbying force and vocal springboard. *n* **2.** legal entity organized and operated on behalf of individual participating dental professionals for the primary purpose of collectively entering into contracts to provide dental services to enrolled populations. Dental professionals may practice in their own offices and may provide care to patients not covered by the contract as well as to IPA patients.

individual retirement account (IRA), *n* a savings certificate exempt from income tax until the time of withdrawal. There are limits to the amount that can be saved annually under this plan, and there are conditions of withdrawal for maximal interest and tax advantage.

individuality, *n* collective characteristics or traits that distinguish one person or thing from all others.

indomethacin/indomethacin sodium trihydrate (in′dōmeth′əsin sō′ dēəm trīhī′drāt), *n brand names:* Indocin, Indocid; *drug class:* nonsteroidal antiinflammatory; *actions:* inhibits prostaglandin synthesis by inhibiting cyclooxygenase needed for biosynthesis; possesses analgesic, antiinflammatory, antipyretic properties; *uses:* rheumatoid arthritis, osteoarthritis, ankylosing rheumatoid spondylitis, acute gouty arthritis, bursitis, tendinitis.

induced, *adj* artificially caused to occur.

induction (induk′shən), *n* **I.** the act or process of inducing or causing to occur. *n* **2.** the process by which the action of one group of cells on another leads to the establishment of the developmental pathway in the responding tissue.

inductive reasoning, *n* analyzing a problem by working from specific facts and discovering general principles. See also deductive reasoning.

indurated tissue (in′dərā′tid), *n* a soft tissue that is abnormally firm because of an influx of exudate transudate or fibrous tissue elements.

induration, *n* **I.** the hardening of tissue, usually because of the accumulation of cells and fluid from an inflamed or infected site. Also called *sclerosis* when caused by inflammation. *n* **2.** an accumulation of hard tissue.

industrial dentistry, *n* **I.** a type of dentistry that is concerned with the dental health of the worker as it affects the working environment. *n* **2.** a dental service provided in the industrial plant, usually restricted to emergency care.

inert (inurt′), *adj* inactive; without the ability to act, move, change, or resist.

inertia (inur′shə), *n* according to Newton's law of inertia, the tendency of a body that is at rest to remain at rest and a body that is in motion to continue in motion with constant speed in the same straight line unless acted on by an outside force.

infant, *n/adj* a child who is in the earliest stage of extrauterine life, a time extending from the first month after birth to approximately 12 months of age, when the baby is able to assume an erect posture. Some extend the period to 24 months of age.

infant mortality, *n* the statistical rate of infant death during the first year after live birth, expressed as the number of such births per 1000 live births in a specific geographic area. Neonatal mortality accounts for 70% of infant mortality.

infant oral health care, n the provision of professional preventive and therapeutic (if necessary) dental treatment to children beginning no later than one year of age. A large portion of the service is designed to prepare caretakers to properly maintain their children's oral health to enhance their opportunity for a lifetime free of preventable oral disease and trauma.

infantilism (infan′tilizəm), n a disturbance marked by mental retardation and retention of childhood characteristics into adult life. Teeth may be delayed in eruption or absent.

infarct (in′färkt), n the death of a tissue caused by partial occlusion of a vessel or vessels supplying the area.

infection (infek′shən), n an invasion of the tissue of the body by disease-producing microorganisms and the reaction of these tissue to the microorganisms and/or their toxins. The mere presence of microorganisms without reaction is not evidence of infection.

infection, atypical mycobacterial, n an infection caused by several types of mycobacteria, similar to the bacteria that causes tuberculosis. These types of infections are very common in those with an abnormally functioning immune system.

infection, adenovirus, n a proliferation of the adenovirus that may cause any number of illnesses, including "swimming pool conjunctivitis" and gastrointestinal or respiratory diseases, among others. It is possible to be infected without manifesting any symptoms.

infection, airborne, n an infection contracted by inhalation of microorganisms contained in air or water particles.

infection control, n.pl procedures and protocols designed to prevent or limit cross-contamination in the health care delivery environment.

infection control, blood bank, and blood transfusion, n.pl the precautions taken to ensure that blood-borne pathogens are not transmitted via donated blood; includes rejection of potential donors whose medical history shows evidence of viral hepatitis, drug addiction, or recent blood transfusions or tattoos, as well as laboratory testing of all donated blood for the presence of hepatitis B and C, syphilis, and the HIV-1 antibody.

infection control, surveillance, n the monitoring of the transmission of a disease in order to limit its occurrence.

infection, focal, n the process in which microorganisms located at a certain site, or focus, in the body are disseminated throughout the body to set up secondary sites, or foci, of infection in other tissue.

infection, hemolytic streptococcal, n **1.** an infection usually caused by Group A hemolytic streptococci. Such infections include scarlet fever, streptococcal sore throat, cellulitis, and osteomyelitis. n **2.** an infection caused by streptococci that produce a toxic substance (hemolysin) that will lyse the erythrocytes and liberate hemoglobin from red blood cells.

infection, inflammatory, n an influx or accumulation of inflammatory elements (cellular and exudative) in the interstices of the tissue as a result of tissue injury by physical, chemical, microbiologic, and other irritants. Cellular elements include lymphocytes, plasma cells, polymorphonuclear leukocytes, and the macrophages of reticuloendothelial origin.

infection, latent, n a lingering infection that may lie dormant in the body for a time but may become active under certain conditions.

infection, local, n the prevention of excitation of the free nerve endings by literally flooding the immediate area with a local anesthetic solution.

infection, nosocomial, n an infection that first occurs during a patient's stay at a health care facility, regardless of whether it is detected during the stay or after.

infection, odontogenic, n a dental infection that involves the teeth or associated tissues.

infection, opportunistic, n an illness or condition that occurs when pathogens are able to exploit a vulnerable host. An infection that is able to take hold because resistance is low.

infection, periapical, *n* infection surrounding the root of a tooth, often accompanied by toothache.

infection, primary, *n* the original outbreak of an illness against which the body has had no opportunity to build antibodies; the originating infection.

infection, recurrent, *n* a reoccurrence of the same illness from which an individual has previously recovered.

infection, submandibular space, *n* a rapidly spreading, bilateral, indurated cellulitis occurring in the suprahyoid soft tissues, the floor of the mouth, and both sublingual and submaxillary spaces without abscess formation.

infection, submasseteric space, *n* infection that occupies the potential space between the lateral border of the mandible and the masseter muscle. Infection in this area is in direct contact with the masseter muscle and usually induces intense spasm in the muscle, resulting in a limitation in mouth opening.

infection, Vincent's, *n.pr* See gingivitis, necrotizing ulcerative.

infection, waterborne, *n* an illness that occurs as the result of drinking contaminated water or of eating fish that has been taken from contaminated waters.

infection resistance, *n* the ability of an individual to fight off the detrimental effects of microorganisms and their toxic products. A complexity involving individual and interacting factors (e.g., antibody formation, adequate nutrition, tissue tone, circulation, emotional stability).

infection susceptibility, *n* the degree of capability of being influenced by or involved in the pathologic processes produced by microorganisms and/or their toxins.

infectious, *adj* contagious; communicable; capable of causing infection.

infectious mononucleosis (mon′ōn oo′klēō′sis), *n* a benign lymphadenosis caused by the Epstein-Barr virus (EBV) and characterized by fever, sore throat, palatal petechiae, enlargement of lymph nodes and spleen, and prolonged weakness with a characteristic shift in the white blood cells during the course of the disease.

inferior, *n* a part of the body located below another; the opposite of *superior* (e.g., the legs are inferior to the hands when facing the body).

inferior alveolar nerve, *n* see nerve, inferior alveolar.

infertile, *adj* unable to produce offspring.

infiltrate (infil′trāt), *n* **1.** the material deposited by infiltration. *v* **2.** to deposit material in a location.

infiltration (in′filtrā′shən), *n* **1.** an accumulation in a tissue of a substance not normal to it. *n* **2.** the placement of a local anesthetic agent. See also anesthesia, infiltration.

inflammation (in′fləmā′shən), *n* the cellular and vascular response or reaction to injury. Inflammation is characterized by pain, redness, swelling, heat, and disturbance of function. It may be acute or chronic. The term is not synonymous with *infection,* which implies an inflammatory reaction initiated by invasion of living organisms.

inflammation, gingival, *n* See gingivitis.

inflammation, granulomatous, *n* a chronic inflammation in which there is formation of granulation tissue.

inflammation, periodontal, *n* See periodontitis and gingivitis.

inflation (inflā′shən), *n* the act of distending with air or a gas.

infliximab *n* brand name: Remicade; *drug class:* monoclonal antibody; *action:* binds to tumor necrosis factor-α (TNF-α) and blocks the binding of TNF-α to its receptors on inflammatory cells; *uses:* Crohn's disease, rheumatoid arthritis, ankylosing spondylitis, severe plaque psoriasis.

influences, local environmental, *n. pl* the factors or agents within the oral cavity that are responsible for the initiation, perpetuation, or modification of a pathologic state within the stomatognathic system.

influences, systemic environmental, *n.pl* the systemic factors that may initiate, perpetuate, or modify disease processes within the stomatognathic system. Generally, the oral manifestations of systemic disease are modified by the influence of local environmental factors.

influenza (in'flooen'zə), *n* a highly contagious infection of the respiratory tract caused by a myxovirus and transmitted by airborne droplet infection. Symptoms include sore throat, cough, fever, muscular pains, and weakness. Fever and constitutional symptoms distinguish influenza from the common cold. Three main strains of influenza virus have been recognized: Type A, Type B, and Type C. New strains of the virus emerge at regular intervals and are named according to geographic origin. Asian flu is a Type A influenza.

influenza-virus vaccine, *n* an active immunizing agent prescribed for immunization against influenza, generally recommended for at-risk populations, such as elderly people.

☐ informed consent, *n* an agreement by a patient, verbal or written, after being told in sufficient detail of possible risks, to have a procedure performed.

infrabony pocket (in'frəbōnē), *n* See pocket, infrabony.

infrabulge (in'frəbulj), *n* the surface of the crown of a tooth cervical to the clasp guide line, survey line, or surveyed height of contour.

☐ infraclusion (in'frəkloo'zhən), *n* the position occupied by a tooth when it has failed to erupt sufficiently to reach the occlusal plane. Also called *infraversion.* See also tooth, ankylosed.

infradentale (in'frədental'ē), *n* the most anterior point of the alveolar process of the mandible.

infrahyoid muscles (in'frəhi'oid), *n. pl* See muscle, suprahyoid and infrahyoid.

infraorbital (in'frəôr'bitəl), *n* pertaining to the area beneath the floor of the bony cavity in which the eyeball is located.

infraorbital foramen, *n* See foramen, infraorbital.

infraorbital region, *n* the region of the head that is located below the orbital region and lateral to the nasal region.

infratemporal crest, *n* a crest that divides each greater wing of the sphenoid bone into temporal and infratemporal surfaces.

infraversion (in'frəvur'zhən), *n* See infraclusion.

infusion (infū'zhən), *n* **1.** the therapeutic introduction of a fluid, such as saline solution, into a vein. In contrast to injection, infusion suggests the introduction of a larger volume of a less concentrated solution over a more protracted period. *n* **2.** a term used in pharmacy for a liquid extract prepared by steeping a plant substance in water.

ingate, *n* See sprue.

inhalant (inhā'lənt), *n* a medicine to be inhaled.

inhalation (inhəlā'shən), *n* the drawing of air or other gases into the lungs.

inhalation, endotracheal, *n* the inhalation of an anesthetic mixture into the lungs through an endotracheal catheter at low or atmospheric pressure.

inhaler, *n* **1.** a device that produces a vapor to ease breathing or is used to medicate by inhalation, especially a small nasal applicator containing a volatile medicament. Also called *nasal inhaler.* *n* **2.** a device that is placed over the nose to permit inhalation of anesthetic agents.

inhibition (in'hibish'ən), *n* a neurologic phenomenon associated with the transmission of an impulse across a synapse. An impulse can be blocked from passing a synapse in a reflex situation by the firing of another, more dominant nerve. It can be achieved directly by preventing the passage of an impulse along an axon, or by liberation of a chemical substance at the nerve ending. This chemical inhibition is demonstrated by the sympathetic-parasympathetic control over smooth muscle activity in a blood vessel. Inhibition is the restraining of a function of a tissue or organ by some nervous or hormone control. It is the opposite of *excitation.*

inhibitor (inhib'itur), *n* a substance that slows or stops a chemical reaction.

inhibitor of cholinesterase (inhib'i tur əv kō'lines'terās), *n* a chemical that interferes with the activity of the enzyme cholinesterase.

inhibitor, proton pump, *n* a pharmacologic agent used to control heartburn by suppressing the production of stomach acid by blocking the action of the proton pump.

inion (in'ēon), *n* the most elevated point on the external occipital protuberance in the midsagittal plane.

initialize, *v* to set counters, switches, and addresses to 0 or other starting values at the beginning of, or at prescribed points in, a computer routine.

initiation stage, *n* the first stage of tooth development.

initiator (inish'ēātur), *n* a chemical agent added to a resin to initiate polymerization.

injection (injek'shən), *n* **1.** the injection of material into an area. *n* **2.** the act of introducing a liquid into the body by means of a needle and syringe. Injections are designated according to the anatomic site involved. The most common injections are intraarterial, intradermal, intramuscular, intravenous, and subcutaneous. The colloquial term is *shot.*

injection, Gow-Gates (GG), *n* See technique, Gow-Gates (GG) anesthetic.

injection, interseptal (in'tersep'təl), *n* an intraosseous injection of a local anesthetic agent in the interseptal bone between two teeth. Often used as a supplemental form of local anesthesia when more anesthesia is needed.

injection, intraosseous (in'trəos 'ēəs), *n* an injection of a local anesthetic agent directly into the alveolar bone. Can include an interseptal injection and periodontal ligament injection.

injection molding, *n* See molding, injection.

injection, periodontal ligament (intraligamentary) (per'ēōdon'təl lig'əmənt in'tralig'əmen'tərē), *n* an intraosseous injection of a local anesthetic agent directly to the alveolar bone surrounding the periodontal ligament. Often used as a supplemental form of local anesthesia when preliminary methods have proved ineffective.

injury, *n* the insult, harm, or hurt applied to tissue; may evoke dystrophic or inflammatory response from the affected part.

injury, root, *n* the damage to the root, especially to the cementum, when an excessive force is placed on the tooth.

injury, toothbrush, *n* the damage to the teeth and associated tissue produced by incorrect toothbrushing.

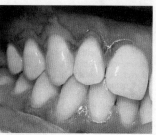

Toothbrush injury. (Sapp/Eversole/Wysocki, 2004)

inlay, *n* **1.** a restoration of metal, fired porcelain, or plastic made to fit a tapered cavity preparation and fastened to or luted into it with a cementing medium. *v* **2.** to perform such a procedure.

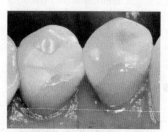

Inlays. (Heymann/Swift/Ritter, 2013)

inlay furnace, *n* See furnace, inlay.

inlay resin, *n* See resin, inlay.

inlay, setting, *n* the procedure of fitting a casting to a preparation; adjusting the occlusal function and contact areas; securing the proper, clean dry field; cementing the cleaned, polished casting in an aseptic, dry prepared cavity; and completing the final finishing and polishing of the restoration.

inlay wax, *n* See wax, inlay.

innervation (in'urvā'shən), *n* the distribution or supply of nerves to a part.

innervation, reciprocal, *n* the simultaneous excitation of one muscle with the inhibition of its antagonist. Rhythmic chewing is achieved efficiently when the masticatory muscles are reciprocally innervated, permitting alternate elevation and depression of the mandible in a smooth, coordinated sequence of actions.

inoculation (ĭnok′ula′shən), *n* a procedure in which a disease-causing substance is introduced into otherwise healthy tissue for the sole purpose of inducing immunity. See also immunization.

inorganic, *adj* having no derivation from living organisms; chemical compounds that generally do not contain carbon.

inositol (inō′sitol), *n* an essential growth factor in tissue culture with no known requirement. It has been used therapeutically in the management of diseases associated with the metabolism of fat.

input, computer, *n* the data to be processed.

input/output control (I/O control), *n* the portion of the central processor of some computer systems that contains software/firmware for supervising data flow between memory and the input/output devices connected to the CPU.

inquiry, *n* a request for information from storage in a computer.

insert, intramucosal (in′trəmūkō′s əl), *n* a nonreactive metal appliance that is affixed to the tissue–bone surface of a denture and offers added retentive qualities to the denture. It consists of a base, cervix, and head. Also known as *mucosal insert and implant button.*

insert, mucosal, *n* See insert, intramucosal.

insertion (insur′shən), *n* **1.** the end of the muscle that is attached to the more movable structure. *n* **2.** the act of implanting or placing materials or introducing the needle into the tissue.

insertion, path of, n the direction in which a prosthesis is inserted and removed.

insidious disease (insid′ēus), *adj* a disease existing without marked symptoms but ready to become active upon some slight occasion; a disease not appearing to be as bad as it really is.

insoluble, *adj* not susceptible to being dissolved.

insomnia, *n* the chronic inability to sleep or remain asleep throughout the night.

Inspection, *n* the visual examination of the body or portions thereof, which

is an integral phase of the physical or dental examination procedure.

inspiration (in′spĭra′shən), *n* the act of drawing air into the lungs.

inspirometer (in′spirom′ətur), *n* an instrument for measuring the force, frequency, or volume of inspirations.

institutionalize, *v* to place a person in a health care or custodial facility for psychologic or physical treatment or for the protection of the person or society.

Instron, *n.pr* an universal testing machine first designed by the Instron company of Canton, MA. The machine allows known forces with differing speeds, frequencies, or other parameters to be applied to materials so as to determine their response.

instruction, *n* a set of characters, together with one or more addresses, that defines a computer operation and, as a unit, causes the computer to operate accordingly on the indicated quantities; a term associated with software operation.

instruction of partial denture patient, n See denture, partial, instruction of patient.

instrument(s), *n* a tool or implement, especially one used for delicate or scientific work. See under the specific type of instrument (e.g., knife). See also instrumenting, instrumentarium.

instrument, air application, n a tool used to apply air to dry teeth, remove debris, and control saliva during treatment or in preparation for a specific procedure.

instrument, biveled cutting (bĭ′bevəld), n an instrument in which both sides of the end of the blade are beveled to form the cutting edge, as in a hatchet.

instrument blade/nib, n the part bearing a cutting edge. it begins at the terminal angle of the shank and ends at the cutting edge.

instrument, blade face, n the innermost surface of a scaler or curet blade.

instrument, carving, n See carver.

instrument, classification of, names, n the classification of instruments by name to denote purpose (e.g., excavator), denote position or manner of use (e.g., hand condenser), describe the form of the point (e.g., hatchet), or describe the angle of the blade in relation to the handle.

instrument, condensing, *n* a handheld device used to adapt dental amalgams to a prepared cavity.

instrument, cutting, *n* an instrument used to cut, cleave, or plane the walls of a cavity preparation; the blade ends in a sharp, beveled edge. Unless otherwise specified, it refers to a hand instrument rather than to a rotary type.

instrument, diamond, *n* a rotary abrasive instrument, wheel, or mounted point. Made of fine diamond chips bonded into a desired form; used to reduce tooth structure.

instrument, double-ended, *n* a handheld tool with two functional ends that are identical or complementary.

instrument, double-plane, *n* an instrument with the curve of the blade in a plane perpendicular to that of the angles of the shank.

instrument, formula name of, *n* a method of naming and describing dental hand instruments. Measurements are in the metric system. The working point is described first; then the formula is given, in three (or sometimes four) units. The first figure denotes the width of the blade, in tenths of millimeters; the second shows the length of the blade, in millimeters; and the third indicates the angle of the blade in relation to the shaft, in centigrades or hundredths of a circle. Whenever it is necessary to describe the angle of the cutting edge of a blade with its shaft, the number is entered in brackets as the second number of the formula. Paired instruments are also designated as right or left. In lateral cutting instruments the one used to cut from right to left is termed right; in direct cutting instruments with right and left bevels, the one having the bevel on the right side of the blade as it is held with the cutting edge down and pointing away from the observer is termed right.

instrument grasp, *n* See grasp, instrument.

instrument, hand, *n* an instrument used principally with hand force.

instrument, holding, *n* an instrument used to support gold foil while a foil restoration is inserted.

instrument, McCall's, *n.pr* a periodontal instrument used for gingival curettage and removing deposits from the tooth surfaces.

instrument nib, *n* the counterpart of the blade in the condensing instrument. The end of the nib is the face.

instrument, parts, *n.pl* the handle or shaft, blade or nib, and shank.

instrument, plastic, *n* an instrument used to manipulate a plastic restorative material.

instrument, rotary cutting, *n* a power-activated instrument used in a dental handpiece, such as a bur, mounted diamond point, mounted carborundum point, wheel stone, or disk.

instrument, screwdriver, *n* an instrument made of surgical alloy; it may have at its tip a screw holder that is designed to drive screws into the bone.

instrument, shaft/handle, *n* the part that is grasped by the clinician's hand while using the instrument.

instrument shank, *n* the part that connects the shaft and the blade or nib.

instrument sharpening, *n* See sharpening, instrument.

instrument, single-beveled cutting, *n* an instrument in which one side of the end of the blade is beveled to form the cutting edge, as in a wood chisel.

instrument, single-plane, *n* an instrument with all its angles and curves in one plane; when the instrument lies on a flat surface, the cutting edge and the blade will parallel the surface.

instrument, sonic, *n* a mechanical tool whose thin tip vibrates at high rates and is used to remove debris, deposits, or dead or damaged tissue.

instrument stop, *n* a device, usually metal, that can be placed on a reamer or file to mark the measurement of the root.

instrument, toe, *n* the tip or terminating end of the blade, may be rounded (blunt) or pointed (sharp).

instrument, universal, *n* a tool that may be used on all types of teeth surfaces.

instrumental values, *n* a person's innermost convictions concerning the means, as opposed to the ends, of a goal.

instrumentarium (in′strəməntar′ē əm), *n* the exact instruments required to perform a specific procedure.

Abbreviation	Meaning
CSF	Cerebrospinal fluid
CSM	Cerebrospinal meningitis
CT	Computed tomography
Cu	Copper
$CuSO_4$	Copper sulfate
CV	Cardiovascular; closing volume
CVA	Cerebrovascular accident; costovertebral angle
CVP	Central venous pressure
CVS	Chorionic villi sampling; clean voided specimen
CXR	Chest x-ray
cyl	Cylinder
D	Dose; vitamin D; right *(dexter)*
d	Day; diem
DAH	Disordered action of the heart
D & C	Dilation (dilatation) and curettage
db, dB	Decibel
DC	Direct current
dc, DC, D/C	Discontinue
DCA	Deoxycorticosterone acetate
Dcg	Degeneration; degree
dg	Decigram
DIC	Disseminated intravascular coagulation
diff	Differential blood count
dil	Dilute or dissolve
dim	One half
DJD	Degenerative joint disease
DKA	Diabetic ketoacidosis
dL	Deciliter
DM	Diabetes mellitus, diastolic murmur
DNA	Deoxyribonucleic acid
DNR	Do not resuscitate
DOA	Dead on arrival
DOB	Date of birth
DOE	Dyspnea on exertion
DPT	Diphtheria-pertussis-tetanus
dr	Dram
DRG	Diagnosis-related groups
DSD	Discharge summary dictated, dry sterile dressing
DT	Delirium tremens
DTR	Deep tendon reflex
D5W	Dextrose 5% in water
Dx	Diagnosis
E	Eye
EAHF	Eczema, asthma, and hayfever
EBV	Epstein-Barr virus
EC	Electroconvulsive therapy
ECF	Extended care facility; extracellular fluid
ECG	Electrocardiogram, electrocardiograph
ECHO	Echocardiography
ECMO	Extracorporeal membrane oxygenation
ECT	Electroconvulsive therapy
ED	Emergency department; erythema dose; effective dose
ED_{50}	Median effective dose
EDD	Estimated date of delivery (formerly EDC, estimated date of confinement)
EEG	Electroencephalogram, electroencephalograph
EENT	Eye, ear, nose, and throat
EKG	Electrocardiogram, electrocardiograph
ELISA	Enzyme-linked immunosorbent assay

Continued

Abbreviation	Meaning
Em	Emmetropia
EMB	Eosin-methylene blue
EMC	Encephalomyocarditis
EMF	Erythrocyte maturation factor
EMG	Electromyogram
EMS	Emergency medical service
ENT	Ear, nose, and throat
EOM	Extraocular movement
EPR	Electrophrenic respiration
ER/ED	Emergency room/department (hospital); external resistance
ERG	Electroretinogiam
ERPF	Effective renal plasma flow
ERV	Expiratory reserve volume
ESR	Erythrocyte sedimentation rate
ESRD	End-stage renal disease
EST	Electroshock therapy
Et	Ethyl
ext	Extract
F	Fahrenheit: field of vision; formula
FA	Fatty acid
FANA	Fluorescent antinuclear antibody lest
F & R	Force and rhythm (pulse)
FAS	Fetal alcohol syndrome
FBS	Fasting blood sugar
FD	Fatal dose; focal distance
Fc	Iron
FeCl₃	Ferric chloride
ferv.	Boiling
FEV	Forced expiratory volume
FH, Fhx	Family history
FHR	Fetal heart rate
Fl, fld	Fluid
fl dr	Fluid dram
fl oz	Fluid ounce
FR	Flocculation reaction
FSH	Follicle-stimulating hormone
ft	Foot
FTT	Failure to thrive
FUO	Fever of unknown origin
fx	Fracture
Gm; g; gm	Gram
GA	Gingivoaxial
Galv	Galvanic
GB	Gallbladder
GBS	Gallbladder series
GC	Gonococcus or gonorrheal
GDM	Gestational diabetes mellitus
GFR	Glomerular filtration rate
GH	Growth hormone
GI	Gastrointestinal
GL	Greatest length (small flexed embryo)
GLA	Gingivolinguoaxial
GP	General practitioner; general paresis
G6PD	Glucose-6-phosphate dehydrogenase
gr	Grain
Grad	By degrees *(gradatim)*
GRAS	Generally recognized as safe
Grav I, II, III, etc.	Pregnancy one, two, three, etc. *(Gravida)*
GSW	Gunshot wound

Abbreviation	Meaning
gt	Drop *(gutta)*
GTT	Glucose tolerance test
gu	Drops *(guttae)*
GU	Genitourinary
Gyn	Gynecology
H	Hydrogen
H+	Hydrogen ion
H & E	Hematoxylin and eosin stain
H & P	History and physical
HAV	Hepatitis A virus
Hb; Hgb	Hemoglobin
H_3BO_3	Boric acid
HBV	Hepatitis B virus
HC	Hospital corps
HCG	Human chorionic gonadotropin
HCHO	Formaldehyde
HCl	Hydrochloric acid
HCN	Hydrocyanic acid
H_2CO_3	Carbonic acid
HCT	Hematocrit
HD	Hearing distance
HDL	High-density lipoprotein
HDLW	Distance at which a watch is heard by the left ear
HDRW	Distance at which a watch is heard by the right ear
He	Helium
HEENT	Head, eye, ear, nose, and throat
Hg	Mercury
Hgb	Hemoglobin
HHC	Home health care
Hib	*Haemophilus influenzae* type B
HIV	Human immunodeficiency virus
HME	Home medical equipment
HNO_3	Nitric acid
h/o	History of
H_2O	Water
H_2O_2	Hydrogen peroxide
HOP	High oxygen pressure
HPI	History of present illness
HR	Heart rate
H_2SO_4	Sulfuric acid
HSV	Herpes simplex virus
Ht	Total hyperopia
HT, HTN	Hypertension
HTLV-III	Human T-lymphotropic virus type III
hx, Hx	History
Hy	Hyperopia
I	Incisive
I	Iodine
^{131}I	Radioactive isotope of iodine (atomic weight 131)
^{132}I	Radioactive isotope of iodine (atomic weight 132)
IA	Inferior alveolar
I & O	Intake and output
IB	Inclusion body
IBW	Ideal body weight
IC	Inspiratory capacity; intracutaneous
ICP	Intracranial pressure
ICS	Intercostal space
ICSH	Interstitial cell-stimulating hormone
ICT	Inflammation of connective tissue

Continued

Abbreviation	Meaning
ICU	Intensive care unit
Id.	The same *(idem)*
IDDM	Insulin-dependent diabetes mellitus
Ig	Immunoglobulin
IH	Infectious hepatitis
IM	Intramuscular; infectious mononucleosis
IO	Infraorbital
IOP	Intraocular pressure
IPPB	Intermittent positive pressure breathing
IQ	Intelligence quotient
IRV	Inspiratory reserve volume
IS	Intercoatal space
IUD	Intrauterine device
IV	Intravenous
IVP	Intravenous pyclogram, intravenous push
IVT	Intravenous transfusion
IVU	Intravenous urogram/urography
JRA	Juvenile rheumatoid arthritis
K	Potassium
k	Constant
Ka	Cathode or kathode
KBr	Potassium bromide
kc	Kilocycle
KCl	Potassium chloride
kev	Kilo electron volts
kg	Kilogram
KI	Potassium iodide
kj	Knee jerk
km	Kilometer
KOH	Potassium hydroxide
KUB	Kidney, ureter, and bladder
kv	Kilovolt
kVp	Kilovoltage peak
KVO	Keep vein open
kw	Kilowatt
L	Left; liter, length; lumbar; lethal; pound
lab	Laboratory
L & A	Light and accommodation
L & D	Labor and delivery
lat.	Lateral
lb	Pound *(libra)*
LB	Large bowel (x-ray film)
LBW	Low birth weight
LCM	Left costal margin
LD	Lethal dose; perception of light difference
LDL	Low-density lipoprotein
LE	Lower extremity; lupus erythematosus
le	Left extremity
l.e.s.	Local excitatory state
LFD	Least fatal dose of a toxin
LGA	Large for gestational age
LH	Luteinizing hormone
Li	Lithium
LIF	Left iliac fossa
lig	Ligament
Liq	Liquor
LLE	Left lower extremity
LLL	Left lower lobe
LLQ	Left lower quadrant

Abbreviation	Meaning
LMP	Last menstrual period
LNMP	Last normal menstrual period
LOC	Level/loss of consciousness
LP	Lumbar puncture
LPF	Leukocytosis-promoting factor
LR	Lactated Ringer's
LTD	Lowest tolerated dose
LTH	Luteotrophic hormone
LUE	Left upper extremity
LUL	Left upper lobe
LUQ	Left upper quadrant
LV	Left ventricle
LVH	Left ventricular hypertrophy
L&W	Living and well
M	Myopia; meter; muscle; thousand
m	Meter
MA	Mental age
mA	Milliamperage
MB	Mental block
Mag	Large (nagnus)
MAP	Mean arterial pressure
MBD	Minimal brain dysfunction
me; mCi	Millicurie
μc	Microcurie
mcg	Microgram
MCH	Mean corpuscular hemoglobin
MCHC	Mean corpuscular hemoglobin concentration
MCV	Mean corpuscular volume
MD	Muscular dystrophy
MDI	Medium-dose inhalants; metered-dose inhaler
Me	Methyl
MED	Minimal erythema dose; minimal effective dose
mEq	Milliequivalent
μEq	Microequivalent
mEq/L	Milliequivalent per liter
ME ratio	Myeloid/erythroid ratio
Mg	Magnesium
mg	Milligram
mcg	Microgram
MHD	Minimal hemolytic dose
MI	Myocardial infarction
MID	Minimum infective dose
ML	Midline
mL	Milliliter
MLD	Median or minimum lethal dose
MM	Mucous membrane
mm	Millimeter, muscles
mm Hg	Millimeters of mercury
mmm	Millimicron
MMR	Maternal mortality rate; measlesmumps-rubella
mμ	Millimicron
μm	Micrometer
μμ	Micromicron
Mn	Manganese
mN	Millinormal
MRI	Magnetic resonance imaging
MS	Multiple sclerosis
MSL	Midsternal line

Continued

Abbreviation	Meaning
MT	Medical technologist; membrane tympani
mu	Mouse unit
MVA	Motor vehicle accident
MW	Molecular weight
My	Myopia
N	Nitrogen
n	Normal
N/A	Not applicable
Na	Sodium
NaBr	Sodium bromide
NaCl	Sodium chloride
Na_2CO_3	Sodium carbonate
$Na_2C_2O_4$	Sodium oxalate
NAD	No appreciable disease
NaF	Sodium fluoride
$NaHCO_3$	Sodium bicarbonate
Na_2HPO_4	Sodium phosphate
NAI	Sodium iodide
N & V, N/V	Nausea and vomiting
$NaNO_3$	Sodium nitrate
Na_2O_2	Sodium peroxide
NaOH	Sodium hydroxide
Na_2SO_4	Sodium sulfate
n.b.	Note well
NCA	Neurocirculatory asthenia
Ne	Neon
NG, ng	Nasogastric
NH_3	Ammonia
Ni	Nickel
NICU	Neonatal intensive cure unit
NIDDM	Non-insulin-dependent diabetes mellitus
NIH	National Institutes of Health
NiTi	Nickel titanium
NKA	No known allergies
nm	Nanometer
NMR	Nuclear magnetic resonance
N.O.	Nursing order
NPN	Nonprotein nitrogen
NPO; n.p.o.	Nothing by mouth *(non per os)*
NRC	Normal retinal correspondence
NS	Normal saline
NSAID	Nonsteroidal antiinflammatory drug
NSR	Normal sinus rhythm
NTP	Normal temperature and pressure
NYD	Not yet diagnosed
O	Oxygen; oculus; pint
O_2	Oxygen; both eyes
O_3	Ozone
OB	Obstetrics
OBS	Organic brain syndrome
OD	Optical density; overdose; right eye *(Oculus dexter)*
OOB	Out of bed
OPD	Outpatient department
OR	Operating room
ORIF	Open reduction and internal fixation
OS	Left eye *(oculus sinister)*
Os	Osmium
OT	Occupational therapy
OTC	Over-the-counter

Abbreviation	Meaning
OTD	Organ tolerance dose
OU	Each eye (oculus uterque)
oz	Ounce
P	Phosphorus; pulse; pupil
P̄	After
P_2	Pulmonic second sound
P-A; P/A; PA	Posterior-anterior
PAB; PABA	Para-aminobenzoic acid
PALS	Pediatric Advanced Life Support
P & A	Percussion and auscultation
Pap test	Papanicolaou smear
Para I, II, III, etc.	Unipara, bipara, tripara, etc.
PAS; PASA	Para-aminosalicylic acid
PAT	Paroxysmal atrial tachycardia
Pb	Lead
PBI	Protein-bound iodine
PCA	Patient-controlled analgesia
PCP	Phencyclidine, *Pneumocystis carinii (jiroveci)* pneumonia, primary care physician, pulmonary capillary pressure
PCV	Packed cell volume
PCWP	Pulmonary capillary wedge pressure
PD	Interpupillary distance
pd	Prism diopter; pupillary distance
PDA	Patent ductus arteriosus
PDR	*Physician's Desk Reference*
PE	Physical examination
PEEP	Positive end expiratory pressure
PEFR	Peak expiratory flow rate
PEG	Pneumoencephalography
PERRLA	Pupils equal, regular, react to light and accommodation
PET	Positron emission tomography
PFF	Protein-free filtrate
PGA	Pteroylglutamic acid (folic acid)
PH	Past history
pH	Hydrogen ion concentration (alkalinity and acidity in urine and blood analysis)
Pharm; Phar.	Pharmacy
PI	Previous illness; protamine insulin
PICC	Percutaneously inserted central catheter
PID	Pelvic inflammatory disease
PK	Psychokinesis
PKU	Phenylketonuria
PL	Light perception
PM	Postmortem; evening
PMB	Polymorphonuclear basophil leukocytes
PME	Polymorphonuclear eosinophil leukocytes
PMH	Past medical history
PMI	Point of maximal impulse
PMN	Polymorphonuclear neutrophil leukocytes (polys)
PMS	Premenstrual syndrome
PN	Percussion note
PND	Paroxysmal nocturnal dyspnea
PNH	Paroxysmal nocturnal hemoglobinuria
PO; p.o.	Orally *(per os)*
PPD	Purified protein derivative (TB test)
ppm	Parts per million
Pr	Presbyopia; prism
PRN, p.r.n.	As required *(pro re nata)*
pro time	Prothrombin time

Continued

Abbreviation	Meaning
PSA	Posterior superior alveolar
PSA	Prostate-specific antigen
PSP	Phenolsulfonphthalein
Pt	Pint
Pt	Platinum; patient
PT	Prothrombin time; physical therapy
PTA	Plasma thromboplastin antecedent
PTC	Plasma thromboplastin component
PTT	Partial thromboplastin time
Pu	Plutonium
PUO	Pyrexia of unknown origin
PVC	Premature ventricular contraction
Px	Pneumothorax
PZI	Protamine zinc insulin
Q	Electric quantity
q	Every
qns	Quantity not sufficient
q.o.d.	Every other day
qt	Quart
Quat	Four (quattuor)
R	Respiration; right; Rickettsia; roentgen
Rx	Take
RA	Rheumatoid arthritis
Ra	Radium
rad	Unit of measurement of the absorbed dose of ionizing radiation; root
RAI	Radioactive iodine
RAIU	Radioactive iodine uptake
RBC; rbc	Red blood cell; red blood count
RCD	Relative cardiac dullness
RCM	Right costal margin
RDA	Recommended daily/dietary allowance
RDS	Respiratory distress syndrome
RE	Right eye; reticuloendothelial tissue or cell
Re	Rhenium
re	Right extremity
Rect	Rectified
Reg umb	Umbilical region
RES	Reticuloendothelial system
Rh	Symbol of rhesus factor; symbol for rhodium
RhA	Rheumatoid arthritis
RHD	Relative hepatic dullness; rheumatic heart disease
RLE	Right lower extremity
RLL	Right lower lobe
RLQ	Right lower quadrant
RM	Respiratory movement
RML	Right middle lobe of lung
Rn	Radon
RNA	Ribonucleic acid
R/O	Rule out
ROM	Range of motion
ROS	Review of systems
RPF	Renal plasma flow
RPM; rpm	Revolutions per minute
RPR	Rapid plasma reagin
RPS	Renal pressor substance
RQ	Respiratory quotient
RR	Recovery room; respiratory rate
RT	Radiation therapy; reading test; respiratory therapy

Abbreviation	Meaning
R/T	Related to
RU	Rat unit
RUE	Right upper extremity
RUL	Right upper lobe
RUQ	Right upper quadrant
S	Sulfur
S.	Sacral
$	Without
S-A; S/A: SA	Sinoatrial
SAS	Sodium acetate solution
SB	Small bowel (x-ray film); sternal border
Sb	Antimony
SD	Skin dose
Se	Selenium
Sed rate	Sedimentation rate
SGA	Small for gestational age
SGOT	Serum glutamic oxaloacetic transaminase
SGPT	Serum glutamic pyruvic transaminase
SH	Serum hepatitis
SI	International system of units (stroke index)
S.L	Soluble insulin
SI	Silicon
SIDS	Sudden infant death syndrome
SLE	Systemic lupus erythematosus
SLP	Speech-language pathology
Sn	Tin
SNF	Skilled nursing facility
SOB	Shortness of breath
sol	Solution, dissolved
SP	Spirit
sp. gr. SG, a.g.	Specific gravity
sph	Spherical
SPI	Serum precipitable iodine
spir	Spirit
SR	Sedimentation rate
Sr	Strontium
s/s	Signs and symptoms
SS	Stainless steel
SSS	Specific soluble substance, sick sinus syndrome
sss	Layer upon layer *(stratum super stratum)*
St	Let it stand *(stet: stent)*
Staph	Staphylococcus
stat	Immediately *(statim)*
STD	Sexually transmitted disease; skin test dose
STH	Somatotrophic hormone
Strep	*Streptococcus*
STS	Serologic test for syphilis
STU	Skin test unit
SV	Stroke volume; supraventricular
sv	Alcoholic spirit *(spiritus vini)*
Sx	Symptoms
Sym	Symmetrical
T	Temperature; thoracic
t	Temporal
T_3	Triiodothyronine
T_4	Thyroxine
TA	Toxin-antitoxin
Ta	Tantalum
TAB	Vaccine against typhoid, paratyphoid A and B

Continued

Abbreviation	Meaning
Tab	Tablet
TAD	Temporary anchorage device
TAH	Total abdominal hysterectomy
TAM	Toxoid-antitoxid mixture
T&A	Tonsillectomy and adenoidectomy
TAT	Toxin-antitoxin, tetanus antitoxin
TB	Tuberculin; tuberculosis; tubercle bacillus
Tb	Terbium
TCA	Tetrachloracetic add
Te	Tellurium; tetanus
TEM	Triethylene melamine
TENS	Transcutaneous electrical nerve stimulation
Th	Thorium
TIA	Transient ischemic attack
TIBC	Total iron-binding capacity
Tl	Thallium
TM	Tympanic membrane
Tm	Thulium; symbol for maximal tubular excretory capacity (kidneys)
TMA	Titanium molybdenum alloy
TMJ	Temporomandibular joint
TNT	Trinitrotoluene
TNTM	Too numerous lo mention
TP	Tuberculin precipitation
TPI	*Treponema pallidum* immobilization test for syphilis
TPN	Total parenteral nutrition
TPR	Temperature, pulse, and respiration
tr	Tincture
Trans D	Transverse diameter
TRU	Turbidity reducing unit
TS	Test solution
TSE	Testicular self-examination
TSH	Thyroid-stimulating hormone
TSP	Trisodium phosphate
TST	Triple sugar iron test
TUR; TURP	Transurethral resection
Tx	Treatment
U	Uranium
UA	Urinalysis
UBI	Ultraviolet blood irradiation
UE	Upper extremity
UIBC	Unsaturated iron-binding capacity
Umb; umb	Umbilicus
URI	Upper respiratory infection
US	Ultrasonic
USP	*U.S. Pharmacopeia*
UTI	Urinary tract infection
UV	Ultraviolet
V	Vanadium; vision; visual acuity
V	Volt
VA	Visual acuity
V & T	Volume and tension
VC	Vital capacity
VD	Venereal disease
VDA	Visual discriminatory acuity
VDG	Venereal disease—gonorrhea
VDM	Vasodepressor material
VDRL	Venereal Disease Research Laboratories (sometimes used loosely to mean venereal disease report)

Abbreviation	Meaning
VDS	Venereal disease—syphilis
VEM	Vasoexciter material
Vf	Field of vision
VHD	Valvular heart disease
VIA	Virus inactivating agent
VLBW	Very low birth weight
VLDL	Very-low-density lipoprotein
VMA	Vanillylmandelic acid
vol	Volume
VR	Vocal resonance
VS	Volumetric solution
VS, v.s.	Vital signs
Vs	Venisection
VsB	Bleeding in arm *(venaesectio brachii)*
VSD	Ventricular septal defect
VW	Vessel wall
VZIG	Varicella zoster immune globulin
W	Tungsten
w	Watt
WBC; wbc	White blood cell; white blood cell count
WD	Well developed
WL	Wavelength
WN	Well nourished
WNL	Within normal limits
WR	Wassermann reaction
wt	Weight
X-ray	Roentgen ray
y, yr	Year
yo	Years old
Z	Symbol for atomic number
Zu	Zinc
Zz	Ginger

Note: Abbreviations in common use can vary widely from place to place. Each institution's list of acceptable abbreviations is the best authority for its records.

Anesthesia Color Codes

Local anesthetic cartridge color codes

Mandated uniform system for local anesthetic cartridges bearing the ADA Seal of Acceptance.*

PRODUCT	COLOR
Lidocaine 2 percent with epinephrine 1:100,000	
Lidocaine 2 percent with epinephrine 1:50,000	
Lidocaine plain	
Mepivacaine 2 percent with levonordefrin 1:20,000	
Mepivacaine 3 percent plain	
Prilocaine 4 percent with epinephrine 1:200,000	
Prilocaine 4 percent plain	
Bupivacaine 1.5 percent with epinephrine	
Articaine 4 percent with epinephrine 1:100,000	
Articaine 4 percent with epinephrine 1:200,000	

* This chart originally appeared in ADA News.

Clinical Oral Structures

Structure	Clinical description	Clinical consideration
LIPS, CHEEKS, AND ORAL MUCOSA		
Philtrum	Midline vertical depression of the skin between the nose and upper lip	Common location for cleft lip
Vermillion zone	Transition area between skin of the face and oral mucosa of the lips; medium pink in light-skinned individuals, and pigmented with melanin in dark-skinned individuals	The junction between the vermillion zone and the skin of the face is a frequent site of herpetic lesions; the lower lip is a frequent site of oral · cancer
		Fordyce's granules or spots (small white spots of ectopic sebaceous material) may be present
Labial commissure	Junction of the upper and lower lips at the corner of the mouth	Frequent site of chafing, herpetic lesions, and cracking (angular cheilitis); avoid pulling with instrument handle
Vestibule	Space bounded by the cheeks, lips, and facial surfaces of the teeth and gingivae	Frequent site of aphthous ulcers
Labial mucosa	Mucosal lining of the inner lip; vascular; small elevations are external manifestation of numerous labial salivary glands	Frequent site of mucoceles, mucus- retention cysts, aphthous ulcers, and scars
Labial frenum (maxillary and mandibular)	Fold of tissue at the midline (maxillary and mandibular) between the inner surface of the lip and the alveolar mucosa	Maxillary fold is sometimes over- developed, which results in a space between the central incisors called a *diastema;* frequently has an extra flap of tissue
		If overextended onto the attached gingiva, mandibular fold may cause recession
Buccal mucosa	Mucous membrane lining of the inner cheek	Frequent site of linea alba, cheek bites, and Fordyce's granules
Parotid papilla	Flap of tissue on the cheek opposite the maxillary first molars; contains the opening of Stensen's duct, which carries saliva from the parotid gland	Large amounts of mainly serous saliva come from this duct; the opening often can be seen as a dark spot

Structure	Clinical description	Clinical consideration
Rugae	Firm irregular ridges of masticatory mucosa on the anterior half of the hard palate	If prominent, rugae may be burned or traumatized more easily
Palatine fovea	Small dimple on either side of the midline at the junction of the hard and soft palates	Touching area posterior to this may initiate the gag reflex
Palatal salivary duct openings	Small dark spots scattered on the hard and soft palates	Represent the duct openings of the minor palatal salivary glands
Palatine raphe	Hard linear elevation along the midline of the hard palate; external manifestation of the palatine suture, which joins the right and left maxillary and palatine bones	Excess bone (tori) or a deep depression may be present there Site of hyperkeratinization or associated nicotinic stomatitis
Maxillary tuberosity	Protuberance of the alveolar bone distal to the last maxillary molar	Erupting third molar may be present there

TONSILLAR REGION

Structure	Clinical description	Clinical consideration
Retromolar area	Triangular area of bone and pad of tissue distal to the last mandibular molar	Erupting third molar may be present, and a flap of tissue (operculum) often is associated with an infection in this area
Pterygomandibular raphe	Fold of tissue from the retromolar area to an area near the maxillary tuberosity; separates the soft palate from the cheek; lies medial to the posterior border of the ramus of the mandible	Covers a ligament from the mandible to the sphenoid bone Used as a guide to identify the posterior border of the ramus of the mandible when targeting the area for needle insertion for inferior alveolar-nerve anesthesia
Anterior or glossopalatine arch	Thin fold of epithelium extending laterally and inferiorly from both sides of the soft palate to the base of the tongue	Marks the entry into the pharynx; the anterior boundary of the tonsillar recess
Posterior or pharyngopalatine arch	Thin fold of epithelium that is more posterior and narrower than the anterior arch	Marks the posterior boundary of the palatine tonsillar recess
Tonsillar recess	Recessed area between the anterior and posterior arches	May or may not contain palatine tonsils
Palatine tonsils	Globules of lymphoid tissue in the tonsillar recess	Vary greatly in size Not visible if removed or atrophied, or may be so large the fauces is very narrow
Uvula	Fleshy tissue suspended from the midline of the posterior border of the soft palate	Closes the opening to the nasopharynx when swallowing Varies in size and shape

Structure	Clinical description	Clinical consideration
Pharyngeal tonsils	Globules of lymphoid tissue on the oropharyngeal wall	Lay term is adenoids Appear as globules of reddish-orange tissue Mucosal secretions from the sinuses may be seen here
Fauces or faucial isthmus	Isthmus (narrowing) of the space from the oral cavity into the pharynx	

From Darby ML: Mosby's comprehensive review of dental hygiene, ed 7, St Louis, 2012, Mosby.

Tooth Designation Systems

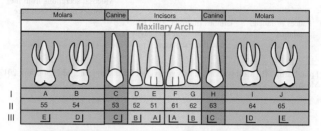

	Molars		Canine	Incisors		Canine	Molars	
	Maxillary Arch							
I	A	B	C	D E	F G	H	I	J
II	55	54	53	52 51	61 62	63	64	65
III	E⌋	D⌋	C⌋	B⌋ A⌋	⌊A ⌊B	⌊C	⌊D	⌊E

	Molars		Canine	Incisors		Canine	Molars	
III	⌉E	⌉D	⌉C	⌉B ⌉A	⌈A ⌈B	⌈C	⌈D	⌈E
II	85	84	83	82 81	71 72	73	74	75
I	T	S	R	Q P	O N	M	L	K
	Mandibular Arch							
	Right				Left			

I Universal tooth designation system

II International Standards Organization designation system

III Palmer Method

	Molars			Premolars		Canine	Incisors				Canine	Premolars		Molars		
	Maxillary Arch															
I	1	2	3	4	5	6	7	8	9	10	11	12	13	14	15	16
II	18	17	16	15	14	13	12	11	21	22	23	24	25	26	27	28
III	8⌋	7⌋	6⌋	5⌋	4⌋	3⌋	2⌋	1⌋	⌊1	⌊2	⌊3	⌊4	⌊5	⌊6	⌊7	⌊8

	Molars			Premolars		Canine	Incisors				Canine	Premolars		Molars		
III	⌉8	⌉7	⌉6	⌉5	⌉4	⌉3	⌉2	⌉1	⌈1	⌈2	⌈3	⌈4	⌈5	⌈6	⌈7	⌈8
II	48	47	46	45	44	43	42	41	31	32	33	34	35	36	37	38
I	32	31	30	29	28	27	26	25	24	23	22	21	20	19	18	17
	Mandibular Arch															
	Right								Left							

I Universal tooth designation system

II International Standards Organization designation system

III Palmer Method

From Bath Balogh M, Fehrenbach MJ: *Illustrated dental embryology, histology, and anatomy*, ed 3, Saunders, 2011, St Louis.

The Use of Dental Implants

INDICATIONS
- Good general physical and mental health to facilitate client acceptance of the dental implant
- A commitment to a daily oral biofilm-control regimen to avoid peri-implantitis
- Manual dexterity to ensure that oral biofilm-control procedures can be performed effectively on a daily basis
- A sufficient quantity and quality of alveolar bone to retain the dental implant
- Continuous cooperation and communication between client and oral health-care team

CONTRAINDICATIONS
- Blood dyscrasias (prevent proper healing and clotting)
- Certain cardiovascular diseases
- Chronic renal diseases
- Corticosteroid use
- Debilitating or uncontrollable disease or compromised healing conditions, such as that resulting from radiation therapy
- Diabetic clients susceptible to gingival and periodontal disease
- Hypersensitivity of tissues to specific implant materials
- Inability of client to maintain optimal daily hygiene care
- Inadequate client motivation
- Local gingival infection
- Metabolic diseases
- Noncorrectable heavy bruxing problem
- Pregnant client
- Psychiatric disorders
- Rheumatoid disease
- Systemic infection
- Unattainable prosthetic reconstruction
- Unrealistic client expectations

BENEFITS
- Improved ability to masticate and speak adequately
- Enhanced self-confidence and esteem because of improved esthetics and function
- Decreased amount of bone resorption
- Decreased tissue ulceration and unnecessary pressure
- Elimination of direct force on the gingival tissue and alveolar crest
- Increased retention of the prosthetic appliance
- Preservation of the remaining bone structure

RISKS

- Failure to osseointegrate
- Improper client selection
- Improper control of immediate stress or load force
- Improper oral hygiene care
- Inadequate allowance of healing time and interface development
- Inadequate control of manufacture quality
- Inadequate implant or prosthetic design
- Periimplantitis
- Surgical complications

From Darby ML, Walsh MM: *Dental hygiene: theory and practice*, ed 3, St. Louis, 2010, Saunders.

Illustration Credits

Abrahams PH, McMinn RMH, Marks SC, et al: McMinn's Color Atlas of Human Anatomy, 5e, Mosby, St. Louis, 2003

Adams JG: Emergency Medicine: Clinical Essentials, 2e, Saunders, Philadelphia, 2014

Aehlert BJ: ACLS Study Guide, 4e, Mosby, St. Louis, 2013

Albert DM, Miller JW, Azar DT, et al: Albert & jakobiec's Principles and Practice of Ophthalmology, 3e, Saunders, Philadelphia, 2008

Andreoli TE, Benjamin I, Griggs RC: Andreoli and Carpenter's Cecil Essentials of Medicine, 8e, Saunders, St. Louis, 2011

Applegate E: The Anatomy and Physiology Learning System, 4e, Saunders, St. Louis, 2011

Avery JK, Chiego DJ: Essentials of Oral Histology and Embryology: A Clinical Approach, 3e, Mosby, St. Louis, 2006

Babbush CA, Hahn JA, Krauser JT, et al: Dental Implants: The Art and Science, 2e, Saunders, St. Louis, 2011

Bagheri SC, Bell B, Khan HA: Current Therapy in Oral and Maxillofacial Surgery, Saunders, St. Louis, Saunders, 2012

Bath-Balogh M, Fehrenbach M: Illustrated Dental Embryology, Histology, and Anatomy, 3e, Saunders, St. Louis, 2011

Berkovitz BKB, Holland GR, Moxham BJ: Oral Anatomy and Embryology, 4e, Mosby, St. Louis, 2010

Block M: Color Atlas of Dental Implant Surgery, 2e, Saunders, St. Louis, 2007

Bird DL and Robinson DS: Modern Dental Assisting, 10e, Saunders, St. Louis, 2012

Bologna JL, Jorizzo JL, Rapini RP: Dermatology, 2e, Mosby, St. Louis, 2008

Bonewit-West K: Clinical Procedures for Medical Assistants, 8e, Saunders, St. Louis, 2008

Bonewit-West K, Hunt S, Applegate E: Today's Medical Assistant: Clinical and Administrative Procedures, 2e, Saunders, St. Louis, 2013

Boyd L: Dental Instruments: A Pocket Guide, 4e, Saunders, St. Louis, 2012

Callen PW: Ultrasonography in Obstetrics and Gynecology, 5e, Saunders, St. Louis, 2008

Casamassimo PS, Fields HW, McTigue DJ, et al: Pediatric Dentistry: Infancy Through Adolescence, 5e, St. Louis, Saunders, 2013

Cobourne M, DiBiase AT: Handbook of Orthodontics, Mosby, St. Louis, 2010

Convissar RA: Principles and Practice of Laser Dentistry, Mosby, St. Louis, 2011

Daniel SJ, Harfst SA, Wilder R: Mosby's Dental Hygiene: Concepts, Cases, and Competencies, 2e, Mosby, St. Louis, 2008

Darby M, Walsh M: Dental Hygiene: Theory and Practice, 3e, Mosby, St. Louis, 2010

Dawson PE: Functional Occlusion: From TMJ to Smile Design, Mosby, St. Louis, 2007

Dean JA, Avery DR, McDonald RE: McDonald and Avery's Dentistry for the Child and Adolescent, 9e, Mosby, St. Louis, 2011

Drake RL, Vogl W, Mitchell AWM: Gray's Anatomy for Students, ed 2, Churchill Livingstone, Philadelphia, 2010

Eley BM, Soory M, Manson JD: Periodontics, 6e, Churchill Livingstone, Philadelphia, 2010

English JD, Peltomäki T, Pham-Litschel K: Mosby's Orthodontic Review, Mosby, St. Louis, 2009

Fehrenbach M, Herring S: Illustrated Anatomy of the Head and Neck, 4e, Saunders, St. Louis, 2012

Finkbeiner BL, Johnson CS: Mosby's Comprehensive Dental Assisting: A Clinical Approach, Mosby, St. Louis, 1995

Flint PW, Haughey BH, Lund VJ, et al: Cummings Otolaryngology – Head and Neck Surgery, 5e, Mosby, St. Louis, 2011

Frazier MS, Drzymkowski J: Essentials of Human Diseases and Conditions, ed 5, St. Louis, Saunders, 2013

Freedman GA: Contemporary Esthetic Dentistry, Mosby, St. Louis, 2012

Frommer HH, Stabulas-Savage JJ: Radiology for the Dental Professional, 9e, Mosby, St. Louis, 2011

Fuller JR: Surgical Technology: Principles and Practice, 5e, Saunders, St. Louis, 2010

Garg AK: Implant Dentistry: A Practical Approach, 2e, Mosby, St. Louis, 2010

Gartner LP, Hiatt JL: Color Textbook of Histology, 3e, Saunders, St. Louis, 2007

Gaylor L: The Administrative Dental Assistant, 2e, Saunders, St. Louis, 2007

Goering R, Dockrell H, Zuckerman M, et al: Mim's Medical Microbiology, 5e, Saunders, St. Louis, 2013

Goldman L, Schafer AI: Goldman's Cecil Medicine, 24e, Saunders, St. Louis, 2012

Graber LW, Vanarsdall RL, Vig KWL: Orthodontics: Current Principles and Techniques, 5e, Mosby, St. Louis, 2012

Gutmann JL, Lovdahl PE: Problem Solving in Endodontics, 5e, Mosby, St. Louis, 2011

Guyot A, Schelenz S, Myint SH: The Flesh & Bones of Medical Microbiology, Mosby, Edinburgh, 2011

Habif T, Campbell JL, Chapman MS, et al: Skin Disease Diagnosis and Treatment, 3e, Saunders, St. Louis, 2012

Halstead CL, Blozis GO, Drinnan AJ, et al: Physical Examination of the Dental Patient, Mosby, St. Louis, 1982

Hargreaves K, Cohen S: Cohen's Pathways of the Pulp, 10e, Mosby, St. Louis, 2011

Hatrick C, Eakle S, Bird W: Dental Materials: Clinical Applications for Dental Assistants and Dental Hygienists, 2e, Saunders, St. Louis, 2011

Henry MCD, Stapleton ER: ENT Prehospital Care, 4e, Mosby, St. Louis, 2012

Heymann HO, Swift EJ, Ritter AV: Sturdevant's Art and Science of Operative Dentistry, 6e, Mosby, St. Louis, 2013

Hibi H, Yamada Y, Ueda Y: Alveolar cleft osteoplasty using tissue-engineered osteogenic material, International Journal of Oral and Maxillofacial Surgery, 35(6):551-555, June 2006

Hockenberry MJ, Wilson D: Wong's Essentials of Pediatric Nursing, 9e, Mosby, St. Louis, 2013

Hockenberry MJ, Wilson: Wong's Nursing Care of Infants and Children, 9e, Mosby, St. Louis, 2011

Hoffbrand AV, Pettit JE: Color Atlas of Clinical Hematology, 3e, Mosby, St. Louis, 2000

Hupp JR, Ellis E, Tucker MR, et al: Contemporary Oral and Maxillofacial Surgery, 6e, Mosby, St. Louis, 2014

Hupp JR, Ellis E, Tucker MR, et al: Contemporary Oral and Maxillofacial Surgery, 5e, Mosby, St. Louis, 2008

Huether SE, McCance KL: Understanding Pathophysiology, 5e, Mosby, St. Louis, 2012

Iannucci J, Howerton L: Dental Radiography Principles and Techniques, 4e, Saunders, St. Louis, 2012

Ibsen O, Phelan J: Oral Pathology for the Dental Hygienist, 5e, Saunders, St. Louis, 2009

Ignatavicious DD, Workman ML: Medical-Surgical Nursing: Patient-Centered Collaborative Care, 6e, Saunders, St. Louis, 2010

James WD, Berger T, Elston D: Andrew's Diseases of the Skin Clinical Dermatology, 11e, Mosby, St. Louis, 2012

Johnson W: Color Atlas of Endodontics, St. Louis, Saunders, 2003

Kaban L, Troulis M: Pediatric Oral and Maxillofacial Surgery, Saunders, St. Louis, 2004

Kock CRD: History of Dental Surgery, vol 1, National Art Publishing, Chicago, 1909

Krouse JH, Derebery MJ, Chadwick SJ: Managing the Allergic Patient (e-book), Saunders, Philadelphia, 2008

Levy MN, Koeppen BM, Stanton BA: Berne & Levy Principles of Physiology, 4e, Mosby, St. Louis, 2006

Liebgott B: The Anatomical Basis of Dentistry, 3e, Mosby, St. Louis, 2011

Little JW, Falace D, Miller C: Dental Management of the Medically Compromised Patient, 7e, Mosby, St. Louis, 2008

Little JW, Falace D, Miller C: Little and Falace's Dental Management of the Medically Compromised Patient, 8e, Mosby, St. Louis, 2013

Logan BM, Reynolds P, Hutching RT: McMinn's Color Atlas of Head and Neck Anatomy, 4e, Mosby, St. Louis, 2010

Lowdermilk DL, Perry SE, Cashion MC: Maternity Nursing, 8e, Mosby, St. Louis, 2011

Malamed SF: Handbook of Local Anesthesia, 5e, Mosby, St. Louis, 2004

Malamed SF: Handbook of Local Anesthesia, 6e, Mosby, St. Louis, 2012

Malamed SF: Medical Emergencies in the Dental Office, 6e, Mosby, St. Louis, 2007

McCance KL, Huether SE: Pathophysiology: the Biologic Basis for Disease in Adults and Children, 6e, Mosby, St Louis, 2010

Mehrotraa D, et al: Random control trial of dermis-fat graft and interposition of temporalis fascia in the management of temporomandibular ankylosis in children, British Journal of Oral and Maxillofacial Surgery, 46(7):521-526, October 2008

Misch CE: Dental Implant Prosthetics, Mosby, St. Louis, 2005

Monahan F, Sands JK, Neighbors M, et al: Phipps' Medical-Surgical Nursing: Health and Illness Perspectives, 8e, Mosby, St. Louis, 2007

Mosby: Mosby's Dictionary of Medicine, Nursing & Health Professions, 9e, Mosby, St. Louis, 2013

Moses KP, Nava PB, Banks JC, et al: Atlas of Clinical Gross Anatomy, 2e, Saunders, St. Louis, 2013

Nanci A: Ten Cate's Oral Histology, 8e, Mosby, St. Louis, 2013

Nelson SJ: Wheeler's Dental Anatomy, Physiology and Occlusion, 9e, Saunders, St. Louis, 2010

Neville BW, Damm DD, Allen C, et al: Oral and Maxillofacial Pathology, 3e, Saunders, St. Louis, 2009

Neville BW, Damm DD, White DK: Color Atlas of Clinical Oral Pathology, 2e, BC Decker, Ontario, Canada, 1999

Newman MG, Takei H, Klokkevold PR, et al: Carranza's Clinical Periodontology, 11e, Saunders, St. Louis, 2012

Nilsson L: A Child is Born, Delacorte Press, New York, 1977

Oleson T: Auriculotherapy Manual: Chinese and Western Systems of Ear Acupuncture, 3e, Churchill Livingstone, Philadelphia, 2002

Parrillo JE, Dellinger RP: Critical Care Medicine: Principles of Diagnosis and Management in the Adult, Mosby, St. Louis, 2008

Patton KT, Thibodeau GA: Anatomy and Physiology, 8e, Mosby, St. Louis, 2013

Patton KT, Thibodeau GA, Douglas MM: Essentials of Anatomy and Physiology, 3e, Mosby, St. Louis, 2012

Perry DA, Beemsterboer PL: Periodontology for the Dental Hygienist, 3e, Saunders, St. Louis, 2007

Prince FP: Mitochondreial cristae diversity in human Leydig cells: a revised look at cristae morphology in these steroid-producing cells, Anat Rec, 254: 534-541, 1999

Proffit WR, White RP, Sarver DM: Contemporary Treatment of Dentofacial Deformities, Mosby, St. Louis, 2003

Proffit WR, Fields, HW, Sarver DM: Contemporary Orthodontics, 5e, Mosby, St. Louis, 2013

Regezi JA, Sciubba JJ, Jordan RCK: Oral Pathology: Clinical Pathologic Correlations, 6e, Saunders, St. Louis, 2012

Regezi JA, Sciubba JJ, Pogrel MA: Atlas of Oral and Maxillofacial Pathology, Saunders, St. Louis, 2000

Rose LF, Mealey B, Genco R: Periodontics: Medicine, Surgery, and Implants, Mosby, St. Louis, 2004

Rosenstiel SJ, Land MF, Fujimoto J: Contemporary Fixed Prosthodontics, 4e, Mosby, St. Louis, 2006

Rothrock JC: Alexander's Care of the Patient in Surgery, 14e, Mosby, St.Louis, 2011

Samaranayake L: Essentials of Microbiology for Dentistry, 3e, Churchill Livingstone, Philadelphia, 2007

Sapp JP, Eversole LR, Wysocki GW: Contemporary Oral and Maxillofacial Pathology, 2e, Mosby, St. Louis, 2004

Sirois M: Principles and Practice of Veterinary Technology, 3e, Mosby, St. Louis, 2012

Smith JA: HIV and AIDS in the adolescent and adult: an update for the oral and maxillofacial surgeon, Oral Maxillofac Surg Clin North Am, 20(4):535-65, Nov 2008

Solomon EP: Introduction to Human Anatomy and Physiology, 3e, Saunders, St. Louis, 2009

Stepp CA, Woods M: Laboratory Procedures for Medical Office Personnel, Saunders, Philadelphia, 1998

Stevens A, Lowe JS: Human Histology, 3e, Mosby, St. Louis, 2005

Stillwell SB: Mosby's Critical Care Nursing Reference, 4e, Mosby, St. Louis, 2007